Reconstructive
Foot and Ankle Surgery
Management of Complications
Second Edition

Reconstructive
Foot and Ankle Surgery
Management of Complications

SECOND EDITION

MARK S. MYERSON, M.D.

Director, Institute for Foot and Ankle Reconstruction
Mercy Medical Center
Baltimore, Maryland

1600 John F. Kennedy Boulevard
Suite 1800
Philadelphia, PA 19103-2899

RECONSTRUCTIVE FOOT AND ANKLE SURGERY   ISBN: 978-1-4377-0923-0
Management of Complications
Copyright © 2010 by Saunders, an imprint of Elsevier Inc.

Notice

Knowledge and best practice in this field are constantly changing. As new research and experience
broaden our understanding, changes in research methods, professional practices, or medical treatment
may become necessary.

Practitioners and researchers must always rely on their own experience and knowledge in evaluating
and using any information, methods, compounds, or experiments described herein. In using such
information or methods they should be mindful of their own safety and the safety of others, including
parties for whom they have a professional responsibility.

With respect to any drug or pharmaceutical products identified, readers are advised to check the most
current information provided (i) on procedures featured or (ii) by the manufacturer of each product to be
administered, to verify the recommended dose or formula, the method and duration of administration,
and contraindications. It is the responsibility of practitioners, relying on their own experience and
knowledge of their patients, to make diagnoses, to determine dosages and the best treatment for each
individual patient, and to take all appropriate safety precautions.

To the fullest extent of the law, neither the Publisher nor the authors, contributors, or editors, assume
any liability for any injury and/or damage to persons or property as a matter of products liability,
negligence or otherwise, or from any use or operation of any methods, products, instructions, or ideas
contained in the material herein.

Library of Congress Cataloging-in-Publication Data or Control Number

Myerson, Mark.
    Reconstructive foot and ankle surgery / Mark S. Myerson. -- 2nd ed.
        p. ; cm.
    Includes bibliographical references and index.
    ISBN 978-1-4377-0923-0 (hardcover : alk. paper) 1. Foot--Diseases--Surgery.
    2. Ankle--Diseases--Surgery. 3. Foot--Abnormalities--Surgery.
    4. Ankle--Abnormalities--Surgery. I. Title.
    [DNLM: 1. Ankle--surgery. 2. Foot--surgery. 3. Reconstructive Surgical
Procedures--methods. WE 880 M996r 2010]
    RD563.M96 2010
    617.5'85059--dc22

Acquisitions Editor: Daniel Pepper
Developmental Editor: Taylor Ball
Publishing Services Manager: Anne Altepeter
Team Manager: Radhika Pallamparthy
Senior Project Manager: Beth Hayes
Project Manager: Preethi Kerala Varma
Design Direction: Lou Forgione

Printed in Canada.

Last digit is the print number: 9 8 7 6 5 4 3 2 1

To my beloved family
This work could not have been possible without your sacrifice.
You have my enduring love, affection, and gratitude.

Preface

Where do new ideas come from? What is original thought, and what can or should be attributed to someone else? The techniques presented in this text are an amalgamation of ideas and approaches that are not all original and certainly not necessarily novel. Some of my procedures have not changed at all over the decades, and indeed it is gratifying to know that although methods of fixation may have improved, the principles of surgical reconstruction remain similar. Certainly, surgical approaches change, but these are driven primarily by the technological advances that abound in our daily practice of medicine.

I have been blessed by those around me. To be an educator is a gift and a wonderful opportunity, and to be a teacher without continuing to learn from others is impossible. The ideas expressed in this book therefore represent the thoughts and techniques that I have accrued from my mentors, my colleagues, and my wonderful fellows. I owe my gratitude to my fellows for constantly challenging me to set the standards in foot and ankle surgery that are essential for our progress.

Mark S. Myerson, M.D.

Contents

Section XI
RHEUMATOID FOOT AND ANKLE SURGERY

Reconstructive
Foot and Ankle Surgery
Management of Complications

SECOND EDITION

The Hallux and Sesamoids

CHAPTER **1**

Chevron Osteotomy

INDICATIONS

Chevron osteotomy is a procedure performed for correction of hallux valgus that is associated with a mild to moderate increase in the intermetatarsal angle. Recent years have seen an increased interest in "pushing" the procedure for correction of more severe deformity. Indeed, with a release of the adductor, a moderate deformity of an intermetatarsal angle between 14 and 17 degrees may be corrected with a more aggressive version of chevron osteotomy. Correction of severe deformity does require moving the metatarsal head laterally by at least 50%, thereby increasing the risk for malunion resulting from poor bone contact. After all, the chevron osteotomy is really just a short version of the scarf osteotomy and, with modifications, can correct multiplanar deformity. In my experience, an adductor release is important for an optimal result, and if any doubt exists regarding the adequacy of the chevron osteotomy for correction, it is preferable to perform a distal soft tissue release. This additional step is even more important in patients who are found to have a greater degree of hallux valgus than that expected on the basis of the radiographic intermetatarsal angle, for whom the soft tissue release is very useful.

The incidence of avascular necrosis of the metatarsal head does not increase when a soft tissue release is performed simultaneously with the osteotomy. Avascular necrosis of the metatarsal head typically results when excessive periosteal stripping is performed along the dorsal lateral metatarsal neck, which really does not need to be exposed. The osteotomy can be performed in conjunction with a closing wedge osteotomy of the hallux proximal phalanx (Akin osteotomy) for patients in whom the distal metatarsal articular angle (DMAA) is abnormal (Figure 1-1). It is preferable, however, to perform a biplanar chevron osteotomy if any doubt remains about the congruency of the articulation achieved with a closing wedge osteotomy. In geometric terms, the improvement obtained in the distal angulation between the first and second metatarsals will correspond to the magnitude of the lateral shift. It is stated that a 1-degree improvement in angulation will take place with a 1-mm shift of the metatarsal. Although this dictum implies that a deformity greater than 14 degrees cannot reestablish the alignment, such limitation is not supported in clinical practice if a soft tissue release is performed.

APPROACH TO A STANDARD CHEVRON OSTEOTOMY

An incision is made medially at the junction of the dorsal and plantar skin, extending proximally for 3 cm from the flare just distal to the metatarsophalangeal joint. This incision is far safer, with more predictable results, than a dorsally based approach, which endangers the nerve and is associated with increased risk for an extension contracture. The incision is deepened through subcutaneous tissue. The soft tissues are dissected carefully to identify the terminal medial cutaneous branch of the superficial peroneal nerve, which is then dorsally retracted (Figure 1-2). It is easier to free the nerve with a hemostat, rather than with a knife or scissors.

I now prefer to use a straight, horizontally oriented capsular incision placed slightly more toward the plantar aspect of the metatarsal head. Although many capsular incisions are possible, the correction of the deformity should be obtained by bone realignment and soft tissue balancing to obtain an optimal result. These essential elements of the surgical correction cannot be replaced by a tight capsulorrhaphy, which never constitutes adequate treatment for hallux valgus. The capsular closure should only gently pull the hallux into neutral alignment. Once the capsule is dissected off the medial eminence and the medial aspect of the metatarsal head, the tibial sesamoid is visible. Inspection of the articular surface for cartilage defects or erosion is important.

The alignment of the first metatarsal is checked with respect to the medial eminence and the hallux, and the exostectomy is performed with a flexible chisel. A saw blade can be used, but with a saw, there is less control over the direction of the cut. The medial eminence must be cut from distal to proximal, to create a smooth transition of the metatarsal head with the metaphyseal flare proximally. Making the cut in the sagittal groove is to be avoided. Such a cut will be too lateral, leading to uncovering of the metatarsal head and medialization of the tibial sesamoid. This altered anatomy will allow irritation of the sesamoid with movement, potentially causing arthritis.

The osteotomy is planned with use of a cautery to mark the apex, approximately 8 mm proximal to the articular surface. I prefer a standard cut at a 60-degree angle, with the dorsal and plantar limbs of the osteotomy equidistant. Although alternative limbs of the osteotomy have been described, use of such alternatives offers

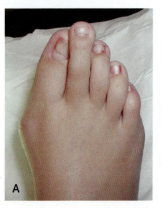 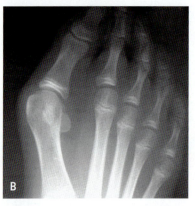 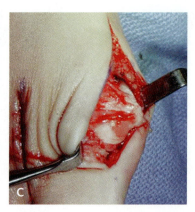

Figure 1-1 A and **B,** The patient was a 14-year-old girl with a hallux valgus angle of 30 degrees and an intermetatarsal angle of 16 degrees on the preoperative radiograph **(B).** A biplanar chevron osteotomy was planned, with a distal soft tissue release. **C,** Note the severe increase in the distal metatarsal articular angle evident intraoperatively, which is not seen as prominently on the radiograph.

no advantages, requires more dorsal exposure and dissection, and is likely to result in further metatarsal shortening. For exposure of the dorsal surface of the metatarsal, the soft tissue is dissected dorsally with limited subperiosteal dissection. Visualizing the dorsal-lateral metatarsal is unnecessary, and only the dorsal and medial aspect of the first metatarsal neck is exposed. Care should be taken not to strip any periosteum on the plantar or dorsal surface more proximal to the level of the osteotomy. A saw blade is used for the osteotomy and aligned perpendicular to the axis of the planned limbs of the osteotomy. It is essential *not* to overperforate the soft tissues laterally; the saw blade should penetrate the lateral cortex only. In cases with a long first metatarsal, slight shortening of the metatarsal may be advantageous, and the saw blade can be oriented or angulated slightly proximally (Figure 1-3). The same concept applies with a short metatarsal, in which case any shortening must be avoided.

The metatarsal neck should be carefully held, because grasping with a clamp can fracture the metatarsal neck. The metatarsal head undergoes a slight disimpaction, is retracted distally, and is then pushed over laterally manually while the metatarsal shaft is held stable. This maneuver is slightly more difficult if a distal soft tissue release has been performed, because the hallux and metatarsophalangeal joint are effectively disarticulated. During this maneuver, the metatarsal head should not be rotated or tilted. The lateral metatarsal shift ideally is approximately 5 mm and should be checked radiographically. If an abnormal DMAA is present, then a biplanar chevron cut is planned (Figure 1-4). Although manually cutting a biplanar wedge is possible, it is not as reliable as use of a mechanical guide. At the completion of the first metatarsal osteotomy, the biplanar jig is inserted into the osteotomy cut, the saw is placed down on the side of the jig itself, and the cut is then made against the surface of the jig. This procedure removes a perfectly formed 1-mm slice of the bone from both the dorsal and the plantar limbs of the osteotomy medially to create the wedge necessary for biplanar corrrection.

Although the metatarsal head often is intrinsically stable, secure internal fixation is preferable. A guide pin is introduced at the dorsal medial border of the metatarsal just proximal to the osteotomy and its position checked radiographically. It is important to insert the screw as far dorsally as possible. With the medial incision the tendency is to insert the screw a little too far medially, which then limits the amount of bone that can be trimmed at the completion of the procedure. In fact, the easiest method of fixation is to use a percutaneously introduced pin, directed from dorsal to plantar, and as much bone as is necessary can then removed from the medial overhang. If a screw is used and inserted too far medially, less medial bone can be trimmed. A drill/countersink is used to prevent fracture of the medial metatarsal neck. The position of the guide pin is checked fluoroscopically, and the length is determined; a screw, usually approximately 20 to 22 mm, is inserted across the guide pin; and compression is obtained. The medial overhanging bone from the osteotomy must be smoothed down with a saw by shaving or back cutting the bone. Once the screw is inserted, an important step is to verify the distal extent of the screw carefully to ensure that it is not in the joint. I have been misled by what initially appears to be a very well-positioned screw, only to find subsequently that the screw is protruding into the joint by 1 mm. Owing to the overlapping shadow of the lesser metatarsal heads, a useful maneuver is to rotate the hallux under fluoroscopy to verify the location of the screw.

Two sutures of 2-0 Vicryl are inserted at an oblique orientation, from the dorsal proximal aspect of the capsule into the plantar distal position, to pull the hallux into slight supination and slight varus. Checking the range of motion of the hallux metatarsophalangeal joint after the capsular repair is important. If the hallux is pulled too far medially or if the range of motion is insufficient, the sutures must be removed and the repair performed again. I prefer to use absorbable sutures for skin closure, with 4-0 Vicryl for the subcutaneous tissue and interrupted 4-0 chromic sutures for skin. Radiographs are obtained at regular intervals after surgery until healing is noted.

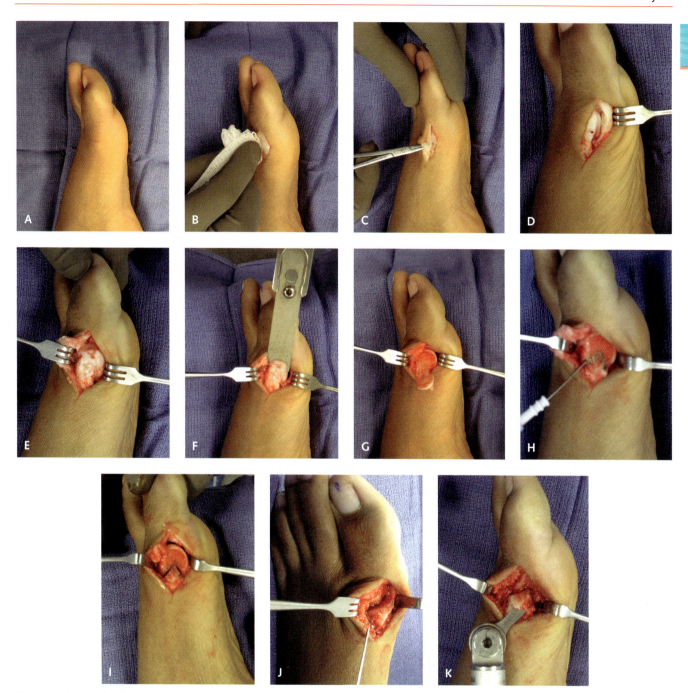

Figure 1-2 Steps in the chevron osteotomy. In this patient, the incision was marked out more distally to perform an additional phalangeal osteotomy. **A** to **C,** After the incision is made **(A),** the dorsal medial cutaneous branch of the superficial peroneal nerve is wiped with a sponge, identified, and retracted **(B** and **C). D** and **E,** After longitudinal capsulotomy **(D),** subperiosteal dissection is performed only medially and dorsally along the metatarsal neck, in the location of the plane of the osteotomy **(E). F** and **G,** The exostectomy is performed; **H,** the osteotomy is marked using an electrocautery. **I,** A fine, small saw blade is used to make the cut at a 60-degree angle. **J,** A small clamp is used to grasp the metatarsal neck, and the head is pushed laterally and fixed with a guide pin and a headless cannulated screw. **K,** The medial overhanging ledge of bone is shaved.

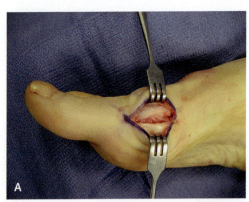 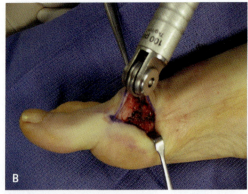

Figure 1-3 A, Note use of the horizontal longitudinal capsular incision. This incision is preferable to vertical and L-shaped incisions, simply because the capsular repair is not adequate for correction of the deformity. **B,** The saw blade is intentionally inclined slightly proximally, to slightly shorten the metatarsal (desirable in this patient).

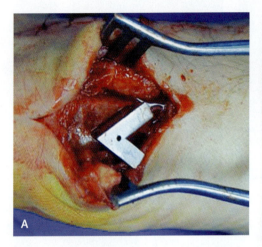 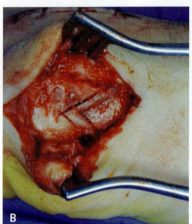

Figure 1-4 Use of the Toomey cutting jig. A K-wire is inserted into the metatarsal head, and the jig position is marked on the metatarsal. **A,** The chevron cut is made according to the shape of the marked fin, and the jig is inserted. **B,** The second saw cut is made, leaving a perfect wedge to be removed to correct the distal metatarsal articular angle. **C,** The final correction is seen on the radiograph.

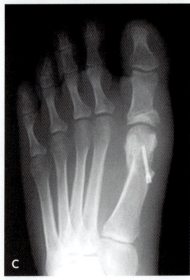

TECHNIQUES, TIPS, AND PITFALLS

- Even though chevron osteotomy is inherently a stable cut, internal fixation of the osteotomy is ideal to prevent malunion. The technique using the double-threaded screw, as described, is reliable, affording stability and allowing early weight bearing and range of motion of the hallux.

- Checking the position of the metatarsal head in relation to the metatarsal shaft intraoperatively is important. The metatarsal head tends to tilt either medially or laterally as impaction is performed. With either of these malpositions, the hallux tends to drift into valgus, although this deviation is worse if any valgus impaction of the head is performed.

- Occasionally, slight varus impaction of the metatarsal head is actually desirable to correct an abnormal DMAA. If this maneuver is deliberately performed, be careful that shortening of the metatarsal does not occur.

- Shortening of the metatarsal may result if metaphyseal bone overlap is created during impaction of the metatarsal head. With this shortening, transfer of weight-bearing pressure to the second metatarsal with metatarsalgia will occur.

- Do not strip the periosteum laterally. The blood supply for the first metatarsal head enters dorsolaterally at the junction of the metatarsal neck. Avascular necrosis of the metatarsal head will not develop unless excessive periosteal stripping on the lateral aspect of the metatarsal neck is performed.

- When exposing the dorsal surface of the metatarsal for the osteotomy, elevate the periosteum over the metatarsal only where it is being cut to insert a soft tissue retractor.

- If intraoperative fracture of the medial edge of the distal metatarsal cortex occurs during screw insertion, either a Kirschner wire (K-wire) or a suture placed around the fractured portion of the metatarsal can be used. A suture applied around the metatarsal is ideal, provided that this repair does not cause any further periosteal stripping.

- In my experience, a variation of the osteotomy cut that features a long dorsal limb confers no advantage over the standard 60-degree cut. Although this long dorsal limb theoretically facilitates the insertion of a dorsal-to-plantar screw, it involves further periosteal stripping, particularly if the incision is made medially.

- Rarely, after a chevron osteotomy, instability of the first metatarsal is present, which may lead to recurrent deformity. This problem can be corrected with a lag-type screw inserted between the first and second metatarsal bases (Figure 1-5). Use of a screw is a good alternative to suturing between the first and second metatarsals distally. The screw is removed between 8 and 10 weeks later, when sufficient scarring has taken place. The other option is to use a mini-tightrope suture at the base of the metatarsal. My own experience to date with this method of fixation has not been favorable, with less than successful results.

- The screw fixation must be carefully planned. If the screw is too medial in position, it will pose an obstruction to the amount of bone that can be trimmed medially, eventually leading to irritation (Figure 1-6).

- A chevron osteotomy can be used successfully to correct metatarsus adductus. Although the deformity may be significant, if the axis of the foot is considered relative to the first metatarsal, the intermetatarsal angle is not significant (Figure 1-7).

- The chevron osteotomy is a useful adjunct to procedures for correction of forefoot deformity including metatarsalgia and lesser metatarsal deformity such as brachymetatarsia. Hallux valgus frequently accompanies brachymetatarsia, and to regain adequate alignment of the forefoot, the hallux deformity must be corrected as well (Figure 1-8).

- A K-wire may be used for fixation if a fracture of the metatarsal occurs during screw insertion. Such fixation will facilitate excellent removal of the overhanging medial bone and permit resection of even more medial bone than would otherwise be possible (Figures 1-9 and 1-10). Use of a medial screw often will be associated with subsequent irritation, necessitating its removal (Figure 1-11).

- Although a dorsal incision has been described for use in a chevron osteotomy and other first metatarsal osteotomies, I caution against its use. Frequently, this incision is associated with dorsal soft tissue contracture, which limits plantar flexion of the metatarsophalangeal joint. Furthermore, the dorsal incision places the dorsomedial cutaneous branch of the superficial peroneal nerve at risk for injury, and scar neuroma formation is more common (Figure 1-12, *A*).

Continued

TECHNIQUES, TIPS, AND PITFALLS—cont'd

- There are many variations in the shape of the osteotomy other than the standard 60-degree-angle cut. It may be preferable to make the plantar cut more horizontal, to increase the stability of the osteotomy. This slight modification also increases the surface area for screw fixation (see Figure 1-12, *B*).

- If a patient has pain in the hallux postoperatively, take adequate radiographs, including oblique views of the joint, to verify the screw location. The importance of such confirmation is illustrated in Figure 1-13; in the case depicted, dorsal collapse of the osteotomy occurred, followed by slight penetration of the screw into the joint, which became symptomatic.

- Correction of hallux valgus associated with any spasticity requires an arthrodesis of the metatarsophalangeal joint. Despite healthy articular cartilage, an osteotomy for mild deformity should not be performed. The recurrence rate after osteotomy for hallux valgus correction in the setting of spasticity of any kind is very high.

- The addition of a distal soft tissue release procedure to a chevron osteotomy improves the position of the hallux and the relationship of the sesamoids to the metatarsal head. This potential for improvement is of particular value in cases characterized by greater valgus deformity of the hallux relative to the intermetatarsal deformity. No increased incidence of avascular necrosis of the metatarsal head, which results from excessive stripping of the dorsolateral periosteum, has been noted with addition of a distal soft tissue release.

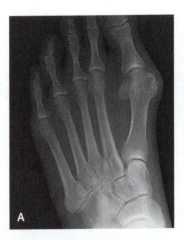
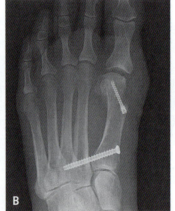
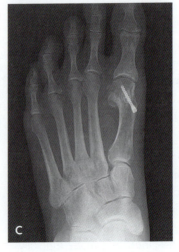

Figure 1-5 A, Correction of a moderate deformity with a 16-degree intermetatarsal angle was performed with a chevron osteotomy with a soft tissue release, but horizontal plane instability was noted at the conclusion of the procedure. **B,** This was corrected with insertion of a stabilization screw between the first and second metatarsals, which was left in place for 8 weeks. **C,** The radiographic appearance at 1 year.

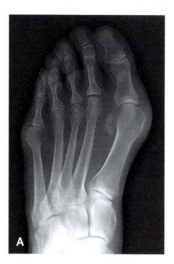 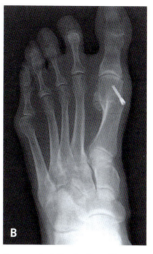

Figure 1-6 A and **B,** Although the overall alignment of the hallux after correction by chevron osteotomy was good, I prefer to perform a more extensive exostectomy medially than was done here. The position of the screw dorsomedially inhibits this medial bone removal.

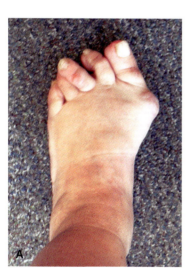 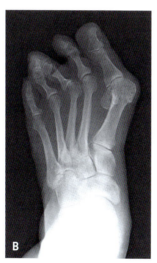 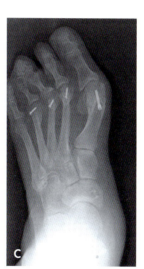

Figure 1-7 A and **B,** The patient demonstrated good range of motion of the metatarsophalangeal joint despite the radiographic appearance suggesting slight arthritis **(B).** A decision was made to perform a chevron osteotomy, although a scarf osteotomy with more shortening of the first and lesser metatarsals might have provided better alignment. **C,** The radiographic appearance 8 years after surgery.

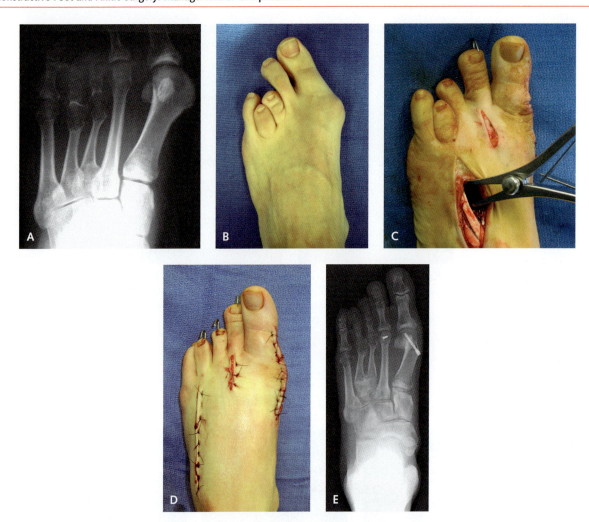

Figure 1-8 A and **B,** The patient presented with brachymetatarsia of the third and fourth metatarsals, along with hallux valgus. **C** and **D,** A single-stage lengthening of the third and fourth metatarsals was performed with structural grafting and K-wire fixation, combined with a biplanar chevron osteotomy and a Weil osteotomy of the second metatarsal. **E,** The radiographic appearance at 4 years after surgery.

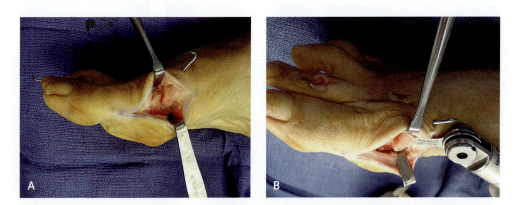

Figure 1-9 A, A K-wire was used for fixation in repair of fracture of the dorsal cortex that occurred with insertion of a screw during osteotomy. **B,** Such fixation also allows resection of more of the overhanging medial bone.

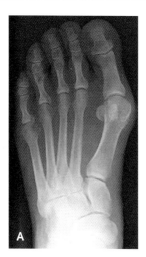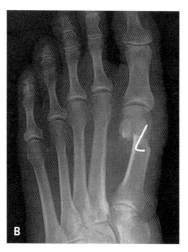

Figure 1-10 A, This moderate deformity (with an intermetatarsal angle of 16 degrees) was corrected with a chevron osteotomy combined with a distal soft tissue procedure. **B,** A K-wire was used for fixation, facilitating increased correction.

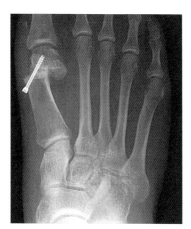

Figure 1-11 Incorrect screw placement is evident here. Despite very good correction of the deformity, the bone prominence caused subsequent pain, necessitating revision with ostectomy.

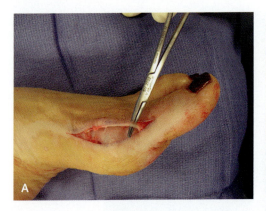
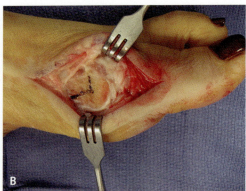
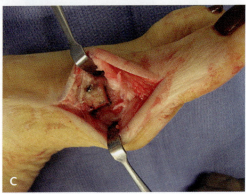

Figure 1-12 A, The identification of the dorsal medial cutaneous nerve is an important step in the procedure. In this case, the patient was noted to have particularly porous bone, raising concern regarding stability. **B** and **C,** Accordingly, a more horizontal plantar cut on the metatarsal was made to increase stability.

Figure 1-13 A, The patient had marked metatarsus adductus, which was treated with a chevron osteotomy, initially with good alignment, as seen on the postoperative radiograph. The development of pain over subsequent months was associated with a malunion of the osteotomy. **B,** As the bone subsided dorsally, the screw penetrated the plantar cortex into the joint, necessitating its removal. **C,** The malunion caused persistent pain with dorsal impingement, subsequently necessitating revision surgery.

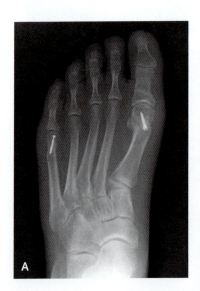
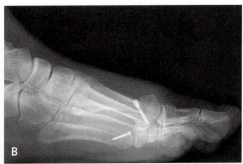
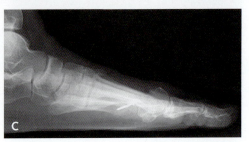

CHAPTER 2

The Modified Ludloff Metatarsal Osteotomy

INDICATIONS AND LIMITATIONS

The indication for a modified Ludloff metatarsal osteotomy is moderate to severe deformity that is not associated with instability of the metatarsocuneiform joint. The procedure is always performed in conjunction with a distal soft tissue release. No limit to the amount of correction that can be achieved with this proximal metatarsal osteotomy has been recognized. This procedure is primarily, however, a rotational or angular osteotomy, and in cases in which the distal metatarsal articular angle (DMAA) is abnormal, an alternative procedure—for example, a scarf osteotomy—is preferable.

As originally described by Ludloff, the osteotomy was made in an oblique plane in the metatarsal, but without fixation. Approximately 15 years ago, while I was performing a long oblique osteotomy of the fifth metatarsal, it occurred to me that a similar rotational osteotomy could be performed on the first metatarsal. One of the problems with many proximally based metatarsal osteotomies is that once the bone is cut, control of the metatarsal position is temporarily lost, and the potential for instability increases. The Ludloff osteotomy is based on the premise that control of the position and fixation is never lost during the procedure. The metatarsal is partially cut, a screw is inserted as far proximally as possible on the metatarsal, and then the osteotomy is completed. Correction of the metatarsal is performed around the axis of the proximal screw, and correction is not lost during fixation. The Ludloff metatarsal osteotomy is a very simple procedure, but with limitations, because it cannot address instability of the first ray, nor can it adequately address deformity of the metatarsophalangeal articulation.

SOFT TISSUE RELEASE

An incision is made in the first web space; the incision extends from the cleft of the web space proximally for a length of 2.5 cm. The terminal branch of the deep peroneal nerve is identified, to avoid injury with consequent numbness in the first web space. A small retractor is inserted into the incision. Then, a small-toothed laminar spreader is inserted between the first and second metatarsals; this insertion places the innominate fascia on stretch to facilitate dissection. The two heads of the adductor tendon are now grasped with a small clamp and then cut sharply off the lateral edge of the fibular sesamoid. The adductor tendon is elevated into the incision, dissected free from the flexor brevis muscle and tendon, as well as

the lateral edge of the sesamoid, and then cut distally. I prefer to cut the adductor tendon completely and not to reattach the tendon to the neck of the metatarsal, as some surgeons describe (Figure 2-1).

Cutting the terminal 1 cm of the adductor tendon prevents any recurrent scarring between the adductor tendon and the sesamoid complex and therefore recurrent deformity. The sesamoid suspensory ligament is cut with a more oblique rotation of the blade. An important consideration is that as the hallux valgus worsens, the sesamoid rotates from a transverse plane to a more oblique or vertical position. With the sesamoid release, the blade must be inserted more obliquely as the deformity increases. The sesamoid is freed from the undersurface of the first metatarsal, the capsule is perforated sharply, and the hallux is manipulated by tearing the capsule into slight varus. It may be necessary to release the deep transverse metatarsal ligament, if the sesamoid is still tethered by the ligament and the ligament is holding the displaced sesamoid laterally. In releasing the ligament, a Metzenbaum scissors is used, working from distal to proximal along the undersurface of the ligament. Care is taken not to injure the common digital nerve, which lies underneath the ligament.

THE CAPSULOTOMY AND OSTEOTOMY

Although the capsulotomy and exposure of the metatarsal are made initially, the exostectomy (bunionectomy) is *not* performed until the metatarsal osteotomy is complete. Subtle rotation of the metatarsal head may occur after the osteotomy, and if the exostectomy is performed first, malrotation of the metatarsal head may occur after the osteotomy. For example, after a minimal exostectomy is performed and correction of the metatarsal is obtained, the plantar surface of the metatarsal may be found to be exposed, and the tibial sesamoid may not be covered adequately by the metatarsal head. A medial incision at the junction of the dorsal and plantar skin is preferable to one more dorsally placed (closer to the extensor hallucis longus tendon). A more dorsal incision may traumatize the nerve, often with consequent dorsal scarring and contracture (Figure 2-2).

The soft tissues are carefully dissected to identify the terminal medial cutaneous branch of the superficial peroneal nerve. The nerve is gradually dissected free using a hemostat and is then retracted dorsally. Although different capsular incisions are possible, I use a straight longitudinal incision extending from the metatarsophalangeal joint proximally along the course of the first metatarsal shaft. This incision is made slightly inferiorly to leave

Figure 2-1 A, The incisions for the osteotomy are marked as noted. **B,** The adductor release is performed with a laminar spreader to place stretch on the transverse metatarsal ligament. **C,** The hallux is manipulated into slight hallux varus after the adductor release.

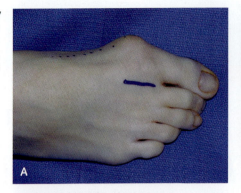

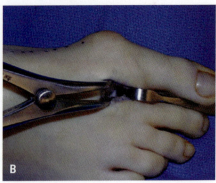

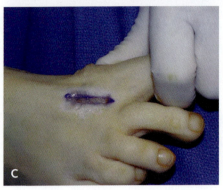

Figure 2-2 A, The medial incision for the procedure is made at the junction of the dorsal and plantar skin, and the capsulotomy is in the plane of the metatarsal. **B,** Only the medial metatarsal is exposed, to minimize soft tissue stripping. **C,** The osteotomy is marked out with cautery.

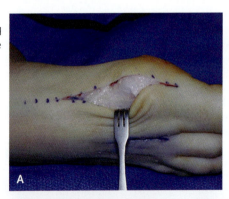

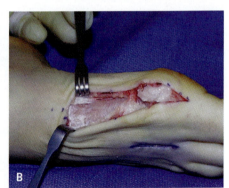

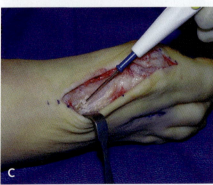

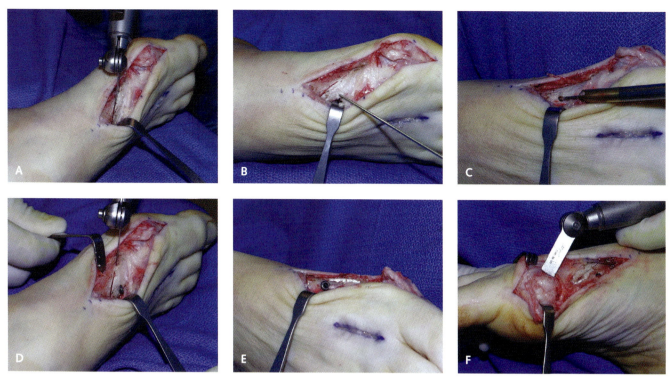

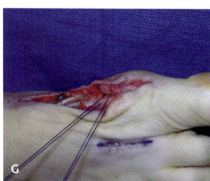

Figure 2-3 A, The osteotomy is begun at approximately a 30-degree angle, with the blade kept perpendicular. **B,** A guide pin is inserted; **C,** the countersink is performed with a burr; and **D,** the first screw is inserted. **E,** The metatarsal is then rotated around the axis of the first screw; **F,** the exostectomy is performed; and **G,** the capsulorrhaphy performed.

abundant capsule dorsally for soft tissue closure. The capsule is now dissected off the medial eminence and medial aspect of the metatarsal head; this dissection exposes the tibial sesamoid. A blunt periosteal elevator is inserted under the metatarsal head to mobilize the sesamoid.

The Osteotomy

The incision is extended proximally along the plane of the first metatarsal, and the subcutaneous dissection is performed proximally to the level of the tarsometatarsal joint. During the dissection, the more proximal terminal cutaneous branch of the superficial peroneal nerve should be retracted dorsally. Only the medial and dorsal surface of the periosteum is dissected off the bone (Figure 2-3). Turning the patient's leg and foot so that the plane of the osteotomy can be precisely identified is helpful.

The osteotomy is marked out using an electrocautery to extend from the dorsal apical surface of the first metatarsal proximally at an angle of approximately 30 degrees distally. The cut is planned to end just proximal to the sesamoid complex. The longer the saw cut, the more likely that it will be too close to the sesamoids distally, thereby making screw fixation more difficult. As the plane of the

osteotomy becomes more vertical, however, it is more unstable. When exposing the proximal dorsal metatarsal, the surgeon should palpate the metatarsocuneiform joint, and the cut should begin 5 mm anterior to the joint. Inserting a retractor into the proximal first web space by drawing back the extensor hallucis longus tendon and the soft tissues is useful.

The saw blade is oriented exactly perpendicular to the axis of the first metatarsal, approximately 4 mm distal to the tarsometatarsal joint dorsally. Tilting the saw blade away from perpendicular is to be avoided because such deviation will affect the rotation as well as the elevation of the metatarsal head. If the saw is inclined in a plantar direction, a corresponding depression of the metatarsal head (which may even be desirable in some cases) will result. As the cut is made more distally, a 1-cm cortical bone bridge is left on the plantar distal surface of the first metatarsal. Slight soft tissue dissection of the dorsal surface of the first metatarsal is performed, and the screw fixation is planned. It is very important to carefully countersink the screw to prevent splitting of the dorsal surface of the first metatarsal, and this may be best accomplished with use of a small burr. The more proximal the screw location, the better the axial rotation around the screw and the greater the control of correction. If the screw is inserted more distally, the metatarsal becomes banana-shaped, and the likelihood of malunion and alteration of the position of the metatarsal head is increased.

The screw is fully inserted but should not compress the osteotomy. The screw is then slightly "backed off" to allow insertion of the saw blade again, and the distal aspect of the first metatarsal osteotomy is completed. A retractor is again inserted proximally between the first and second metatarsals. When the proximal aspect of the proximal first metatarsal is pushed medially and the first metatarsal head is simultaneously directed laterally, the metatarsal direction is corrected.

The value of this osteotomy is that at no time does the surgeon lose control of the plane and position of the metatarsal. Once the position of the metatarsal is corrected, with good coverage of the metatarsal head achieved distally, a second screw is introduced from plantar to dorsal to complete fixation. If the second screw does not give excellent stable fixation, then I add a small plate medially to improve fixation. The overhanging bone is now shaved down proximally, dorsally, and medially with a saw blade. The stability of the metatarsal must be checked, and the exostectomy and capsulorrhaphy must be performed.

This concept of metatarsal stability is important. Approximately 5% of the time, after an excellent correction of the metatarsal, transverse plane instability is found to be present. This instability may not have been noted preoperatively, because the ideal operation would then have been a Lapidus procedure. To some extent, this instability may be controlled postoperatively with tight bandaging, but I prefer not to rely on bandaging and instead use added fixation to control the position of the metatarsal. Some surgeons use a suture to stabilize the metatarsal (a mini-tightrope suture [Arthrex, Naples, Florida]), but I have not had good experience with this method of fixation and prefer to use a screw, which is left in for 2 to 3 months.

An exostectomy does not always have to be performed. However, even with excellent correction of the metatarsal head, gently abrading the medial head with a saw blade to facilitate stable healing of the capsule is useful. Before the exostosis cut is made, correct alignment of the first metatarsal with respect to the medial eminence and the hallux is checked fluoroscopically. With a saw blade, the medial eminence is cut from dorsal to plantar, to leave the proximal aspect of the ostectomy flush with the metaphyseal flare. To prevent overcorrection, hallux varus, and sesamoid arthritis, it is essential not to resect too much bone off the medial head.

The capsulorrhaphy is performed with the plantar capsular tissue using two sutures of 2-0 Vicryl. These are inserted in oblique orientation, from the dorsal proximal capsule into the plantar distal position, to pull the hallux into very slight varus and supination. During the capsular repair, the hallux is maintained in a neutral position in terms of both alignment and rotation of the axial plane. Before closure, it is important to ensure that the range of motion of the hallux metatarsophalangeal joint is adequate without clicking or locking, which may indicate joint incongruency. Any clicking or locking may indicate that the distal metatarsal articular angle is not satisfactory and that an osteotomy of the hallux proximal phalanx may need to be performed.

POSTOPERATIVE COURSE AND RECOVERY

Patients may begin weight bearing as tolerated on the foot immediately after surgery; however, heel weight bearing is preferable. If there is any concern regarding the stability and rigidity of the fixation, then a boot, rather than a postoperative shoe, is used. The foot is immobilized for approximately 4 weeks, and then weight bearing in a firm accommodative shoe, as tolerated, can begin. Physical therapy with massage, strapping, and exercise of the forefoot is useful and can begin at 6 weeks after surgery.

TECHNIQUES, TIPS, AND PITFALLS

- Malunion and nonunion are rare with the modified Ludloff metatarsal osteotomy. The major advantage of this osteotomy is that at no point during the procedure is control of the metatarsal position lost. Nonunion is a possible complication if primary bone healing fails to occur, in which case periosteal bone formation will be evident on radiographs obtained in the early postoperative phase. If periosteal new bone formation around the osteotomy site is noted, it is more than likely loose, and although union of the osteotomy will occur, slight elevation and dorsal malunion also may occur simultaneously. If periosteal bone formation is noted, weight bearing should be controlled in a boot, and the foot carefully strapped.

- The type of fixation used is important to facilitate primary bone healing. Because of the plane of this osteotomy, bone-to-bone contact can be limited, and the plane of screw fixation is critical.

- Rotation of the metatarsal occurs around a single axis point of the more proximal screw. Because this is an angular or rotational and not a translational osteotomy, the geometry of correction must be fully appreciated. The further proximal the osteotomy is performed or the closer the axis of rotation is to the tarsometatarsal joint, the less the angular deformity of correction is distally. For example, if the center of rotation is in the center of the metatarsal, the metatarsal will be banana-shaped, and the likelihood is that even with good correction, the metatarsal head will be facing more laterally. Accordingly, a banana-shaped metatarsal can predispose the patient to recurrent hallux valgus.

TECHNIQUES, TIPS, AND PITFALLS—cont'd

- The plane of the osteotomy itself is important. The saw blade must be exactly perpendicular to the axis of the metatarsal. If the saw blade is raised, the first metatarsal head will depress, and the metatarsal head will rotate into slight supination, which is desirable. The converse applies with a plane of the osteotomy in which the saw blade is dropped down, whereupon the metatarsal head will tilt up. The result may be a dorsal malunion with pronation of the metatarsal head, associated with an increased likelihood of recurrent hallux valgus.

- Occasionally, after a well-performed osteotomy, intraoperative deformity between the first and second metatarsals may still be present. Patients with this deformity have clinically unrecognized instability of the tarsometatarsal joint, in which this instability may be in the transverse and not the sagittal plane. Unfortunately, the tarsometatarsal joint cannot be stabilized with arthrodesis at this late stage. I have used two alternative techniques for this purpose. The first is to insert sutures between the first and second metatarsals distally. This technique has been well described for both proximal and distal metatarsal osteotomies in conjunction with the distal soft tissue release. The second technique consists of insertion of a transverse screw between the first and second metatarsals proximally; the location of the screw does not interfere with fixation of the osteotomy. This second technique is less reliable and carries an increased risk for stress reaction of bone and possible stress fracture of the second metatarsal. Strapping of the foot at weekly intervals is important to stabilize the overall alignment of the first and second metatarsals postoperatively.

- Be aware of the possibility of a contracture of the extensor hallucis longus tendon, which may be present with even moderate deformity, as noted. A contracted tendon must be lengthened.

- Unrecognized preoperative instability of the first metatarsal may be present, which may lead to failure of the osteotomy with recurrence of deformity. This instability occurs in the transverse and not the sagittal plane. Some surgeons use firm taping of the foot postoperatively and consider this strapping to provide sufficient support, in the belief that this instability will not cause a problem. If the metatarsal instability is not corrected after the osteotomy, however, my own observations suggest that taping will not be adequate to hold the correction. I use a lag screw (the syndesmosis screw) to secure the first to the second metatarsal (Figures 2-4 and 2-5).

- The axis of rotation of the metatarsal must be as proximal as possible to facilitate correction. If the screw is inserted too far distally, the corrected metatarsal will have a banana shape, and although the alignment of the hallux with the center of the metatarsal head may be adequate, the result may be an incongruent center of rotation, with subsequent development of arthritis (Figure 2-6).

- The angle of the osteotomy must be as oblique as possible without entering the sesamoid apparatus distally and the tarsometatarsal joint proximally. An angle that is too steep results in an irregular correction, associated with an increased incidence of delayed union (Figure 2-7).

- Primary bone healing of the osteotomy is expected (Figure 2-8); if periosteal new bone formation around the osteotomy is noted during healing, it can be inferred that movement is taking place at the osteotomy, which may retard bone healing.

- If the ability of screws to keep the osteotomy stable is of concern, then the screws should be supplemented by K-wires or a plate. At present, if I have any doubt about the quality of the bone or the stability of the fixation, I use a small plate (Figure 2-9).

- The key to this osteotomy procedure is the ability to rotate the metatarsal around a single axis of the proximal screw. This should therefore be a stable osteotomy, with good control of the metatarsal position maintained throughout the operation. This technique is therefore an angular or rotational osteotomy (Figure 2-10).

- If no medial bone overhang is observed after screw fixation, the reduction may have been lost as the compression was applied to the screw.

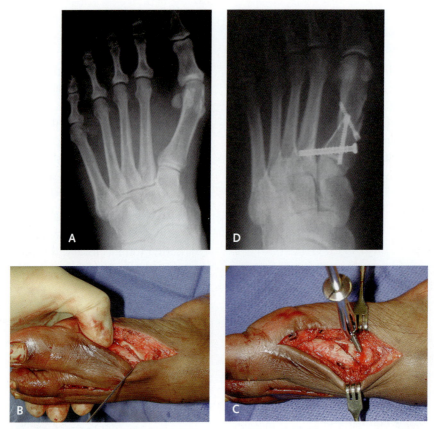

Figure 2-4 The patient had undergone a previous simple bunionectomy with failure. **A,** Hypermobility that was apparent on the first radiograph film was not appreciated preoperatively, and, **B,** a Ludloff osteotomy was performed. **C,** The sequence of the screw fixation was standard, but gross transverse plane instability was noted after initial screw fixation, until a syndesmosis screw was inserted between the first and second metatarsals **(D)**.

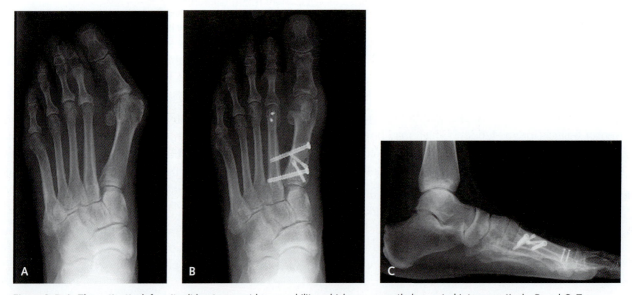

Figure 2-5 A, The patient's deformity did not suggest hypermobility, which was nevertheless noted intraoperatively. **B** and **C,** Two syndesmosis screws were inserted and left in for 4 months postoperatively.

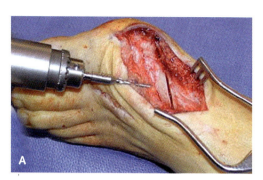
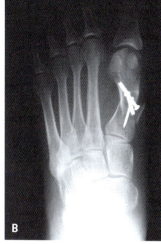

Figure 2-6 A, The axis of rotation in this osteotomy is too distal, and the plane of the osteotomy is too vertical. **B,** Note the postoperative banana shape of the first metatarsal, which is incorrect.

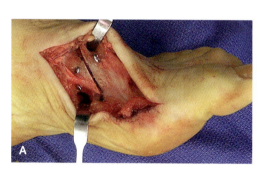
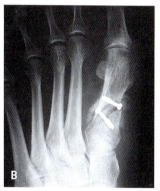

Figure 2-7 A, The plane of the osteotomy in this patient is too vertical, increasing the likelihood of delayed union. **B,** Radiographic appearance of a delayed malunion at 5 weeks after surgery. Compare with that in the postoperative radiograph in Figure 2-8, *B,* in which primary bone healing occurred as expected.

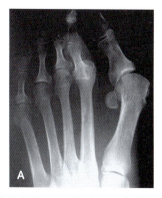
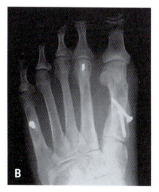

Figure 2-8 A, Preoperative image. **B,** Primary bone healing has occurred in a patient who underwent the Ludloff osteotomy. The healing indicates stable fixation and, indirectly, the correct plane of the osteotomy.

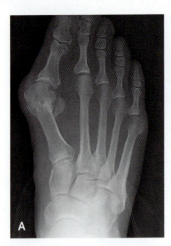 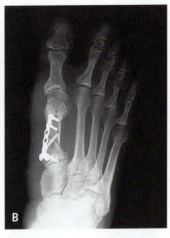 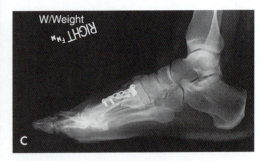

Figure 2-9 The fixation obtained after Ludloff osteotomy in an older patient was not stable. To compensate for the osteopenia, seen best in **A,** a plate was added for increased stability of fixation, as shown in **B** and **C.**

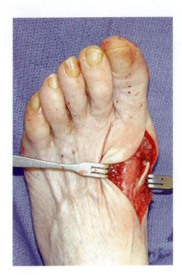

Figure 2-10 The rotation of the osteotomy around the axis of the screw is highlighted here. A few millimeters of bone should remain on the medial and proximal dorsal metatarsal, indicating adequate rotation of the osteotomy.

CHAPTER **3**

The Modified Lapidus Procedure

OVERVIEW

It is important to distinguish between the procedure as originally described by Paul Lapidus, which included an arthrodesis between the base of the first and second metatarsals, and the modified Lapidus procedure, which stabilizes only the first metatarsocuneiform (MC) joint. The true Lapidus procedure is indicated primarily when significant transverse plane instability is present. This instability may be at the MC joint, or between the medial and middle columns, extending into the interspace between the medial and middle cuneiforms. Generally, I perform the modified Lapidus procedure, with addition of stabilization between the first and second metatarsals only if persistent instability is present after arthrodesis of the MC joint. The indications for the Lapidus bunionectomy therefore include hypermobility and instability of the first metatarsal in *either* the sagittal or the transverse plane.

Examination for sagittal plane instability or hypermobility is best performed by stabilizing the lateral aspect of the foot and then manipulating the medial column in a dorsal or plantar direction (Figure 3-1). There is obviously a "feel" to this examination, and although objective interobserver reliability may not be achievable among surgeons who examine the foot for instability, each surgeon should establish personal criteria for what is normal and what is abnormal. An important component of this test for increased first ray mobility is to establish that it is only the first metatarsal and not the entire medial column that is mobile. By pushing the lateral column into maximum dorsiflexion and then testing the first ray, a more accurate result will be obtained. Radiographic parameters of instability are helpful but unreliable in planning this operation; however, instability in the transverse plane is easy to document (Figure 3-2).

Patients with arthritis of the first or second metatarsal cuneiform joint associated with hallux valgus are best treated with an extended Lapidus procedure to include the metatarsocuneiform joints. Arthritis of the second tarsometatarsal (TMT) joint usually is the result of the instability of the first metatarsal, with hypermobility leading to overload of the second metatarsal and, ultimately, arthritis. Frequently, patients with arthritis of the second metatarsal cuneiform joint have associated arthritis of the first metatarsal cuneiform joint as well, but the Lapidus procedure is indicated nonetheless in the absence of arthritis of the first metatarsal cuneiform joint.

The Lapidus procedure is an important adjunct to the correction of the flatfoot deformity when instability of the first metatarsocuneiform joint is present.

INCISION AND DISSECTION

I used to perform the procedure using three incisions, one for the distal soft tissue release, one for the exostectomy and the capsulorrhaphy, and one for the arthrodesis. I have found that one long dorsal incision is cosmetically preferable, and indeed, the exostectomy can be performed through the same incision or may not be needed at all (Figure 3-3). After the distal soft tissue and adductor release, the incision is extended proximally, lateral to the extensor hallucis longus tendon, without injury to the deep peroneal nerve. In my experience, this single midline incision is more cosmetically acceptable and facilitates exposure of the TMT joint proximally. The exostectomy is *not* performed at this time, because subtle rotation of the metatarsal may occur after arthrodesis, changing the axis of the exostectomy, and if the arthrodesis is performed correctly, it is often not necessary to do an exostectomy. The extensor hallucis longus tendon is retracted medially, and with subperiosteal dissection, the dorsal surface of the articulation is identified and opened. The key to the joint debridement is *restraint*, because only the articular cartilage and minimal subchondral bone should be removed.

Although the first metatarsal is moved laterally during the procedure, such movement is not performed through removal of any wedges of bone, which shortens the metatarsal. Instead, translation and rotation of the metatarsal base are preferable. The ease of this manipulation will depend on the configuration of the articulation, which typically is saddle-shaped and may not be amenable to this translational movement. A smooth laminar spreader is inserted into the TMT articulation, and the joint is distracted to provide visualization of the plantar surface of the first metatarsal. The joint is much deeper than might be expected, and for prevention of a dorsal malunion, the entire joint must be denuded. I prefer to use a chisel instead of a saw blade to denude the articular cartilage, and then I perforate the joint multiple times using a small drill bit down to healthy bleeding subchondral bone on both the metatarsal and cuneiform surfaces (Figure 3-4). The perforation of the joint surfaces probably is the most important component of the procedure, and with this minor change to technique, I have rarely encountered a nonunion over the recent past.

CORRECTION OF DEFORMITY

The metatarsal deformity is corrected with a maneuver that includes adduction and simultaneous supination. To plantar flex the metatarsal and prevent dorsal malunion, I dorsiflex the hallux to force

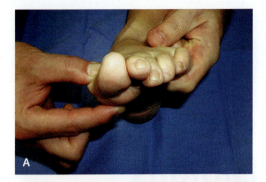

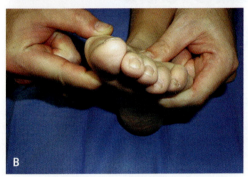

Figure 3-1 Hypermobility associated with hallux valgus is revealed by moving the first metatarsal in a plantar **(A)** and then a dorsal **(B)** direction after firmly stabilizing the lateral column of the foot. There is a "feel" for this maneuver, and all patients with hallux valgus should undergo this test for instability in the sagittal plane. Examination specifically for instability in the transverse plane (between the first and second metatarsals) also is indicated.

the first metatarsal into slight plantar flexion. The first metatarsal is then squeezed to the second metatarsal, and the combination of hallux dorsiflexion and adduction of the metatarsal serves to correct the deformity. The articular surface should be nicely impacted, and both the base of the first metatarsal and the articular surface of the medial cuneiform should be well apposed. If the alignment is corrected and no instability remains, then the fixation is planned between the first metatarsal and the medial cuneiform only. Two guide pins are inserted: The first one, which is inserted from the dorsal proximal aspect of the medial cuneiform, is aimed in a distal and plantar direction in the first metatarsal, and the screw is inserted. Before insertion of the second guide pin, a burr hole is made in the dorsal cortex of the first metatarsal to function as a countersink maneuver. The second guide pin is inserted from the first metatarsal dorsally and is directed in a slightly proximal, plantar, and lateral direction relative to the first guide pin. This articulation should now be checked fluoroscopically to ascertain the position of the first metatarsal head in relation to the sesamoid and to ensure that overcorrection is not present. I use two 4-mm partially threaded cancellous cannulated screws. Countersinking the medial cuneiform is unnecessary, but this maneuver must be carefully performed in the metatarsal to prevent fracture and splitting of its proximal dorsal

apical surface. If instability is noted between the first and second metatarsals, or even between the medial and middle TMT columns (i.e., between the first and second metatarsals and the medial and middle cuneiforms), an extra screw is inserted between the first metatarsal and the medial cuneiform. The third screw is introduced from the base of the first metatarsal and introduced obliquely into the second metatarsal or middle cuneiform, depending on the plane of the metatarsal and the ability to avoid the first two screws. Performing a formal arthrodesis between the first and second metatarsals, as originally described by Lapidus, is unnecessary unless gross instability is present and this is part of a more extensive arthrodesis procedure of the TMT joints (Figures 3-5 and 3-6).

EXOSTECTOMY AND CAPSULAR REPAIR

The alignment of the first metatarsal is checked with respect to the medial eminence and the hallux. Occasionally, an exostectomy is unnecessary because the alignment is already perfect. If an exostectomy is performed unnecessarily, the hallux may become unstable, with resultant hallux varus. The incision is extended from the flare just distal to the metatarsophalangeal joint and carried proximally. The capsulotomy can be made in a longitudinal direction, but I prefer a more standard inverted L shape with the apex proximal and dorsal, which leaves the capsule mobile for soft tissue closure.

With a saw blade, the medial eminence is cut from dorsal to plantar to create the proximal aspect of the exostectomy flush with metaphyseal flare. It is important not to resect too much bone relative to the first metatarsal shaft axis, because the extent of such resection will affect the position of the tibial sesamoid relative to the hallux. With the hallux in a well-aligned position relative to the first metatarsal, the capsulorrhaphy is performed, with absorbable 2-0 sutures inserted in oblique orientation, from the dorsal proximal aspect of the capsule into the plantar distal position, to pull the hallux into slight supination.

MANAGEMENT OF COMPLICATIONS

Whether nonunion or malunion is present, correction of residual or recurrent deformity is an essential aspect of revision surgery. As previously noted, plantar flexing the first metatarsal is important during the fixation; this is best accomplished by dorsiflexion of the hallux to force the first metatarsal into plantar flexion. If dorsal malunion occurs, then revision with osteotomy or interposition bone grafting is necessary (Figure 3-7). Management of nonunion is more difficult, because sclerosis and some avascular change of the joint surfaces usually are present, and in order to debride the joint to healthy bleeding bone surfaces, a defect frequently is created, requiring use of a bone graft (Figure 3-8). Contributing factors in the development of nonunion are inadequate or incorrect apposition of the bone surfaces at the TMT joint, inappropriate fixation, premature weight bearing after surgery, and inadequate joint preparation. As noted earlier, the most important change in my technique over the years has been the creation of multiple perforations in the metatarsal and cuneiform with a small drill bit, to produce bleeding and a slurry of bone at the joint interface.

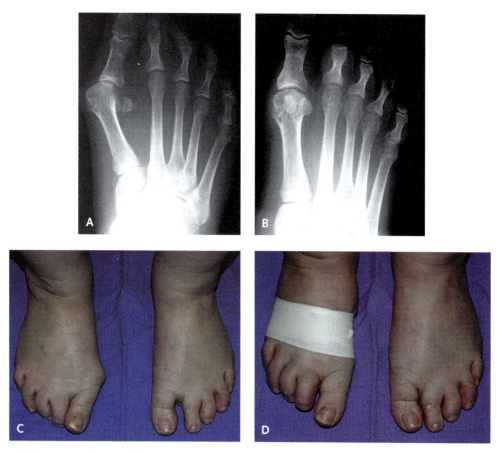

Figure 3-2 Transverse plane instability, demonstrated in **A** and **B,** is correctable with strapping of the forefoot, as shown in **C** and **D.** Radiographs taken with and without the strapping will confirm the presence of such excessive mobility. This is an ideal deformity to correct with the modified Lapidus procedure.

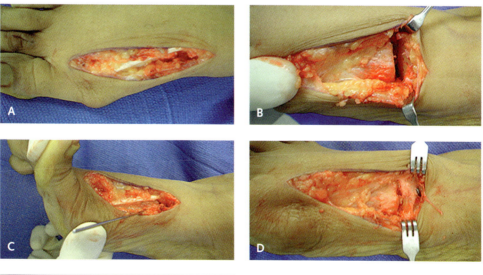

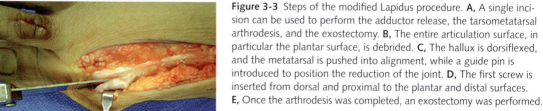

Figure 3-3 Steps of the modified Lapidus procedure. **A,** A single incision can be used to perform the adductor release, the tarsometatarsal arthrodesis, and the exostectomy. **B,** The entire articulation surface, in particular the plantar surface, is debrided. **C,** The hallux is dorsiflexed, and the metatarsal is pushed into alignment, while a guide pin is introduced to position the reduction of the joint. **D,** The first screw is inserted from dorsal and proximal to the plantar and distal surfaces. **E,** Once the arthrodesis was completed, an exostectomy was performed.

Figure 3-4 A and **B,** Preoperative radiographs showing an unstable hallux deformity in a 21-year-old patient. Elevation of the first metatarsal is evident on the lateral view **(B). C,** A 2-mm drill bit was used to perforate the joint surfaces, creating a slurry in the joint. **D** and **E,** No transverse plane instability was noted intraoperatively, so only axial screw fixation was used in a modified Lapidus procedure. No exostectomy or capsulorrhaphy was performed.

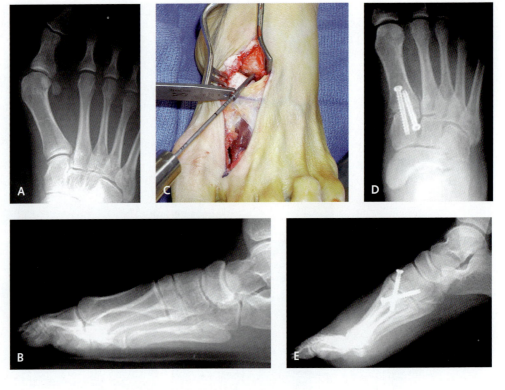

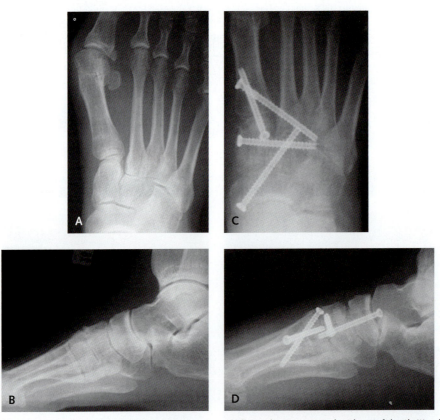

Figure 3-5 A and **B,** The patient was treated for recurrent hallux valgus associated with painful arthritis of the tarsometatarsal and naviculocuneiform joints. **C** and **D,** An extended arthrodesis was performed. Note the oblique screws that were inserted across the first and into the second metatarsal.

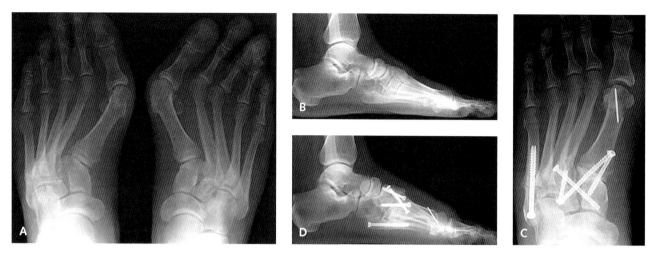

Figure 3-6 A and **B,** The patient had severe multiplanar deformity associated with marked metatarsus adductus and painful arthritis of the second metatarsocuneiform joint. **C** and **D,** The deformity was corrected with an extended tarsometatarsal arthrodesis and a biplanar chevron osteotomy. The stress fracture of the fifth metatarsal was fixed simultaneously.

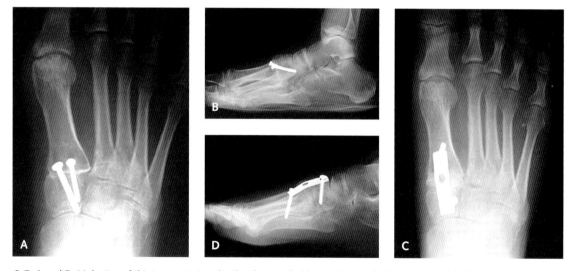

Figure 3-7 A and **B,** Malunion of this tarsometatarsal arthrodesis probably was the result of inadequate debridement of the base of the articulation. Note elevation of the first metatarsal. **C** and **D,** Revision surgery included use of a structural triangular graft, with restoration of the declination angle of the first metatarsal.

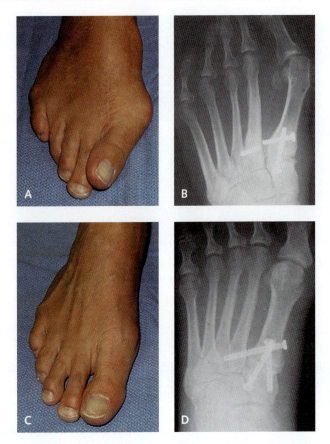

Figure 3-8 A and **B,** The patient was referred for treatment of nonunion after an attempted Lapidus procedure. Note the severe deformity associated with pronation and hallux valgus. **C** and **D,** Correction was accomplished with a revision that included bone graft and arthrodesis of the intermetatarsal space between the first and second metatarsals. Of note, no osteotomy of the hallux phalanx was required for correction.

TECHNIQUES, TIPS, AND PITFALLS

- Be careful with the soft tissue (adductor) release with this procedure. Correction of deformity with arthrodesis is excellent, and with excessive adductor release, hallux varus will occur. Consider that a "modified" or "minimal" adductor release is performed for this procedure.

- Exostectomy may not be necessary and is not performed until completion of the realignment and arthrodesis.

- The correct positioning of the first metatarsal in the sagittal plane is imperative during this procedure. Using a dorsal incision makes exposure of the base of the first MC joint more difficult. Furthermore, when the joint surface is debrided, more cartilage may be removed dorsally than on the plantar surface, and this asymmetrical removal leaves the apex of the joint intact inferiorly. Leaving bone on the plantar surface of the joint automatically dorsiflexes the metatarsal, creating a dorsal malunion. A lamina spreader facilitates full exposure of the joint surface.

- Rotation of the first metatarsal head must be avoided with stabilization. Ideally, the metatarsal head should be slightly supinated during the stabilization and arthrodesis. Because of the plane of inclination of the first metatarsal, as it is being pushed over toward the second metatarsal, the first metatarsal tends to undergo slight pronation, rather than supination, and this must be avoided.

- The fixation of the TMT joint can be done in one plane (from the first metatarsal into the cuneiform, and vice versa) or in two planes (to control transverse plane instability as well). Generally speaking, sagittal plane instability must be corrected primarily, and if additional instability is noted in the mediolateral (transverse) plane, then an additional screw must be inserted obliquely from the first metatarsal into the second metatarsal or middle cuneiform.

- The Lapidus procedure is a logical choice for correction of hallux valgus associated with a chronic nonunion of a stress fracture of the second metatarsal base (Figure 3-9).

- Screw fixation of the arthrodesis generally is sufficient; however, I use a plate if a fracture of the metatarsal is present or if the bone quality is not ideal (Figure 3-10).

- Arthrodesis between the first and second metatarsals and the intercuneiform space may be unnecessary. However, if the arthrodesis is being performed as part of a procedure for correction of arthritis and deformity in which the second metatarsal cuneiform joint is included in the arthrodesis, then fusion between the medial and middle columns is advisable as well (Figure 3-11).

- A formal Lapidus procedure also can be used for correction of a nonunion of the base of the second metatarsal, where bone graft is inserted between the first and second metatarsals (Figure 3-12).

- Shortening of the metatarsal will occur if a wedge from the MC joint is resected. Depending on the shape of the articulation, the correction should be done by translation and not by resection of a bone wedge. If a bone wedge *has* to be resected, make sure that that this shortening is compensated by plantar flexing the first metatarsal.

- Not all patients with a nonunion have symptoms. If a revision is performed, the goal should be a solid arthrodesis, but in the *correct position*. Union may occur, but this may be at the expense of length, and a malunion does not help the patient either.

- Revision is required for shortening of the first metatarsal, malunion, or a painful nonunion. Although revision can be accomplished with screw fixation, a small, dorsally applied two-hole plate is the most useful, with bone graft inserted to realign or lengthen the first metatarsal, as needed.

- An increase in the distal metatarsal articular angle (DMAA) is not always anatomically correct and, certainly, may constitute a rotational anomaly for some patients. The Lapidus procedure is an excellent choice for correction of failed hallux valgus surgery even when the DMAA is apparently increased (Figure 3-13).

- The Lapidus procedure is very useful as part of a more global correction of severe metatarsus adductus with associated arthritis of the MC joints (Figure 3-14).

- The Lapidus procedure is an important adjunct to the correction of a flatfoot deformity associated with instability of the first MC joint (Figure 3-15).

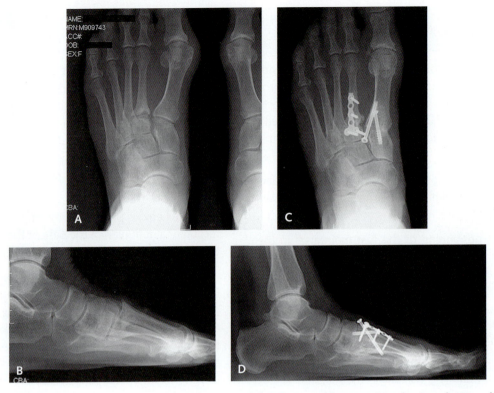

Figure 3-9 A and **B,** Although the patient's hallux valgus deformity was mild, a nonunion of a stress fracture of the second metatarsal was present. **C** and **D,** The Lapidus procedure was performed to address both problems.

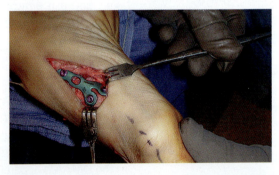

Figure 3-10 Because of the patient's extremely poor bone quality, a dorsomedial plate (Orthohelix, Akron, Ohio) was used in addition to an axial screw for fixation.

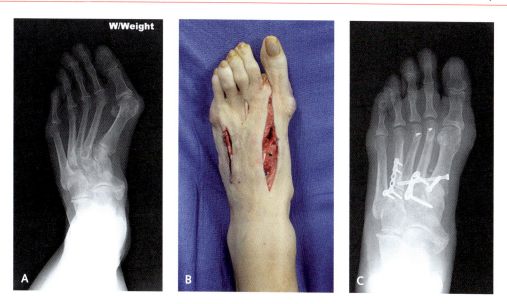

Figure 3-11 A, Marked metatarsus adductus associated with arthritis in a 52-year-old patient. **B,** The Lapidus procedure was performed in combination with arthrodesis of the second and third metatarsocuneiform joints, as well as shortening osteotomies of the second and third metatarsals to realign the toes.
C, Postoperative radiograph.

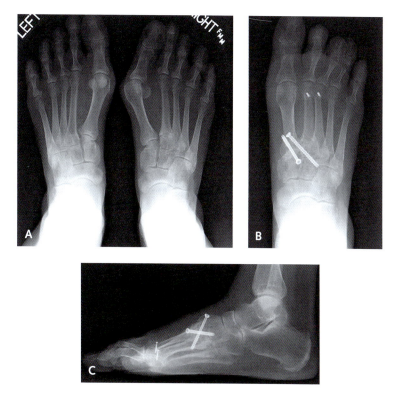

Figure 3-12 A, This chronic nonunion of the base of the second metatarsal was treated with a Lapidus procedure. **B** and **C,** The base of the second metatarsal was included in the bone graft but without fixation.

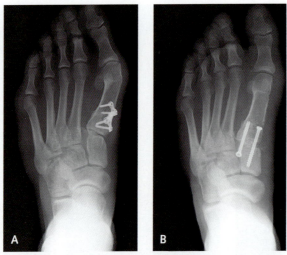

Figure 3-13 A and **B,** Despite the apparent increase in the distal metatarsal articular angle (DMAA) after a previous failed correction with an opening wedge plate, no additional correction beyond stabilization using a Lapidus procedure with screw fixation was needed for the distal metatarsal deformity.

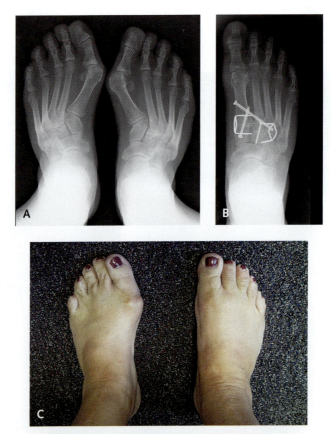

Figure 3-14 A-C, The Lapidus procedure was performed for treatment of diffuse forefoot deformity associated with metatarsus adductus. The patient also had arthritis of the second and third metatarsocuneiform joints.

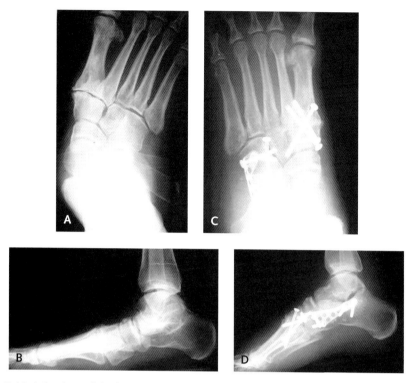

Figure 3-15 Arthrodesis of the first metatarsocuneiform joint is an important adjunct to correction of a flatfoot deformity. **A** and **B**, The patient had marked abduction of the forefoot associated with a flexible flatfoot. **C** and **D**, Correction was obtained with a lateral column lengthening arthrodesis of the calcaneocuboid joint and a modified Lapidus procedure.

SUGGESTED READING

Faber FW, Kleinrensink GJ, Mulder PG, Verhaar JA: Mobility of the first tarsometatarsal joint in hallux valgus: A radiographic analysis, *Foot Ankle Int* 22:965–969, 2001.

Myerson M, Allon S, McGarvey W: Metatarsocuneiform arthrodesis for management of hallux valgus and metatarsus primus varus, *Foot Ankle* 13:107–115, 1992.

Myerson MS: Metatarsocuneiform arthrodesis for treatment of hallux valgus and metatarsus primus varus, *Orthopedics* 13:1025–1031, 1990.

Myerson MS, Badekas A: Hypermobility of the first ray, *Foot Ankle Clin* 5:469–484, 2000.

Sangeorzan BJ, Hansen ST Jr: Modified Lapidus procedure for hallux valgus, *Foot Ankle* 9:262–262, 1989.

CHAPTER **4**

Proximal Phalangeal Osteotomy (Akin Osteotomy)

A commonly performed adjunctive procedure for correction of hallux valgus is an osteotomy of the proximal phalanx of the hallux—the Akin osteotomy. By itself, this procedure has few indications. When the Akin osteotomy is performed alone, the recurrence rate for hallucal deformity is exceedingly high because the biomechanical deformity and imbalance around the metatarsophalangeal (MP) joint are uncorrected. When closing wedge phalangeal osteotomy is used as an adjunctive procedure with other osteotomies for correction of hallux valgus, however, the outcome is predictable and reliable.

Although used predominantly for correction of symptomatic hallux valgus, this osteotomy is useful in conjunction with correction of a crossover second toe deformity, even when the hallux valgus is asymptomatic. The second toe is difficult if not impossible to realign if the hallux is abutting it laterally, because there is no room to correct the toe deformity and reposition the toe without underriding of the toe by the hallux, leading to recurrent deformity. Correction of the mechanical axis of the hallux MP joint also is important, for example, with an abnormal distal metatarsal articular angle. Correction of the MP joint alignment abnormality with a biplanar osteotomy of the distal first metatarsal is preferable. With the addition of the phalangeal osteotomy, however, the hallux shortens slightly. As a result, tension on the extrinsic tendons decreases, and correction of the pronation is easier. Although the closing wedge phalanx osteotomy is of secondary importance, it does improve the cosmetic appearance of the toe. The phalangeal osteotomy is very useful to correct fixed pronation of the hallux. This deformity does not correct well with any osteotomy, and trying to pull the capsule using the capsulorrhaphy to correct the pronation does not work (Figure 4-1).

The traditional use of the phalangeal osteotomy is to function as an adjunctive procedure for the correction of hallux valgus. As discussed further on, this osteotomy is performed in the metaphysis at the base of the proximal phalanx. A far more important use of the phalangeal osteotomy, however, is the correction of hallux valgus interphalangeus (Figures 4-2 and 4-3). Other than an arthrodesis of the hallux interphalangeal (IP) joint, the only method of correction that will work is an osteotomy through the distal portion of the proximal phalanx.

The incision is made along the medial aspect of the proximal phalanx, extending from the capsule distally toward the IP joint, and the periosteum is split. The attachment of the capsule to the base of the proximal phalanx must be preserved to facilitate the capsulorrhaphy. After subperiosteal dissection, small retractors are inserted subcutaneously to expose the bone. Because supinating the hallux is usual, a biplanar osteotomy generally is performed, in addition to the closing wedge phalanx osteotomy. Two sets of pilot holes are now made on either side of the osteotomy with a Kirschner wire (K-wire). These are unicortical holes inserted at a 45-degree angle with respect to the plane of the phalanx. The proximal set is made in line with the medial aspect of the phalangeal shaft, and then the distal set is drilled more plantarward so that when the osteotomy is closed, the hallux is supinated, and the two sets of holes line up with each other. The distal holes are approximately 2 mm inferior to the proximal holes (Figure 4-4).

The osteotomy is made in metaphyseal bone just distal to the metaphyseal flare. When the proximal cut is made, it must be exactly parallel with the base of the proximal phalanx. Because of the orientation of the phalanx, the surgeon's tendency is to aim laterally, and because of the hallux valgus, this cut has a tendency to be too close to the articular surface. The osteotomy is made in the middle of these holes, and a 2-mm wedge of bone is removed. Preserving the lateral cortex of the phalanx is important. The osteotomy should not cross the cortical surface but should be pried open with a small osteotome, with the lateral cortex cracked. The hinged cortex can then be used for closure. Once the osteotomy is complete, the hallux is supinated and secured in position with two fixation sutures placed across it and inserted through the pre-drilled holes. Absorbable 2-0 suture material on a tapered needle is used for closure of the osteotomy. To maintain the result, neither screws nor staples are needed; reliable correction can be obtained simply with the suture technique. The hallux should be in the neutral position with respect to the axis of the metatarsal and in slight supination at the completion of the osteotomy. If the hallux is very pronated, the osteotomy can be intentionally supinated. In this case, the suture holes are made eccentrically, and once the wedge is removed, the hallux is supinated and secured with suture fixation (Figure 4-5).

As noted, this is the traditional method used for the phalangeal osteotomy. If the hallux is already short, however, this osteotomy is not an ideal repair, because it will shorten the phalanx even more. In this situation, I perform a dome osteotomy of the phalanx, which can be proximally or distally based. The incision must be made dorsally, and if the incision for the bunionectomy

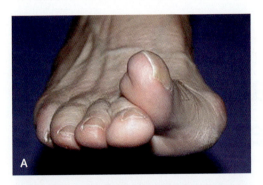
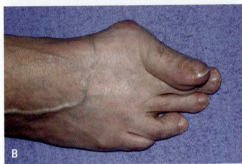
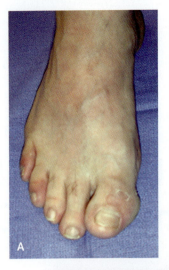
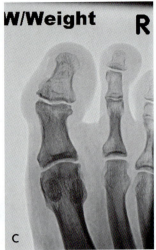

Figure 4-1 A and **B,** The phalangeal osteotomy is a very useful adjunct to correct a severely pronated hallux, as in this case, regardless of which osteotomy procedure is chosen for correction of the metatarsal deformity.

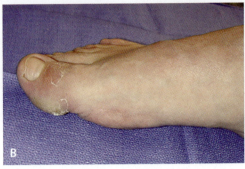

Figure 4-3 The patient had suffered an injury to the hallux, followed by development of arthritis of the interphalangeal joint. **A-C,** The bulbous interphalangeal joint and the fixed deformity are evident both clinically and radiographically. Correction was accomplished with a distal phalangeal osteotomy, although an arthrodesis would have been an acceptable procedure.

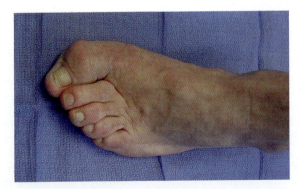

Figure 4-2 The phalangeal osteotomy is very useful to correct an interphalangeal deformity, even in the presence of arthritis. The slight shortening with the osteotomy can correct a rigid contracture of the interphalangeal joint, as seen here.

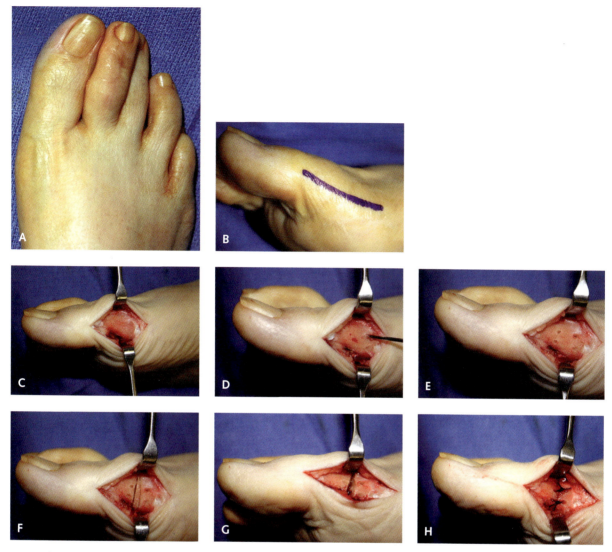

Figure 4-4 A, The patient had asymptomatic hallux valgus accompanied by a deformity of the second toe that could not be corrected without realignment of the hallux. **B,** The incision is marked out almost to the interphalangeal joint. **C,** The medial phalanx is then exposed. **D** and **E,** Four pilot holes are introduced with a 0.062-inch K-wire at a 45-degree angle in two pairs. **F** and **G,** A wedge of bone approximately 1 to 2 mm thick is removed in between the pilot holes. **H,** The osteotomy is secured with two 2-0 absorbable sutures.

is made medially, then the incision must be curved dorsally, medial to the EHL for exposure. The EHL is retracted laterally, and the dome saw blade is directed from dorsal to plantar. The phalanx is then rotated around its axis until correction is obtained (Figure 4-6). The phalangeal osteotomy can be added to any

metatarsal osteotomy or a Lapidus procedure to improve the alignment of the hallux (Figure 4-7). In order to avoid an arthrodesis of the IP joint, the phalangeal osteotomy also can be used as an adjunctive procedure—for example, with an arthrodesis of the hallux MP joint (Figure 4-8).

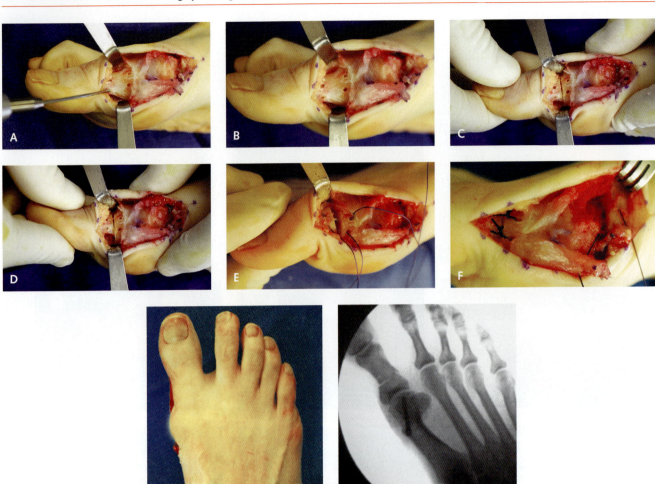

Figure 4-5 The steps of the closing wedge osteotomy of the proximal phalanx of the hallux in a case in which the hallux has to be supinated. **A** and **B,** The two sets of pilot holes are offset in order to rotate the phalanx. **C-E,** The 1-mm wedge of bone is removed and the osteotomy is closed. The hallux is then supinated to line up the pilot holes (**C** and **D**). and sutures are inserted (**E**). **F,** The capsule was repaired through a K-wire hole in the metatarsal cortex. **G** and **H,** The final appearance in a clinical photograph and on a fluoroscopic image.

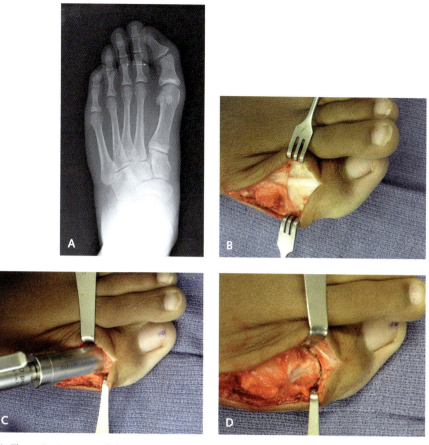

Figure 4-6 A, The patient was an adolescent who presented with severe hallux valgus interphalangeus in addition to mild hallux valgus. The hallux was very short and underriding the second toe. **B-D,** A dome distal phalangeal osteotomy was used to correct the deformity, to avoid further shortening of the hallux.

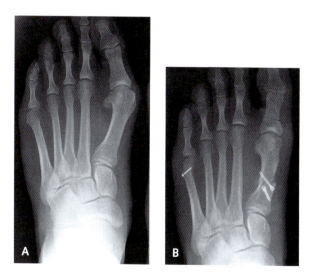

Figure 4-7 A, A Ludloff osteotomy was combined with a closing wedge phalangeal osteotomy for correction of this seemingly straightforward deformity that was, however, far more rigid than radiographically apparent. **B,** Despite adequate adductor release, the hallux remained in valgus, perhaps because of an incongruent metatarsophalangeal joint.

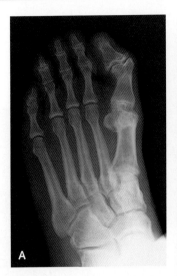 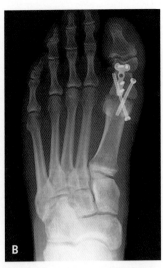

Figure 4-8 A, The patient had hallux rigidus in addition to hallux valgus interphalangeus—a difficult combination to treat, because an arthrodesis of the metatarsophalangeal and interphalangeal joints is not ideal. **B,** This combination deformity was corrected with an arthrodesis of the hallux metatarsophalangeal joint and a simultaneous osteotomy of the phalanx using a closing wedge distal osteotomy and fixation with a mini-T plate (F3 plate, DePuy Orthopaedics, Inc., Warsaw, Indiana).

CHAPTER 5

Management of Complications After Correction of Hallux Valgus

GENERAL PRINCIPLES OF MANAGING COMPLICATIONS

As the saying goes, the best way to treat a complication is to avoid one to begin with, and this applies in particular to correction of hallux valgus, for which many treatment approaches carry an increased risk of failure. Some very simple principles or rules should be followed in planning hallux valgus surgery. The presence of soft tissue problems, including scarring, contracture, and neuritis, must be taken into consideration with any revision of forefoot procedures. Unfortunately, further scarring and stiffening at the metatarsophalangeal (MP) joint are likely with many revision metatarsal procedures. Regardless of the bone correction and the ultimate alignment obtained, the potential for failure due to stiffness of the MP joint must be considered. Stiffness can be global and may include not only the MP joint but also the sesamoid apparatus. Although healed bones and improved alignment are worthwhile goals, the potential for worsening of any scarring, neuritis, and stiffness of the MP joint must be a primary consideration.

Because of this concern, arthrodesis is an appealing choice for some revision procedures. This is particularly the case when the deformity and disease involve the MP joint only. If the hallux interphalangeal (IP) joint is contracted or deformed, then MP arthrodesis may not be the preferred procedure.

In any case, the following general principles should be addressed in surgical planning:

- Do not overextend the indications for a procedure.
- Identify deformity of the metatarsal in more than one plane, if present.
- Be cognizant of the effect of the hallux on the lesser toes, and vice versa (Figure 5-1).
- Be familiar with the concept of hypermobility and increased motion of the first metatarsal in both the sagittal and the horizontal planes.
- Evaluate the functional status of the sesamoid apparatus and the extrinsic tendons, and identify any contracture of the extensor hallucis longus.

- Avoid incisions that can cause neuroma formation.
- Avoid a dorsal incision, which is associated with increased stiffness of the hallux postoperatively and, in particular, with an inevitable decrease in plantar flexion.
- Maintain an awareness of the blood supply to the first metatarsal.
- Recognize the effect of the hindfoot on the forefoot, because correction of hallux valgus may fail if a flatfoot deformity is present, causing increased pronation on the hallux (Figure 5-2).
- Avascular necrosis occurs as a result of excessive stripping of the periosteum—for no other reason. If avascular necrosis occurs, too much exposure of the metatarsal was performed; if it occurs more than once in a specific surgeon's clinical practice, the need for changes in surgical technique should be considered, because something is wrong (Figure 5-3).
- Fixed pronation of the hallux of the hallux cannot be corrected with the metatarsal osteotomy, and an osteotomy of the phalanx should be performed.
- Recognize the occasional association of hallux valgus with more rigid and arthritic deformity of the metatarsophalangeal joint. The patient will be far happier with a fused MP joint with a corrected deformity than one that is painful with recurrent hallux valgus (Figure 5-4).
- A primary arthrodesis for correction of hallux valgus is a good operation. Anticipate the need for arthrodesis in selected patients.
- Because arthrodesis works well for patients with rheumatologic deformity, it undoubtedly merits increased use in corrective foot and ankle surgery. Dislocation of the MP joint can be realistically corrected only with arthrodesis (Figure 5-5).
- The lesser toe deformities associated with hallux valgus always require correction, and if abducted or adducted toes are not straightened (generally with shortening osteotomies of the metatarsals), recurrent deformity of the hallux will develop (Figure 5-6).
- A soft tissue release should be performed for many hallux valgus deformities. Although this may not be perceived as necessary with use of a distal metatarsal osteotomy, the results with a distal chevron osteotomy, for example, have been demonstrated to be better when the release is performed.

Figure 5-1 A and **B,** Even with optimal correction of the hallux deformity, unless the lesser toes are realigned, recurrent hallux valgus will develop. Abduction of the toes cannot be corrected adequately with soft tissue release only. Shortening of the lesser metatarsals is required.

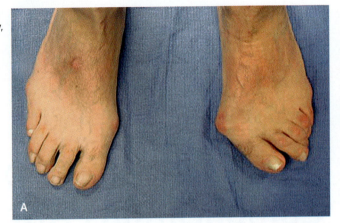
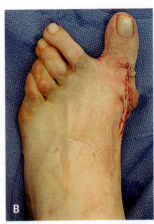

Figure 5-2 A and **B,** With hallux valgus associated with a very flexible flatfoot deformity, as shown here, surgical correction must be because postoperative recurrence of hallux valgus is likely unless the hindfoot deformity is corrected simultaneously.

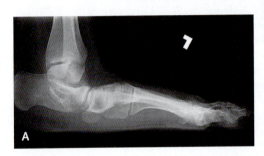
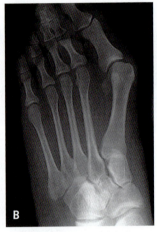

Figure 5-3 A, Avascular necrosis with hallux varus developed after treatment with a distal metatarsal osteotomy. **B,** Treatment was with an arthrodesis, using a structural bone graft to lengthen the avascular shortened metatarsal.

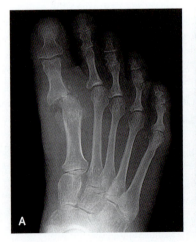
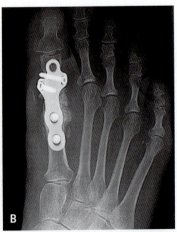

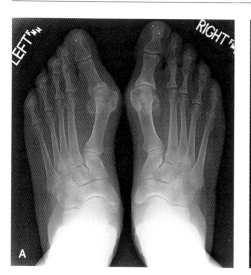
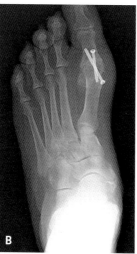

Figure 5-4 Arthrodesis for correction of hallux valgus is a good option for management of severe deformity, with or without arthritis. **A** and **B,** In these radiographs, the valgus deformity is accompanied by evidence of arthritis.

5

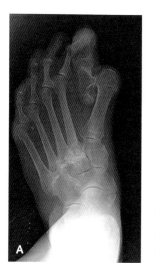
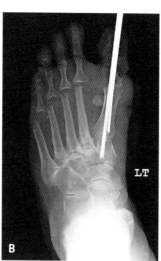
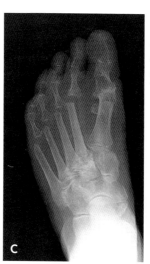

Figure 5-5 A, Dislocation of the metatarsophalangeal joint seen in this radiograph was not associated with rheumatologic deformity. **B** and **C,** Treatment was with arthrodesis using threaded pins for fixation.

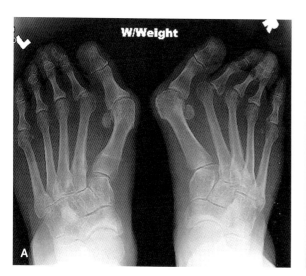
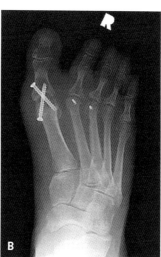

Figure 5-6 A, Although arthritis was not severe, the deformity was significant. **B,** The opposite foot had been treated unsuccessfully with a crescentic osteotomy, resulting in recurrence, and an arthrodesis was selected as the ideal procedure for correction of the hallux deformity.

- Lengthening the first metatarsal does not make anatomic or biomechanical sense. Increasing the tension on the intrinsic muscles can only increase the likelihood of recurrent deformity or stiffness of the MP joint.

- For an optimal result, some relaxation of the intrinsic musculature around the hallux should be obtained with correction.

- Fixation should always be stable. Periosteal new bone formation around the osteotomy indicates motion, inadequate fixation, and an increased likelihood of delayed or nonunion.

- Spasticity, such as that associated with cerebral palsy, does not lend itself to management with osteotomy; an arthrodesis of the MP joint gives a more reliable result.

NONUNION

Nonunion generally is the result of inadequate fixation, excessive stripping and exposure, or incorrect placement of the osteotomy cut. With any nonunion, an avascular segment of bone at the nonunion interface is likely, with shortening of the metatarsal, but further shortening also is likely once debridement has been performed. Debridement is required to obtain bone bleeding and healing but inevitably leads to further shortening and the likelihood of increasing lateral metatarsalgia. Therefore the approach to correction will depend on the presence of existing metatarsalgia, the amount of shortening already present in the first metatarsal, the presence of any arthritis in the MP joint, and any associated soft tissue problems.

Accordingly, with repair of a nonunion, the issues are whether a structural bone graft can be used to restore length or whether primary bone healing can be obtained through supplementation of a cancellus bone graft. It generally is easier to obtain fixation of the diaphysis but easier to obtain bone healing in the metaphysis. Nonunion of a distal metatarsal osteotomy is unusual. However, simultaneous repair of the nonunion and adequate fixation of the metatarsal head in appropriate alignment is difficult to achieve.

During the operation, the surgeon must establish the correct length of the metatarsal with a laminar spreader after debridement at the osteotomy nonunion site (Figure 5-7). In restoring length to the metatarsal, it is important to ensure that too much stress is not present on the hallux MP joint, because this will decrease motion of the hallux considerably. Once I have stretched the metatarsal back out to its appropriate length, multiple Kirschner wires (K-wires) are inserted transversely among the first, second, and third metatarsals to stabilize the first metatarsal in the desired position while fixation options are explored. The same applies to repair of a malunion or nonunion of the metatarsal head after a distal metatarsal osteotomy, although here, the risk of stiffness is markedly increased. Salvage of a distal metatarsal nonunion must be considered as an alternative to an arthrodesis. If arthrodesis is performed, however, most of the metatarsal head will need to be excised, and a very large bone graft must be used to restore length. For this reason, I am always prepared to attempt salvage of the distal metatarsal nonunion with restoration of length, and then, if painful arthritis develops, to perform an arthrodesis later on (Figure 5-8). A more proximal metatarsal nonunion is often the result of inadequate fixation or excessive patient activity in the postoperative period without adequate immobilization. It is important to restore the length of the metatarsal, and as noted earlier, avascular bone generally is present on either side of the osteotomy, necessitating use of a bone graft (Figures 5-9 and 5-10). Depending on the orientation of the nonunion, a structural bone graft usually is necessary to lengthen the metatarsal. Perhaps

these complications can be anticipated if periosteal new bone formation develops in the early postoperative period (see Figure 5-10). This finding is an indicator of excessive motion at the osteotomy, and immobilization may be sufficient at this stage. If the bone heals, it often will do so with some dorsiflexion, and a malunion will be the result. This complication is, however, easier to treat than a nonunion.

AVASCULAR NECROSIS

As noted, AVN is the result of too-aggressive exposure with excessive soft tissue stripping. If the patient presents with pain in the hallux or the MP joint in the postoperative period, AVN should be the primary diagnostic consideration. It can be treated with high-energy shock wave therapy; I use 3000 cycles at 24 kV, applied to the medial and dorsal aspects of the metatarsal head. The AVN may of course be progressive, in which case collapse of the metatarsal head with or without arthritis will occur (Figure 5-11). Correction of avascular necrosis depends on the extent of MP joint arthritis and the shortening of the metatarsal. The decision to perform an arthrodesis depends on the extent of the avascular necrosis, but under most circumstances, this operation will be required. More important is the decision to lengthen the first metatarsal and restore the appropriate weight bearing to the hallux with an interpositional structural graft (Figures 5-12 and 5-13). An important consideration is that because bone often has to be resected until bleeding is obtained, the metatarsal further shortens. Whenever possible, I prefer to perform an arthrodesis without any structural graft because the rate of fusion is slightly lower with use of grafting techniques. The decision is based on the extent of the shortening and the presence of metatarsalgia. Additional procedures may need to be performed for correction of metatarsalgia, such as shortening osteotomies or resection of all of the lesser metatarsal heads. The latter salvage procedure, in conjunction with an arthrodesis (a rheumatoid-type forefoot operation), should be reserved only for patients with severe forefoot deformity with involvement of the lesser metatarsal heads and MP joints. This procedure does, however, give excellent relief despite the decrease in function of the lesser toes (see Figure 5-13).

INFECTION

The approach to correction of infection depends on the extent of the bone involvement. If the infection involves the MP joint, arthroplasty or arthrodesis ultimately needs to be performed. The only problem with these single-stage procedures is the predictable need for eradication of infection before resection arthroplasty or arthrodesis is performed. For this reason, I use antibiotic-impregnated bone cement in a staged procedure and then return at 6 weeks to perform the definitive arthrodesis or arthroplasty (Figure 5-14). As with treatment of other infected joints, before the definitive procedure, a biopsy of the synovium is performed and a frozen section obtained to determine the number of white blood cells per high-power field. If this cell count is less than 5, then the arthrodesis is performed; otherwise, a second cement block is inserted as part of a staged procedure. If arthroplasty is to be performed, then once the cement is removed, realignment of the MP joint can be performed as an interposition arthroplasty. An example of this approach is illustrated in Figure 5-15: A patient with neuropathy had been treated with previous metatarsal head resections for ulceration and infection. Owing to the length of the first metatarsal relative to the lesser toes, some

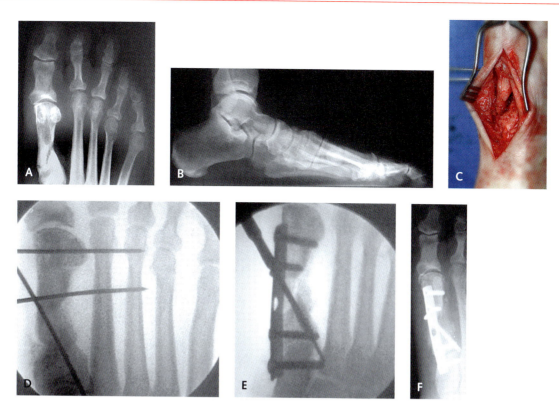

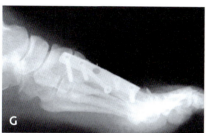

Figure 5-7 **A** and **B,** Symptomatic nonunion of a proximal metatarsal osteotomy. Note the radiographic appearance, with elevation and shortening of the first metatarsal. **C,** The nonunion was identified and its osseous components were loosened. **D,** The metatarsal was then distracted distally to restore length. **E,** Next, cancellous bone graft was inserted. Placement of a cannulated screw and plate fixation was performed. **F** and **G,** The final radiographic appearance.

shortening was felt to be necessary, and although the shortening could have been performed with an arthrodesis, because of the neuropathy, an attempt at correction by arthrodesis was considered to carry an increased risk for failure. A resection arthroplasty was performed, and the joint became infected. The infection was treated with insertion of an antibiotic-impregnated cement block, removal of all necrotic bone, which included most of the metatarsal head, and then placement of a threaded Steinmann pin to achieve realignment, followed by removal once stability was obtained.

For some patients with severe infection and bone loss, it may not be possible to restore function in one or even two stages. This limitation was apparent in the patient whose radiographs are presented in Figure 5-16, who was referred for treatment for infection of the entire metatarsal head. Once complete debridement of the metatarsal was performed, there was gross shortening of the metatarsal, which could not be restored even with a large bone block graft. A lengthening of the metatarsal was first performed using a mini-external fixator, gaining approximately 17 mm of length. The bone block arthrodesis was then subsequently performed (see Figure 5-16). Another treatment option for managing infection (or, for that matter, avascular necrosis of

the metatarsal head) is with a fresh osteoarticular allograft. Once infection is under complete control, an antibiotic-impregnated cement spacer is inserted. Provided the articular surface of the base of the proximal phalanx is healthy, the procedure can be considered. Bone healing at the margin of the metatarsal graft is excellent, although the range of motion of the MP joint may be somewhat restricted. Nonetheless, this is a very suitable option for treating bone loss with a well-maintained phalangeal articular surface (Figure 5-17).

DORSAL MALUNION AND RECURRENT DEFORMITY

The management of a dorsal malunion of the proximal metatarsal osteotomy can be difficult. Although performing a plantar flexion osteotomy of the first metatarsal may seem logical, this osteotomy is not easy to perform because of dorsal soft tissue contracture. Usually the dorsal malunion is accompanied by a shortening of the hallux extensors (Figure 5-18). With a plantar flexion osteotomy of the first metatarsal, further tightening occurs with the potential for recurrent deformity and development of a cock-up deformity.

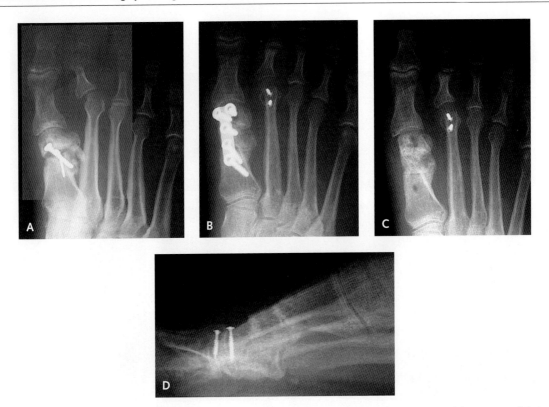

Figure 5-8 A, Nonunion after distal metatarsal osteotomy was associated with marked bone loss and shortening of the metatarsal, but with preservation of the blood supply to the hallux. **B,** Lengthening of the first metatarsal with use of interposition structural allograft was performed with a small T-plate to hold the position of the reduction; this was combined with slight shortening of the second metatarsal. **C** and **D,** Adequate bone healing of the osteotomy occurred, and despite the radiographic appearance, no symptomatic arthritis was present, with 45 degrees of motion at the metatarsophalangeal joint after plate removal.

The alternative procedures for correction of a dorsal malunion are an opening wedge osteotomy with bone graft, a closing wedge osteotomy through resection of a plantar-based wedge, and a dome osteotomy. A dome osteotomy can be performed from the medial aspect of the metatarsal with a crescentic saw blade inserted perpendicular to the metatarsal. This is an excellent technique because no further shortening of the metatarsal occurs. However, the radius of curvature of the blade is not large enough to accommodate the plain of the metatarsal. For this reason, the crescentic saw blade can be used on the plantar three quarters of the metatarsal. Then the osteotomy can be completed dorsally with a vertical step cut, through which a screw can be inserted for fixation. The other option is an opening wedge osteotomy with insertion of graft, as shown for a malunion after a Lapidus procedure (Figure 5-19).

Malunion occurs for many reasons, including incorrect use of a metatarsal osteotomy, undercorrection, inappropriate use of fixation of the osteotomy, the inherent nature or potential for instability based on the geometry of the osteotomy, and instability of the first tarsometatarsal (TMT) joint. In Figure 5-20, an unusual case of delayed union and then malunion resulted from unrecognized neuropathy. The correction of malunion can be frustratingly difficult because of soft tissue contracture, scarring, neuritis, bone loss, and multiplanar deformity. The combination of a malunion with a nonunion, as shown in Figure 5-21, is an especially difficult problem to treat, owing to the associated arthritis of the MP joint. In the case illustrated, the first metatarsal obviously has been overcorrected, creating a negative intermetatarsal angle. Correction of this malunion did establish the MP joint alignment, but because significant arthritis was present, an arthrodesis was required.

5

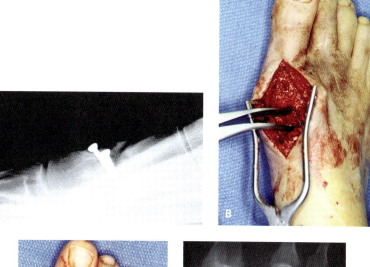

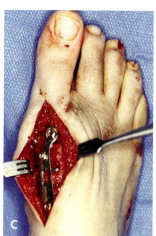
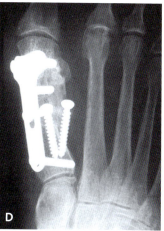

Figure 5-9 A, Nonunion occurred after metatarsal osteotomy of unknown type. Shortening and elevation of the first metatarsal are evident. **B,** A laminar spreader was used to establish the length of the metatarsal after debridement of the nonunion. **C** and **D,** This was followed by insertion of a tricortical bone graft and a plate to maintain the alignment.

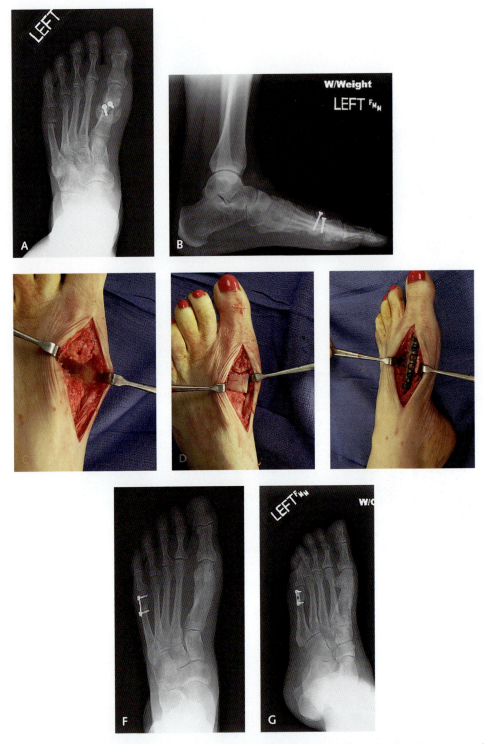

Figure 5-10 Nonunion in this case probably occurred as a result of the osteotomy in the metatarsal diaphysis. **A** and **B,** Note the periosteal new bone formation, indicative of motion at the osteotomy during healing. **C-E,** After removal of all necrotic avascular bone, marked shortening was present; this was treated with a structural graft and plate fixation. **F** and **G,** The radiographic appearance after plate removal.

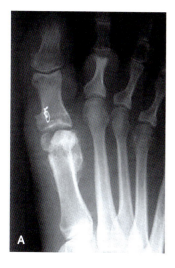

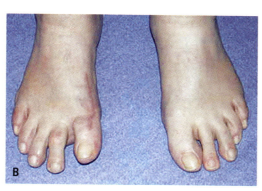

Figure 5-11 **A** and **B,** Avascular necrosis occurred after a distal metatarsal osteotomy of unknown type. Severe shortening and necrosis were present, with a cock-up deformity of the hallux. Salvage was accomplished with a bone block arthrodesis of the metatarsophalangeal joint with insertion of a structural allograft.

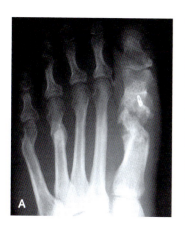

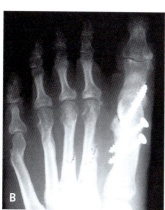

Figure 5-12 **A,** Avascular necrosis with shortening of the first metatarsal occurred after a distal metatarsal osteotomy of unknown type. Severe metatarsalgia of the second and third metatarsals was present (note that an osteotomy of the fourth and fifth metatarsals also had been performed previously). **B,** An arthrodesis of the hallux metatarsophalangeal joint was performed with structural bone graft and screw fixation. An oblique proximal shortening osteotomy of the second and third metatarsals was performed simultaneously.

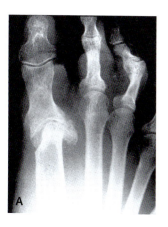

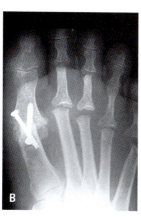

Figure 5-13 **A,** Avascular necrosis was associated with severe metatarsalgia and toe deformities in an elderly patient. **B,** An arthrodesis was performed in situ with resection of the lesser metatarsal heads, instead of a lengthening of the first metatarsal with a graft.

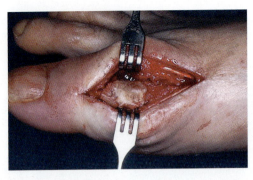

Figure 5-14 Infection after an implant arthroplasty with osteomyelitis was treated with staged interposition of antibiotic cement.

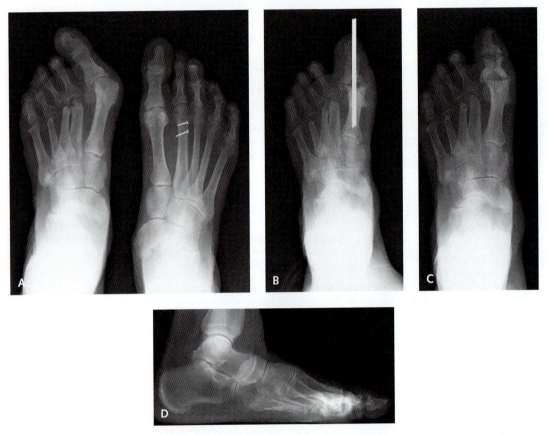

Figure 5-15 A, A patient with neuropathy who presented for treatment of irritation of the hallux on the shoe had undergone metatarsal head resection to treat lesser metatarsal ulceration. **B-D,** Owing to the presence of neuropathy, a resection arthroplasty was selected over arthrodesis but was complicated by infection of the metatarsal head. The infection was successfully treated with realignment, further bone removal, and stabilization with a threaded Steinmann pin.

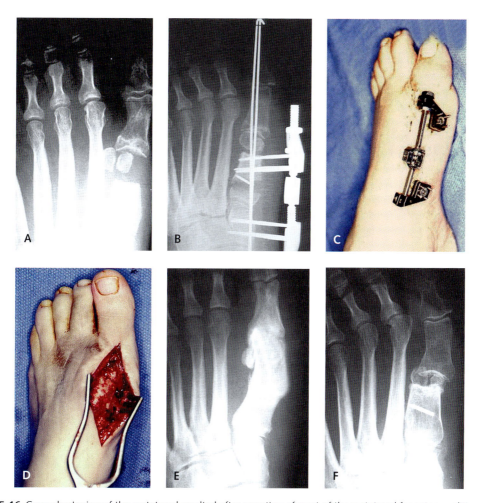

Figure 5-16 Gross shortening of the metatarsal resulted after resection of most of the metatarsal for osteomyelitis consequent to a distal metatarsal osteotomy. **A,** The metatarsal was so short that even with an interpositional structural graft, it was considered too short for adequate function. **B** and **C,** For this reason, staged operations were performed, first with a lengthening with a mini-external fixator. **D,** This procedure gained 17 mm of length. **E** and **F,** Insertion of a structural allograft completed the revision.

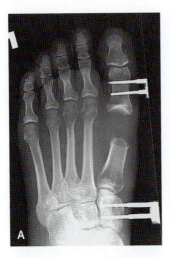
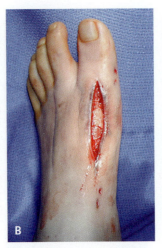
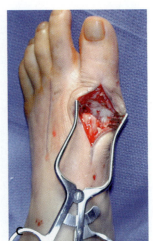
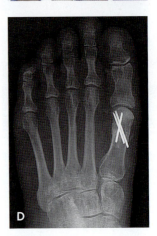

Figure 5-17 A, The patient underwent treatment after resection of the metatarsal head for presumed infection consequent to a distal metatarsal osteotomy. The fixator had been applied elsewhere, and drainage from the incision persisted. **B** and **C,** After repeated bone and joint debridement, an antibiotic-impregnated cement spacer was inserted to maintain length, and placement of a fresh osteoarticular allograft followed 4 months later. **D,** The radiographic appearance of the hallux 6 years later.

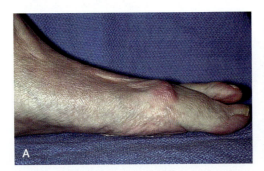
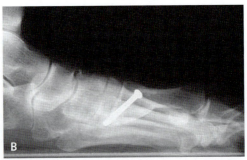

Figure 5-18 A and **B,** Dorsal malunion after a proximal crescentic osteotomy occurred in a patient who subsequently underwent treatment for painful limitation of motion of the hallux and metatarsalgia of the second metatarsal with a dome crescentic osteotomy at the base of the first metatarsal.

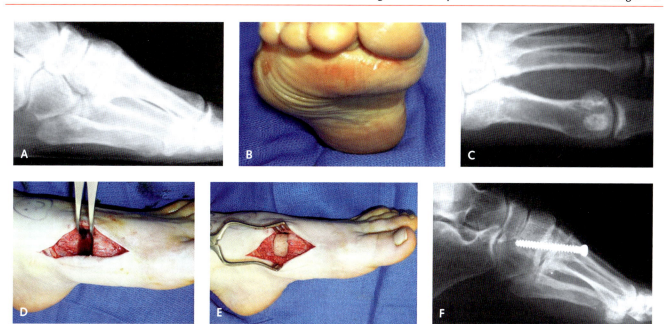

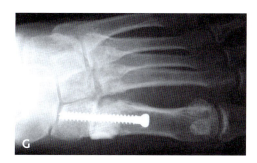

Figure 5-19 **A-C,** The patient presented with painful limitation to motion of the hallux metatarsophalangeal joint and second metatarsalgia associated with shortening and elevation of the first metatarsal, a dorsal bunion, limitation of motion of the hallux, and metatarsalgia of the second metatarsal. Excessive bone had been removed to perform this procedure. The type of fixation originally used was unknown. **D** and **E,** The revision was performed with an osteotomy through the malunion at the level of the original first tarsometatarsal joint, with a triangular structural allograft and preservation of the plantar cortical base of the osteotomy as a hinge. **F** and **G,** Radiographs showing the final correction, with good restoration of the length of the first metatarsal, improvement of the declination, and relief of metatarsalgia.

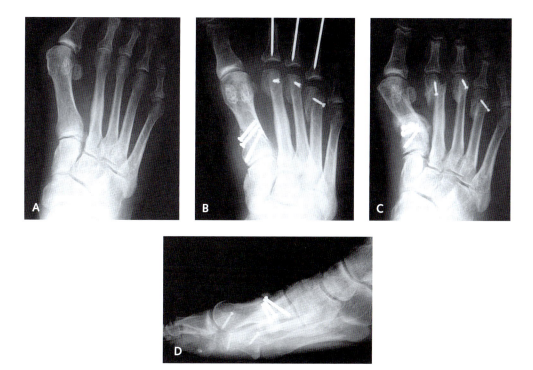

Figure 5-20 **A** and **B,** The patient was treated with a proximal metatarsal osteotomy for correction of deformity in conjunction with Weil osteotomies of the lesser metatarsals. **C** and **D,** The patient had unrecognized neuropathy, and despite adequate immobilization, delayed union and ultimately severe malunion occurred.

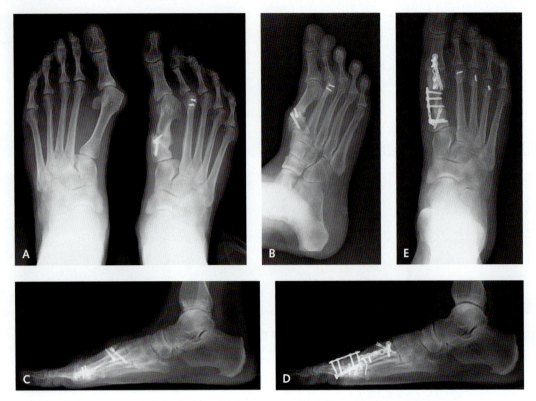

Figure 5-21 A and **B,** This severe malunion and nonunion was associated with hallux varus and a negative intermetatarsal angle. **C-E,** The metatarsophalangeal (MP) joint was adequately corrected with restoration of the metatarsal alignment, but arthritis was present, so a simultaneous arthrodesis of the MP joint was performed.

TECHNIQUES, TIPS, AND PITFALLS

- The use of a dorsal incision for correction of hallux valgus is associated with very high postoperative rates of dorsal capsular contracture, scarring, and limitation of plantar flexion (Figure 5-22).

- Salvage of the failed joint replacement is accomplished with either a soft tissue interposition arthroplasty or an arthrodesis. If the joint range of motion is very good but the joint is painful, then an arthroplasty may be preferable. In Figure 5-23, relief of joint pain in a patient with bilateral failure of implant arthroplasty required removal of previously placed implants and insertion of a balled-up tendon graft.

- Various percutaneous techniques for correction of hallux valgus gained some popularity a few years ago, but an unacceptable incidence of complications has since been demonstrated. Reported rates for nonunion, joint stiffness, arthritis, and, in particular, malunion have been unacceptably high to warrant continued use of this procedure (Figure 5-24).

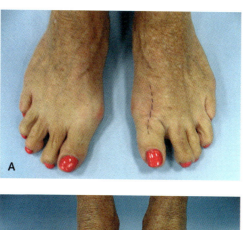

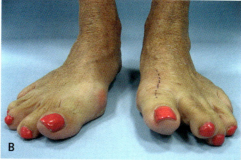

Figure 5-22 A and **B,** The patient presented with a cock-up hallux after distal metatarsal osteotomy. Limited dorsiflexion of the hallux was present. The likely cause of the restricted motion was the use of a dorsal incision to approach the metatarsophalangeal joint.

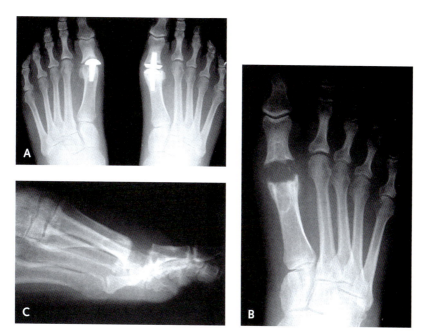

Figure 5-23 The patient received treatment for severe bilateral metatarsophalangeal joint pain with limited motion after bilateral implant arthroplasties. **A,** Only the right foot was infected. **B** and **C,** The right foot was treated first with removal of the implant and a staged interposition arthroplasty with a rolled up tendon graft.

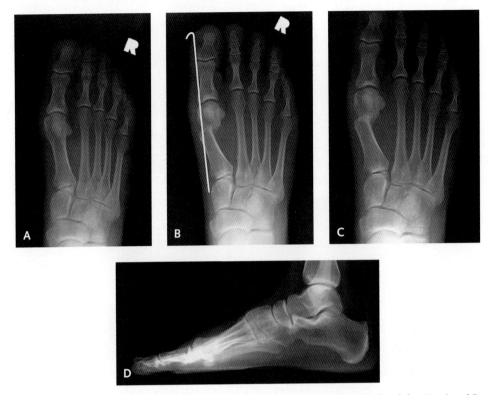

Figure 5-24 A and **B,** A percutaneous distal metatarsal osteotomy was used to correct this deformity. **C** and **D,** The metatarsophalangeal joint was very stiff after removal of the Kirschner wire, and a dorsal malunion was present, probably the result of inadequate fixation of the osteotomy.

SUGGESTED READING

Easley ME, Kelly IP: Avascular necrosis of the hallux metatarsal head. *Foot Ankle Clin* 5:591–608, 200.

Edwards WH: Avascular necrosis of the first metatarsal head, *Foot Ankle Clin* 10:117–127, 2005.

Myerson MS, Miller S, Henderson MR, Saxby T: Staged arthrodesis for salvage of the septic hallux metatarsophalangeal joint, *Clin Orthop* 307:174–181, 1994.

Myerson MS, Schon LC, McGuigan FX, Oznur A: Result of arthrodesis of the hallux metatarsophalangeal joint using bone graft for restoration of length, *Foot Ankle Int* 21:297–306, 2000.

Richardson EG: Complications after hallux valgus surgery, *Instr Course Lect* 48:331–342, 1999.

Sammarco GJ, Idusuyi OB: Complications after surgery of the hallux, *Clin Orthop* 391:59–71, 2001.

Vianna VF, Myerson MS: Complications of hallux valgus surgery. Management of the short first metatarsal and the failed resection arthroplasty, *Foot Ankle Clin* 3:33–49, 1998.

CHAPTER **6**

Hallux Varus

DECISION MAKING FOR CORRECTION

The type of treatment for correction of hallux varus is determined by the flexibility of the metatarsophalangeal (MP) and interphalangeal (IP) joints. Imbalance is always present between the flexor hallucis brevis (FHB) and the extensor hallucis brevis (EHB) muscles and between the abductor hallucis and adductor hallucis muscles. As with any muscle imbalance, the deformity will generally gradually increase, causing a spectrum of fixed and flexible deformities of the MP and IP joints, with or without arthritis of either joint. Fortunately, the IP joint remains flexible in most hallux varus deformities. Over time, however, with increasing imbalance of the FHB and EHB muscles, a contracture of the IP joint develops. If this contracture is rigid or if arthritis of the IP joint is present, an arthrodesis of this joint is usually necessary (Figure 6-1). If an IP contracture is present but the joint is fairly flexible, then I try to manipulate the joint and determine if a tendon transfer without arthrodesis is possible. Release of this contracture generally is not successful because of the contracture of the FHL in addition to tightness of the plantar capsule. Once an arthrodesis of the IP joint is performed, the MP joint deformity must be corrected either dynamically with a tendon transfer or statically through restoration of ligament stability with a tenodesis.

Maintaining MP joint mobility is ideal but not always possible because of arthritis or rigid contracture. Obviously, for a tendon transfer or tenodesis to obtain balance, the joint must be mobile and reducible. At times, however, the flexibility of the MP joint is not clear, and passive correction with manipulation does not clarify the situation. An example is seen in Figure 6-2; in the case depicted, hallux varus is present, and strapping of the hallux into valgus confirmed the flexibility of the joint. This joint reduction must be confirmed radiographically as well as clinically. It is not sufficient to push the hallux into neutral position or even valgus while the patient is seated—the same maneuver should be performed with the patient standing. This assessment will give a far better idea of the dynamic extent of the contracture, when weight-bearing forces are brought to bear on the hallux.

In the presence of a rigid deformity with contracture of the MP joint in both varus and extension, it is unlikely that soft tissue balance can be achieved with a tendon transfer, and an arthrodesis of the MP joint is preferable. In some patients, however, a resection arthroplasty of the MP joint may be a useful alternative, because arthrodesis of the MP joint should not be performed if both the MP and the IP joint are deformed. This situation requires a difficult treatment decision in the occasional patient who has arthritis of the MP joint and rigid contracture of the IP joint, or vice versa. In such cases, an arthrodesis of the IP joint can be combined with a resection arthroplasty of the MP joint.

Accordingly, whenever possible, tendon transfer should be used to correct the deformity. However, tendon transfer is contraindicated if either arthritis or rigidity of the MP joint is present. In certain clinical situations, despite apparent flexibility of the MP joint, correction of deformity by restoring soft tissue balance seems implausible. In the case illustrated in Figure 6-3, the patient had a very long first metatarsal with imbalance of the abductor and adductor hallucis muscles. Although an arthrodesis or a resection arthroplasty of the joint can be considered in such instances, my preference would be to shorten the first metatarsal with an osteotomy (a scarf osteotomy is useful here), thereby relaxing the intrinsic contractures, and obtaining further soft tissue balance with a tendon transfer if necessary.

TENDON TRANSFER AND TENODESIS

I divide the surgical approaches for correction of hallux varus into those procedures that primarily address the soft tissues (abductor hallucis tendon release or transfer, extensor hallucis longus or brevis tendon transfer, or tenodesis), the bone (first metatarsal osteotomy, hallux proximal phalangeal osteotomy), or the joint (arthrodesis of the IP joint and arthrodesis or resection arthroplasty of the MP joint). If a soft tissue procedure is performed, the postoperative result must include balance around the hallux MP joint. Therefore the abductor hallucis tendon should be lengthened, cut, or transferred, and a medial capsulotomy should be performed in conjunction with the lateral stabilizing procedure. If hallux varus is seen immediately postoperatively as a result of overplication of the medial capsule and the metatarsal is well aligned, simple strapping of the hallux into valgus may suffice to stretch the tight medial capsule. If hallux valgus persists in the early postoperative period, release of the abductor tendon or capsule may be sufficient to correct deformity. For all other situations, tendon and soft tissue balancing needs to be performed.

Tendon Transfers

Various tendon transfers are available for correction of dynamic deformity. The use of the entire extensor hallucis longus (EHL) tendon in conjunction with arthrodesis of the IP joint has been described in the literature, but this is not my preferred procedure.

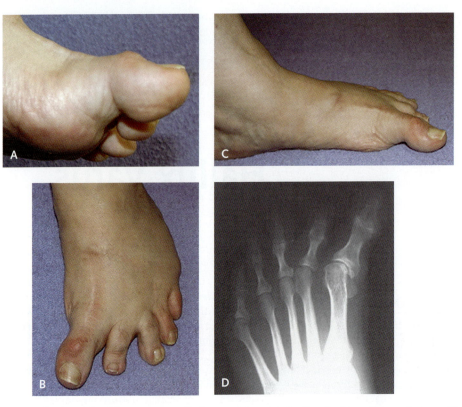

Figure 6-1 The clinical **(A-C)** and radiographic **(D)** appearance of hallux varus associated with a flexible metatarsophalangeal joint but a fixed contracted interphalangeal joint. Despite the radiographic appearance, because of the flexibility, the patient is a good candidate for an interphalangeal joint fusion and either a split extensor hallucis longus or extensor hallucis brevis tenodesis.

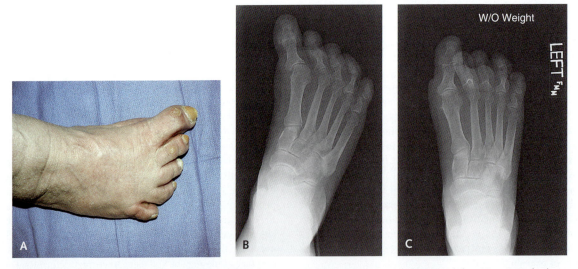

Figure 6-2 **A** and **B,** The patient presented with flexible hallux varus associated with lesser toe adduction deformities. **C,** To further evaluate the flexibility of the metatarsophalangeal joint, the hallux was strapped into valgus. Good joint correction was obtained.

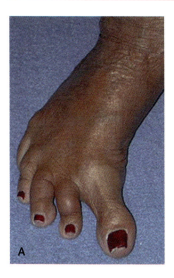
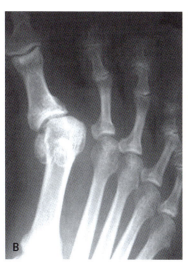

Figure 6-3 **A,** This deformity was flexible; however, irreversible changes have taken place in the hallux metatarsophalangeal (MP) joint, precluding correction with a tendon transfer. Either a shortening osteotomy of the first metatarsal or an arthrodesis or arthroplasty of the MP joint is required, in addition to correction of the lesser toe deformities. **B,** Even though the hallux is flexible and will be well realigned after arthrodesis, the toes will not necessarily return to a neutral position and further correction will be required.

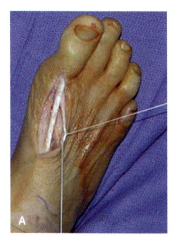
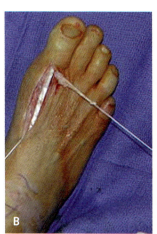
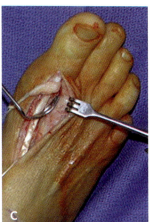

Figure 6-4 Tendon transfer. **A,** The extensor hallucis brevis is isolated proximally, and a stay suture is inserted into the tendon. **B,** The tendon is cut proximally, and tension is applied to be sure that this does not tear distally. **C,** A tapered aneurysm needle is passed from proximal to distal, through which the suture is passed, to grasp the suture and pull the tendon proximally.

Even if rigid deformity of the IP joint is present and an IP arthrodesis is necessary, I prefer to use half of the EHL for the transfer, maintaining the remaining half as a dorsiflexor of the hallux. If the IP joint is flexible, fusing the joint is unnecessary, and transfer of either a portion of the EHL tendon (a split transfer of the EHL tendon) or the entire EHB tendon is performed (Figures 6-4 and 6-5). Distinguishing a *tendon transfer*, which has the potential for dynamic correction of deformity, from a *tenodesis*, in which the tendon is used statically, is relevant here (see Figure 6-5). Both procedures apply to the EHL and EHB tendon transfer, because both may function as either a tenodesis or a dynamic transfer.

One of the problems I have experienced with the split EHL tendon transfer is that when the tendon is split from proximal to distal and the lateral half of the tendon is used for the transfer, the medial half of the EHL tendon never retains adequate tension. This imbalance and loss of tension in the remaining half of the tendon are unavoidable. This type of transfer effectively lengthens the medial half of the tendon, leading to dorsiflexion weakness. An alternative would be to use the EHL tendon in a tenodesis procedure by splitting the tendon from distal to proximal in the same way as for the EHB tenodesis. In general, however, I prefer to keep the EHL tendon intact, and in the presence of flexible IP and MP joints, I prefer to use the EHB tendon in a tendon transfer or tenodesis procedure.

Through a dorsal longitudinal incision, lateral to the EHL tendon, the EHB tendon is identified and carefully dissected from the EHL tendon and extensor retinaculum. Proximally, the EHB tendon is transected just distal to the musculotendinous junction at the level of the base of the first metatarsal. The EHB tendon must be carefully dissected distal to the MP joint through the release of the extensor hood. The worst that can happen is that the EHB tendon is transected distally, and if the distal attachment of the EHB tendon is tenuous, a suture is inserted to maintain its attachment to the extensor hood. A 2-0 suture is inserted at the end of the transected EHB tendon with a fine needle, and the tendon is then passed under the deep transverse metatarsal ligament from distal to proximal. A blunt-tipped curved tapered needle (an aneurysm needle) works well for this purpose. It is not absolutely necessary to pass the tendon under the deep transverse metatarsal ligament, and any firm tether from scar tissue in the first web space is sufficient.

If a tendon transfer of the EHB is to be performed, the tendon is sutured back onto itself using 4-0 nonabsorbable sutures under the appropriate tension. A dynamic tendon transfer is always preferable to a tenodesis, and the latter is used only if the EHB tendon ruptures or if insufficient length is present to permit suturing it back onto itself. For a tenodesis, a drill hole is then made from medial to lateral in the distal neck of the first metatarsal, and the tendon is

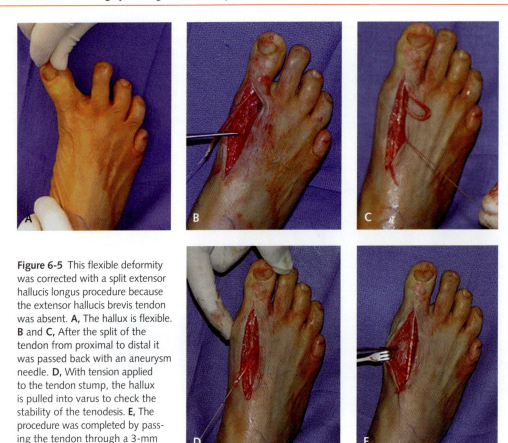

Figure 6-5 This flexible deformity was corrected with a split extensor hallucis longus procedure because the extensor hallucis brevis tendon was absent. **A,** The hallux is flexible. **B** and **C,** After the split of the tendon from proximal to distal it was passed back with an aneurysm needle. **D,** With tension applied to the tendon stump, the hallux is pulled into varus to check the stability of the tenodesis. **E,** The procedure was completed by passing the tendon through a 3-mm drill hole in the metatarsal.

passed through the drill hole and secured under tension. Before the tendon is tightened, adequate balance must be restored. I prefer to see that the hallux is lying in a neutral position after release of the medial capsule and contracted abductor tendon. The length of the EHB tendon is always sufficient to permit suturing it back down over the dorsal periosteum with a nonresorbable suture. I use the EHL tenodesis procedure when the EHB tendon is scarred, torn, or absent. It is performed the same way as that described for the EHB tendon. More tendon length from the split EHL tendon usually is available, and the tendon can be passed back onto itself over the dorsal surface of the metatarsal after passage through the drill hole.

After these tenodesis procedures, the hallux should rest in a neutral position, and it should not have to be pushed over at all. Fixing the MP joint with a Kirschner wire during surgery should not be necessary. I like to tape the hallux in a slightly overcorrected position in slight valgus for 2 months (Figure 6-6). The patient is allowed to bear weight immediately after this procedure while wearing a postoperative walking shoe. After 4 weeks, the patient is allowed to use a stiff-soled shoe. Toe-off with bending of the MP joint should not be allowed for 8 weeks.

Transfer of the abductor hallucis tendon is a logical procedure to perform if the availability of either the EHL or the EHB is compromised. It would be a good option, for example, if the MP joint remains flexible and a previous attempt at correction of the hallux varus has already been made using either the EHB or the EHL. If both the EHL and the EHB are not functioning, the hallux is very weak, and the patient will complain about the lack of active dorsiflexion (Figure 6-7). The use of the abductor tendon should always

be considered, because medial joint contracture, unless the joint is very flexible, requires a medial capsular release as well as a release of the abductor tendon. If the abductor is going to be released, then why not use it for a more dynamic transfer? The tendon is released from its attachment to the base of the proximal phalanx with as much length of the tendon as possible. It must be carefully dissected off the flexor brevis so as to leave the attachment of the sesamoid complex intact. The tendon is then passed below the metatarsal head either deep or superficial to the sesamoid complex and pulled laterally, where it is attached to the base of the proximal phalanx. I use a small bone anchor into the lateral base of the proximal phalanx and then establish appropriate tension on the tendon.

HALLUX VARUS AFTER FIRST METATARSAL OSTEOTOMY

Deformity of the first metatarsal is another contraindication to correction of hallux varus by means of tendon transfer alone (Figure 6-8). Of interest, hallux varus can occur after a distal metatarsal osteotomy that is complicated by either a varus or a valgus malunion, although typically, when a valgus malunion is present, the hallux "falls off the joint" medially as the abductor tightens (see Figure 6-8, *A*). Hallux varus may follow either a distal (see Figure 6-8, *A*) or a proximal (see Figure 6-8, *C*) metatarsal osteotomy, and the deformity may be either flexible or rigid. This deformity can be the result of overcorrection of the metatarsal with a negative intermetatarsal angle, leading to medial subluxation of the MP joint and hallux varus. If the malunion of the first metatarsal is left

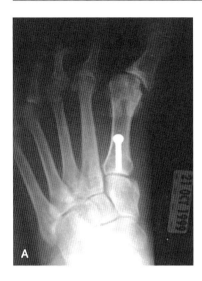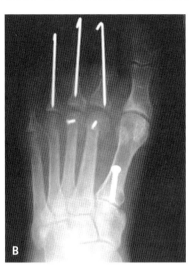

Figure 6-6 This deformity was flexible. Neither crepitus nor pain was elicited by range-of-motion manipulation of the hallux metatarsophalangeal (MP) joint. **A,** Dislocation of the second toe MP joint and severe subluxation of the third and fourth MP joints were present. **B,** These were corrected with a tenodesis procedure of the extensor hallucis brevis tendon; arthrodesis of the second, third, and fourth proximal interphalangeal joints; and osteotomies of the second and third metatarsals. The Kirschner wires were removed from the toes at 4 weeks after surgery.

uncorrected, the tendon transfer will not correct the soft tissue imbalance. Correction of the metatarsal alignment with osteotomy must then be performed in conjunction with a tendon transfer, which can be accomplished simultaneously.

Regardless of the magnitude of the deformity, I always try to obtain correction of the first metatarsal alignment. Invariably this correction has a beneficial effect on the alignment of the hallux, although the range of motion of the joint may be permanently compromised. For example, the deformity in Figure 6-9 was flexible at the MP joint, fixed at the IP joint, and associated with a valgus malunion of the distal metatarsal osteotomy. A medial incision was used to approach the MP joint, and the abductor hallucis tendon dissected sharply off its attachment to the phalanx. The capsule was incised and the neck of the metatarsal marked out under fluoroscopic guidance, and a small (2-mm) wedge was removed using a saw. This was fixed using a mini L-plate, and then the abductor hallucis was transferred under the neck of the metatarsal to the lateral aspect of the joint, where it was attached to the proximal phalanx with sutures.

Hallux varus that occurs in the immediate postoperative period can be corrected easily, provided that a malunion of the first metatarsal is not present. For many of these deformities, the varus is a result of overrelease of the adductor complex or overtightening of the medial capsule. In either instance, provided that the joint remains flexible, taping the hallux into valgus will resolve the problem. The hallux should be strapped tightly into valgus for 3 months. Recurrent valgus deformity is not likely to develop owing to the alignment of the first metatarsal, which typically is quite straight (Figure 6-10). If the varus deformity is the result of overtightening of the capsule and the joint is not easily reduced, then a simple release of the medial capsule and perhaps the abductor can be successful. This procedure will work only if the joint is reducible and flexible, and no malunion of a metatarsal osteotomy occurs (Figure 6-11). The hallux should be taped into valgus for 2 months after this capsulotomy.

Arthrodesis and Resection Arthroplasty

For correction of either arthritis or rigid deformity at the MP joint, I prefer to use an arthrodesis. Occasionally, either because of a fixed, contracted IP joint or patient preference, I perform a resection arthroplasty (Figures 6-12 to 6-14). With either of these procedures, further soft tissue balancing usually is not required.

For the *resection arthroplasty*, the cut of the base of the proximal phalanx must be vertical. The surgeon should be careful with the plane of the cut to prevent any further inadvertent dorsiflexion of the MP joint, and the hallux varus deformity can be addressed with a cut perpendicular to the long axis of the proximal phalanx or with a slight valgus inclination. This arthroplasty needs to be performed in conjunction with complete release of the medial joint contracture. When *arthrodesis* is used for correction, the aberrant position of the metatarsal head, the previous medial exostectomy, and the malunion of the first metatarsal pose additional challenges. I have found that accurate positioning of the hallux is difficult as a result of various deformities around the MP joint. The normal landmarks for positioning the phalanx on the first metatarsal are not always present, and using the clinical position of the hallux to guide the final position for the arthrodesis often is easier.

It is important to note the effect of the hallux varus on the rest of the forefoot, particularly the lesser toes. If the hallux is in marked varus, over time it will pull the lesser toes into varus as well. The toes will not return to a normal position even after excellent correction of the hallux deformity and must be realigned with the hallux. Standard correction of lesser toe deformity such as capsulotomy with release of the medial collateral ligament is not sufficient, even if followed by prolonged immobilization with a K-wire. I have found that the shortening of the metatarsal (which indirectly lengthens the intrinsic muscles and thereby releases the contracture) is ideal.

A good example of correction of a first metatarsal malunion is seen in Figure 6-13. Owing to the severity of the malunion of the metatarsal in this case, positioning the hallux for an arthrodesis would be quite difficult. Although this approach is technically feasible, the resultant position of the hallux would never be normal, and it is preferable to correct the deformity with an osteotomy and soft tissue balance, which was performed in this case. With many of these distal metatarsal deformities, the osteotomy can be performed using a dome-shaped saw—in this case, from the dorsal aspect of the metatarsal. This approach minimizes further shortening of the metatarsal, which would occur if a wedge was removed, and allows for a biplanar correction.

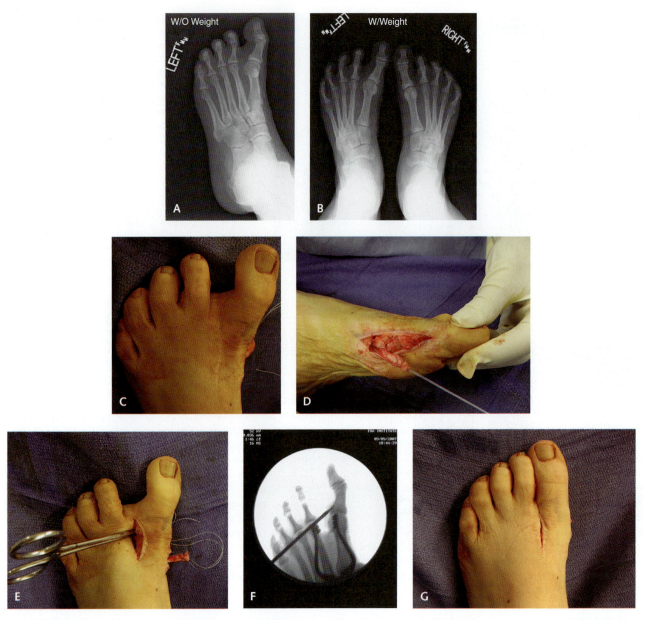

Figure 6-7 The patient required treatment for hallux varus resulting from a previous fibular sesamoidectomy and associated with a partial footdrop from previous spine surgery. **A-C,** Note the varus of the hallux and the overall position of the foot. **D** and **E,** The abductor hallucis was detached **(D).** and then passed under the metatarsal head and retrieved laterally with a clamp **(E). F,** The tendon was attached to the base of the proximal phalanx with a suture anchor. **G,** The intraoperative radiographic appearance.

6

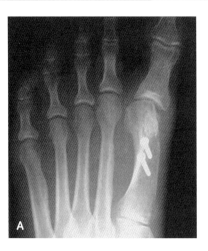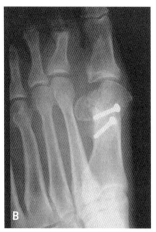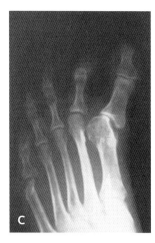

Figure 6-8 A-C, In each of these examples, malunion after a metatarsal osteotomy is causing the hallux varus. In **A** and **B,** a tendon transfer was performed after correction of the malunion. In **C,** An arthrodesis was performed.

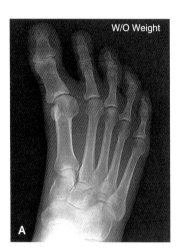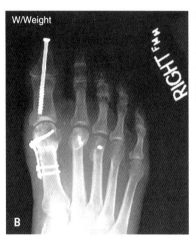

Figure 6-9 A, A valgus malunion of a distal metatarsal osteotomy in addition to a fibular sesamoidectomy caused the hallux deformity, which was fixed at the interphalangeal (IP) joint and flexible at the metatarsophalangeal joint. **B,** This was corrected with a closing wedge medial osteotomy, an arthrodesis of the IP joint, a transfer of the abductor hallucis, and osteotomies of the second and third metatarsals.

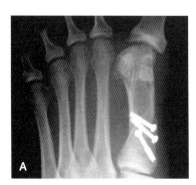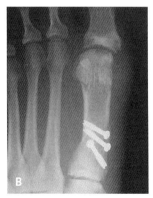

Figure 6-10 A, A Ludloff metatarsal osteotomy was performed for correction of hallux valgus, followed by hallux varus, seen at the first postoperative evaluation. **B,** Taping of the hallux into valgus for 8 weeks resulted in excellent alignment, with good scarring of the lateral joint capsule.

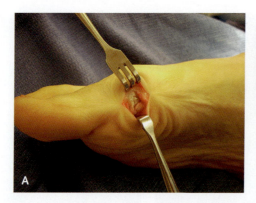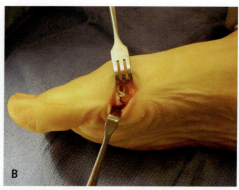

Figure 6-11 The release of the abductor hallucis **(A)** is performed with a medial joint capsulotomy **(B)** in a patient with mild postoperative hallux varus caused by an overtight capsulorrhaphy.

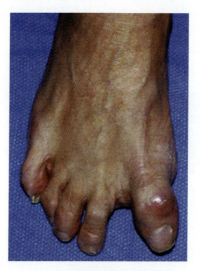

Figure 6-12 Fixed contracture of the interphalangeal (IP) joint in this patient was corrected with an arthrodesis of the IP joint, along with a resection arthroplasty of the metatarsophalangeal joint.

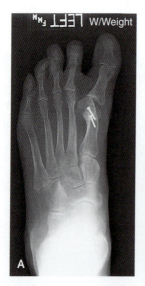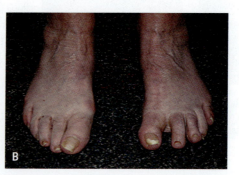

Figure 6-13 A and **B,** This malunion of a distal metatarsal osteotomy was so severe that even an arthrodesis could not be considered for correction.

Continued

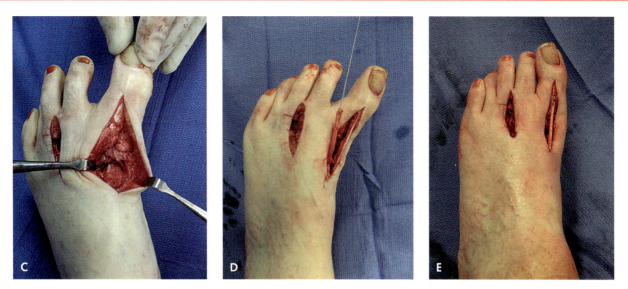

Figure 6-13—cont'd C and **D,** A dome distal osteotomy was marked out through a dorsal incision **(C)** followed by a transfer of the extensor hallucis longus **(D). E,** The intraoperative appearance after the tendon transfer with second and third metatarsal osteotomies.

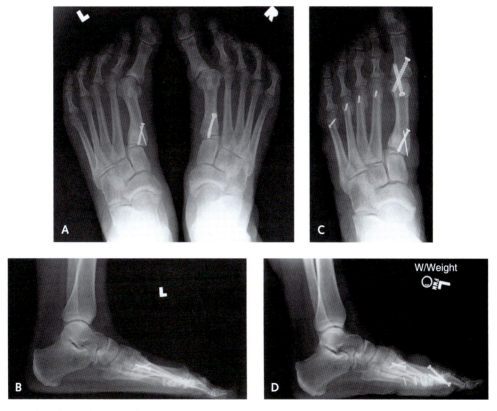

Figure 6-14 Bilateral complications after a proximal crescentic osteotomy. **A** and **B,** Note bilateral overcorrection of the first metatarsal **(A),** with marked dorsal malunion of the first metatarsal **(B). C** and **D,** An arthrodesis of the metatarsophalangeal joint with lesser metatarsal osteotomies was performed.

TECHNIQUES, TIPS, AND PITFALLS

- No procedure adequately corrects a hallux varus if a malunion of a metatarsal osteotomy is present, even when an arthrodesis of the MP joint is performed. The malunion must first be corrected.

- If hallux varus occurs immediately postoperatively as a result of either an excessively tight capsulorrhaphy or soft tissue release, correction can be effected with prompt taping of the hallux into valgus for 8 weeks.

- If the hallux IP joint is fixed in flexion, an arthrodesis of the IP joint must be performed. At the MP joint, however, an array of procedures may be performed, ranging from arthroplasty to tendon transfer. Simultaneous arthrodesis of the IP and MP joints is not desirable.

- A soft tissue correction of idiopathic hallux varus associated with a flatfoot deformity should not be undertaken without due consideration. The intrinsic contracture is severe, and other than a transfer of the abductor hallucis, which may work, an arthrodesis of the MP joint is necessary (Figure 6-15).

- It is always worth trying to correct the alignment of the hallux with revision of a malunion of a first metatarsal osteotomy. Arthrodesis or resection arthroplasty should be a salvage procedure for management of painful arthritis.

- It is obviously critical to determine the flexibility of the MP joint before any correction, because a tendon transfer or tenodesis will not yield a functional result in the presence of a rigid joint.

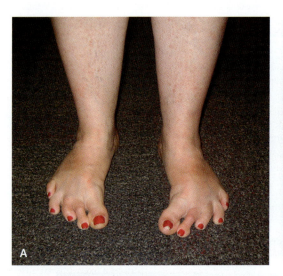 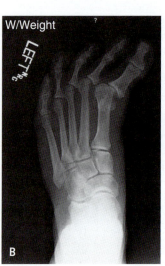 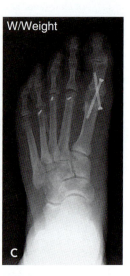

Figure 6-15 A, Bilateral hallux varus associated with a flexible flatfoot. **B,** Note the effect of the intrinsic muscle contractures on all of the metatarsophalangeal (MP) joints. **C,** This was treated with arthrodesis of the MP joint and lesser metatarsal osteotomies.

SUGGESTED READING

Donley BG: Acquired hallux varus, *Foot Ankle Int* 18:586–592, 1997.

Juliano PJ, Myerson MS, Cunningham BW: Biomechanical assessment of a new tenodesis for correction of hallux varus, *Foot Ankle Int* 17:17–20, 1996.

Lau JT, Myerson MS: Modified split extensor hallucis longus tendon transfer for correction of hallux varus, *Foot Ankle Int* 23:1138–1140, 2002.

Myerson M: Hallux varus. In Myerson MS, editor: *Current Therapy in Foot and Ankle Surgery*, St. Louis, 1993, Mosby–Year Book, pp 70–73.

Myerson MS: Hallux valgus. In Myerson MS, editor: *Foot and Ankle Disorders*, Philadelphia, 2000, WB Saunders.

Myerson MS, Komenda GA: Results of hallux varus correction using an extensor hallucis brevis tenodesis, *Foot Ankle Int* 17:21–27, 1996.

Skalley TC, Myerson MS: The operative treatment of acquired hallux varus, *Clin Orthop* 306:183–191, 1994.

Trnka HJ, Zettl R, Hungerford M, et al: Acquired hallux varus and clinical tolerability, *Foot Ankle Int* 18:593–597, 1997.

CHAPTER 7

Claw Hallux Deformity

EVALUATION AND CLINICAL DECISION MAKING

Claw hallux deformity occurs with a variable degree of severity. Clinical presentations may range from milder forms characterized by flexible interphalangeal (IP) and metatarsophalangeal (MP) joints to fixed deformities with severe subluxation of the MP joint. In other variants of claw deformity of the hallux, the MP joint is in neutral, but a fixed flexion contracture of the IP and or the MP joint is present as a result of tethering of the flexor hallucis longus or the intrinsic muscles, or both. This tethering may arise as a result of scarring in the distal third of the leg associated with a tibia fracture, the consequence of a compartment syndrome in the foot, or associated with various neurologic processes. The approach to correction is based entirely on the flexibility of the hallux at either joint and whether or not dynamic function of the hallux is present. With each of these variants, a different approach to treatment is indicated—for example, a flexible IP joint may be associated with a rigid MP joint, or a rigid IP joint associated with a flexible MP joint, with corresponding implications.

In simplistic terms, the number of procedures that can be performed at either joint level is limited. Fusion of the IP joint can be accomplished with or without a lengthening or a transfer of either the extensor hallucis longus (EHL) or flexor hallucis longus (FHL) tendon, or the joint can be left alone, with only a tendon lengthening or transfer performed. Either the MP joint contracture is released completely or an arthrodesis can be performed. It is surprising how well the hallux works despite some stiffness, provided that the digit is straight, so an arthrodesis of either the IP or MP joint should not be routinely performed.

CLAW HALLUX DEFORMITY SECONDARY TO A COMPARTMENT SYNDROME

For example, in the setting of severe fibrosis of the intrinsic muscles secondary to a compartment syndrome, the approach would be very different from that in which an intrinsic minus deformity is a result of intrinsic muscle weakness associated with a neuromuscular disorder. In patients in whom the hallux is significantly stiff at the IP and MP joints, it is important to identify the specific components of the contracture. In the example in the following section, the contracture is predominantly in the extrinsic FHL, and not in the intrinsic muscles, although clearly a component of this deformity also is present. Correction of a claw hallux deformity secondary to a compartment

syndrome can be extremely difficult. In such cases, there usually is a fixed flexion contracture at both the MP and IP joints. The extensor hallucis longus typically is functioning, but because of the fixed flexion contracture it has little power to dorsiflex the hallux.

I have attempted various soft tissue releases and ultimately have come to the conclusion that the only way this deformity can be repaired is by completely releasing the sesamoid complex. The approach is through a medial incision similar to that for a sesamoidectomy, and the branch of the medial plantar nerve is identified and retracted. The abductor tendon as well as the volar plate is now cut, identifying the flexor hallucis longus. Once the flexor hallucis is retracted, then the volar plate ligament is cut completely, allowing the sesamoids to retract proximally. The hallux is then passively dorsiflexed. At this time, at least 45 degrees of passive dorsiflexion with the ankle in neutral should be possible. If this is not present or if the hallux is starting to contract at the IP joint, then a lengthening or transfer of the flexor hallucis longus needs to be performed. It is preferable to perform this lengthening proximally, proximal to the medial malleolus either through a fractional lengthening at the musculotendinous junction or by a standard Z-lengthening of the tendon. If a step-cut Z-lengthening is performed, at least 60 degrees of passive dorsiflexion of the hallux must be achieved, because some recurrent contracture is to be expected postoperatively. Once the volar plate has been completely released, the effect of the contracture on the interphalangeal joint must be observed. Is this is a fixed contracture, or is there a passive tenodesis effect of the FHL that is eliminated with plantar flexion of the ankle? In order to determine this, plantar flex the foot and assess the amount of dorsiflexion that occurs through the interphalangeal joint. If the IP joint can be straightened completely with the foot plantar flexed but flexion of the hallux at the IP joint is observed with the foot in neutral or dorsiflexion, then a tenodesis effect is present. If a fixed flexion contracture is present, then an arthrodesis of the interphalangeal joint can be performed or the FHL transferred into the base of the proximal phalanx of the hallux (Figure 7-1).

In many patients with deformity secondary to injury, the contracture responsible for clawing of the hallux is caused by fibrosis of the intrinsic musculature. This is far more difficult to treat, and although the hallux will function, it will never be normal. Most affected patients present with a fixed flexion at the MP joint, with some remaining function and flexibility at the IP joint. I have tried numerous procedures to release the hallux MP joint contracture and have found that a complete release allowing the sesamoid

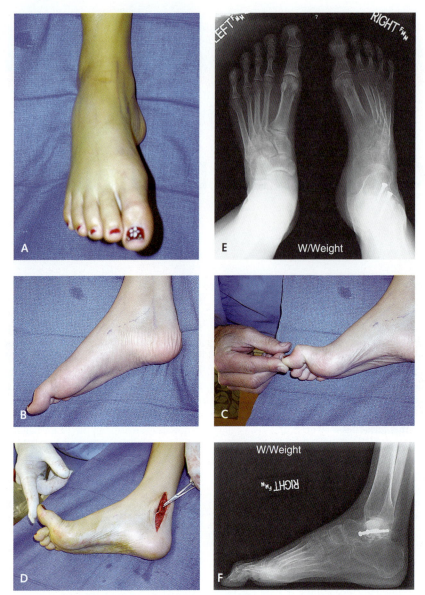

Figure 7-1 A, This severe contracture deformity of the hallux developed after the patient suffered a talus fracture. The deformity was attributed to sequelae of an associated compartment syndrome, including contracture of the flexor hallucis longus (FHL). **B,** The deformity was present predominantly in the interphalangeal joint. With the foot in plantar flexion, the hallux is in flexion at the IP joint and extension at the metatarsophalangeal joint. **C,** With any dorsiflexion of the foot, however, a severe flexion contracture of the IP joint becomes evident. The latter finding indicates a tethering of the FHL, which is more likely to be present in the distal leg. **D,** Accordingly, the release was accomplished with lengthening of the FHL behind the ankle. **E** and **F,** The preoperative appearance on weight-bearing radiographs.

complex to retract proximally is the only realistic option. This application is well illustrated in Figure 7-2, in which the patient's severe forefoot deformity was the result of a compartment syndrome that developed after an ankle arthroscopy. Very fixed flexion and adduction deformity of all of the MP joints is evident on the preoperative weight-bearing radiographs. A good aesthetic and functional result was achieved with extensive surgical release as described.

Correction of Neuromuscular Hallux Deformity

There are patients with a flexible hallux IP joint and a fixed MP joint for whom the solution is more difficult. Depending on the severity

of the deformity as well as the flexibility, a number of procedures can be considered. If both the IP and MP joints are contracted but reasonably flexible, then a transfer of the flexor hallucis longus to the base of the proximal phalanx can be considered (Figure 7-3). Alternatively, if the contracture at the MP joint is severe, the appearance will be that of a severe hallux rigidus associated with a fixed elevation of the first metatarsal, in which case the only option is an arthrodesis of the hallux MP joint (see Figure 7-3, *C*). In such cases, special care is indicated in planning and execution of the arthrodesis, because the sesamoid complex still needs to be completely released and allowed to retract proximally.

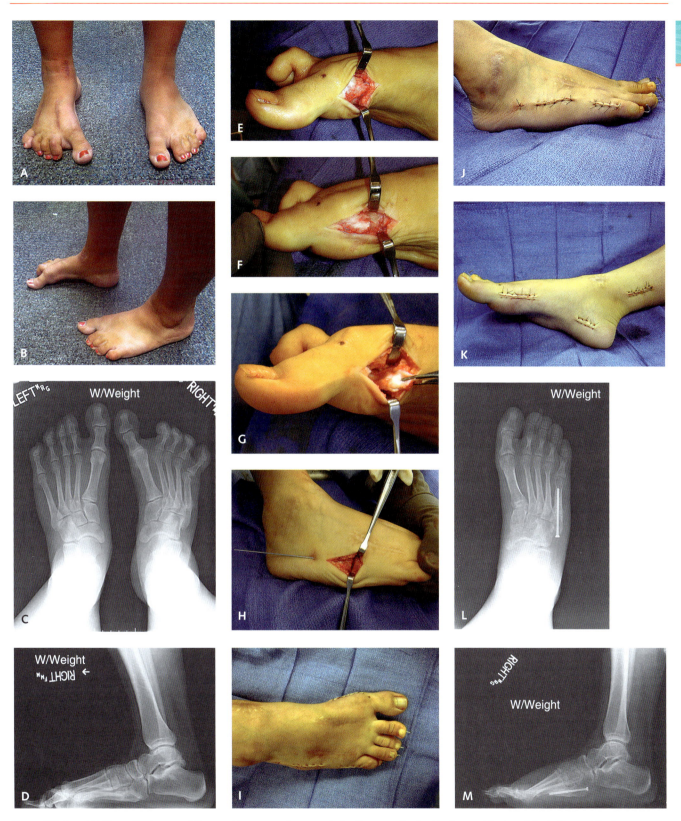

Figure 7-2 **A** and **B,** The patient was an 18-year-old woman who presented with severe fixed adduction and flexion of the hallux and the lesser metatarsophalangeal (MP) joints. **C** and **D,** The fifth MP joint is dislocated laterally as a result of contracture of the abductor digiti quinti. Note the fixed, elevated position of the first metatarsal. **E** and **F,** The abductor hallucis tendon was exposed (**E**) and then cut, exposing the MP joint (**F**). **G,** The abductor and flexor brevis muscles were then stripped out completely to release the MP joint contracture, allowing the sesamoids to retract proximally. **H-J,** In order to correct the dislocation of the fifth MP joint, a closing wedge osteotomy of the base of the fifth metatarsal was performed in conjunction with stripping of the abductor digiti quinti muscle and reduction of the MP joint dislocation. **K,** The medial correction was completed with fractional lengthening of the posterior tibial tendon at the musculotendinous junction and stripping of the plantar fascia. **L** and **M,** The final radiographs after correction of the forefoot deformity. Note in particular the reduction of the first metatarsal elevatus deformity and the realignment of all of the MP joints.

CORRECTION OF SEVERE METATARSOPHALANGEAL JOINT DEFORMITY

There are some deformities in which the MP joint is severely hyperextended, and a decision has to be made whether or not a fusion would be preferable to a soft tissue release. The latter may be a reasonable approach, but subsequent function of the hallux is never good. However, the dilemma arises in which both the MP and IP joints are fixed, because arthrodesis at both the MP and IP joints is not ideal. If I go through with a soft tissue release for correction of severe claw hallux, then in addition to an EHL lengthening or transfer (to the metatarsal neck as a Jones procedure), the dorsal capsule as well as the collateral ligaments are completely released and a curved periosteal elevator inserted into the joint in order to forcibly plantar flex it and release the sesamoids. Motion after this procedure is never very good, but still may be preferable for the patient who needs an IP fusion for correction of a severe fixed claw hallux deformity. With severe claw hallux deformities, there are usually dysplastic changes that take place in the MP joint, because the head is compressed slightly dorsally and adequate range of motion may never be regained. Nonetheless, it is important to perform a complete transverse dorsal capsulotomy and then an EHL lengthening or tendon transfer as necessary. It may be necessary to strip the undersurface of the volar plate and the sesamoid apparatus to loosen the attachment to the metatarsal neck such that the sesamoid will slide more proximally under the head with plantar flexion of the hallux, which was previously blocked as a result of the extension contracture. Therefore it is useful to look at the type of motion at the MP joint in plantar flexion. Ideally, one wants a gliding motion, and not to have the joint "booking" open as the hallux is plantar flexed (Figure 7-4). The extension at the MP joint may not be severe, and if this is associated with a flexible hallux IP joint, then all that may need to

be performed is a lengthening of the EHL. In general, lengthening of the tendon will weaken its strength, but in this type of problem the hallux only needs to make contact with the floor and avoid rubbing on the shoe (Figure 7-5).

EXTENSOR HALLUCIS LONGUS TRANSFER

If the IP joint is fixed in flexion, an arthrodesis of that joint needs to be performed. Flexion of the hallux then occurs through the long flexor tendon (if functioning), and does not rely on the flexor hallucis brevis, which is usually compromised in these claw hallux deformities. The correction of the MP joint depends on the flexibility and the position of the first metatarsal. If the MP joint is reasonably flexible, and more dorsiflexion power of the foot is required (a common problem, for example, in patients with Charcot-Marie-Tooth disease), then an IP fusion is performed with a transfer of the EHL to the first metatarsal (Figure 7-6).

FLEXOR HALLUCIS LONGUS TRANSFER

If a cock-up deformity is present with the IP joint in flexion (but not severely fixed and contracted), in addition to performing an IP arthrodesis, I transfer the FHL around or through the base of the proximal phalanx to improve MP flexion strength. This maneuver moves the axis point for flexion of the hallux more proximally. The transfer has to be combined with a lengthening of the EHL and a capsulotomy of the MP joint (Figure 7-7).

INTERPHALANGEAL JOINT ARTHRODESIS

Arthrodesis of the IP joint is performed through a longitudinal incision over the dorsal aspect of the hallux medial to the EHL tendon. Distally, it is not as important to attempt to preserve the attachment of the EHL as it is not to injure the germinal matrix at the base of

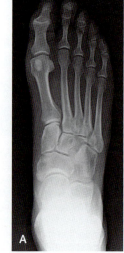
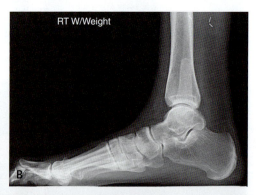
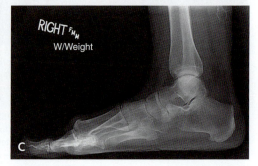

Figure 7-3 The deformities in these feet, all secondary to a compartment syndrome, are very different. In **A** and **B**, both the interphalangeal (IP) and metatarsophalangeal (MP) joints are flexible, and a transfer of the flexor hallucis longus tendon can be considered. The alternative would be to perform an arthrodesis of the IP joint. In **C**, the MP joint deformity is fixed, and the sesamoid complex must be released (cut distal to the sesamoids through the volar plate) and allowed to retract proximally. The MP joint may ultimately require an arthrodesis.

the nail. The incision can be cut in either an L or a T shape in order to facilitate exposure and then retract the EHL. I pull the EHL over to one side with a skin hook, after incising the extensor hood. The EHL always remains partly tethered to the extensor retinaculum and will not retract far proximately even if cut at the level of the IP joint.

A longitudinal incision is made medial to the extensor hallucis longus tendon dorsally and then the subcutaneous tissue retracting the tendon laterally. If a fixed deformity of the hallux is present with a severe hyperextension deformity, then the EHL does not need to be preserved and is transferred proximally into the first metatar-

sal. Generally, however, the EHL will be retracted laterally and an attempt made to preserve the tendon. Even with slight extension at the MP joint, once the IP joint is fused, there will be an increased force across the MP joint in plantar flexion through the IP arthrodesis and the flexor hallucis longus. In order to facilitate exposure of the arthrodesis of the interphalangeal joint, the incision is turned laterally to create an L or T shape. The distal corner of the attachment of the EHL and extensor hood to the base of the proximal phalanx is incised and then the soft tissue flap elevated to raise the EHL and move it laterally. This is best done by using a small skin hook and then with subperiosteal dissection, the collateral ligament is cut, and the

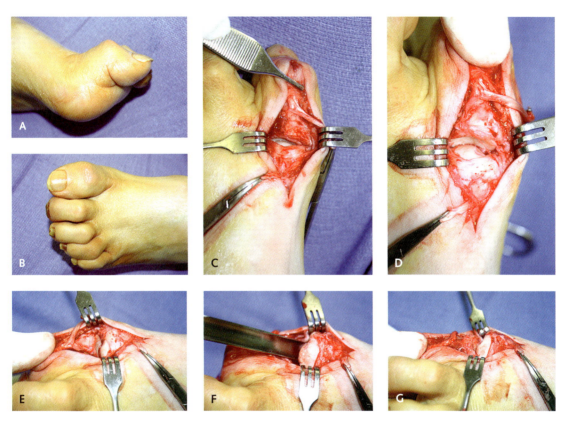

Figure 7-4   The hallux interphalangeal (IP) and metatarsophalangeal (MP) joints were both quite rigid in this patient. **A** and **B,** A decision was made to fuse the IP joint, lengthen the extensor hallucis longus (EHL), and salvage the MP joint with a complete soft tissue release. **C,** Note the lengthening of the EHL and exposure of the MP joint. **D** and **E,** With attempts to flex the MP joint, instead of rotating as a ball and socket, it hinges open as a result of severe subluxation of the sesamoid complex. **F** and **G,** The only way to improve flexion at the MP joint is to completely strip the undersurface of the sesamoid complex with a curved periosteal elevator and allow the volar plate to slide proximally.

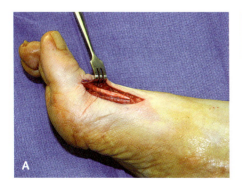

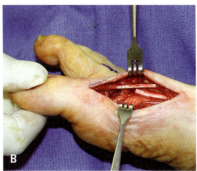

Figure 7-5   A cock-up extension deformity of the hallux without interphalangeal joint deformity was associated with a flexible extension contracture at the metatarsophalangeal joint. **A** and **B,** The deformity was simply corrected with a lengthening of the extensor hallucis longus and a dorsal joint capsulotomy.

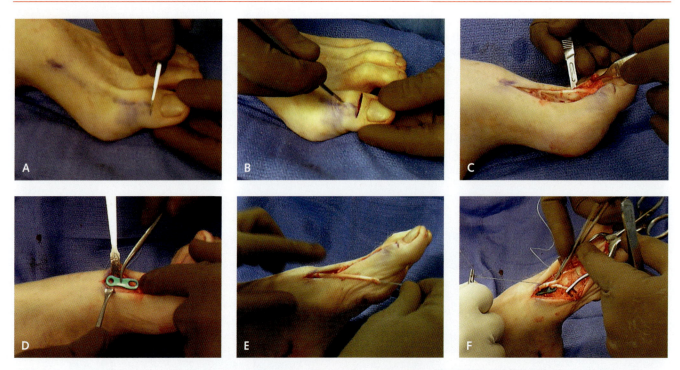

Figure 7-6 A, The interphalangeal (IP) joint of the hallux was very rigid, but the metatarsophalangeal (MP) joint is flexible. **B,** An IP joint arthrodesis was performed. **C,** In addition, the extensor hallucis longus was transferred to the first metatarsal. **D,** An osteotomy of the first metatarsal was performed, followed by application of a locking compression plate. **E** and **F,** The tendon was then transferred into the metatarsal neck after the MP joint release and the IP fusion.

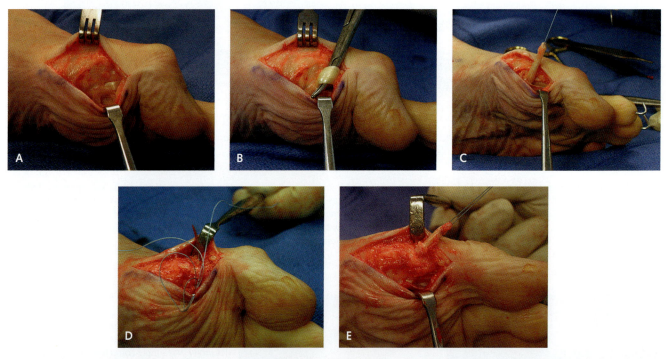

Figure 7-7 The interphalangeal (IP) and metatarsophalangeal (MP) joints were flexible enough in this patient to consider a transfer of the flexor hallucis longus (FHL) to the base of the proximal phalanx. **A,** An incision is made medially at the junction of the dorsal and plantar skin. **B,** The FHL sheath is opened and the tendon identified. **C,** The tendon is cut as far distally as possible and sutured; **D,** a 2.5-mm drill hole is then made in the medial phalanx from dorsal to plantar, and the tendon is passed through from plantar to dorsal using a large curved needle. **E,** The tendon is pulled through and then sutured back on to itself or to the dorsal periosteum.

joint finally exposed. The EHL can be lifted up off the proximal phalanx and then retracted laterally while the head of the proximal phalanx is completely delivered into the incision. The proximal phalanx is then cut, removing only the articular surface. This can be cut slightly obliquely so as to create some dorsiflexion into the arthrodesis, but usually I will do this once a second cut on the base of the distal phalanx has been made when I know how much bone to resect.

The cut on the distal phalanx is not as easy, because laterally the attachment of the EHL is now at risk. If the tendon is detached, it can be repaired, because it does not slide proximally, as a result of the attachment of the EHL to the extensor hood. The base of the distal phalanx curves slightly proximally under the proximal phalanx, so this cut will always include slightly more bone on the plantar than on the dorsal surface even if it is made perpendicular to the axis of the hallux. Once the bone surface is cut, the apposition distal to the proximal phalanx is checked and fixation performed using a single cannulated 4.0-mm partially threaded screw. A fully threaded screw also can be used if the hallux is compressed manually during insertion of the screw. A guide pin is inserted antegrade distally out the distal phalanx and then back across into the proximal phalanx, ensuring that the hallux is well centered over the middle of the phalanx in doing so. A skin incision is now made over the guide pin but must be made transversely in line with the skin creases. By contrast, an incision that is made vertically creates more of a scar, which can be potentially painful. While the screw is being introduced, there may be a tendency for it to push the distal phalanx away from the proximal phalanx, so the correction should be held firmly in position. If a slight gap is observed, I take out the screw, appose the phalangeal segments manually, and then reinsert the screw while maintaining the apposition under manual compression.

If a tendency for the hallux to cock up at the MP joint is noted after the arthrodesis, then an EHL lengthening or transfer must be performed. Caution is advised regarding a decision to transfer the entire EHL if the EHB is not functioning well. Such malfunction is common in severe claw hallux deformity, and the best one could hope for is a hallux that functions passively but lies in a more neutral position with respect to the metatarsal on the weight-bearing surface of the floor.

TECHNIQUES, TIPS, AND PITFALLS

- It is preferable to retain movement of either the MP or IP joint whenever possible. An arthrodesis should be used for more severe and fixed deformity.

- I prefer to transfer the FHL rather than perform an IP arthrodesis. The FHL can then be used to increase plantar flexion of the MP joint rather than through a more distal fulcrum at the IP joint.

- Correction of severe hyperextension of the MP joint requires more than a capsular release. The collateral ligaments on both sides of the joint must be released, followed by stripping of the sesamoid complex under the metatarsal head.

- Transfer of the EHL may leave the hallux quite weak, because the EHB rarely functions well. Patients do not often complain about this weakness. If the hallux remains flexible in dorsiflexion, passive movement in toe-off is sufficient.

- Fixed flexion of the MP joint cannot be effectively corrected without an extensive sesamoid–volar plate release. The FHL can be transferred to the base of the proximal phalanx to increase MP joint plantar flexion strength.

- When performing an IP arthrodesis, make sure that no medial or lateral translation of the distal phalanx has occurred. The resultant malunion in such instances is not well tolerated. Place two fingers on either side of the joint while inserting the screw to ensure correct positioning.

SUGGESTED READING

Steensma MR, Jabara M, et al: Flexor hallucis longus tendon transfer for hallux claw toe deformity and vertical instability of the metatarsophalangeal joint, *Foot Ankle Int* 27(9):689–692, 2006.

CHAPTER **8**

Hallux Rigidus

OVERVIEW OF SURGERY AND DECISION MAKING

Surgical correction of hallux rigidus gives fairly predictable results, and patient acceptance and aesthetic and functional outcomes should be good. Many surgical alternatives are available to choose from, all based on considerations of the underlying anatomy, the pathologic changes, and the severity of the arthritis. Patient needs for activities and shoe wear will also influence the decision making for the type of surgery. In my own practice, the cheilectomy, with or without an osteotomy at the base of the proximal phalanx (the Moberg procedure), is the most predictable operation for correction of hallux rigidus. For management of the more severe grades of arthritis, although I perform arthrodesis frequently, I have obtained excellent results with interposition arthroplasty. Despite efforts with various implants, I have achieved less than desirable results with any type of implant arthroplasty. Arthrodesis continues to be a mainstay of treatment in the management of severe arthritis associated with deformity or in cases in which other salvage procedures in the forefoot need to be performed simultaneously.

In planning surgery, the range of motion of the metatarsophalangeal (MP) and interphalangeal (IP) joints of the hallux is important. I examine the foot while the patient is seated, as well as standing, because additional contracture, particularly of the flexor hallucis brevis, may become evident with standing. The ability of the patient to passively dorsiflex the hallux while standing also is noted.

Occasionally, osteotomy of the first metatarsal is advantageous. Elevation of the first metatarsal may not have a significant role in the pathogenesis of hallux rigidus (Figure 8-1). Nevertheless, a most definite correlation exists between metatarsus elevatus and severe grades of hallux rigidus. In such cases, however, the elevation of the first metatarsal may be secondary to the severe contracture of the intrinsics and retraction of the volar plate, rather than a primary condition. Although osteotomy may be required for correction of primary or congenital metatarsus elevatus, one has to be careful with the notion that an osteotomy of the metatarsal is routinely necessary to alleviate dorsal impingement from hallux rigidus. Clearly, certain deformities will benefit from an osteotomy—for example, a long first metatarsal or one that is abnormally elevated. Other deformities require more care with decision making about the corrective procedure. Regardless of the extent of its deformity, an arthrodesis of the MP joint will not be successful in a patient with a fixed elevated first metatarsal and hyperextension of the hallux IP joint. The result will be only to create additional load on the IP joint, ultimately causing pain with further subluxation and extension. The hallux will have to be cocked up significantly to position the arthrodesis in order to unload it from the plantar weight-bearing surface. This cocked-up position in turn will cause rubbing of the tip of the hallux on the shoe. Note that in Figure 8-2, the patient had already undergone an unsuccessful cheilectomy. In the standing position, the hallux is rigidly on the ground and the IP joint is hyperextended. Further attempts at passive dorsiflexion of the joint only worsened the IP hyperextension.

What is the condition of the sesamoids? Is there arthritis between the sesamoids and the metatarsal head? It is useful to perform a compression test or "grind test" by pressing under the sesamoids while attempting to dorsiflex the hallux. If such testing causes pain, even if radiographic degenerative changes are minimal, a cheilectomy may not work. A long metatarsal with the hallux in slight fixed flexion is associated with scarring and tightening of the sesamoid complex, and a cheilectomy will not work here either. In this latter situation, I would prefer to slightly shorten the metatarsal to take the pressure off the sesamoid apparatus and improve dorsiflexion.

CHEILECTOMY

Historically, cheilectomy has been used for patients with early- or intermediate-stage arthritis. An increasing trend over the past few years, however, has been to extend the indications for a cheilectomy to more advanced forms of arthritis. In clinical practice I have encountered many a patient who returns some years after a successful cheilectomy for treatment of hallux rigidus on the opposite foot. Radiographs of both feet typically demonstrate that the operated asymptomatic foot looks worse than the symptomatic foot. This finding may have something to do with denervation of the joint, but certainly, it is common enough that a cheilectomy may be performed for more advanced arthritis of the MP joint.

An incision is made dorsomedial to the extensor hallucis longus (EHL) tendon extending for 3 cm over the MP joint (Figure 8-3). The dorsal medial cutaneous branch of the superficial peroneal nerve must be avoided and retracted laterally. The capsule is incised, preserving a cuff of at least 5 mm medially for later closure. The capsule and periosteum are reflected off the metatarsal neck to expose the hypertrophic osteophytes dorsally. It can be difficult to expose the joint in the presence of large osteophytes, but the entire dorsal head must be exposed. Adequate exposure can be a problem in the foot with a large medial eminence as well as hallux rigidus, in which case the exostectomy will need to be performed with preservation of as much of the capsule medially as possible for closure. Alternatively, a medial incision with a medial capsulotomy can be used to approach cheilectomy in the presence of hallux valgus.

Figure 8-1 A, Although the first metatarsal is elevated, a metatarsal osteotomy was judged not to be of any potential benefit to the patient. The metatarsophalangeal (MP) joint was quite mobile, as was the first metatarsal. **B,** A standard cheilectomy was performed, with good results, including improved motion at the MP joint after surgery.

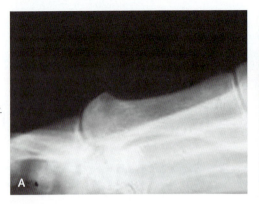 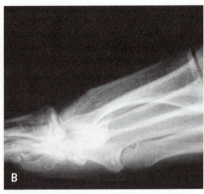

Figure 8-2 Elevation of the first metatarsal in a patient who already underwent an unsuccessful cheilectomy. **A,** With the patient standing, the tip of the hallux is noted to be extended. **B,** On pushing up further under the hallux, dorsiflexion of the metatarsophalangeal joint does not occur; only further extension of the interphalangeal joint is seen.

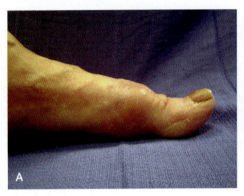 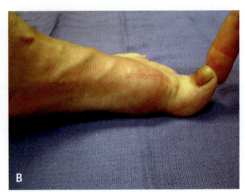

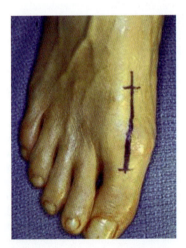

Figure 8-3 The dorsomedial incision for cheilectomy.

I prefer to use a chisel to remove the dorsal apical surface of the metatarsal head, because this gives me better control than that possible with an osteotome or a saw. The chisel is placed in the center of the metatarsal head, and one third of the dorsal surface of the metatarsal head is removed (Figure 8-4). At this point in the procedure, it always seems that too much of the metatarsal head is being removed, but the amount of bone that should be removed is almost always underestimated. When the head is viewed from above, one third of its volume seems like a large amount of bone to resect until an intraoperative

radiograph is obtained, whereupon how little has actually been removed becomes evident. The ostectomy must be performed from distal to proximal, with removal of the dorsal osteophytes, and then the medial and lateral margins of the metatarsal head are contoured. If cysts are present in the metatarsal head, the ostectomy can be performed just dorsal to the erosion, or the head drilled with a Kirschner wire (K-wire), which may improve the fibrocartilaginous surface (Figure 8-5). Rounding off of the metatarsal head is performed using a rongeur and chisel, but care is taken not to dissect too far proximally. If the marginal osteophytes need to be removed, this can be done with the chisel, but again, it is essential not to go too far proximally on the lateral aspect of the head, which can result in avascular necrosis. The capsular attachment to the medial aspect of the first metatarsal head should be left intact. Range of dorsiflexion of the MP joint should be at least 65 degrees after the cheilectomy.

OSTEOTOMY OF THE PROXIMAL PHALANX (MOBERG OSTEOTOMY)

Osteotomy of the proximal phalanx—the Moberg osteotomy—is an easy operation to perform, with a predictable outcome. The hallux is dorsiflexed approximately 10 degrees off the floor. This operation does not increase range of motion of the hallux but simply facilitates clearance of the hallux so that at the starting point, the MTP joint is already in slightly greater dorsiflexion. I use this operation frequently, mostly for grade II arthritis. It is useful in cases in which additional "movement" is desirable, and, in particular, for patients who need an increased dorsiflexion of the hallux because of athletic and shoe wear needs (Figure 8-6). In patients with combined hallux

8

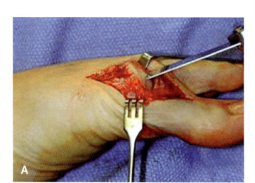
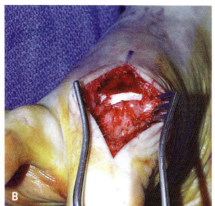

Figure 8-4 A, The dorsal one third of the metatarsal head is removed with a chisel. **B,** The intraoperative appearance of the articulation after the cheilectomy.

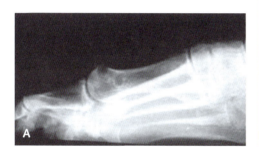
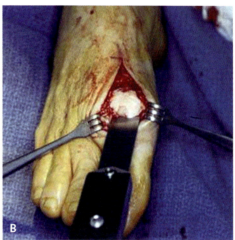

Figure 8-5 A, Note cyst formation in the metatarsal head, indicating a more advanced form of arthritis. **B,** At surgery, a central defect in the metatarsal head was present, and a cheilectomy was performed. Note position of the chisel blade immediately under the central cartilage erosion.

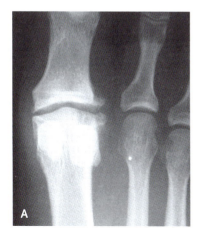
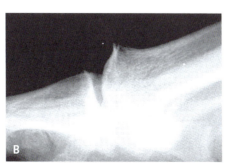
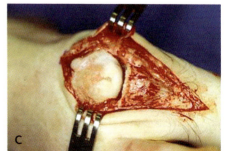

Figure 8-6 A, Flattening out of the metatarsal head and proximal phalanx is a common change associated with hallux rigidus. **B,** Reasonable preservation of the joint space is evident, and a cheilectomy was planned. **C,** The patient was a runner and desired more hallux dorsiflexion, so a Moberg osteotomy was added to the cheilectomy.

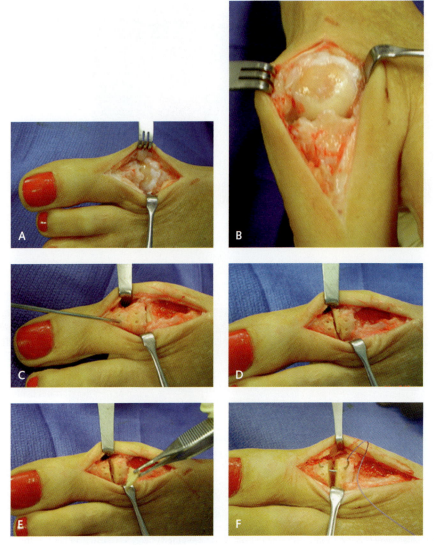

Figure 8-7 The Moberg osteotomy is demonstrated for arthrosis involving the dorsal one third of the metatarsal head in a 41-year-old female athlete. Limited range of dorsiflexion was present. **A** and **B,** Note the erosion of the dorsal one third of the metatarsal head, with preservation of the deeper cartilage. **C,** After a cheilectomy, two sets of pilot holes are made in the proximal phalanx with a 2-mm Kirschner wire at a 45-degree angle. **D** and **E,** A 2-mm triangular wedge of bone is removed with a saw. Note that the bone wedge is slightly dorsal and medial, allowing the hallux to be set in dorsiflexion, to correct very slight valgus. **F,** The osteotomy is secured with two 2-0 absorbable sutures.

rigidus and mild hallux valgus, a biplanar phalangeal osteotomy is performed to adduct and dorsiflex the hallux simultaneously, combining an Akin with a Moberg procedure. The surgery usually is performed in the setting of hallux rigidus, in conjunction with a cheilectomy, and the incision is simply extended more distally over the base of the proximal phalanx. The EHL must be retracted laterally and protected completely during the osteotomy.

The dorsal aspect of the cortex must be well exposed, and two sets of pilot holes are now inserted into the dorsal surface of the proximal phalanx. These are made obliquely at a 45-degree angle with respect to each other. The first set is made just distal to the articular surface and a second set approximately 1.5 cm more distally. These are unicortical pilot holes to be used for later suture fixation, and the osteotomy is planned in between these holes. A 1.5-mm slice of bone is removed with a saw. Once the bone wedge is removed, the base of the osteotomy is quite a bit more than 1.5 mm because of the width of the saw blade, and the osteotomy wedge must therefore be limited to prevent a cock-up deformity.

A margin of 2.0 mm must be maintained on either side of the predrilled holes after the osteotomy, to prevent fracture through the hole and loss of fixation. The plantar cortex of the osteotomy is maintained intact, and a greenstick-type fracture of the osteotomy is created by first plantar flexing and then dorsiflexing the phalanx to completely close down the osteotomy. I open the osteotomy first using an osteotome, which loosens the plantar cortex but not the periosteal hinge. The osteotomy is secured with two sutures introduced through the predrilled holes using a curved tapered needle that fits the contour of the holes. These sutures will provide excellent stability, and screw, wire, or plate fixation is not necessary (Figure 8-7).

INTERPOSITION ARTHROPLASTY

Indications

Interposition arthroplasty is a good procedure that reliably increases the range of motion of the MP joint. Regardless of the technical aspects of this procedure, the interposition of soft tissue is a good

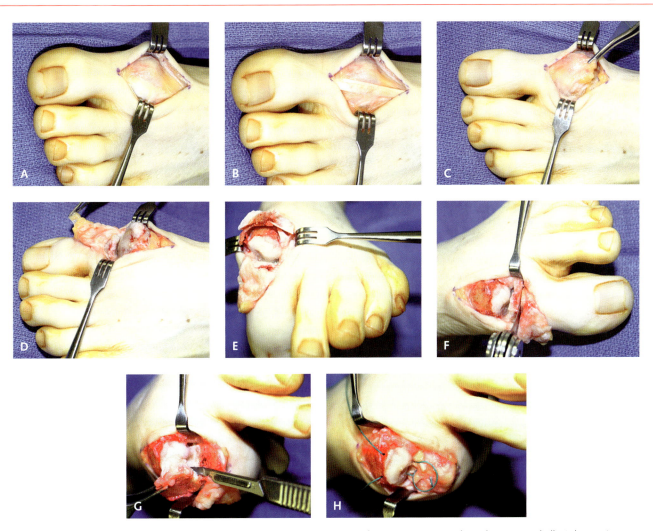

Figure 8-8 A, The incision for an interposition arthroplasty is performed and the soft tissues are retracted. **B,** The extensor hallucis longus is identified and retracted laterally. **C** and **D,** The flap of capsule and extensor hallucis brevis is cut and elevated distally. **E,** After the complete elevation of the soft tissue flap, the cheilectomy is performed with rounding off of the metatarsal head. **F** and **G,** The base of the proximal phalanx is cut with a saw **(F)** and carefully peeled off to preserve the attachment of the plantar plate **(G)**. **H,** The soft tissue flap is inserted under the metatarsal head using sutures passed through drill holes in the metatarsal head.

concept. This technique has been described using autogenous as well as allogeneic tissue, harvested either locally from the dorsal MP joint or from other adjacent autogenous tissue. Generally, I use a turndown soft tissue flap from the dorsal metatarsal neck, but I also have created an interposition graft as a large "anchovy" rolled up into a ball, which is then sutured in place into the joint. Either allograft or autograft tendon is suitable for this purpose.

I use interposition arthroplasty preferably as a salvage procedure when the joint is severely distorted or eroded from prior surgery, avascular necrosis, or cyst formation from a previous implant arthroplasty. In general, an interposition arthroplasty is contraindicated in patients who already have a short hallux, short metatarsal, or adjacent metatarsalgia. Clearly, some weakening and obvious shortening of the hallux will occur as a result of this operation. Regardless of how the procedure is performed, plantar flexion strength is compromised.

Technique

The incision is made dorsomedial to the extensor hallucis longus tendon and extends over the MP joint for approximately 3 cm. The dorsomedial cutaneous branch of the superficial peroneal nerve must be identified and retracted. Once the dissection through the subcutaneous tissue is complete, the extensor retinaculum is cut approximately 5 mm medial to the extensor hallucis longus (EHL) tendon to maintain an adequate cuff of tissue for later closure. The EHL is retracted, exposing the extensor hallucis brevis (EHB) tendon as well as the dorsal soft tissue and capsule over the metatarsal neck. This exposed tissue is now cut transversely as far proximally at the level of the metatarsal neck as one thick layer. The entire flap is now gradually mobilized and should include the periosteum, the EHB tendon, and the dorsomedial and dorsolateral aspect of the capsule. The flap is gradually dissected sharply off the dorsal osteophytes toward the base of the proximal phalanx (Figure 8-8).

The hallux is plantar flexed, and with complete subperiosteal dissection the osteophytes over the dorsal aspect of the metatarsal head are visualized; this is followed by a cheilectomy of the metatarsal head. It is important to resect the dorsal one third of the metatarsal head, and I use a chisel and not a saw to perform this cheilectomy. In addition to the dorsal osteophytes, the medial and lateral margins of the metatarsal head are contoured (see Figure 8-8, *E*). Rounding off of the metatarsal head is now performed using a rongeur. It is difficult to maintain the capsular attachment to the medial aspect

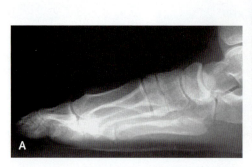
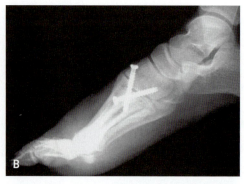

Figure 8-9 The patient was a 27-year-old female athlete who had previously undergone an unsuccessful cheilectomy to relieve pain at the metatarsophalangeal (MP) joint on toeing-off. Pain persisted with walking and particularly with running. She had good passive range of motion of the MP joint, with pain at maximum dorsiflexion. **A,** Although no arthrosis of the metatarsophalangeal joint was present, dorsiflexion was markedly limited. **B,** An arthrodesis of the first tarsometatarsal joint was performed, with the metatarsal in plantar flexion and the hallux in dorsiflexion.

to the metatarsal head with this dissection if the medial eminence is removed, and if it is disrupted, a repair of the abductor and capsule must be done later. Usually, however, the hallux rigidus is not associated with hallux valgus, so this is not a common problem.

At the completion of the cheilectomy, the capsular flap is carefully elevated by holding the flap dorsally with skin hooks using a knife to dissect off the base of the proximal phalanx. The saw cut is made from dorsal to plantar approximately 8 mm distal to the articular surface, almost at the metaphyseal flare. Awareness of the actual position of the joint is essential to precise placement of the cut on the phalanx. The cut can be made slightly obliquely so as to leave intact the attachment of the volar plate on the plantar surface of the proximal phalanx. Preservation of this attachment may result in slight elevation of the hallux off the ground at rest, but I generally prefer a vertical cut to maintain better contact of the hallux with the ground. The base of the proximal phalanx is very gradually and sharply detached from the soft tissue, to prevent stripping of the attachment of the plantar plate to the remnant of the base of the proximal phalanx.

The prepared capsular flap must now be interposed under the surface of the metatarsal head. This can be done with sutures inserted through drill holes with a K-wire or with a bone suture anchor inserted into the undersurface of the metatarsal head. The anchor should be well impacted into the metatarsal head, and the sutures from the anchor are used to bring the dorsal soft tissue flap plantarward and line the entire MP joint. Good tension on the flap must be maintained, but the range of motion of the MP joint must be at least 60 degrees with this interposition.

METATARSAL OSTEOTOMY AND ALTERNATIVE PROCEDURES

I also determine if hypermobility or metatarsus elevatus of the first ray is present, because this may be pathologic in some patients with hallux rigidus. Hypermobility is a very unusual cause of hallux rigidus but can occur in some individuals who are not able to activate the normal windlass mechanism, with consequent jamming of the MP joint in toe-off. If a patient presents with MP joint pain, and the radiographic appearance is normal, I confirm the location of the problem with infiltration of 1 mL of lidocaine (Xylocaine) into the MP joint. If necessary, a magnetic resonance imaging (MRI) or computed tomography (CT) study of the joint also may be helpful to ensure that the pain is not intraarticular or the result of sesamoid pathology.

In Figure 8-9, a previous cheilectomy was unsuccessful in relieving the patient's symptoms of pain at the MP joint on toe-off, with persistence of the pain with walking and particularly with running. The first metatarsal was markedly elevated (see Figure 8-9, *A*). An arthrodesis of the first tarsometatarsal joint was performed, with the metatarsal in slight plantar flexion.

Occasionally, osteotomy of the first metatarsal is necessary. Elevation of the first metatarsal does not have a well-defined role in the pathogenesis of hallux rigidus; as noted, however, a correlation exists between metatarsus elevatus and severe grades of hallux rigidus. In these patients the elevation of the first metatarsal is either primary or secondary to the severe contracture of the intrinsics and retraction of the volar plate. Although osteotomy or even a first tarsometatarsal arthrodesis may be required for correction of primary metatarsus elevatus, a metatarsal osteotomy is not a commonly performed procedure. There are patients, however, who have a long first metatarsal, and in this defined group, a shortening osteotomy may be a better procedure (Figure 8-10).

For patients with a long and elevated first metatarsal, a cheilectomy may not be the ideal treatment, despite the somewhat minimal radiographic changes present in the MP joint. It has been demonstrated in numerous studies that one of the factors in the pathogenesis of hallux rigidus is a long first metatarsal. If grade I or grade II changes are noted on the radiograph with a long first metatarsal, some shortening of the metatarsal may be indicated, either along with or instead of a cheilectomy. On the basis of the success of a similar osteotomy of the lesser metatarsals for treatment of joint arthrosis, I began to perform first metatarsal osteotomy for treatment of hallux rigidus, but under specific circumstances: a documented long first metatarsal, grade I or II radiographic changes, or an elevated first metatarsal.

The technique of performing the osteotomy also has evolved. Initially, based on experience with the Weil osteotomy, a similar type of cut was made on the first metatarsal head. The osteotomy is performed after a (minimal) cheilectomy, because less dorsal bone resection is necessary than when the cheilectomy is the only procedure. The osteotomy is made at an angle to shorten and displace plantarward the head of the metatarsal. The angle may vary depending on the amount of elevation of the first metatarsal, such that a steeper angle could be used if compensation for elevation is needed. In this way, the head is displaced slightly plantarward as well as shortened (Figure 8-11). Much like the Weil osteotomy of the lesser metatarsal, however, this technique leaves a small ridge

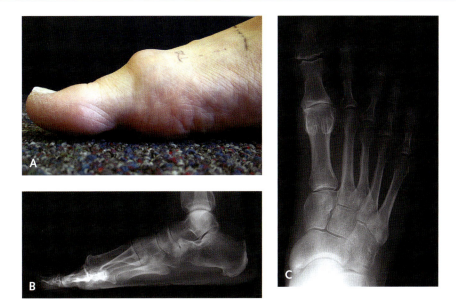

Figure 8-10 The patient was a 48-year-old woman with severe restriction of motion in dorsiflexion of the hallux metatarsophalangeal (MP) joint. **A-C,** Note the dorsal bunion **(A)** and the markedly elevated first metatarsal **(B)**, as well as the increased length of the first metatarsal **(C)**. This is not a good foot for an interposition arthroplasty and certainly not ideal for an arthrodesis of the MP joint. Either a proximally based plantar flexion osteotomy or an arthrodesis of the first tarsometatarsal joint is the preferred procedure to plantar flex and slightly shorten the first metatarsal.

of cancellous bone exposed over the dorsal aspect of the articulation. This may cause impingement or irritation of the phalanx in dorsiflexion, particularly if the dorsal articular base of the proximal phalanx is not normal.

On the basis of increasing experience, I changed the geometry of the osteotomy more in keeping with an osteotomy originally described for the lesser metatarsal by Ernesto Maceira. After a minimal cheilectomy, the first cut is made at a 30-degree angle with respect to the first metatarsal, commencing not at the articular surface but just above it. The desired amount of shortening of the metatarsal should be determined preoperatively from the radiograph, and the bone can now be precisely shortened intraoperatively. The second cut is made vertically from dorsal to plantar, usually approximately 4 to 5 mm proximal to the apex of the first osteotomy. Instead of translating the metatarsal proximal and plantarward as in the Weil osteotomy, a small wedge is now removed from the distal metatarsal and the head is then slightly shortened and angulated dorsally so that there is articular cartilage and not bone on the dorsal articular surface. This maneuver has the advantage of being precise, maintaining articular contact throughout the range of motion, and removing the pathologic dorsal rim of the joint. The potential disadvantage of this osteotomy is that the plantar surface of the joint is slightly rotated forward so that the sesamoids may not articulate perfectly under the crista of the metatarsal head. This type of osteotomy cannot be performed if the metatarsal is already elevated.

As noted previously, the indications for metatarsal osteotomy in the setting of hallux rigidus are quite precise. If a patient has metatarsus primus elevatus and gross elevation of the first metatarsal, limited dorsiflexion, and no arthritis, then a proximal plantar flexion osteotomy or an arthrodesis of the first tarsometatarsal joint can be performed. Remember, however, that as the metatarsal head is angulated in a plantar direction, the dorsal aspect of the metatarsal head, which is pathologic to begin with, may limit and com-

promise the effectiveness of this type of osteotomy. If a proximal osteotomy must be performed, I use a closing wedge procedure with the base of the wedge approximately 5 mm in width. A medial incision is used to perform this osteotomy, and after elevation of the periosteum, the entire base of the metatarsal is visible. The plantar base wedge is now removed, and the dorsal cortex is kept intact. Only approximately 4 mm should be removed during the initial part of this wedge osteotomy. With the wedge resected, the hallux is dorsiflexed, and as it dorsiflexes, pressure is exerted on the metatarsal head and the distal metatarsal is pushed down into plantar flexion. With increasing dorsiflexion of the hallux, greater plantar flexion force is exerted on the metatarsal, and vice versa. From here, the fine adjustments can be made to the amount of bone removed by the wedge osteotomy. If limitation and dorsiflexion are still present, then the saw blade can be inserted again into the partially closed osteotomy so that it will just access the saw blade. Then, with the saw blade repeatedly passing through the closed osteotomy, an increase in the plantar flexion of the distal metatarsal occurs with a reciprocal increase in the dorsiflexion of the hallux. Rarely does a cheilectomy need to be performed in conjunction with this procedure.

The premise for this operation is to decrease the intrinsic contracture that is present as a result of the elevation of the first metatarsal. With primary metatarsus elevatus, the short flexor contracts and the gliding of the volar plate apparatus is restricted. Through resection of the wedge, the relaxation that occurs in the plantar musculature and ligaments facilitates motion. Fixation is performed with the components under tension. I have tried to use dorsally inserted K-wires and screws in the past, but these seem insufficient to maintain the metatarsal in the plantar flexed position and to keep the osteotomy closed. A small two-hole compression plate works well, particularly if it is applied more on the plantar surface of the first metatarsal. Patients need to be kept non–weight-bearing for approximately 6 weeks after surgery until the osteotomy

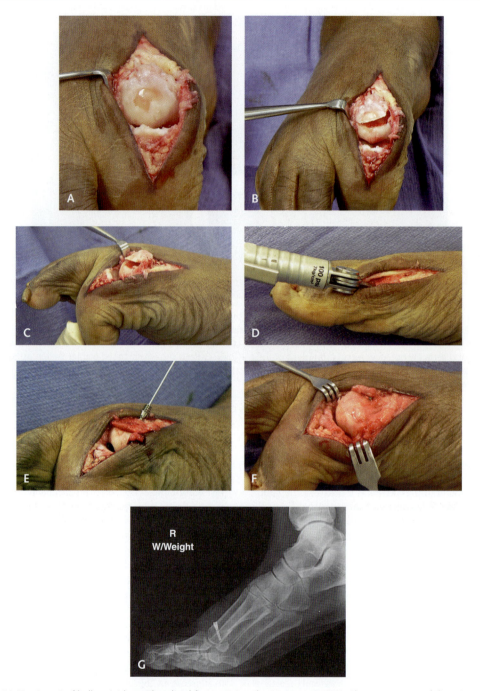

Figure 8-11 Treatment of hallux rigidus with a distal first metatarsal osteotomy. **A,** Note the appearance of the joint at surgery with dorsal erosion of the metatarsal head. **B** and **C,** A cheilectomy was performed; **D,** then the metatarsal osteotomy was performed at approximately 30 degrees. **E** and **F,** The osteotomy was secured with a small headless cannulated screw. **G,** Range of motion of the hallux at 5 weeks after surgery.

is healed, to prevent any gaps in the osteotomy and any malunion with recurrent dorsal impingement.

TAKEDOWN OF ARTHRODESIS

Finally, although arthrodesis is an excellent procedure for correction of hallux rigidus and deformity, some patients do not tolerate the accompanying stiffness and the load on the hallux IP joint, despite a good position of the arthrodesis. Illustrated in

Figure 8-12 is the case of a patient who was treated for arthritis and severe deformity with arthrodesis but 5 years later desired motion in the MP joint. The fused joint was approached through a dorsal incision and an osteotomy of the metatarsophalangeal joint performed. Once the hallux was completely plantar flexed, the periosteum under the metatarsal was stripped and a conical burr used to remove a 1.5-cm defect on either side of the metatarsophalangeal joint. The joint was distracted with a laminar spreader, and once it was completely loose, a balled-up tendon graft (in this

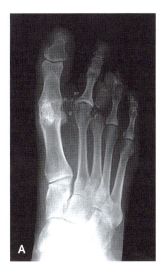
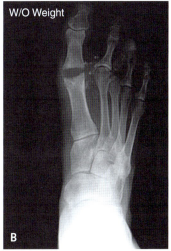
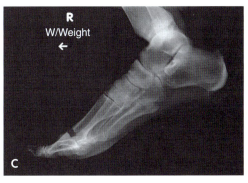

Figure 8-12 A, The patient underwent an arthrodesis of the hallux metatarsophalangeal joint to treat severe recurrent hallux valgus deformity with avascular necrosis of the first metatarsal head and lesser toe deformity. Although the arthrodesis was technically successful, she experienced progressively worsening pain under the hallux interphalangeal joint over the next 8 years. **B** and **C,** The hallux was already very painful at the tip of the toe under the nail, and further dorsiflexion of the fusion was not possible, so resection of the fusion with interposition of a free tendon graft was performed.

case a hamstring allograft tendon was used) was loosely sutured into place. At 3 years after this procedure, 40 degrees of motion including 30 degrees of dorsiflexion was present, which was more than adequate for function. One of the problems associated with this procedure is the gradual development of osteophytes on either side of the joint, ultimately limiting motion and causing pain as a result of impingement.

OSTEOCHONDRAL GRAFTS

Perhaps one of the more frustrating lesions of the metatarsal head to treat is a central osteochondral defect. The etiology of these central defects is clearly different from that in a majority of patients with idiopathic hallux rigidus, and such defects are likely to be the result of trauma or compression of the joint. Because dorsal joint impingement is not always present, the ideal treatment for this lesion would be to preserve the articulation, however possible. This is all the more important because the mechanics of the joint usually is normal: There is no associated arthritis or fibrosis of the sesamoids, the range of motion of the joint usually is good, dorsal impingement is unlikely, and the length and metatarsal declination angle also are normal. Debridement with drilling of the lesion is an option but cannot restore normal cartilage and should therefore be performed only if some type of graft procedure cannot be used. If the presence of an osteochondral defect in the center of the head can be anticipated preoperatively, then a fresh osteochondral graft is a good treatment. The other options are to take an autograft from the dorsal surface of the ipsilateral metatarsal head (Figure 8-13) and to use a synthetic biphasic osteochondral plug (Figure 8-14).

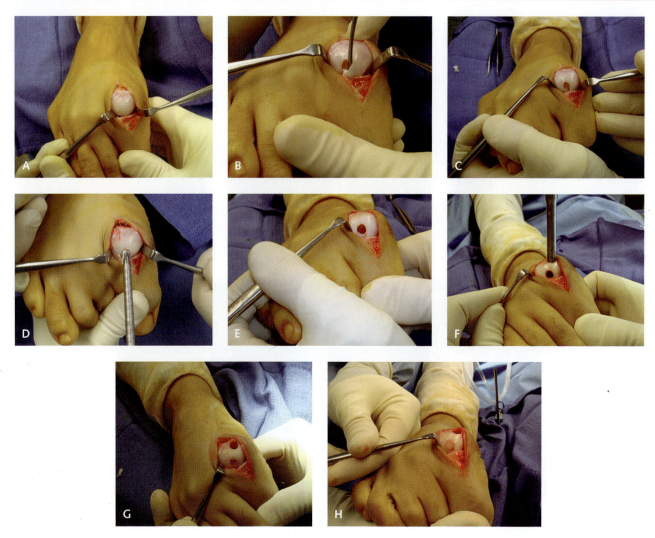

Figure 8-13 The patient was a 34-year-old woman with pain in the joint and limited range of motion. **A,** At surgery a central osteochondral defect of the metatarsal head was noted. **B-E,** This was debrided (**B** and **C**) and then drilled, leaving a central contained defect (**D** and **E**). **F-H,** An osteochondral autograft was then harvested from the dorsomedial metatarsal head (**F** and **G**) and inserted into the central metatarsal head defect (**H**).

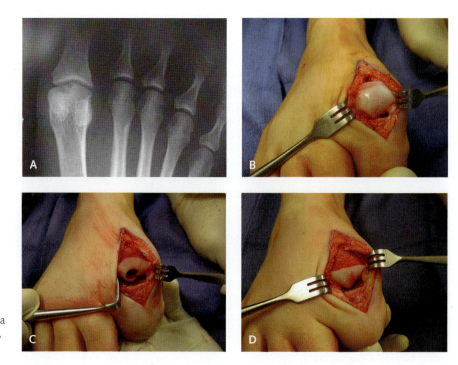

Figure 8-14 A 39-year-old patient presented with decreased range of motion and deep pain in the metatarsophalangeal joint, noted particularly with compression of the joint in the midrange of motion. **A,** The plain radiograph confirmed the presence of a central osteochondral defect. **B,** The defect in the center of the metatarsal head was identified at surgery. **C,** and **D,** A cheilectomy was performed and the defect excised with drilling of the central metatarsal head, which was then grafted using a synthetic bone graft (OsteoCure, Tornier, Edina, Minnesota).

TECHNIQUES, TIPS, AND PITFALLS

- Always note the presence of pain in the sesamoid articulation. Sesamoid-metatarsal arthritis may decrease the function of the MP joint and increase pain postoperatively.

- The goal of cheilectomy is to decrease pain. While an increase in the range of motion is desirable, it should not be the goal for surgery.

- The range of motion obtained during cheilectomy will not persist after surgery, and decreases approximately 30%.

- It is difficult to remove too much bone during the cheilectomy. A lateral intraoperative radiograph is helpful to confirm adequate bone removal.

- A cheilectomy is a reversible procedure; because there are other surgical alternatives if arthritis worsens, this is the procedure of choice for grade II and sometimes even grade III arthritis. It is surprising how well patients will do over the years after this surgery, despite the radiographic appearance.

- The use of a nonsteroidal antiinflammatory medication postoperatively will decrease the inflammation and extent of fibrosis.

- A series of hyaluronate injections commencing at 4 weeks postoperatively also may improve the outcome after cheilectomy.

- In the presence of a central osteochondral defect, I try to remove the defect in the metatarsal head and then, if necessary, drill or microfracture the exposed bone.

- A patient with little range of motion preoperatively will appreciate any increase in motion postoperatively, regardless of the procedure. Conversely, it is not desirable to treat a patient with good motion preoperatively with an arthrodesis.

- Management of hallux valgus and associated hallux rigidus is difficult. If the valgus deformity is mild, and the medial eminence needs to be removed, this resection can be done as part of the cheilectomy. If the deformity is more severe, an arthrodesis may have to be performed.

- I prefer a dorsomedial and not a medial incision for correction of hallux rigidus. The medial incision has the advantage of permitting good visualization of the sesamoid complex but is associated with the marked disadvantage of scarring and a need to protect the hallux during recovery from moving into valgus while the capsule is healing.

SUGGESTED READING

Altman A: Nery C: Osteochondral injury of the hallux in beach soccer players, *Foot Ankle Int* 29:919–921, 2008.

Coughlin MJ, Shurnas PS: Hallux rigidus: Demographics, etiology, and radiographic assessment, *Foot Ankle Int* 24:731–743, 2003.

Coughlin MJ, Shurnas PS: Hallux rigidus. Grading and long-term results of operative treatment, *J Bone Joint Surg Am* 85-A:2072–2088, 2003.

Lau JT, Daniels TR: Outcomes following cheilectomy and interpositional arthroplasty in hallux rigidus, *Foot Ankle Int* 22:462–470, 2001.

Haddad SL: The use of osteotomies in the treatment of hallux limitus and hallux rigidus, *Foot Ankle Clin* 5:629–661, 2000.

Hamilton WG, Hubbard CE: Hallux rigidus. Excisional arthroplasty, *Foot Ankle Clin* 5:663–671, 2000.

Horton GA, Park YW, Myerson MS: Role of metatarsus primus elevatus in the pathogenesis of hallux rigidus, *Foot Ankle Int* 20:777–780, 1999.

Malerba F, Milani R, Sartorelli E, Haddo O: Distal oblique first metatarsal osteotomy in grade 3 hallux rigidus: A long-term followup, *Foot Ankle Int* 29:677–682, 2008.

Mann RA: Intermediate to long term follow-up of medial approach dorsal cheilectomy for hallux rigidus, *Foot Ankle Int* 21:156, 2000.

Schenk S, Meizer R, Kramer R, et al: Resection arthroplasty with and without capsular interposition for treatment of severe hallux rigidus, *Int Orthop* 33:145–150, 2009.

CHAPTER 9

Disorders of the Sesamoids

EVALUATION

Making the correct pathologic and clinical diagnosis of sesamoid disorders can be difficult, although distinguishing between an acute and a chronic pathologic process involving the sesamoids, as required to identify a bipartite sesamoid, for example, is fairly straightforward. In the case illustrated in Figure 9-1, the patient was a 27-year-old runner who presented with acute pain around the hallux metatarsophalangeal (MP) joint, and it was difficult to determine whether the pain was in the joint or reflected a sesamoid problem. The plain radiograph demonstrated a bipartite morphology for both the tibial and the fibular sesamoids.

A bipartite sesamoid may be painful, the result of acute injury, with diastasis between the fragments. Figure 9-2 is the forefoot radiograph of a 29-year-old marathon runner who presented for treatment of acute pain under the sesamoids. Note that the tibial sesamoid is bipartitite and is slightly larger than the normal-sized fibular sesamoid. The fibular sesamoid, which was painful, demonstrates a diastasis of the distal pole (the sum of the two parts of the fibular sesamoid is normal, whereas the sum of the two parts of the tibial sesamoid is greater than it should be). This finding helps in diagnosis, and in the case illustrated, the acutely fractured fibular sesamoid was excised.

When the diagnosis is in doubt, additional imaging studies such as computed tomography (CT), magnetic resonance imaging (MRI), and technetium bone scan may be helpful, as in the case depicted in Figure 9-3. The patient was a professional tennis player with diffuse pain under the first metatarsal, and on the plain radiograph, neither sesamoid was normal: the tibial sesamoid was bipartite, and the fibular sesamoid appeared to be avascular. Bone scan, CT scan, and MRI confirmed avascular necrosis of the fibular sesamoid, which was excised.

Further imaging studies may be helpful in other circumstances as well. In Figure 9-4, the patient was a 44-year-old woman who presented with significant pain associated with hallux rigidus. The alternative of an arthrodesis and interposition arthroplasty was discussed with her, but the radiographic appearance was worrisome because of the arthritic changes in the sesamoid-metatarsal complex. If arthritis is present, arthroplasty may not be the correct procedure, because pain under the hallux MP joint may persist postoperatively. A CT scan confirmed presence of arthritis (see Figure 9-4), so an arthrodesis of the MP joint was recommended.

In evaluating the sesamoids and the hallux MP joint, assessment of the dynamic range of motion is important: At what point does the joint become painful? Where exactly is the pain located? Is the pain reproduced with pressure? In Figure 9-5, the patient was

a 31-year-old recreational runner with a cavus foot who presented with the complaint of pain under the tibial sesamoid. The passive range of motion of the MP joint was excellent, with good dorsiflexion, but pain was present at the midrange of motion of the hallux. Significant equinus of the first metatarsal, with increased pressure under the first metatarsal head, was demonstrated on the pedobarogram (see Figure 9-5, C). If a sesamoidectomy is performed in a patient with a cavus foot, the pressure will shift to the adjacent fibular sesamoid or the undersurface of the metatarsal head. Thus a tibial sesamoidectomy is not a good option for this patient, regardless of the underlying pathologic process. After orthotic management failed to provide pain relief, a dorsiflexion osteotomy of the first metatarsal was recommended.

Dynamic range of motion of the MP joint is important to assess after injury, with determination of the location of pain in particular and of the position of the sesamoids with passive dorsiflexion. Figure 9-6 illustrates the case of a patient with chronic pain under the first metatarsal head, with bipartite tibial and fibular sesamoids. Pain was present during passive dorsiflexion of the hallux and simultaneous application of pressure on the sesamoids. With this more diffuse pain, a sesamoidectomy is contraindicated, because removal of one sesamoid will only increase the pain under the remaining sesamoid. The focus of management must therefore be on use of orthotic support; if this fails to provide clinical improvement, then an osteotomy of the first metatarsal can be performed if its position at rest is in plantar flexion or equinus. If the metatarsal is in neutral position and therefore is not the source of the increased pressure, it may be necessary to remove the more symptomatic of the two sesamoids. Bone grafting of the abnormal bipartite sesamoid also could be considered.

After injury, the static and dynamic positioning of the sesamoids must be determined with radiographs taken during weight bearing. Retraction of one or both sesamoids or half of the fractured or bipartate sesamoid must be recognized if present. In Figure 9-7, the patient was a professional football player who presented with acute pain after a hyperextension injury to the left hallux. Subtle proximal retraction of both sesamoids with such injuries is suggestive of a rupture of the plantar plate (see Figure 9-7, A). This was confirmed on passive dorsiflexion lateral radiographs of both feet (see Figure 9-7, B and C). Note the position of the sesamoids in the right foot (see Figure 9-7, B) relative to their more proximal location in the left foot (see Figure 9-7, C). The sesamoids in the left foot clearly are not moving with the sesamoid complex in passive dorsiflexion of the hallux, thereby confirming rupture of the volar plate complex. In the case shown in Figure 9-8, a similar diagnosis

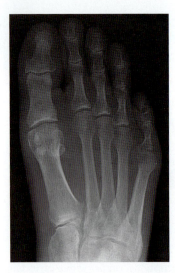

Figure 9-1 The patient was a 27-year-old runner who presented with acute pain around the metatarsophalangeal joint of the hallux. It was difficult to determine whether the pain was in the joint or reflected a sesamoid problem because the radiograph demonstrated bipartite tibial and fibular sesamoids.

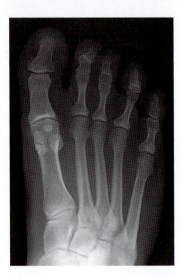

Figure 9-2 The patient was a 29-year-old marathon runner who presented for treatment of acute pain under the sesamoids. Note that the tibial sesamoid is bipartitite and is slightly larger than the normal-sized fibular sesamoid. The fibular sesamoid, which was painful, exhibits a diastasis of the distal pole.

was made of an acute volar plate injury, also in an American football player. The plain radiograph (see Figure 9-8, *A*) demonstrates the fracture of the tibial sesamoid and the slightly proximal position of the fibular sesamoid. This is a more difficult diagnosis, because chronic problems may already have been present in the fibular sesamoid, as was confirmed on MRI scan (see Figure 9-8, *B*) in this patient.

TIBIAL SESAMOIDECTOMY

When sesamoid disease is present, I am more inclined to perform a sesamoidectomy than to attempt other procedures, such as sesamoid shaving, bone grafting of the sesamoid, or removal of one pole of the sesamoid. Regardless of whether a tibial or a fibular sesamoidectomy is performed, it is essential to be aware of the

mechanical changes that take place around the hallux. After *tibial* sesamoidectomy, the hallux tends to drift into slight hallux valgus with a weakness in push-off strength; even dorsiflexion contracture may occur. After *fibular* sesamoidectomy, hallux varus, as well as a weakness in push-off strength, may develop. Bone grafting of the sesamoid (e.g., in the setting of a chronic nonunion of the sesamoid) can work. Because of the morbidity associated with this particular procedure, with requirements for non–weight bearing and the potential for persistent nonunion after prolonged rehabilitation, however, sesamoidectomy is a more appealing procedure. The only clinical situation in which I do not perform a sesamoidectomy for sesamoid disease is after acute fracture with diastasis of the end of the sesamoid (e.g., in the setting of a severe "turf toe" injury in which the volar plate has retracted proximally and a cerclage suture technique is used around the sesamoid to facilitate healing), assuming that comminution is not present. If sesamoid comminution exists, then I perform a sesamoidectomy. Figure 9-9, *A*, shows an acute fracture of the tibial sesamoid in a 34-year-old competitive squash player. This finding, however, was against a background of intermittent chronic aching of the hallux MP joint, confirmed on bone scan by some uptake in the fibular as well as in the predominant acute process involving the tibial sesamoid. For this reason, excision of the tibial sesamoid was not performed, and the fracture was repaired using a cannulated screw inserted percutaneously in a retrograde manner from the distal pole of the sesamoid.

To begin the tibial sesamoidectomy, an incision is made over the medial aspect of the MP joint just dorsal to the plantar skin. Following this landmark is essential to avoid injury to the cutaneous nerve. This incision must be carefully deepened, and skin hooks are then inserted into the plantar skin flap and retracted inferiorly. With a hemostat, the subcutaneous tissue is gradually divided down to the fascial layer, which is perforated and spread until the common digital nerve to the hallux is identified and retracted. A longitudinal incision is made directly above the abductor tendon and through the medial joint capsule to enter the articulation of the MP joint. Identifying the abductor tendon is important because this may be used later for repair and reconstruction of the plantar medial ligament deficit (Figure 9-10).

The sesamoid is not easy to excise because the periosteal fibers (Sharpey fibers) are adherent and no simple plane for dissection exists. The sesamoid is grasped with a small skin hook, and with a distal to proximal approach, the sesamoid is gradually dissected free. Grasping the sesamoid with a clamp followed by twisting it in one direction or another to mobilize it is a helpful maneuver. Usually, I detach the distal portion of the sesamoid first and then peel it away, trying to preserve the layer of the fibers of the flexor hallucis brevis tendon (Figure 9-11).

The remaining attachment of the medial head of the flexor hallucis brevis tendon must be imbricated. At times, there is sufficient tissue for imbrication with a simple suture and for attachment to the base of the proximal phalanx, while the integrity of the volar plate is maintained (Figure 9-12). If the defect is more substantial, it must be repaired to prevent hallux valgus. I use the abductor hallucis tendon to strengthen the plantar-deficient flexor hallucis brevis ligament. The tendon can be detached from the medial aspect of the base of the proximal phalanx and then advanced into the plantar aspect of the base of the proximal phalanx with a suture anchor. The medial joint capsule must then be reinforced with 2-0 nonabsorbable sutures to maintain the joint in neutral position. If the flexor hallucis brevis complex is repairable, then the abductor and capsular tissue is carefully tightened with interrupted, overlapping figure-of-eight 2-0

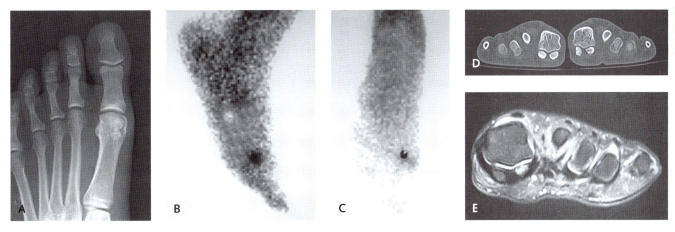

Figure 9-3 Neither sesamoid was normal in a 31-year-old professional tennis player with diffuse pain under the first metatarsal. **A,** The tibial sesamoid is bipartite, and the fibular sesamoid has an avascular appearance on the plain radiograph. These findings were confirmed as representing avascular necrosis of the fibular sesamoid on additional imaging studies: **B** and **C,** bone scan; **D,** computed tomography scan; and **E,** magnetic resonance imaging study.

nonabsorbable sutures. Tension is applied during repair of the abductor and capsule flaps to preserve the hallux in slight plantar flexion and in a neutral position in the transverse plane.

The metatarsal head and the flexor hallucis longus must always be inspected for chronic injury. Splits of the flexor hallucis longus tendon occasionally will be noted, which should be repaired. The undersurface of the metatarsal head may be arthritic or eroded, and presence of such tissue changes will have relevance to the outcome and recovery of the sesamoidectomy (Figure 9-13). Inspecting the flexor hallucis longus tendon and making sure that it is completely intact are important (Figure 9-14).

The hallux is taped into slight varus for the first 3 weeks and then taped with a figure-of-eight strap for an additional 6 weeks into a neutral position. Weight bearing may begin immediately after surgery in a surgical shoe and in a thick-soled running shoe worn at 3 weeks. Exercise may start at 4 weeks without use of any push-off strength, because passive dorsiflexion of the hallux must not take place for 8 weeks. Cycling and other static exercise machines may be used as tolerated, but again, no dorsiflexion of the hallux must occur.

FIBULAR SESAMOIDECTOMY

The main issue with respect to fibular sesamoidectomy is the surgical approach—specifically, dorsal versus plantar. Usually, the diseased sesamoid sits directly underneath the metatarsal head, and a dorsal approach is difficult. On the other hand, the potential morbidity from a plantar incision is an important consideration, so a dorsal incision may at times be used. From this dorsal incision, however, it is far more difficult to repair the sesamoid complex. Provided that the nerve on the plantar aspect of the foot is protected, use of the plantar incision is the preferred approach.

Figure 9-15, *A* and *B*, shows the radiographic and CT features an acute fracture of the fibular sesamoid. Because fracture of the fibular sesamoid is not as common as that of the tibial sesamoid, and owing to the presence of the changes noted in both sesamoids, a bone scan and an MRI study were performed (see Figure 9-15, *C* and *D*), confirming the acute nature of the fibular sesamoid injury. The sesamoid was excised using a plantar approach (Figure 9-16).

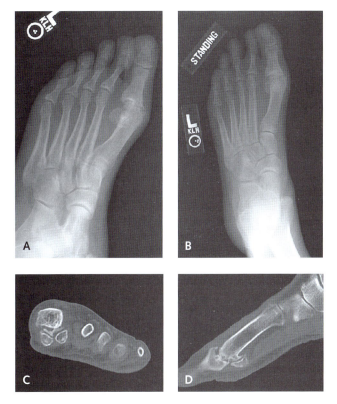

Figure 9-4 The patient was a 44-year-old woman who presented with metatarsophalangeal joint pain associated with hallux rigidus and radiographic changes of arthritis of the sesamoid complex (**A** and **B**); presence of arthritis was confirmed by computed tomography (**C** and **D**). The arthritis precluded use of arthroplasty for correction, and an arthrodesis was performed.

To begin the fibular sesamoidectomy, the sesamoid is approached through a vertical incision made lateral to the weight-bearing surface of the first metatarsal head. The incision is therefore made almost under the first web space, and with dissection, the plantar aspect of the fatty tissue is gradually retracted until the

Figure 9-5 The patient was a 31-year-old recreational runner with a cavus foot who presented with a complaint of pain under the tibial sesamoid. **A** and **B,** The passive range of motion of the metatarsophalangeal joint was evaluated. **C,** Note the equinus of the first metatarsal on the pedobarogram, with increased pressure under the first metatarsal head.

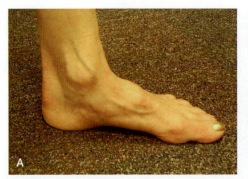
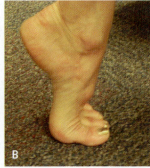
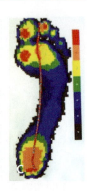

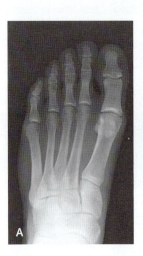
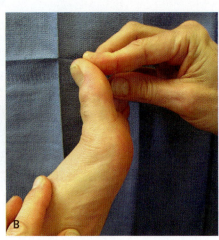
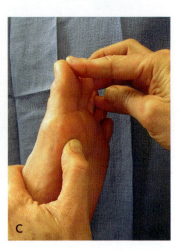

Figure 9-6 The patient presented with chronic pain under the first metatarsal head. **A,** Bipartite tibial and fibular sesamoids are evident on the plain radiograph. **B** and **C,** Pain was present during passive dorsiflexion of the hallux with simultaneous pressure exerted on the sesamoids.

plantar terminal hallucal nerve is identified. The nerve is larger than might be expected and can be found by sweeping a curved hemostat under the tissue until it delivers the nerve into the incision. The nerve generally is retracted laterally with a retractor and should be protected through the rest of the dissection.

Figure 9-17 presents an example of acute-on-chronic fibular sesamoid pain in a ballet dancer, showing the appearance of the pathologic process on plain radiograph and CT scan, the plantar approach to the excision, and the chronic changes in the sesamoid articular surface associated with avascular necrosis. The sesamoid is encased in periosteum and surrounded by the adductor complex and the attachments of the lateral head of the flexor hallucis brevis tendon. I incise the periosteum, and then, with as much protection as possible of the lateral head of the flexor hallucis brevis tendon and the adductor tendon, the sesamoid is gradually removed. The attachment of the sesamoid to the intersesamoid ligament has to be cut before removal of the sesamoid. The size of the defect is unpredictable, but a repair should be attempted. For some patients with mild hallux valgus, the hallux is less likely to drift into hallux varus, and a repair is unnecessary. If a defect is present, however, the adductor tendon should be sutured into the short flexor tendon, and a cerclage suture should be placed between the flexor hallucis brevis tendon and the volar plate and the distal aspect of the intersesamoid ligament. In this way, the slight plantar flexion and valgus positioning of the hallux is maintained.

The dorsal incision should be used sparingly and only when the sesamoid is accessible in the web space; otherwise, a repair of the sesamoid sling as previously described is difficult. A dorsal 2.5-cm incision is made in the first web space. The terminal branch of the deep peroneal nerve is identified and retracted laterally, and the soft tissues are gradually dissected. Use of a small retractor facilitates exposure, and the innominate fascia is cut to expose the adductor complex in the deeper soft tissues. The plane of the sesamoid depends on the presence of hallux valgus and associated disease. A knife is inserted between the sesamoid and the undersurface of the metatarsal head, and the sesamoid suspensory ligament is cut. The sesamoid is grasped with a clamp and is then gradually dissected free of the attachment to the intersesamoid ligament. Once the sesamoid is detached from its soft tissue attachments, the adductor complex must be repaired. The distal stump of the adductor tendon is grasped and reattached to the distal head of the flexor hallucis brevis tendon using 2-0 braided Dacron suture on a tapered needle. Checking the stability of the hallux and noting any absence of deformity (in varus) with stress applied to the hallux are important.

The key to successful excision of the fibular sesamoid is the identification of the plantar nerve and the flexor hallucis longus, the inspection of the articular surface of the hallux metatarsal, and the repair of the adductor complex, as shown in Figure 9-18. Figure 9-19 illustrates the case of a patient referred for management of chronic

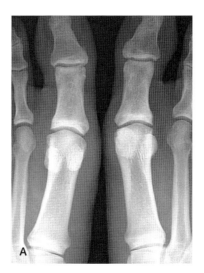

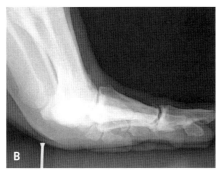
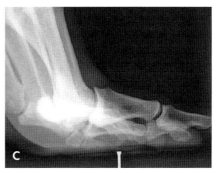

Figure 9-7 A hyperextension injury of the hallux in a professional football player. **A,** The retraction of both sesamoids on the left hallux is indicative of a rupture of the plantar plate. **B** and **C,** This was confirmed on passive dorsiflexion lateral radiographs of the hallux on both feet. Note the position of the sesamoids on the right foot **(B)** relative to the more proximal location of the sesamoids in the left foot **(C)**.

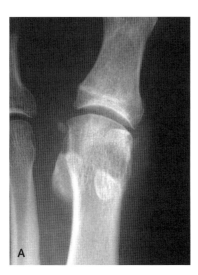

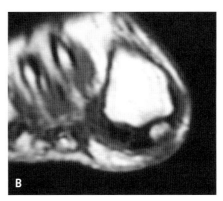

Figure 9-8 An acute volar plate injury, otherwise known as a turf toe injury, in a professional American football player. **A,** Note the fracture of the tibial sesamoid and the slightly proximal position of the fibular sesamoid. **B,** This is a more difficult diagnosis, because chronic problems also may have been present in the fibular sesamoid, as confirmed in this case by magnetic resonance imaging.

Figure 9-9 Acute fracture of the tibial sesamoid in a squash player with chronic soreness of the sesamoids. **A,** The fracture is apparent on the plain radiograph. **B,** Presence of underlying pathologic change was confirmed on bone scan by some uptake in the fibular sesamoid as well as in the predominant acute process involving the tibial sesamoid.

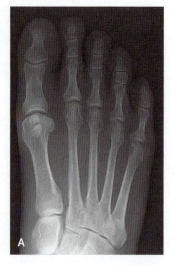
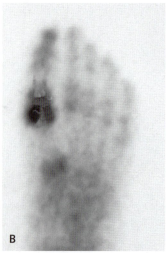

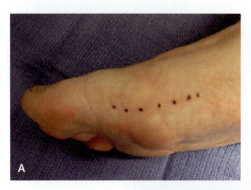
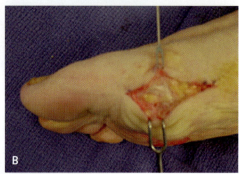
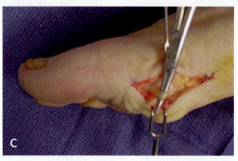

Figure 9-10 The steps in a tibial sesamoidectomy: **A,** the skin incision; **B,** superficial dissection; and **C,** identification of the medial hallucal nerve.

pain after an incorrectly performed sesamoidectomy. The terminal branch of the medial plantar nerve had been cut (see Figure 9-19), leaving a very painful stump neuroma. This lesion was excised, and the stump of the nerve passed dorsally through a separate incision in the first web space and buried in the interosseous muscle.

MANAGEMENT OF TURF TOE INJURY AND RECONSTRUCTION

Management of the acute hyperextension injury of the hallux can be challenging. The diagnosis may be clear, but the extent of the problem is never fully recognized until the surgical pathology report. MRI is very helpful in this regard (Figure 9-20), and all radiographs should be obtained with weight bearing to assess the position of the sesamoids relative to the MP joint. Dynamic flexion and extension radiographs of the hallux also should be obtained, noting the movement of the sesamoids with the hallux with dorsiflexion. As noted earlier (see Figure 9-9), there is marked variation in the pathologic findings, which may include a partial or a complete rupture of the volar plate, a fracture of one sesamoid associated with a rupture of the adjacent volar plate, fractures through both sesamoids, or tears or splits of the flexor hallucis longus. If not diagnosed, retraction of the sesamoid complex occurs, making it more difficult to repair the volar plate and advance the sesamoids to the corrected position if the muscle is scarred. It is not clear when the retraction is of such an extent that a repair should *not* be performed. If the retraction is severe and chronic, and a repair is performed to advance the sesamoids distally, the hallux loses passive dorsiflexion.

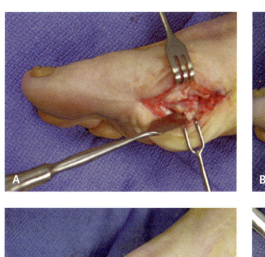
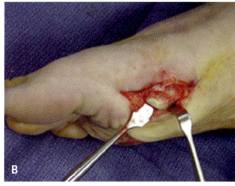
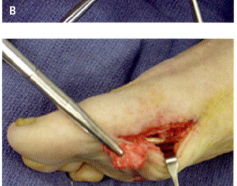
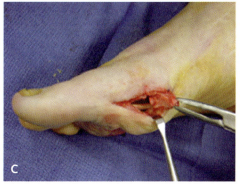

Figure 9-11 **A,** The tibial sesamoid is removed with periosteal stripping performed using a small, sharp elevator. **B-D,** The sesamoid attachment is broken by twisting it on its pedicle.

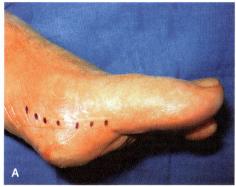
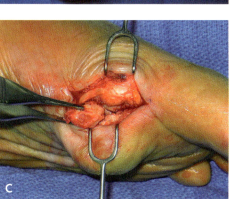
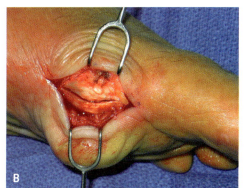
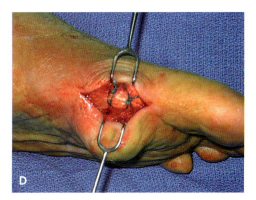

Figure 9-12 Excision of the tibial sesamoid for intractable bursitis associated with recurrent ulceration in a patient with diabetes. **A,** Slight hyperextension of the hallux is evident, along with the enlarged bursa. The incision is marked out. **B,** The abductor tendon is incised longitudinally. **C** and **D,** The abductor and flexor hallucis brevis tendons are sharply divided from the sesamoid, which is removed **(C),** and the abductor tendon is repaired **(D).**

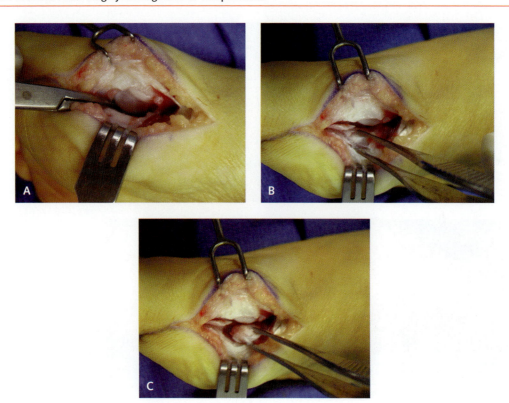

Figure 9-13 A-C, The undersurface of the metatarsal head was arthritic and eroded. **A,** The sesamoid is grasped in the forceps **(B)** and removed **(C).**

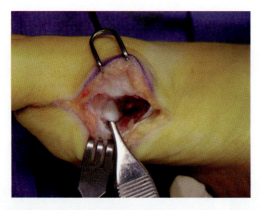

Figure 9-14 The flexor hallucis longus must be identified and examined at the completion of the sesamoidectomy. Injury to this tendon can occur during surgery, and longitudinal splits or tears may be present as a result of trauma.

Further compression of the joint may occur, causing articular chondrolysis and arthritis. The abductor hallucis may be torn along with the medial aspect of the volar plate, causing an acute hallux valgus deformity, as seen in Figure 9-21. The patient was a professional soccer player who sustained this complex injury 2 months previously, which was associated with pain, hallux valgus, and weakness of the hallux. At surgery, the tear of the abductor hallucis and the medial half of the volar plate was identified. The base of the proximal phalanx was debrided with a burr to freshen up the cortical rim, and a suture anchor inserted. The volar plate and the abductor were advanced distally using the suture anchor, followed by a closing wedge osteotomy of the hallux to realign the toe.

The incision to repair the torn volar plate depends on the extent of the injury. I use a medially based incision and then examine the sesamoid complex. If I need more exposure, I extend the incision under the proximal flexion crease of the hallux MP joint to further expose the plantar surface of the joint. This has the advantage of a direct exposure of the joint from the medial side but requires a lot of retraction on the nerves. An alternative is to start with the medial incision, evaluate the joint, and then use an accessory longitudinal incision as described for excision of the fibular sesamoid. Illustrated in Figure 9-22 is an example of a torn volar plate injury, along with the approach used for correction, in a professional American football player. The medial incision is made just dorsal

9

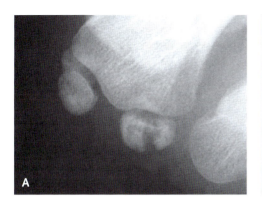

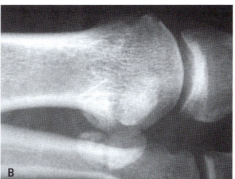

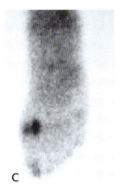

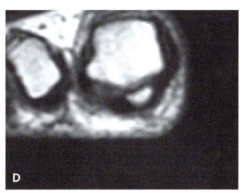

Figure 9-15 Acute fracture of the fibular sesamoid. **A** and **B,** Radiographic changes are apparent in both sesamoids. **C** and **D,** A bone scan and magnetic resonance imaging study confirmed the acute injury to the fibular sesamoid.

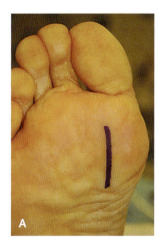

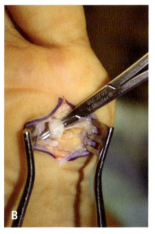

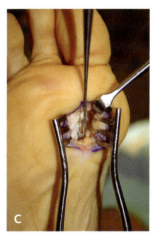

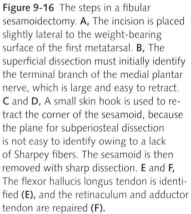

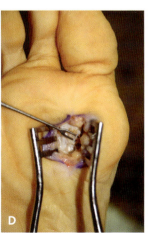

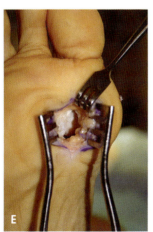

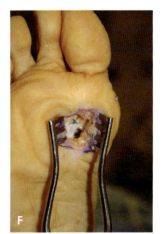

Figure 9-16 The steps in a fibular sesamoidectomy. **A,** The incision is placed slightly lateral to the weight-bearing surface of the first metatarsal. **B,** The superficial dissection must initially identify the terminal branch of the medial plantar nerve, which is large and easy to retract. **C** and **D,** A small skin hook is used to retract the corner of the sesamoid, because the plane for subperiosteal dissection is not easy to identify owing to a lack of Sharpey fibers. The sesamoid is then removed with sharp dissection. **E** and **F,** The flexor hallucis longus tendon is identified **(E),** and the retinaculum and adductor tendon are repaired **(F).**

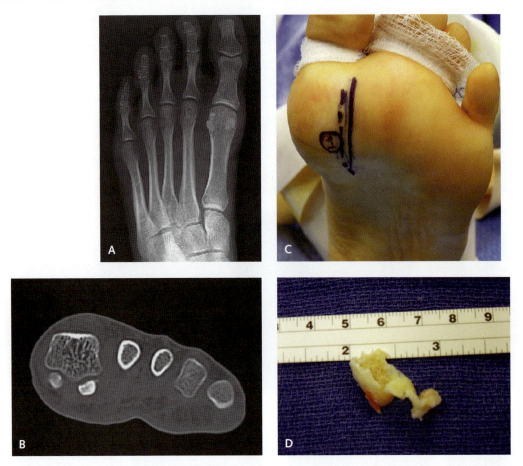

Figure 9-17 Acute injury to the fibular sesamoid in a ballet dancer who also had experienced years of pain. Appearance of the injury on plain radiograph **(A)** and computed tomography scan **(B)**, respectively. **C,** A plantar approach to the excision is used. **D,** The chronic changes in the sesamoid articular surface associated with avascular necrosis.

to the terminal branch of the medial plantar nerve. The joint was opened once the nerve had been identified and retracted, with no normal anatomy observed. The flexor hallucis longus was retracted and inspected, revealing longitudinal splits in the tendon. A complete rupture of the volar plate was found with retraction of both sesamoids. The lateral aspect of the joint could be reached, and a small stump of the distal ligamentous attachment of the volar plate remnant was present and used for the suture repair. The sutures were inserted but the lateral repair was not tightened until the flexor hallucis longus and the medial volar plate ligament also were repaired. If adequate tissue is present medially at the base of the phalanx, a suture anchor is not necessary. Slight flexion of the joint is required to maintain the correction at the appropriate tension. Rehabilitation after repair of this injury is similar to that outlined for excision of the tibial sesamoid.

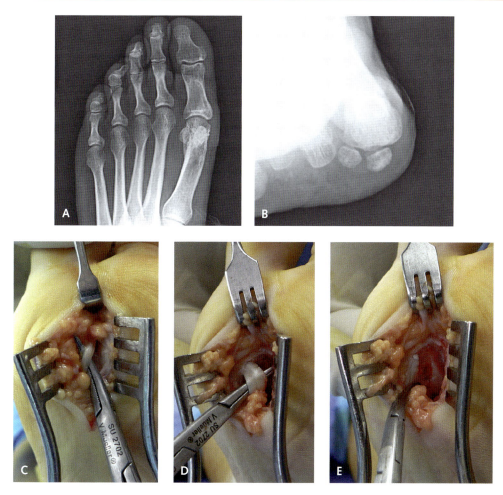

Figure 9-18 A and **B,** Pain localized to the fibular sesamoid was the presenting complaint in a patient who previously had undergone a bunionectomy and distal metatarsal osteotomy. **C** and **D,** The plantar nerve was identified **(C)** and the flexor hallucis longus inspected **(D). E,** The articular surface can be seen to be eroded.

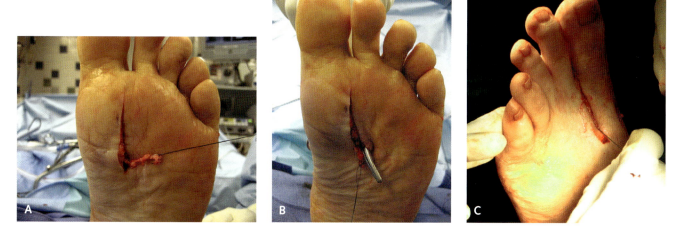

Figure 9-19 The patient presented with chronic pain after undergoing a fibular sesamoidectomy. **A,** The terminal branch of the medial plantar nerve had been cut, leaving a very painful stump neuroma. **B** and **C,** This lesion was excised, and the stump of the nerve passed dorsally through a separate incision in the first web space and buried in the interosseous muscle.

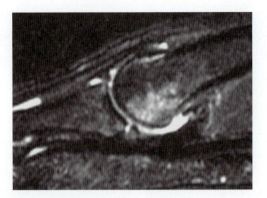

Figure 9-20 An acute hyperextension injury to the hallux associated with compression was correctly diagnosed, but the extent of the problem was revealed only by magnetic resonance imaging.

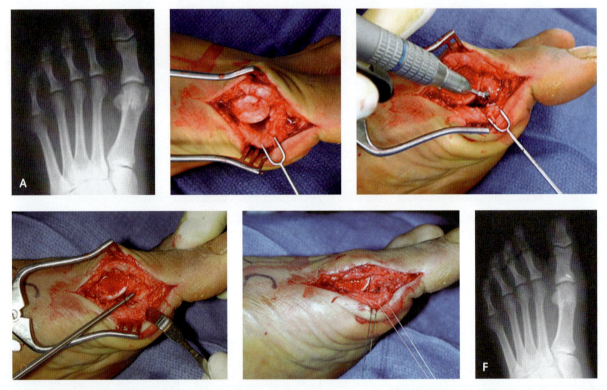

Figure 9-21 A traumatic rupture of the medial collateral ligament and the medial aspect of the volar plate off the hallux in a professional football player. **A,** The patient presented with pain and weakness of the hallux, with a hallux valgus deformity. **B,** Note the defect in the volar plate and the detachment of the abductor hallucis tendon. **C-F,** The base of the proximal phalanx was burred to create a bleeding bed for reattachment of the ligament **(C),** and a suture anchor was inserted (**D** and **E**). **F,** The repair was performed and was followed by an osteotomy of the base of the proximal phalanx to improve the rotation of the hallux.

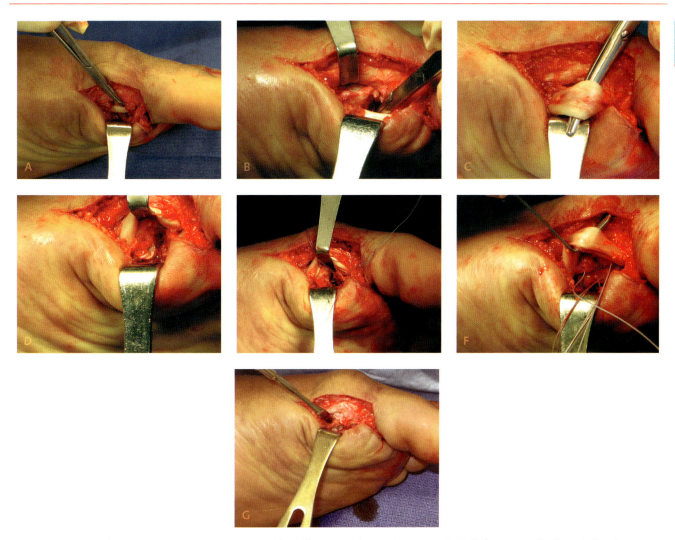

Figure 9-22 An acute hyperextension compression injury of the hallux in a professional American football player. **A-C,** The flexor hallucis longus (FHL) was retracted and inspected, revealing longitudinal splits in the tendon. A complete rupture of the volar plate was found with retraction of both sesamoids. **D** and **E,** The lateral aspect of the joint could be reached, and a small stump of the distal ligamentous attachment of the volar plate remnant was present, and used for the suture repair. **F,** The FHL was repaired. **G,** Note the slight flexion of the joint required to maintain the correction at the appropriate tension.

TECHNIQUES, TIPS, AND PITFALLS

- Protecting the terminal branch of the medial plantar nerve to the hallux is essential. Injury to this nerve will result in the formation of a debilitating neuroma. Once the nerve has been identified, it must be retracted and protected.

- After tibial sesamoidectomy, strapping of the hallux is essential postoperatively. This should be done to produce slight hallux varus and slight plantar flex-ion. Limitation of dorsiflexion for the first 2 months is important. Wearing a stiff-soled shoe, with an orthosis including a Morton extension, also is helpful.

- Be cautious in undertaking a sesamoidectomy in a patient with a forefoot cavus or fixed plantar flexion of the first metatarsal. Although the pain from the symptomatic sesamoid may abate, pressure under the first metatarsal may result, with transfer of pain to the fibular sesamoid.

SUGGESTED READING

Cohen BE: Hallux sesamoid disorders, *Foot Ankle Clin* 14:91–104, 2009.

Jahss MH: The sesamoids of the hallux, *Clin Orthop* 157:88–97, 1981.

Leventen E: Sesamoid disorders and their treatment, *Clin Orthop 269*:236–240, 1991.

McCormick JJ, Anderson RB: The great toe: Failed turf toe, chronic turf toe, and complicated sesamoid injuries, *Foot Ankle Clin* 14:135–150, 2009.

Richardson EG, Brotzman SB, Graves SC: The plantar incision for procedures involving the forefoot. An evaluation of one hundred and fifty incisions in one hundred and fifteen patients, *J Bone Joint Surg Am* 75:726–731, 1993.

Watson TS, Anderson RB, Davis WH: Periarticular injuries to the hallux metatarsophalangeal joint in athletes, *Foot Ankle Clin* 5:687–713, 2000.

CHAPTER **10**

Correction of Lesser Toe Deformity

CLAW TOE AND HAMMERTOE CORRECTION

I follow a simple algorithm for correction of claw toe and hammertoe:

Is the deformity fixed or flexible?

Is the deformity at the proximal interphalangeal (PIP) joint, the metatarsophalangeal (MP) joint, or both?

In most patients with claw toe or hammertoe deformities, I perform a *resection arthroplasty* of the PIP joint. *Arthrodesis* is performed in patients with the following indications:

1. Recurrence of deformity
2. Deformity of the PIP joint in the transverse plane
3. Neuromuscular etiology of the deformity
4. Inadequate flexion strength at the MP joint when stiffness of the IP joint will be acceptable to the patient
5. Requirement for a degree of predictability of surgery when the patient may not object to a stiff toe

In terms of the functional result, there does not appear to be much difference between arthroplasty and arthrodesis of the IP joint. Strength is improved with an arthrodesis because the force of the long flexor tendon is then transmitted to the MP joint to improve plantar flexion of the MP joint. The grip strength of the toe at the level of the PIP joint is better with an arthroplasty, provided that the toe remains flexible. However, the toe is rarely flexible. The potential for complications of both arthroplasty and arthrodesis also has to be considered. Although arthrodesis leaves the toe rigid, it is indeed straight, and depending on how the operation is performed, arthrodesis can avoid the toe shortening that is inherent with some arthroplasty procedures. An important potential complication of a PIP arthrodesis is a fixed flexion deformity of the distal interphalangeal (DIP) joint. Because a mallet toe occurs in approximately 10% of patients as a result of overpull or contracture of the flexor digitorum longus (FDL) tendon on the DIP joint.

In establishing the optimal approach to a claw toe or hammertoe deformity, it is important to distinguish a vertical plane deformity from a horizontal plane deformity such as the crossover toe deformity. The latter can never be corrected with an interphalangeal joint arthroplasty, because the apex of the deformity is not the IP but the MP joint (Figure 10-1). Certain deformities are very difficult to correct as a result of intrinsic contracture. These include, for example, the deformities associated with the complications of crush injuries of the forefoot or secondary to a compartment syndrome. The muscle fibrosis and intrinsic contractures shorten the flexor brevis muscle, and tenotomy is never sufficient. Correction of the fixed IP joint deformity will straighten the toe but will not improve flexibility at the MP joint, and the stiffness frequently is more debilitating. If indeed the toe is straightened, and the MP joint is stiff, toe pain will be worse, because the pressure on the tip of the toe increases. Typically, the toe can be extended slightly with the MP joint in flexion, but if the toe is extended, then the fixed, contracted nature of this deformity becomes more apparent (Figure 10-2). In addition to correction of the fixed contracture at the PIP joint, the MP joint requires release by shortening the metatarsal and relative lengthening of the intrinsic muscles. Even this procedure is not always sufficient, and metatarsal head resection may be necessary, particularly after crush injuries of the forefoot. What is the best approach to toe deformities in the elderly associated with asymptomatic hallux valgus? Clearly, the incidence of recurrent deformity of the toes will be high if the hallux is not simultaneously corrected. It frequently is the second or third toe, however, that is markedly dislocated or fixed at the PIP joint. Can an isolated toe procedure be performed with any expectation of a predictable result? If the hallux is overriding the second toe, it is possible to perform the toe surgery without correcting the hallux deformity, as illustrated in Figure 10-3. In this case, the patient had bilateral painful second and third toe deformities, but the hallux was fairly rigid after a previous resection arthroplasty. After the corrective surgery, the toes are straight and the hallux lies dorsal to the toes.

Another option for surgical management of the painful second toe is amputation (Figure 10-4). This is an excellent treatment in the presence of an isolated painful toe deformity or a fixed asymptomatic hallux valgus, or cases in which the hallux cannot realistically move into any further valgus because it is already abutting the third or fourth toes (see Figure 10-4, *B*). Toe amputation also may work well in the patient who has undergone an arthrodesis of the hallux MP joint (see Figure 10-4, *C*). This approach is a good alternative, particularly with a grade IV crossover second toe dislocation. When the amputation of the second toe is performed,

it is very important to eliminate all sources of pain, including the plantar surface of the metatarsal head. A logical assumption might be that with amputation, there is no pressure on the metatarsal, so metatarsalgia will be relieved. This is not the case, however, and I have encountered a patient who experienced persistent pain under the metatarsal head after amputation. The likely cause is subluxation of the fat pad from under the metatarsal head, so that even after amputation, pain under the head can persist. In such patients, I always remove the plantar condyles at the same time as the amputation.

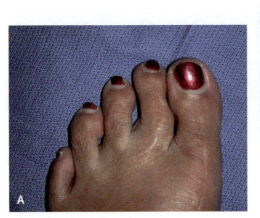 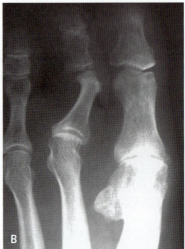

Figure 10-1 **A** and **B**, Recurrent deformity in a patient who underwent a bunionectomy and distal metatarsal osteotomy for correction of hallux valgus and a second proximal interphalangeal resection arthroplasty for correction of a presumed claw toe. This is a crossover toe deformity and cannot be treated in the same way as for a claw toe.

Figure 10-2 **A** and **B**, Typical appearance of the forefoot after a compartment syndrome. Mild contractures of the proximal interphalangeal (PIP) and metatarsophalangeal (MP) joint seem to be present, but with no dorsiflexion at the MP joint. **C** and **D**, With the MP joint extended as far as it can go, the flexor brevis is so fibrosed that the contracture of the PIP joint is exacerbated. Shortening osteotomies of the metatarsals were performed in conjunction with percutaneous flexor tenotomy at the PIP joint.

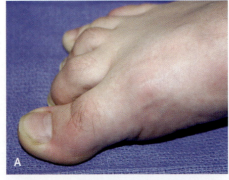 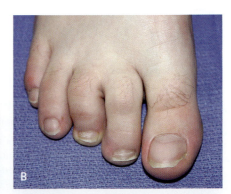
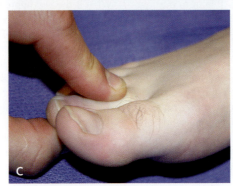 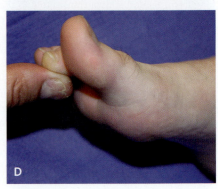

CORRECTION OF THE METATARSOPHALANGEAL JOINT CONTRACTURE

I approach the MP joint release sequentially. The procedure begins with a release of the long and short extensor tendons, followed by a transverse dorsal capsulotomy. If a contracture still persists, I release the collateral ligaments dorsally and then, finally, release the volar plate contracture, if present. If the joint is unstable or dislocated, soft tissue releases as described for a contracture are not sufficient, and a shortening osteotomy of the metatarsal needs to be performed. If the MP release is performed as an isolated procedure, in the absence of correction of the IP joint, then a decision has to be made whether to secure the MP joint with a Kirschner wire (K-wire), which should be used judiciously. There is always the potential for breakage of the wire, and in particular, infection with consequent chronic swelling may be a problem (Figure 10-5). These infections

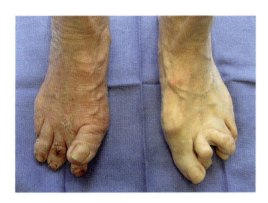

Figure 10-3 Corrective surgery normally would not be restricted to only the deformity of the lesser toes, while leaving the hallux untouched. In this case, however, the hallux deformity was asymptomatic, and the hallux was riding over the lesser toes, so a recurrent deformity of the lesser toes was less likely.

take a very long time to settle down, and the toe may remain swollen for months. If I detect any unusual swelling or inflammation in the toe after placement of a K-wire, it is removed promptly, and a debridement of the joint performed if necessary. The K-wire should never be used to reduce an unstable joint, because the subluxation will recur promptly once the wire is removed. In other words, the K-wire can facilitate scarring of the MP joint, but it should not be relied on to correct deformity.

PROXIMAL INTERPHALANGEAL RESECTION ARTHROPLASTY AND ARTHRODESIS

Either a longitudinal or a transverse elliptical incision is made over the posterior interphalangeal (PIP) joint, over a length of approximately 1 cm. I use small hooks to retract the skin and then incise the extensor hood either longitudinally or transversely. Choice of the incision depends on whether arthroplasty or arthrodesis is performed and whether K-wire fixation of the joint is used. In elderly patients, I prefer to use strapping instead of a K-wire to stabilize the toe, and in these patients, I use a transverse ellipse over the PIP joint and can close the ellipse to help with the alignment of the toe. This transverse incision does, however, cause some thickening of the PIP joint, which is permanent. Once the distal portion of the PIP joint is identified, the collateral ligaments on either side are cut. The cut is directed inward toward the joint, to prevent accidental laceration of the neurovascular bundle. A curved periosteal elevator (named a *shmogler* by Dr. Melvin Jahss) is inserted into the IP joint to strip the soft tissue from the medial lateral surface and undersurface of the phalangeal neck (Figure 10-6).

Either a small bone cutter or a saw can be used to remove no more than the distal one quarter of the proximal phalanx. A bone cutter will, however, cause minor crushing of the edges of the condyle, leading to painful ridges on the margins of the point unless these are trimmed; my preference is to use a saw. A smooth contour of the distal remnant of the proximal phalanx should be created, and a saw may be preferable for this purpose. The PIP joint must be stabilized,

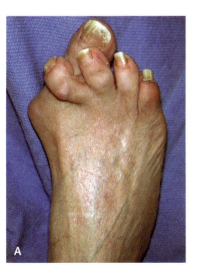 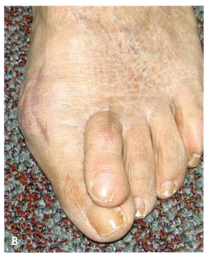 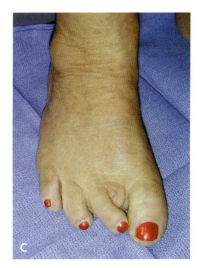

Figure 10-4 Amputation may be appropriate management for severe lesser toe deformity and pain. **A,** Severe pain in the second toe and asymptomatic hallux valgus were associated with a rigid hallux metatarsophalangeal (MP) joint with arthritis in an elderly patient. An amputation of the second toe was selected. **B,** In another patient, although the hallux deformity was not as severe as in some cases, it was less likely to worsen because of the rigidity of the MP joint. The patient had undergone previous operations on both the hallux and the second toe, with recurrence of deformity. Although the hallux is in severe valgus, it was asymptomatic, and a second toe amputation was performed. **C,** A third patient had severe painful arthritis of the hallux MP joint with an unreconstructable recurrent deformity of the second toe, for which an amputation was performed in conjunction with an arthrodesis of the hallux MP joint.

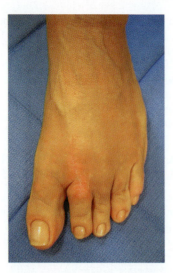

Figure 10-5 This second toe was infected at 5 weeks after surgery. The Kirschner wire had been removed 2 weeks earlier. Inflammation of the tip of the toe persisted for 2 weeks until the pin was removed. Débridement of the metatarsophalangeal joint followed by intravenous antibiotic therapy was necessary for treatment.

and this stability can be achieved with a suture placed in the extensor hood or a K-wire. If the MP joint has been opened, the K-wire is best introduced antegrade from the MP joint distally through the PIP joint arthroplasty, out through the toe, and then driven back retrograde into the metatarsal. Depending on the need for MP stability, the K-wire can be left in the phalanx or driven across the MP joint. If a K-wire is used, the condyles over the PIP joint are palpated through the skin to ensure that no minor mediolateral deviation of the joint is present; such deviation is associated with chronic postoperative pain. If palpation reveals deviation, then the K-wire must be redirected, or the spur must be trimmed with a burr. The alignment of the toe is, however, more important, and if any transverse plane deviation is detected, then the K-wire must be repositioned. If a K-wire is not used, then the toe must be stabilized with a suture placed through the extensor hood and capsule. I use two figure-of-eight sutures of 4-0 absorbable material. I prefer to use absorbable 5-0 chromic sutures for the skin closure. If a K-wire is not used, then the toe must be held stable with a bandage or splint for 3 weeks postoperatively.

I use an arthrodesis of the PIP joint to correct fixed contracted deformity such as that secondary to a compartment syndrome, neuromuscular disease–related deformity, instability associated with good IP joint flexion, and some recurrent deformities. The goal of the procedure is to realign the toe and make use of the long flexor tendon to improve plantar flexion of the MP joint. If an arthrodesis of the PIP joint is performed, then I prefer to use a 3-mm burr and not a saw to cut and fashion the joint into a cup and cone shape. Use of a burr minimizes bone loss and does not widen the toe at the PIP joint (Figure 10-7). The condyles and the articular cartilage are removed, but the medial and lateral cortical margins are preserved. The burr is then compressed into the middle phalanx to create a reciprocal cup shape for the phalanx.

A number of alternatives are available for stabilization of the PIP joint. If the MP joint is unstable, then a K-wire is used. It is introduced from the MP joint distally and then is moved retrograde across both the PIP and MP joints. Alternatively, if only the toe is be fixed, a guide hole is first prepared with a K-wire in the proximal phalanx and is then introduced antegrade across the IP joint and then retrograde across the previously drilled K-wire hole. The reason for the predrilled hole in the proximal phalanx is to facilitate

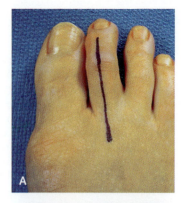

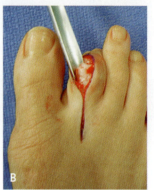

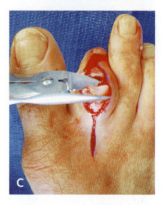

Figure 10-6 **A,** The proximal interphalangeal arthroplasty incision is marked out to be performed with release of the metatarsophalangeal joint. **B,** A curved periosteal elevator (a *shmogler*) is inserted into the edge of the joint to release the collateral ligament; **C,** 4 mm of bone is then removed with a bone cutter.

the correct passage of the wire across the IP joint. If it is not perfectly in the center of the toe, then a malunion of the fusion results, with painful medial or lateral deviation. Arthrodesis of the PIP joint creates a toe that is straight, which for some patients may not be physically or cosmetically acceptable. Slight flexion is preferable but not easy to accomplish with standard methods of fixation.

Over the past several years, I have tried to avoid longitudinal K-wire fixation for lesser toe arthrodesis. This alternative approach is very appealing because the presence of a K-wire is a nuisance for the patient and, as noted, increases the risk for infection postoperatively. I therefore use intramedullary fixation if possible. The ideal screw is one that can be inserted from the tip of the toe antegrade through the distal phalanx and buried into the middle phalanx while compressing the PIP joint. The headless cannulated screws are ideal for this purpose. After preparation of the joint surfaces, the guide pin hole is made in the proximal phalanx, and

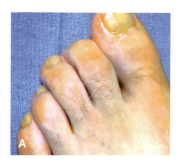
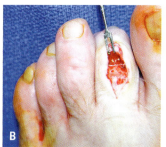
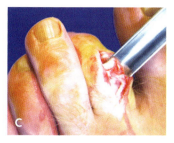
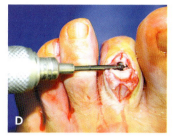
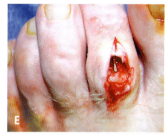

Figure 10-7 A, Arthrodesis of the proximal interphalangeal joint of the second toe was performed for a fixed claw deformity secondary to a compartment syndrome. **B,** After exposure through a dorsal longitudinal incision, a curved *shmogler* is inserted into the edge of the joint to free up the collateral ligament. **C,** A 4-mm burr is then used to contour the edges of the proximal phalanx, followed by creation of a reciprocal defect in the middle phalanx. **D,** A pilot hole is now made in the center of the proximal phalanx with a Kirschner wire. **E,** The wire is inserted out of the tip of the toe and then moved retrograde into the predrilled hole in the proximal phalanx.

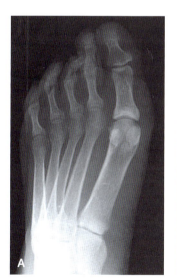
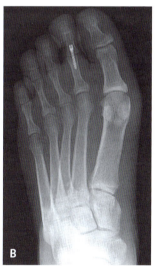

Figure 10-8 A and **B,** Asymptomatic mild hallux valgus with a fixed contracture of the proximal interphalangeal joint was treated with an arthrodesis using an intramedullary screw **(B)**.

then another guide pin hole from proximal to distal in the middle phalanx and delivered out the toe distally. The toe is then drilled, and a screw between 22 and 26 mm in diameter is used for fixation (Figure 10-8). The alternative locking compression screws that are inserted from inside the joint will work to hold the joint aligned, but if there is a problem with the toe after surgery, the screw cannot be removed, presenting a terrible problem with the revision because the PIP joint or phalanx has to be cut and the toe completely distracted in order to retrieve the implant. Such a case is illustrated in Figure 10-9. The patient was referred for treatment of a failed toe surgery, and although the arthrodesis was successful, and the toe was straight, the patient experienced pain at the interphalangeal

joint, and the implant had to be removed. This entailed a formidable surgical procedure because an osteotomy of the toe was required to break the toe and remove the implant.

COMPLICATIONS OF LESSER TOE SURGERY

If I did not have to perform lesser toe surgery, I would never do it. The rate of complications and patient dissatisfaction is unfortunately high. The outcome of a routine arthroplasty or arthrodesis is not predictable, and the exact same technique and procedure on one toe on the same patient may not yield the same result on the adjacent toe. Therefore, for both the surgeon and, more important, the patient, preoperative expectations must be realistic. It is never possible to make a toe with deformity completely normal, no matter what type of surgery is performed. Whether the correction is accomplished using arthroplasty or arthrodesis, fixation or no fixation, a K-wire or a screw, or a transverse or a longitudinal incision, the potential for various problems is always present. To begin with, the appearance of the toe may not be satisfactory to the patient because of postoperative swelling, which may be the result of infection or reactive fibrosis; the latter condition may take many months to resolve. It is important to recognize that the more bone that is removed, the shorter and the fatter the toe will be, and the thickness of the toe may never return to "normal" (Figure 10-10). Excessive shortening of the toe is avoidable, and no more than 4 mm of bone should be removed (this amounts to approximately the thickness of the distal condyles plus the distal end of the proximal phalanx).

If after removal of the distal part of the proximal phalanx the PIP joint remains stiff and cannot be easily straightened, then more bone should be removed. Fixed toe deformities should not be corrected with a manual manipulation of the joint. If the toe is stretched, then ischemia will result (Figure 10-11). Ischemia is particularly prone to occur with use of a larger K-wire, with correction of a more severe fixed deformity, and in cases in which the circulation is impaired to begin with. Such impairment is not always

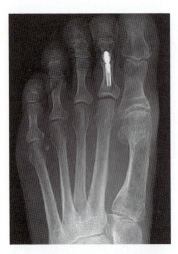

Figure 10-9 Radiograph of the forefoot of a patient referred for treatment of persistent pain after an arthrodesis with compression screw fixation. Although the toe was straight, the patient experienced pain at the interphalangeal joint. The implant therefore had to be removed, which was a very difficult procedure, necessitating osteotomy of the phalanx.

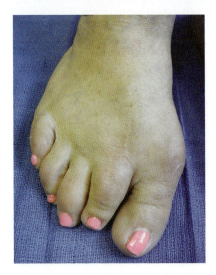

Figure 10-10 Appearance of the second toe at 5 months after metatarsophalangeal and proximal interphalangeal joint surgery. No infection had been noted, although minor infection is the most likely cause of chronic swelling of this nature and resolution of the swelling took 4 more months, with use of taping and massage of the digits.

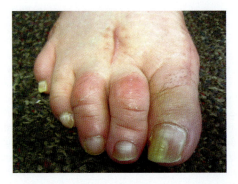

Figure 10-11 Extensive swelling due to infection at 2 weeks after a proximal interphalangeal arthrodesis with placement of an intramedullary screw, performed for correction of fixed deformity of the second toe. The screw was removed, and additional bone was resected. The toe was taped into neutral for 6 more weeks while the swelling and infection resolved.

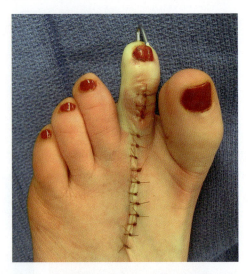

Figure 10-12 Intraoperative ischemia was noted after insertion of a K-wire to secure the reduction of the proximal interphalangeal and metatarsophalangeal joint dislocation. The K-wire was bent into flexion to improve perfusion to the toe.

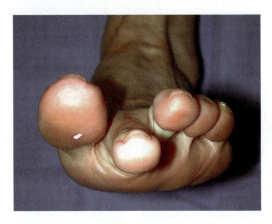

Figure 10-13 This fixed contracture was present at 6 weeks after surgery. The K-wire had been left in place for too long. The patient was returned to the operating room a week later (at 7 weeks after surgery) for corrective manipulation of the metatarsophalangeal joint, followed by injection of corticosteroid.

detectable preoperatively, because ischemic change may be present despite perfectly normal and palpable digital pulses. If ischemia is noted intraoperatively with the K-wire in place, the first thing I do is to bend the K-wire slightly (Figure 10-12). The toe often is too straight, and with addition of some flexion to the deformity, less stretch is placed on the vessels. At the same time, I smear nitroglycerin paste on the toe to improve the circulation. If these measures do not improve the perfusion within 5 minutes, the pin is removed. I prefer to remove the pin, if necessary, during surgery, rather than later in the recovery unit, because I may have to adjust the tension on the skin incision accordingly to maintain the toe in a corrected position.

Caution is advised regarding how long these K-wires are left in position. Use of K-wires is advantageous to add to some stability to both the PIP and MP joints, but if such fixation is prolonged, irreversible stiffness of the MP joint may result. In the example shown in Figure 10-13, the patient was returned to the operating room at 7 weeks after surgery and a manipulation of the MP joint was performed, followed by injection of corticosteroid.

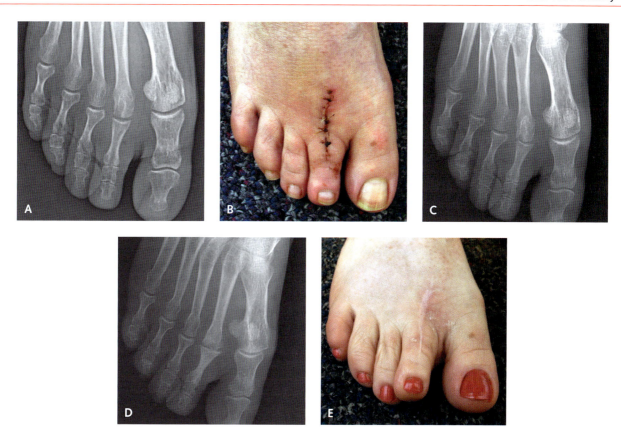

Figure 10-14 A 52-year-old patient presented for treatment of chronic pain after surgery to the toe of unknown type. The toe and the metatar-sophalangeal (MP) joint were very swollen and inflamed, with crepitus elicited by range-of-motion manipulation. **A,** A large bioresorbable pin was found to be present and had caused an erosion of the metatarsal head, as well as reactive osteolysis of the phalanx. **B,** The pin was removed, the synovitis of the MP joint debrided, and the toe stabilized with taping. **C** and **D,** The radiographic appearance at 1 and 4 years after revision surgery, respectively. **E,** The clinical appearance with arthritis of the MP joint.

Other types of fixation devices that are buried in the phalanges are appealing but must be used only after careful consideration, particularly the buried bioresorbable pin, which is very thick and does not resorb as anticipated. In the case illustrated in Figure 10-14, the patient was referred for treatment of chronic pain after surgery to the toe of unknown type. The toe was very swollen and inflamed, and the MP joint demonstrated inflammation with crepitus elicited by range-of-motion manipulation. Radiographic evaluation confirmed the presence of a large bioresorbable pin, which had caused an erosion of the metatarsal head, as well as reactive osteolysis of the phalanx (see Figure 10-14, A). The pin was removed, the synovitis of the MP joint debrided, and the toe stabilized with taping (see Figure 9-14, B), with overall good results despite arthritis of the MP joint (see Figure 9-14, C and D).

Shortening of the toe after resection arthroplasty is a common complication. As noted, only enough bone should be removed that the toe can be straightened, and this generally is approximately 4 mm. The shortened toe can be very floppy, unstable, painful, and cosmetically unacceptable to the patient. Salvage procedures are limited and include lengthening plus bone grafting and screw fixation. The screw fixation is technically easier, but I am always concerned that if this approach fails, the toe has suffered additional bone loss, making further salvage impossible. The surgery is performed through a dorsal incision, opening the joint and exposing the bone margins. Because an arthrodesis is not being performed, it is not necessary to debride the bone margins any

further (Figure 10-15). The toe is distracted, and at the end of distraction when the toe is out to length, perfusion must be checked. A fully threaded headless screw is then inserted from distal to proximal while holding the toe out to length. The other option is to use the same implant device demonstrated in Figure 10-9, which also can control the length of the toe without arthrodesis. My preference for obtaining length is to perform an arthrodesis with insertion of a small bicortical bone block graft. The joint is opened dorsally, and the bone margins are cleaned with a small burr. It is important to try to preserve as much of the length of the remaining bone as possible. The middle phalanx in particular must be kept to length, and the burr can be used to flatten and contour the middle phalanx without shortening.

The bone graft is then prepared. I use a small bicortical graft from either the ipsilateral calcaneus or an iliac crest (autograft or allograft). The graft is then cut to shape and generally will be longer than it is wide. The graft is held with a small hemostat clamp to ensure that it will fit in the phalanx. The key to the procedure is then to create a channel in the graft for fixation, because it is very difficult to insert a K-wire accurately through the graft and the toe at the same time. The graft is then predrilled with a small smooth K-wire, simply to make a guide hole. The pin is then removed from the graft, and the same smooth K-wire is then drilled antegrade out the tip of the toe. From here a larger threaded K-wire is inserted retrograde from the tip of the toe through and into the graft (Figure 10-16). The toe is then manipulated with the graft in place, the graft is inserted, and the threaded K-wire is advanced

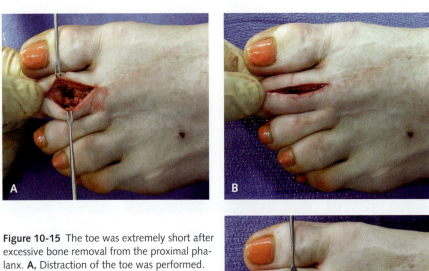

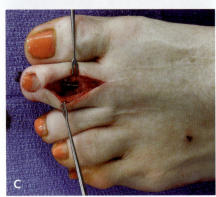

Figure 10-15 The toe was extremely short after excessive bone removal from the proximal phalanx. **A,** Distraction of the toe was performed. **B,** Perfusion was found to be normal with the toe held out to length. **C,** A fully threaded headless screw was then inserted from distal to proximal while the toe was held out to length.

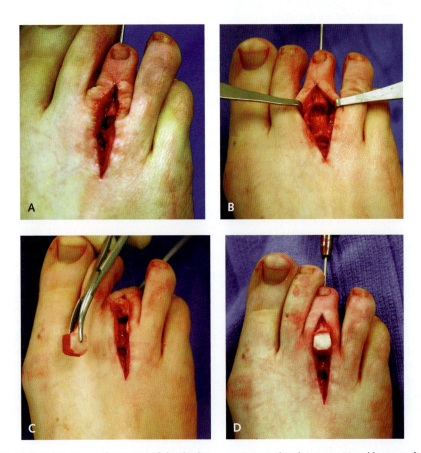

Figure 10-16 A and **B,** Severe shortening of the third toe was corrected with interpositional bone graft arthrodesis. The threaded K-wire is inserted retrograde into the toe, and the graft is predrilled with a small smooth K-wire, simply to make a guide hole. **C** and **D,** The threaded K-wire is inserted retrograde from the tip of the toe through and into the graft.

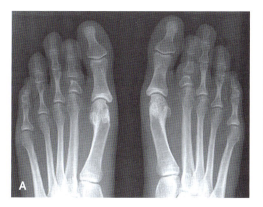
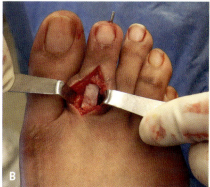
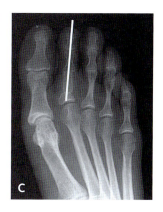
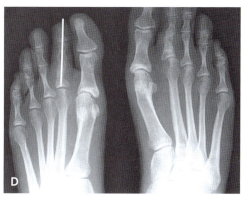
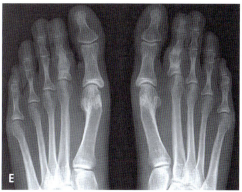

Figure 10-17 A, Bilateral floppy toes, with a cosmetic defect resulting from excessive bone removal from the proximal phalanx. **B,** The right second toe defect was treated first with interpositional grafting. **C** and **D,** The left toe defect was treated 6 months later. **E,** The final result 3 years later.

under fluoroscopic guidance into the base of the proximal phalanx. It is important to use a threaded K-wire here, because the graft will rotate on a smooth pin, which will loosen up over time. The K-wire is left in place for 8 weeks, which is not possible with a smooth pin.

The results of this procedure have been very satisfying, even when very little phalanx is available to work with (Figures 10-17 and 10-18). In Figure 10-18, the very short toe demonstrates horizontal plane deviation as well. It was not felt that all of the required surgery could be performed on the toe simultaneously, and the first phase was to lengthen the toe. This step was followed 6 months later with a shortening osteotomy of the metatarsal to realign the joint and address the arthritis already present in the MP joint (see Figure 10-18).

Certain deformities are beyond salvage, and all that can be offered to the patient is amputation (Figures 10-19 and 10-20). For these toes, a functional correction generally is impossible. To some extent, the cosmesis may be improved if there is a good adjoining toe, so that a syndactyly can be performed between the unstable and the stable toes. This solution is far from desirable, however, and although a syndactyly may give some modest stability, it remains quite ugly and generally is not cosmetically acceptable to the patient. The floppy toe catches on stockings, and barefoot walking is difficult.

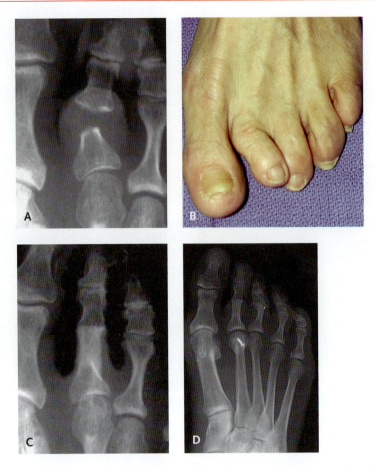

Figure 10-18 Recurrent deformity of the second toe after attempted resection arthroplasty. **A,** The toe is short, curved, and painful. **B,** Note the excessive bone resection, the medial deviation of the metatarsophalangeal (MP) joint, and the slight MP joint subluxation. An interpositional bone graft harvested from the ipsilateral calcaneus was used to lengthen the toe fixed with a single threaded K-wire. **C,** The final appearance shows good alignment of the toe and improved length. **D,** A shortening osteotomy of the second metatarsal was performed 6 months later.

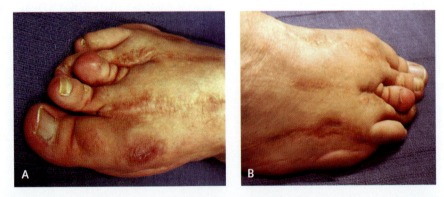

Figure 10-19 A, Severe deformity after multiple failed surgical corrective procedures in a 37-year-old man with a cavus foot deformity. **B,** The toes were floppy, unstable, and painful in shoes or barefoot. No further treatment was provided.

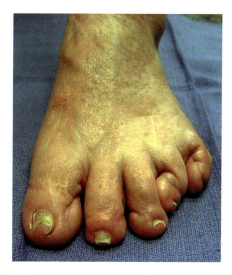

Figure 10-20 Floppy toes in a 46-year-old woman. The patient could not tolerate the difficulties posed by the deformity, and because insufficient bone was left to permit reconstruction, amputation at the proximal interphalangeal joints was performed.

TECHNIQUES, TIPS, AND PITFALLS

- Bone loss after excessive resection arthroplasty of the PIP joint can be corrected with arthrodesis. This procedure will shorten the toe even further, and therefore an arthrodesis with interpositional structural bone grafting is necessary.

- A longitudinal incision over the PIP joint leaves the toe narrower, and the toe can be further tapered through excision of a longitudinal ellipse from the PIP joint. However, if a longitudinal skin incision is used, then some sort of fixation of the IP joint is required. The fixation can be with a K-wire or through placement of a suture in the extensor hood. Alternatively, a transverse ellipse can be made through the skin, subcutaneous tissue, and extensor hood; when closed, this type of incision facilitates restoration of the position of the toe. However, this type of approach will lead to a slight widening of the toe, which may be undesirable.

- Arthrodesis of the PIP joint results in a straight toe. This outcome is not always well tolerated, so if possible, slight flexion should be incorporated into the arthrodesis. With the antegrade-retrograde technique using the K-wire, this flexion is not possible, and an alternative form of fixation must be used. Small threaded K-wires can be introduced obliquely across the PIP joint and either buried flush with the bone or left out percutaneously.

- If infection of the PIP joint occurs postoperatively, this may lead to a swollen inflamed toe, which always remains slightly thickened and uncomfortable. Interstitial fibrosis occurs, so even with resolution of the infection, permanent widening of the toe is present. This may necessitate revision surgery with scar resection and realignment.

- Some patients benefit from correction of hammertoe, but the correction cannot be accomplished without realignment of the hallux. The decision regarding realignment is difficult, for example, in elderly patients who have an asymptomatic bunion but a painful fixed deformity of the second toe. For these patients, I advocate an amputation of the second toe. It is quick, recovery is easy, and the procedure is remarkably well accepted by patients, particularly elderly patients. Usually, the hallux has already drifted as far as it can go—it is abutting the third toe, and the second toe is no longer functional. Amputation improves shoe wear and decreases pain without compromising forefoot function.

- The presence of rigid deformities of all of the lesser toes, with or without MP joint dislocation, warrants caution in surgical decision making. Such deformities may be seen not only in some elderly persons but also in patients after crush injuries. In the patient with

TECHNIQUES, TIPS, AND PITFALLS—cont'd

severe contracture without dislocation, the tendency is to perform a soft tissue release with realignment of the PIP joint. This approach seems reasonable; however, the wound complication rate is high in these patients because of stretching of the skin. The other option is to shorten the metatarsal, with either a metatarsal head resection or a Weil osteotomy. Even these operations, however, are associated with an increased frequency of skin healing problems.

- Amputation of the second toe is an excellent procedure for management of fixed deformity, particularly in elderly patients, when the toe is dislocated and the hallux deformity is asymptomatic.

- Some toe deformities are severe although asymptomatic. These often require correction, not necessarily for cosmetic purposes but for prevention of recurrent deformity of the hallux.

- Fixed toe deformity at both the MP and IP joints should be corrected with shortening of the toe or metatarsal. Frequently, the deformity is of such a magnitude that even metatarsal shortening osteotomy is not realistic, and metatarsal head resection is preferable.

SUGGESTED READING

Cohen I, Myerson MS, Weil LS Sr: Flexor to extensor tendon transfer: A new method of tensioning and securing the tendon, *Foot Ankle Int* 22:62–63, 2001.

Gallentine JW: Removal of the second toe for severe hammertoe deformity in elderly patients, *Foot Ankle Int* 26:353–358, 2005.

Jones S, Hussainy HA, Flowers MJ: Re: Arthrodesis of the toe joints with an intramedullary cannulated screw for correction of hammertoe deformity, *Foot Ankle Int* 26:1101, 2005.

Kaz AJ, Coughlin MJ: Crossover second toe: Demographics, etiology, and radiographic assessment, *Foot Ankle Int* 28:1223–1237, 2007.

Myerson MS, Shereff MJ: The pathological anatomy of claw and hammer toes, *J Bone Joint Surg Am* 71:45–49, 1989.

O'Kane C, Kilmartin T: Review of proximal interphalangeal joint excisional arthroplasty for the correction of second hammer toe deformity in 100 cases, *Foot Ankle Int* 26:320–325, 2005.

Trnka HJ, Nyska M, Parks BG, Myerson MS: Dorsiflexion contracture after the Weil osteotomy: Results of cadaver study and three-dimensional analysis, *Foot Ankle Int* 22:47–50, 2001.

CHAPTER 11

Correction of Crossover Toe Deformity

SURGICAL APPROACH

Crossover toe deformity cannot be corrected in the same way as for a claw toe or hammertoe. If correction is undertaken using a standard metatarsophalangeal (MP) joint release with arthroplasty of the interphalangeal (IP) joint, the deformity will invariably recur, because the associated contracture is in the transverse plane. Ideally, stability in the transverse plane should be enhanced, but at the same time, flexibility of the MP joint and control of any sagittal plane instability should be maintained. To some extent, the success of the operation will depend on the cause of the deformity. The pathogenesis of this condition is assumed to involve a rupture of the lateral collateral ligament, followed by some degree of rupture of the plantar lateral volar plate, followed by dorsomedial deviation.

If the crossover deformity is associated with a long second metatarsal, then the second metatarsal should be shortened. Shortening the metatarsal relieves the medial joint contracture because pressure is taken off the intrinsic tendons, as illustrated in Figure 11-1. In this case, the patient presented for treatment 1 year after bilateral hallux valgus correction. An interesting observation is that recurrent hallux valgus did not develop, despite the lack of anatomic barriers to valgus drift of the hallux (see Figure 11-1, *A* and *B*). The lesser toe deformities were treated with shortening osteotomies of the lesser metatarsals. The alignment initially was not ideal but improved somewhat with taping of the toes into varus for 3 months after surgery (see Figure 11-1, *C*).

Treating a crossover toe deformity as a claw toe will lead to prompt recurrence of deformity (Figure 11-2). Repair of the ruptured lateral collateral ligament and volar plate is technically difficult and probably unrealistic. For the repair to be performed, the suture must be inserted into the lateral collateral ligament without restraint of the joint and creation of a dorsiflexion contracture. To approach the plantar aspect of the MP joint with a transverse or longitudinal incision is very difficult, because the plantar joint does not correspond with the plantar skin crease. Techniques for repair of the lateral collateral ligament have been described; an important consideration in the surgical evaluation, however, is the underlying cause of the ligament rupture. If the rupture is the result of wear against the base of the third toe phalanx or from a long metatarsal, will a simple repair correct the deformity? This outcome is very unlikely, and an attempt at an anatomic repair, versus a simpler procedure such as a tendon transfer or a shortening of the metatarsal head, is not worth the effort. In elderly patients, when the MP joint is severely subluxated,

with crossover of the toe on the hallux and asymptomatic hallux valgus, amputation of the toe may be a very reasonable option. The hallux does not drift further, because it typically is abutting the third toe already, and the removal of the painful second toe generally is a very successful procedure for the patient (Figure 11-3).

COMPONENTS OF SURGICAL CORRECTION

Incision and Dissection

The incision begins at the MP joint, with an adequate soft tissue release of the dorsal and medial contracture. The extensor hood is identified and is incised longitudinally medial to the extensor digitorum longus tendon, which is retracted laterally. The attachment of the extensor hood to the base of the proximal phalanx must be maintained, and a transverse dorsal capsulotomy is performed. On the dorsal-medial aspect of the MP joint the collateral ligament is now released. This can be cut at its attachment to the proximal phalanx or the metatarsal head, but the volar plate ligament should be maintained.

Extensor Digitorum Brevis Tendon Transfer

If the instability of the toe is predominantly in the transverse and not the sagittal plane, then the extensor digitorum brevis (EDB) tendon transfer, rather than a flexor-to-extensor tendon transfer, is preferred. The EDB tendon and the extensor digitorum longus tendon are identified proximally and dissected free of each other by means of a longitudinal split of the extensor hood with Metzenbaum scissors, as shown in Figure 11-4. In this case, after the proximal interphalangeal (PIP) arthroplasty, the toe is seen sticking up in the air and crossing over the hallux—a classic example of why some decompression of the MP joint is necessary. Some increase in the strength of plantar flexion of the toe is necessary using either a flexor-to-extensor tendon transfer or an extensor brevis tendon transfer. A 6-cm length of the EDB tendon is selected, and before division of the tendon, two nonabsorbable 4-0 sutures are inserted on either side of the tenotomy to stabilize the tendon after its division for transfer. A tenotomy is now performed in between these two sutures, and the distal portion of the EDB tendon is now gradually mobilized. It is dissected free more distally from the extensor hood. Its attachment to the extensor hood overlying the base of the proximal phalanx must be maintained (see Figure 11-4).

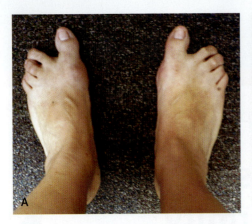 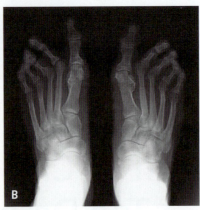 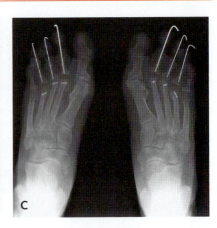

Figure 11-1 A and **B,** Valgus deformity at 1 year after bilateral hallux valgus correction. Of note, recurrent hallux valgus did not develop in this time period, although there was nothing to stop the valgus drift of the hallux. The lesser toe deformities were treated with shortening osteotomies of the metatarsals. **C,** The alignment was not ideal, but taping of the toes into varus for 3 months postoperatively resulted in some additional improvement.

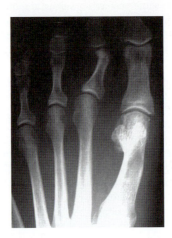

Figure 11-2 Recurrent second toe deformity in a patient who underwent a bunionectomy and distal metatarsal osteotomy for correction of hallux valgus and a second proximal interphalangeal joint resection arthroplasty for correction of a presumed claw toe. This was a crossover toe deformity, however, and cannot be treated in the same way as for a claw toe.

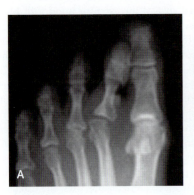 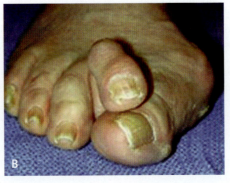 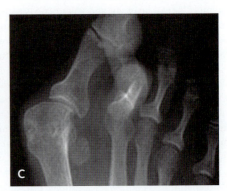

Figure 11-3 A and **B,** The patient was a 77-year-old woman who presented with a grade IV crossover toe deformity associated with a painless hallux valgus. **C,** The second toe was amputated without worsening of the hallux deformity.

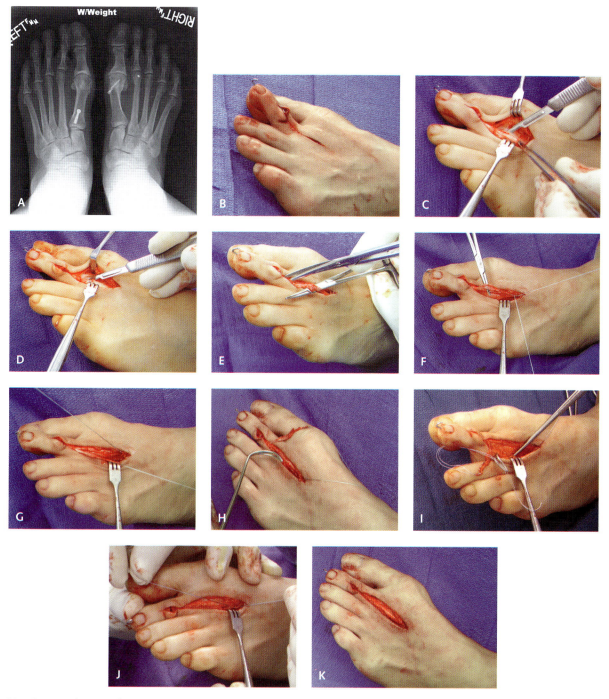

Figure 11-4 Extensor digitorum brevis (EDB) tendon transfer was performed for correction of a grade II crossover toe deformity. **A** and **B,** A proximal interphalangeal (PIP) arthrodesis was performed, and the Kirschner wire was inserted across the PIP but not the metatarsophalangeal (MP) joint. **C-E,** The EDB tendon is exposed with more proximal dissection. **F** and **G,** Two 4-0 stay sutures are inserted, and the tendon is cut in between the sutures. **H** and **I,** A curved tapered needle is passed under the deeper soft tissue in the second web space. **J,** When the EDB tendon is pulled, the toe now assumes a more normal position under tension. **K,** Final appearance of the repair.

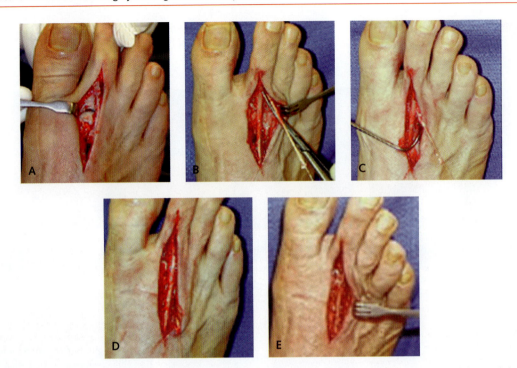

Figure 11-5 Correction of moderate crossover toe deformity. **A,** Release of the dorsal medial capsule and the medial collateral ligament. **B** and **C,** The extensor brevis tendon was dissected (**B**) and passed under the deep transverse metatarsal ligament with an aneurysm needle (**C**). **D** and **E,** The tendon was not long enough to suture back onto itself as a dynamic transfer, so a tenodesis to the metatarsal was performed by suturing the tendon into the periosteum.

If the EDB tendon tears or looks as if it will separate from the extensor hood, then a stay suture can be inserted between the distal tendon and the extensor hood. With the work now being done in the lateral web space, a curved, blunt-tipped (aneurysm) needle is passed from proximal to distal and below the deep transverse metatarsal ligament. The needle is then curved up into the soft tissue, and the suture attached to the EDB tendon is passed through the needle, which is then delivered proximally. The EDB tendon is now pulled deep to the soft tissue tether and passed proximally. As the tendon is pulled, the toe should assume a normal alignment, with good correction in both the transverse and the sagittal planes. Because of the axis of the tendon transfer, the toe may supinate slightly, and this supination must be noted (see Figure 11-4).

At this point, two options are available for stabilization: either a dynamic transfer of the EDB tendon or the use of the transferred tendon for a tenodesis. Generally, I prefer a more dynamic use of the EDB tendon, and the proximal stay suture is now used to tie the tendon transfer back down onto itself for this tendon transfer. If the tendon suture does not hold, then the EDB tendon can be inserted either into the dorsolateral periosteum or through a drill hole in the metatarsal neck. Once the toe is aligned, a Kirschner wire (K-wire) may be placed temporarily across the MP joint for additional stabilization of the toe.

Oblique Metatarsal Head Osteotomy (Maceira Osteotomy)

The indication for oblique metatarsal head osteotomy (the Maceira osteotomy) is instability of the MP joint in either the sagittal or the transverse plane. In this section the the osteotomy procedure is described for correction of a transverse plane deformity such as

the crossover toe. The Weil or Maceira osteotomy also is necessary for correction of any other medial or lateral deviation of the lesser toes off the metatarsal head, such as with severe valgus or abduction of the toes or with generalized varus or adductus of the toes associated with hallux varus. The goal of the operation is to slightly shorten the metatarsal head, releasing the intrinsic contracture on either side of the MP joint. This procedure also is performed in conjunction with treatment of subluxation or dislocation of the MP joint, occasionally in the setting of metatarsalgia, when instability is present in addition to the crossover or varus deformity (Figure 11-5).

Despite the popularity of the Weil osteotomy and indeed my own extensive experience with this procedure, its unpredictability with respect to the axial alignment of the toe after the surgery is a recognized problem. It has certain advantages: Decompression of the joint is excellent, and shortening can be readily accomplished. Nevertheless, this type of osteotomy has been shown in both clinical and laboratory settings to result in slight elevation of the axis of the intrinsic tendons dorsal to the center of the metatarsal head. The force exerted by the extensor tendons is then augmented by the slight dorsal shift in the intrinsic tendons, which do not as effectively plantarflex the MP joint. The toe is therefore slightly shortened and also slightly elevated off the ground, causing what has been referred to as the "floating toe deformity."

To some extent, this elevation can be limited but not reversed entirely with vigorous plantar flexion exercises of the MP joint that begin soon after surgery. The flexor-to-extensor transfer is not the definitive operation for correction of instability, because it too may be associated with complications, including stiffness and patient dissatisfaction with the use of the toe. Nonetheless, in the presence

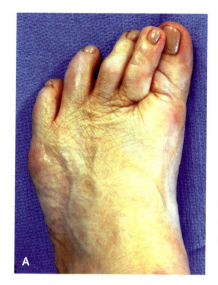

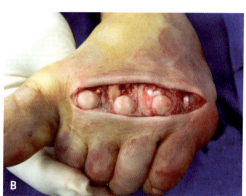

Figure 11-6 A, Osteotomies of the second to the fourth metatarsals were performed for adducted varus toe deformities. **B,** The transverse incision was used to expose all of the adducted toes. It is important to protect the veins, superficial nerve branches, and extensor tendons with this incision. Otherwise, during the osteotomy, the tendons may be accidentally cut with the saw.

of a dislocated MP joint, a shortening osteotomy of the metatarsal of some type is necessary, and the Weil osteotomy is an effective procedure to reduce this dislocation. It is not an ideal procedure for correction if isolated metatarsalgia is present, however, because alternative osteotomies are available that do not result in elevation of the toe. Surprisingly, in view of the plane of the osteotomy, avascular necrosis of the metatarsal head is extremely rare, and although arthritis of the MP joint may occur, it is uncommon.

The role of the flexor-to-extensor transfer in treatment of a crossover toe deformity is not clear-cut. This procedure was used fairly frequently a decade ago but was associated with problems of sufficient magnitude, including recurrence of deformity, that I do not often use this transfer for a crossover toe. Instead, I use an osteotomy when needed and then the extensor brevis transfer for deformities of lesser severity. If the extensor brevis procedure fails intraoperatively, I use the flexor-to-extensor transfer procedure. If the MP joint is dislocated as opposed to subluxated, again I am more inclined to use the flexor-to-extensor transfer.

The incision for the metatarsal osteotomy is made and located according to the number of metatarsals to be cut. If the correction is focused on a single metatarsal, an incision is made directly over the MP joint. If two adjacent metatarsals require osteotomies, then the incision is made between them (e.g., in the second interspace). Although performance of the central three metatarsal osteotomies through a single incision located over the third MP joint is possible, it entails too much stretching of the skin with the potential for wound breakdown. I therefore prefer to use either two incisions, one medial to the second MP joint and then one slightly lateral to the fourth, or a single transverse incision (Figure 11-6). The incision is deepened through the subcutaneous tissue, and the extensor tendons are lengthened, particularly in the setting of any subluxation, dorsiflexion contracture, or dislocation. A dorsal capsulectomy is performed to expose the metatarsal head, and a curved periosteal shmogler is inserted into the MP joint *if it is dislocated*. As it is levered down, the metatarsal head becomes visible. Care is taken not to injure the articular surface as the shmogler is inserted. If the joint is dislocated, the volar plate must be stripped off the underside of the metatarsal head, to facilitate scarring down of the volar plate under the neck.

With the metatarsal head visible, the cut is planned at the apex of the metatarsal head. The cut must avoid the articular surface and

must be at the level of the neck dorsal to the articular surface. The cut is made at a 30-degree angle, but the angle will vary according to the declination of the metatarsal. It typically is extended for approximately 2 cm, which corresponds to the length of the saw blade used. The cut is completed, and a second cut is made just vertically perpendicular to the axis of the metatarsal. This second cut, according to Maceira, allows precise measurement of the amount of shortening required for the osteotomy. The third cut is then made as a slice or with resection of a small wedge of bone along the axis of the metatarsal. The metatarsal head now is reduced directly onto the distal end of the metatarsal osteotomy, without any overhang of the dorsal surface of the metatarsal on the articular surface as seen with the Weil osteotomy (Figure 11-7).

The metatarsal is held firmly with the clamp, and a K-wire hole is predrilled into the metatarsal, and a screw is inserted with a small threaded twist-off screw from the dorsal aspect of the distal metatarsal. Rarely, two screws are used. The screw should be aimed into the metatarsal head, and not directly plantarward, so that the screw threads are buried and not protruding. Any protrusion can cause metatarsalgia or irritation of the volar plate with limitation and dorsiflexion.

Depending on the remaining stability, further procedures can be performed, including a flexor-to-extensor tendon transfer or an EDB tendon transfer. Although a K-wire can be used, the plane of the osteotomy is such that the K-wire can displace the metatarsal head during insertion, so I prefer not to use a K-wire after this osteotomy if at all possible. Positioning the toe in the axis of the metatarsal is difficult, because the toe protrudes into the shoe. If stability is essential and the use of a K-wire is thought to be important, the toe must be plantar-flexed in line with the metatarsal; then an appropriate cutout of the shoe is made to support the pulp of the toe and prevent it from getting irritated on the shoe itself. The K-wire is left in for approximately 3 weeks to stabilize the volar plate and prevent recurrent instability. Leaving the K-wire in place also facilitates scarring down of the volar plate and the intrinsic tendons, so that dorsal subluxation is less likely to occur. Of note, the shortening osteotomy should be performed for any transverse plane deviation, as in Figures 11-8 and 11-9. The osteotomy may be performed using longitudinal or transverse incisions, depending on the deformity and the number of metatarsals involved. The only issue with the transverse incision is the need for excellent and

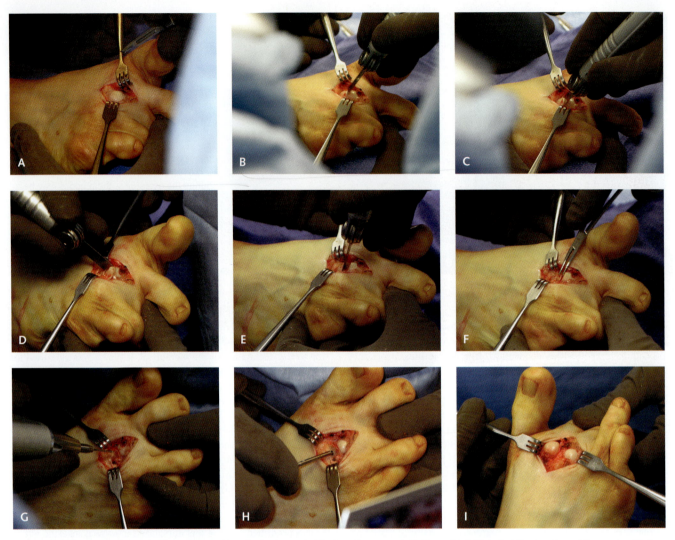

Figure 11-7 The steps of the Maceira metatarsal head osteotomy. **A,** The head is exposed. **B,** The cut is initiated at the junction of the neck with the metatarsal head. **C,** The cut is completed at a 30-degree angle. **D,** The second cut is measured at a specific length for shortening and marked, then cut perpendicular to the metatarsal, removing only a wedge down to the first cut. **E** and **F,** The third cut is made under the tip of the distal metatarsal, removing a slice of bone. **G** and **H,** The head is moved proximally to align up precisely against the metatarsal shaft **(G)** followed by standard fixation **(H)**. **I,** The third metatarsal was corrected in an identical manner from the same dorsal longitudinal incision.

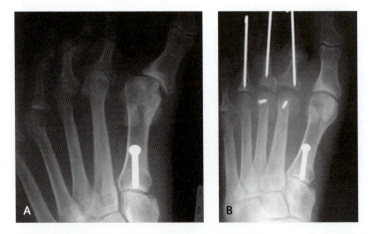

Figure 11-8 A and **B,** Adductus of these toes associated with hallux varus and proximal interphalangeal (PIP) deformities was corrected with metatarsal shortening osteotomies, an extensor hallucis brevis transfer, and PIP arthroplasties.

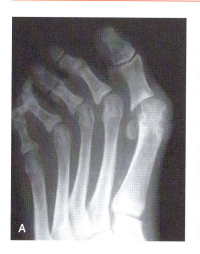
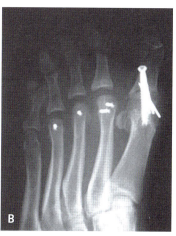

Figure 11-9 A and B, Abducted valgus toe deformities also can be treated with shortening osteotomies here performed with standard Weil osteotomies.

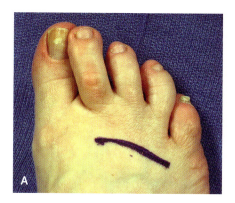
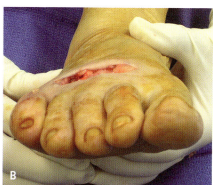

Figure 11-10 A and B, With osteotomy of more than two metatarsals, a transverse incision is quite helpful to delineate accurately the alignment and the shortening required.

vigorous therapy on the MP joints to prevent scarring. With use of the transverse incision, the nerves and veins as well as the extensor tendons are preserved. Usually, sufficient relaxation of the extensor tendons is obtained after the shortening osteotomy that lengthening is not necessary, but this aspect of function should be monitored as needed (Figure 11-10).

The Flexor-to-Extensor Tendon Transfer

At the completion of the soft tissue release as previously described, the stability of the MP joint is evaluated. If the joint is unstable in both the sagittal and the horizontal planes, then a flexor-to-extensor tendon transfer can be performed. A flexor-to-extensor tendon transfer can be used for other indications, but instability, subluxation, or dislocation of the MP joint should be present. Two methods are used for performing the flexor-to-extensor transfer: one that splits the tendon and sutures it dorsally and another in which the tendon is passed through a drill hole in the phalanx and sutured dorsally. The latter method is biomechanically sound, because the force on the MP joint is more proximal and located more precisely. The problem with the transfer in which the tendon is split and passed on either side of the phalanx is that the axis of force is slightly distal to the MP joint, and further subluxation of the base of the proximal phalanx may occur.

For the split tendon technique, a short transverse incision is made on the plantar surface of the proximal flexion crease, and the small vein in the center in the incision is cauterized. Small soft tissue retractors are inserted on either side of the incision, medially and laterally (Figure 11-11). The flexor tendon sheath is identified when the fatty tissue is pulled out of the way. The sheath is cut longitudinally from proximal to distal, with the tendons exposed. A curved hemostat is inserted through and under both flexor tendons, and when they are placed on stretch, the distal phalanx is flexed. A percutaneous tenotomy of the longus flexor tendon is performed at the level of the distal interphalangeal (DIP) joint.

A second hemostat is now passed under the long flexor tendon proximally, and the tendon is pulled into the incision. The distal tendon stump is grasped on both sides with two hemostats, and the tendon is split in half along the median raphe. This split can be made using a knife or by pulling the clamps to separate the tendon. The split tendon is now passed from plantar to dorsal with a small clamp, which is then passed from dorsal to plantar along the base of the proximal phalanx and out the plantar incision. The clamp must hug the edge of the phalanx to prevent vascular injury. Each end of the flexor tendon is inserted into the tip of the clamp and then passed from plantar to dorsal on each side of the phalanx. The tendon ends are then looped superficially to the extensor hood, and a knot is tied in the tendon (see Figure 11-11, C). By tensioning the knot (pulling on the medial slip of the tendon pulls the phalanx more laterally), the surgeon can correct the frontal plane alignment into a neutral position. Immediately before the suture is

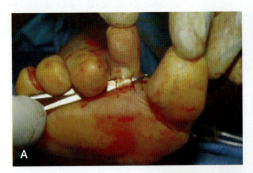
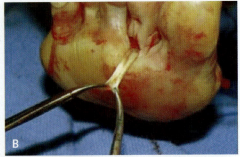
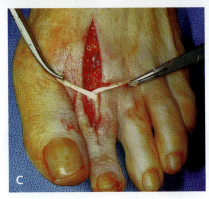

Figure 11-11 A-C, The flexor-to-extensor tendon transfer is demonstrated with the split tendon technique. To correct the crossover of the second toe, the knot in the tendon was pulled eccentrically to align the second toe into neutral.

tensed, a K-wire is introduced antegrade across the MP joint and out the tip of the toe. Once the suture has been tied and the tension on the flexor tendon transfer is corrected, the K-wire is then inserted retrograde back across the MP joint to stabilize the toe further. To establish appropriate tension of the transfer and to prevent tightness of the MP joint, the tendon is sutured with the toe in approximately 30 degrees of dorsiflexion while the ankle is held in neutral dorsiflexion. The tendon is now secured with two interrupted nonabsorbable 4-0 sutures both to itself and to the extensor hood.

For the drill tunnel technique, the exposure of the tendon is performed similarly on the plantar surface, but the tendon is not split. From the dorsal aspect of the base of the proximal phalanx, a drill hole is made obliquely from dorsal and proximal to distal and plantar. The drill hole does not exit exactly at the point at which the exposure of the tendon has been performed, because the plantar incision is distal to the base of the phalanx. A cannulated guide pin or a large tapered needle is inserted through the phalanx from dorsal to plantar, and the sutures on the flexor tendon are placed in the needle and pulled dorsally. The tendon is then sutured as outlined previously.

TECHNIQUES, TIPS, AND PITFALLS

- The flexor-to-extensor tendon transfer works well to increase flexion strength of the toe when the intrinsic muscles are weak or atrophied. In Figure 11-12, note the resting position of the second toe in slight elevation, the dorsiflexion of all of the toes, but most importantly, the grip strength of the second toe following the flexor-to-extensor transfer (see Figure 11-12, *C*).

- Transverse plane deformity cannot be treated without shortening osteotomy of the metatarsal. This may be performed distally at the level of the metatarsal head, as with a Weil or Maceira osteotomy, or in the shaft with plate fixation (Figure 11-13).

- The problem with the Weil osteotomy at the articular surface is illustrated in Figures 11-14 and 11-15. Depending on the location of the cut, the osteotomy will leave a ledge of cancellous bone overhanging the dorsal rim of the metatarsal head. This ridge of bone does not articulate well with the base of the proximal phalanx and must be removed, as shown in Figure 11-14, *B* and *C*. In Figure 11-15, all of the metatarsal heads demonstrate the cancellous bone ridge on their dorsal aspect.

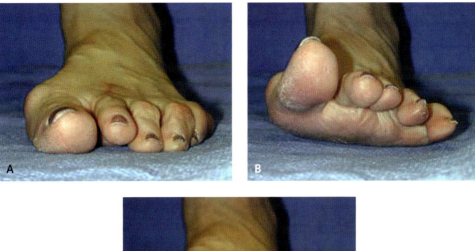

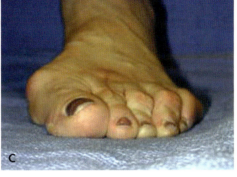

Figure 11-12 Note the resting position of the second toe in slight elevation **(A),** the dorsiflexion of all of the toes **(B),** but, most important, the grip strength of the second toe after the flexor-to-extensor transfer **(C).**

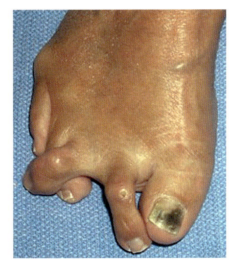

Figure 11-13 A shortening osteotomy of either the distal metatarsal head or the midshaft is necessary to correct this deformity.

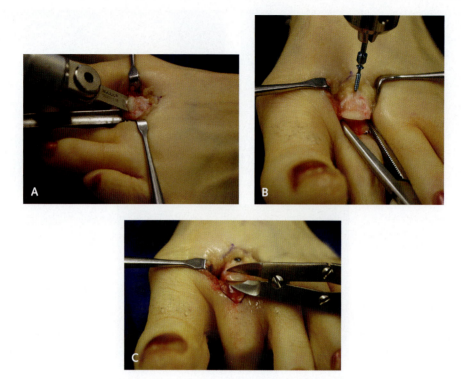

Figure 11-14   The steps of the Weil osteotomy. **A,** The first cut is made 1 mm inferior to the dorsal surface of the metatarsal head. **B,** The head is shifted proximally by the desired amount and secured with a twist-off screw. **C,** The dorsal bone lip is removed with a bone cutter.

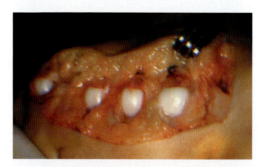

Figure 11-15   After Weil osteotomies of the second to the fourth metatarsals, a cancellous bone ridge can be seen dorsally interfering with the metatarsophalangeal joint articulation.

CHAPTER 12

Management of Metatarsalgia

OSTEOTOMIES FOR METATARSALGIA

A dorsal wedge osteotomy of the lesser metatarsals is performed for specific conditions of isolated metatarsalgia. Although alternatives for correction of metatarsalgia are available, such as the Weil or Maceira osteotomy, a shortening diaphyseal osteotomy, and a shortening proximal metatarsal osteotomy, each procedure is associated with potential problems. I have found that the Weil osteotomy can be used for correction of isolated metatarsalgia, but results are not very predictable because of the variable position of the metatarsal after osteotomy in the sagittal plane. When performed for specific relief of metatarsalgia, a dorsal wedge osteotomy gives a very predictable result; however, the potential for subsequent "transfer metatarsalgia" must be considered. Although no osteotomy is so precise that transfer of weight can be avoided, the dorsal wedge osteotomy of the metatarsal neck remains a reasonable procedure for correction after a previous fracture, stress fracture, or previous osteotomy of an adjacent metatarsal. With the more proximal metatarsal osteotomy at the base, the result is very unpredictable, and accurate control cannot be achieved.

Dorsal Wedge Osteotomy

An incision is made over the neck of the metatarsal, and the dorsal aspect of the metatarsal head is visualized. The soft tissues, including the periosteum and extensor tendons, are retracted, and two pilot holes are inserted. These are unicortical holes, made with a 1-mm Kirschner wire (K-wire) and at a 45-degree angle to each other and placed approximately 1 cm apart. The osteotomy is performed in between these pilot holes. Not more than 1 mm of bone must be removed. Accordingly, the actual base of the osteotomy, including the thickness of the saw blade, is approximately 0.5 mm deep. A greenstick cut is performed, and the plantar cortex *must* be left intact. I prefer to complete the osteotomy with a fracture maneuver that actually opens up the initial cut using manual dorsal pressure on the head of the metatarsal. This maneuver preserves a nice periosteal bridge on the plantar surface, thereby preventing excessive dorsal shift of the metatarsal head. Fixation of the osteotomy is performed with a stout suture of 2-0 absorbable material on a tapered needle, which is easily passed through the predrilled holes. More extensive fixation is not necessary (Figure 12-1).

Although I have performed this for more than one metatarsal at a time, multiple dorsal wedge osteotomies need to be carefully planned, because the risk for transfer metatarsalgia increases with the number of these osteotomies performed, and multiple Weil or Maceira osteotomies are preferable.

Lengthening of one metatarsal may need to be combined with shortening of another. This is a common problem with brachymetatarsia, in which one or more of the lesser metatarsals are short and metatarsalgia is present on the adjacent metatarsal (Figure 12-2). For these cases of brachymetatarsia, I prefer to use a single-stage lengthening of the involved metatarsals, combined with shortening of the adjacent metatarsals using a Maceira osteotomy. I correct brachymetatarsia according to the age of the patient and the number of metatarsals involved. Although gradual distraction of the metatarsal can be performed successfully, I prefer, wherever possible, to perform a single (nonstaged) lengthening using interpositional graft. This is certainly preferable when more than one metatarsal is involved because the application of distraction to two adjacent lesser metatarsals is impractical. Nonetheless, gradual distraction is a reliable technique, provided it is tolerated by the patient.

If isolated brachymetatarsia is present, correction of the dorsiflexed and extended lesser toe must be performed simultaneously. This operation usually is done with an extensor tendon lengthening and metatarsophalangeal (MP) joint release with percutaneous stabilization of the toe across the MP joint with a K-wire if it is rigid. If the toe is not stabilized at the MP joint, gradual hyperextension of the MP joint may occur with worsening deformity of the toe during lengthening. Lengthening as a single-stage procedure with insertion of structural bone graft has an advantage in that the exact length of the toe can be attained in one setting. The only limiting factor is the actual length that can be obtained without the potential for ischemia of the toe, but I usually am able to obtain approximately 18 mm of length of a single metatarsal without jeopardizing perfusion to the toe. A laminar spreader is inserted while the circulation to the toe is checked as the spreader is gradually distracted. Once the desired length has been attained, then temporary K-wires are inserted in multiple planes across the metatarsals for temporary fixation to keep it out to length with insertion of the graft. The graft can be held secure with a small dorsal plate or with K-wires inserted

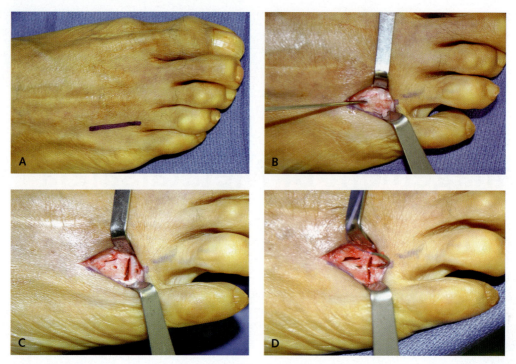

Figure 12-1 A dorsal wedge osteotomy of the fourth metatarsal was performed for treatment of isolated fourth metatarsalgia secondary to a stress fracture to the third metatarsal. **A,** The incision is marked along the distal metatarsal. **B,** Two unicortical pilot holes are made in the neck of the metatarsal at an angle of 45 degrees to the metatarsal. A saw is used to resect a 1-mm wedge of bone. **C** and **D,** The metatarsal neck is then pushed up across an intact plantar cortex, and a suture is inserted through the predrilled holes for fixation.

externally, inserted through the tip of the toe. Function of the toes, however, is good on resolution, and rarely is a flexion contracture of the toe present.

In general, shortening osteotomies of the lesser metatatarsals are very useful to correct diffuse metatarsalgia, particularly that associated with transverse plane deformity of the toes (Figure 12-3). In cases with second metatarsal overload, it is important to identify the source of the increase in the forefoot pressure, and the concept of the metatarsal rocker is very useful. It would be a serious error, for example, to shorten a second metatarsal if the source of the problem was an elevated first metatarsal, particularly if the elevation was from a malunion after fracture or previous surgery. For these cases, instead of trying to correct the overload of the second metatarsal, the first ray must be addressed. This may involve a plantar flexion osteotomy or an arthrodesis of the first tarsometatarsal joint in plantar flexion (Figure 12-4). The plantar flexion osteotomy of the first metatarsal may be performed as an opening wedge with a small bone graft inserted dorsally. Alternatively a dome osteotomy is performed with the saw directed from the medial aspect of the metatarsal, rotating the metatarsal into the corrected position. I do not favor a closing wedge osteotomy performed from the plantar aspect of the metatarsal because this is not as stable. The exact opposite scenario exists with a rigid plantar flexed first metatarsal associated with pain under the sesamoids. Figure 12-5 illustrates a case in which I inadvertently fused the medial column in too much plantar flexion. The patient was a 70-year-old woman who had undergone a triple arthrodesis 20 years previously, with arthritis and deformity of the tarsometatarsal joints developing in combination with abduction deformity of the midfoot. Although an arthrodesis was obtained, with the abduction corrected, the forefoot was now in too much plantar

flexion, which was not tolerated, and a dorsal wedge osteotomy of the first metatarsal was required. This was accomplished with a long oblique wedge resection from the dorsal base of the metatarsal (see Figure 12-5, *E-G*).

Other situations may arise in which the outlook appears to be almost hopeless, whether the pain is under the first or the lesser toe metatarsals. In Figure 12-6, the patient had undergone nine previous forefoot surgeries, including various lesser metatarsal osteotomies with revisions, with continued scarring and pain under multiple metatarsals. Eventually, the implant was removed from the hallux MP joint, an arthrodesis was performed with bone grafting, and the lesser metatarsal heads were resected.

Classic Triangular and Weil/Maceira Osteotomies

The classic osteotomy of the metatarsal head is performed for management of osteochondrosis, using a triangular osteotomy through the metatarsal head itself. It is quite remarkable how good these metatarsals look after this type of osteotomy (Figure 12-7). The Weil and Maceira osteotomies are variations of this triangular metatarsal head osteotomy, whereby the direction of the saw cut is angled more obliquely into the metatarsal shaft instead of the head of the metatarsal. I find that these latter osteotomies are very helpful for managing metatarsalgia, but the utmost care is required in surgical decision making, because balancing the forefoot is difficult, and transfer of pain to an adjacent metatarsal is common.

The Weil or the Maceira osteotomy is indicated for many conditions, ranging from subluxation and dislocation of the MP joint, to crossover toe deformity, correction of rheumatologic deformity of the MP joint, and metatarsalgia. For treatment of metatarsalgia, I routinely remove a 2-mm slice of bone from the metatarsal head for the Weil osteotomy, and shorten the metatarsal further using

12

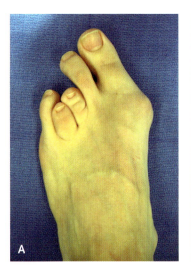
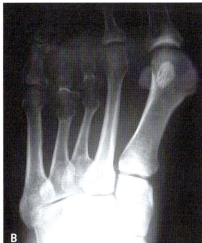
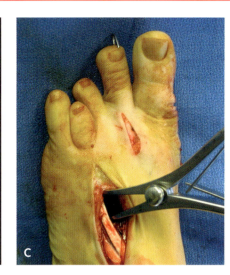
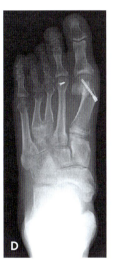
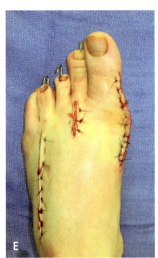

Figure 12-2 A and **B,** Brachymetatarsia of the third and fourth toes associated with metatarsalgia of the fourth and fifth toes and hallux valgus in a 30-year-old patient. **C-E,** Correction was obtained with a single-stage lengthening of the third and fourth metatarsals using a structural graft and a shortening Maceira osteotomy of the second metatarsal, combined with a chevron osteotomy.

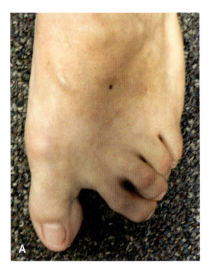
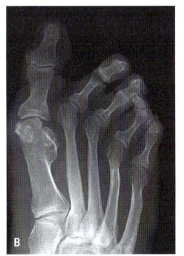
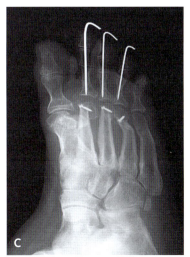

Figure 12-3 A and **B,** It is unknown why recurrent hallux valgus did not occur in association with such severe abduction deformity of the lesser toes. **C,** Correction of this transverse plane deformity was obtained with shortening Weil osteotomies.

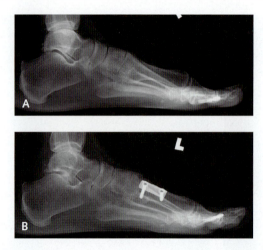

Figure 12-4 A, Elevation of the first metatarsal, with transfer of weight bearing and pain under the second metatarsal, was noted after a proximal crescentic osteotomy. **B,** The first metatarsal was lengthened and plantar flexed simultaneously using a small triangular structural bone graft and plate fixation.

the Maceira technique. Numerous anatomic cadaveric studies have been performed in which the pressures under the metatarsal heads were checked. The osteotomy can cause a change in pressure under either the operated or the adjacent metatarsal. The issue arises as to whether an isolated second metatarsal osteotomy should be done or whether the third and possibly the fourth should be included for management of metatarsalgia. The decision depends, of course, on the preexisting disease. If only the second metatarsal is to be cut, then the incision is centered over this joint. If the second and third metatarsals are to be cut, then the incision is based in the second web space. If the second, third, and fourth metatarsals are to undergo osteotomy, I use a transverse incision as outlined in Chapters 10 and 11. Before the osteotomy, the metatarsal head must be fully exposed and the collateral ligaments cut. They do not need to be completely transected, but are released dorsally and then stretched as the joint is subluxated inferiorly. If the joint is dislocated, then it must be reduced with a curved periosteal elevator (i.e., a shmogler); the proximal phalanx should be pushed under the head to expose the head for the osteotomy (Figure 12-8). If no subluxation is present, then the phalanx can be bent downward to expose the dorsal surface for the osteotomy. The cut in the metatarsal head is made at the dorsal

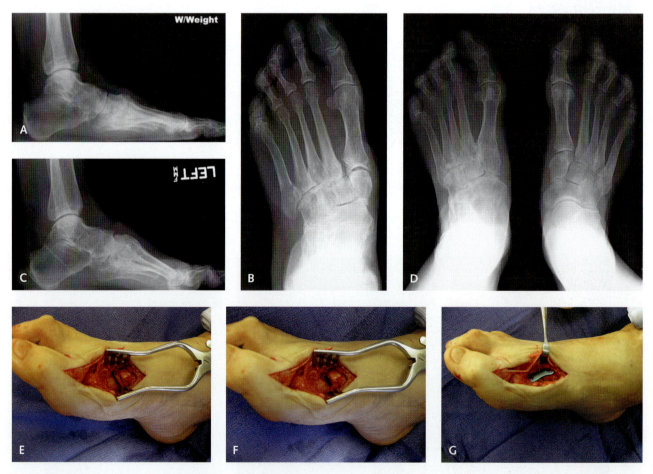

Figure 12-5 A and **B,** The patient was a 70-year-old woman who had undergone a triple arthrodesis 20 years previously, with subsequent development of arthritis and deformity of the tarsometatarsal joints in combination with abduction deformity of the midfoot. **C** and **D,** Although an arthrodesis was obtained and with the adduction corrected, the forefoot was now in too much plantar flexion, which was not tolerated. **E-G,** A dorsal wedge osteotomy of the first metatarsal was performed: A long oblique wedge was resected from the dorsal base of the metatarsal, and the osteotomy was secured by a locking compression plate (Orthohelix, Akron, Ohio).

apical surface of the head just inferior to the dorsal joint cartilage. The cut is made with a saw at an angle approximately 25 degrees with respect to the metatarsal shaft. The appropriate angle will vary, however, according to the declination angle of the metatarsal. Thus, if a 25-degree cut is used and the second metatarsal is in equinus, the metatarsalgia will worsen. The angle of the osteotomy has to increase toward the more lateral metatarsals, which are always "flatter" than the declination of the second metatarsal.

The cut is not completed, and a second saw cut is made just inferior to the first cut so that a wedge or slice of bone is now resected measuring approximately 1 to 2 mm. The slice of bone is then removed, and the first cut is completed on the more dorsal surface of the metatarsal. Recognizing that the osteotomy has been completed is easy because when the metatarsal is perforated on its plantar surface, the head suddenly shifts and retracts to a more proximal position.

The metatarsal head must be held securely in the desired position; for this purpose, a clamp can be used or the phalanx can be pushed up under the head to compress the osteotomy. The head should be shortened by approximately 5 mm, although the

appropriate amount will depend entirely on the underlying disease. While the metatarsal head is held in the corrected position, a twist-off screw (DePuy Orthopaedics, Inc., Warsaw, Indiana) is inserted through the metatarsal neck. Usually a 12-mm screw is the correct length (Figure 12-9). The dorsal overhanging bone shelf of the metatarsal head osteotomy is now trimmed with either a small bone cutter or a saw until the shelf is smooth.

Complications of healing of this osteotomy are uncommon, being in fact quite rare. It is remarkable that an osteotomy directed through the metatarsal head does not cause avascular necrosis, yet I have rarely seen this complication.

Nonunion similarly is very rare but, when present, is quite difficult to treat, as illustrated in Figure 12-10. In this case, the patient had undergone unsuccessful surgery for metatarsalgia and hallux rigidus, with nonunion of the osteotomy, and subsequently presented for treatment of pain, mostly in the second MP joint. In addition to lengthening of the metatarsal head, positioning the second toe into plantar flexion was required; both corrections were accomplished with the use of bone graft and a small contoured plate, which eventually was removed.

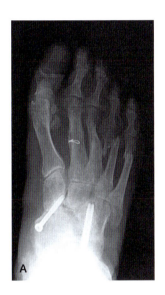
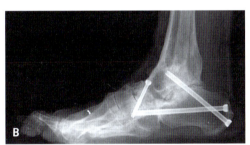

Figure 12-6 The patient was a 66-year-old man with gout and painful arthritis of the second metatarsophalangeal joint. A, Note the arthritis and absence of joint space. Correction was accomplished with a triangular osteotomy through the metatarsal head. The wedge was 9 mm at the base and extended to the center of the articular surface of the metatarsal head. B, The result at 2 years after surgery.

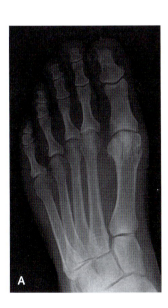
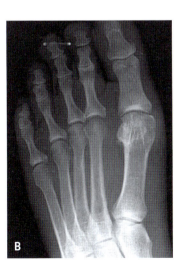

Figure 12-7 The classic osteotomy of the metatarsal head is performed for management of osteochondrosis (A), using a triangular osteotomy through the metatarsal head itself (B).

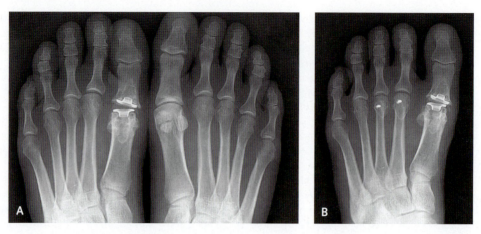

Figure 12-8 The patient had undergone an implant arthroplasty for correction of hallux rigidus 3 years previously. **A,** Despite shortening and dysfunction of the hallux, it was not painful. **B,** Pain was present under the second and third metatarsals; correction was accomplished by means of a shortening Maceira osteotomy.

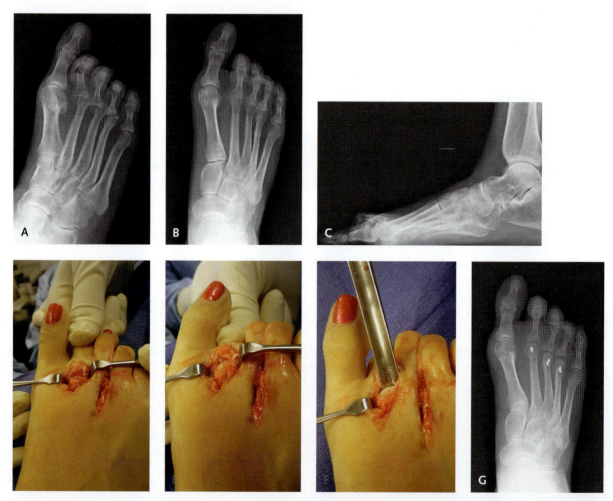

Figure 12-9 A-C, The patient had undergone surgery for a resection of a neuroma of the third web space, but the initial diagnosis was incorrect; in fact, the metatarsophalangeal (MP) joints were dislocated. **D** and **E,** The revision surgery was performed through two longitudinal incisions, with sequential reduction of each MP joint. **F** and **G,** Joint reduction was accomplished using a curved periosteal elevator; this was followed by a shortening Maceira osteotomy.

12

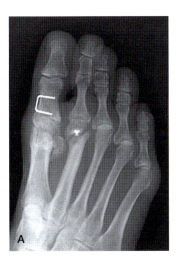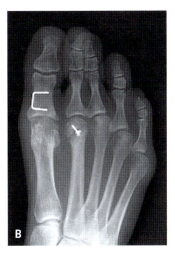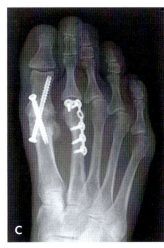

Figure 12-10 A and **B,** The patient was referred for treatment of metatarsalgia and hallux rigidus, which previous surgery had failed to correct. Note the nonunion of the second metatarsal and arthritis of the hallux metatarsophalangeal (MP) joint. The patient complained of pain in the second MP joint and under the third metatarsal. **C,** In addition to lengthening of the second metatarsal head, establishing plantar flexion was required, both accomplished with the use of bone graft and a small contoured plate, which was ultimately removed.

OSTEOTOMY IN MANAGEMENT OF ARTHRITIS

Management of arthritis of the lesser metatarsal head associated with osteochondrosis does not mandate resection arthroplasty or metatarsal head resection (Figure 12-11). Even for severe arthritis, an osteotomy of the metatarsal head itself can invariably be performed (Figures 12-12 and 12-13). With this triangular osteotomy, a wedge is removed from the metatarsal head, the avascular sclerotic bone is resected, and the intact cartilage is rotated from the undersurface of the head. The plantar cartilage is almost always healthy, and this is shifted up into an anterior-facing position so that the plantar surface of the metatarsal head now articulates anteriorly with the proximal phalanx. The size of the osteotomy is based on the extent and location of the avascular necrosis. Generally, the arthrosis and avascular bone are in the dorsal anterior aspect of the metatarsal head. I start the osteotomy just inferior to this and aim the saw blade back plantar and posterior, preserving at least 5 mm of the articular surface of the metatarsal head. The wedge is then resected from the more dorsal aspect of the head, and a triangular piece with a base that measures approximately 4 to 6 mm is removed. Fixation of the head is performed with a suture. I drill the dorsal distal metatarsal with a single small K-wire hole and then insert an absorbable suture first through the articular cartilage and then out the predrilled hole to secure the metatarsal head. The head does not require any more fixation than this, and I do not suggest using a K-wire, which can spin the small segment of the head right off. The osteotomy always heals, the blood supply always seems to be sufficient either through the articular surface itself or through the distal metatarsal head to nourish the small osteochondral piece.

Surgical management of arthritis of the lesser toe MP joint, particularly the second toe, has to be approached as a salvage operation, because little can be done to maintain a healthy, flexible joint. The goals should therefore be to relieve pain, to maximize range of motion and, most important, not to compromise the stability of the joint. The arthritis frequently develops after a previous operation of the toe or joint (Figure 12-14). Treatment options include a complete

metatarsal head resection, a partial metatarsal head resection, and shortening of the metatarsal head or shaft. I use an interposition arthroplasty combined with partial shaving of the anterior aspect of the metatarsal head when the joint cannot be preserved. This is an operation that works well and accomplishes the goals previously described through maintenance of motion and stability. This operation must be used cautiously in the setting of a dislocation of the MP joint associated with arthritis, however, because subluxation may persist.

The key to the interposition arthroplasty is to resect the appropriate amount of the metatarsal head, leaving the undersurface of the condyles of the head intact, to maintain a plantigrade weight-bearing surface (Figure 12-15). Clearly, if too much of the head is removed, adjacent metatarsalgia will result. The long extensor tendon is dissected off the bone and retracted. Then a transverse cut is made in the periosteum, the capsule, and the extensor brevis tendon as far proximally on the metatarsal neck as possible. This entire soft tissue flap is then lifted up and raised in a U shape, with a distal base that remains attached to the base of the proximal phalanx. Once the flap has been elevated off the metatarsal head, the joint must be completely reduced using a shmogler. The joint is then exposed, and the metatarsal head is cut with a saw, with the cuts contoured to maintain a circular shape of the head. I remove approximately 4 mm of the metatarsal head. The amount resected must, however, be adequate to permit motion without compression on the head with range of motion. Provided that the condyles are left intact, more of the metatarsal head can, in fact, be removed. The soft tissue flap that has been raised is now used for an interposition and is anchored underneath the metatarsal head in one of two ways: Either a small suture anchor is inserted into the undersurface of the metatarsal head, or two K-wire holes are made in the head. A U-shaped suture is inserted through the K-wire holes to capture the flap. The flap is then pulled underneath the metatarsal head at the appropriate tension. The remaining tissue of the flap must sit underneath the metatarsal head so that the flap can then function as a tenodesis maintaining the reduction of the MP joint.

Why a Weil osteotomy would work in the setting of arthritis is puzzling, but clearly, the shortening of the metatarsal through

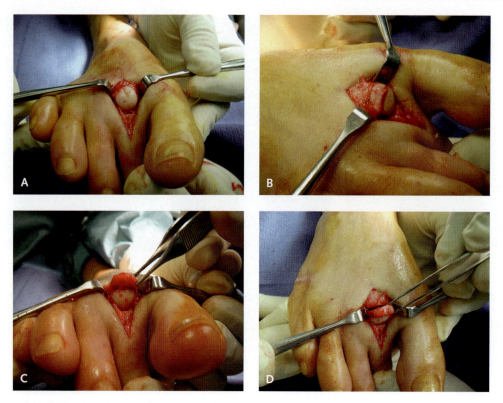

Figure 12-11 A, In addition to arthritic changes in the second metatarsophalangeal joint, a central erosion of the metatarsal head is evident. **B** and **C,** This defect was treated with a triangular wedge resection osteotomy of the metatarsal head. The osteotomy was not completed on the plantar metatarsal surface, and a greenstick-type osteotomy that kept the plantar metatarsal head intact was performed. **D,** After removal of the bone wedge, the osteotomy was secured with two absorbable sutures.

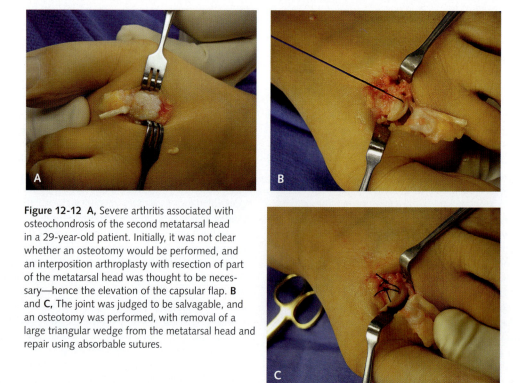

Figure 12-12 A, Severe arthritis associated with osteochondrosis of the second metatarsal head in a 29-year-old patient. Initially, it was not clear whether an osteotomy would be performed, and an interposition arthroplasty with resection of part of the metatarsal head was thought to be necessary—hence the elevation of the capsular flap. **B** and **C,** The joint was judged to be salvageable, and an osteotomy was performed, with removal of a large triangular wedge from the metatarsal head and repair using absorbable sutures.

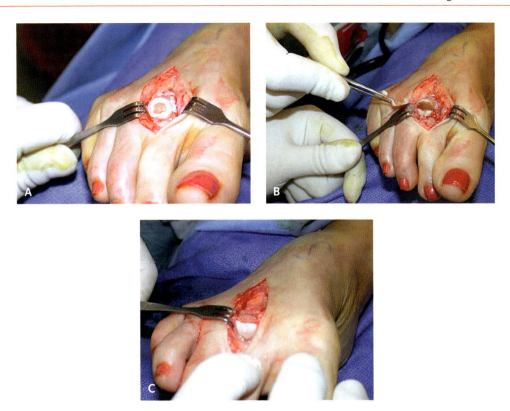

Figure 12-13 A, Severe arthritis with a massive central defect of the metatarsal head in a 42-year-old woman with osteo-chondrosis. **B** and **C,** A triangular wedge was removed from the metatarsal head, the avascular sclerotic bone was resected, and the intact plantar cartilage was rotated from the undersurface of the head.

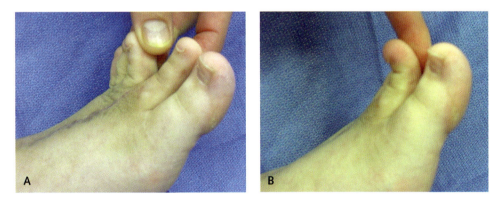

Figure 12-14 Posttraumatic arthritis in the second metatarsophalangeal (MP) joint in a 24-year-old patient. **A** and **B,** Note the limited dorsiflexion of the MP joint and the hyperextension of the distal interphalangeal joint with passive dorsal pressure.

release of the pressure on the intrinsic tendons decompresses the pressure on the joint. The Weil osteotomy has a role in the treatment of joint arthritis for the described conditions and in the setting of rheumatologic deformity. Metatarsal head resection is never a good choice for surgical management of arthritis of a single joint. With involvement of multiple lesser toes, however, resection of *all* of the lesser metatarsal heads may be appropriate. Such resection constitutes a salvage operation; accordingly, it usually is performed to treat more diffuse metatarsalgia and arthritis and not arthritis affecting an isolated joint. Amputation of a digit is an obvious alternative for management of intractable metatarsalgia, particularly in the elderly patient (Figure 12-16).

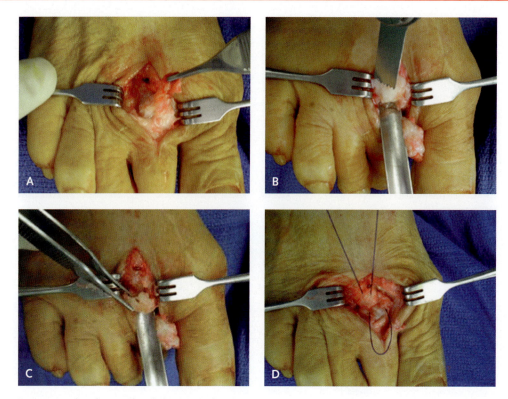

Figure 12-15 Resection arthroplasty with soft tissue capsular interposition in a 42-year-old patient who had been treated with numerous previous surgeries for second metatarsophalangeal joint synovitis. **A,** The dorsal capsule and periosteum including the extensor brevis tendon are elevated as a single flap and retracted distally. **B** and **C,** The bone is cut with a saw, removing the distal 5 mm of the head and maintaining the contour of the metarsal head. **D,** The interposition of the flap is performed with sutures inserted through drill holes in the metatarsal head.

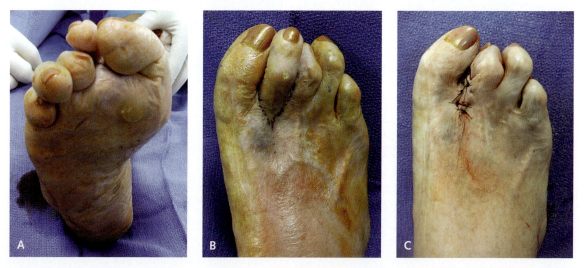

Figure 12-16 Painless hallux valgus with severe metatarsalgia of the second toe **(A)** in a 76-year-old patient. The metatarsalgia was treated with amputation of the second toe, performed through an elliptical incision **(B** and **C).**

SUGGESTED READING

Barouk LS, Barouk P: The joint preserving surgery, *Foot Ankle Int* 30:284, 2009.

Dalal R, Mahajan RH: Single transverse, dorsal incision for lesser metatarsophalangeal exposure, *Foot Ankle Int* 30:226–228, 2009.

Davies M, Saxby TS: Metatarsal neck osteotomy with rigid internal fixation for the treatment of lesser toe metatarsophalangeal joint pathology, *Foot Ankle Int* 20:630–636, 1999.

Espinosa N, Maceira E, Myerson MS: Current concept review: Metatarsalgia, *Foot Ankle Int* 29:871–879, 2008.

Feibel JB, Tisdel CL, Donley BG: Lesser metatarsal osteotomies. A biomechanical approach to metatarsalgia, *Foot Ankle Clin* 6:473–489, 2001.

Garg R, Thordarson DB, Schrumpf M, Castaneda D: Sliding oblique versus segmental resection osteotomies for lesser metatarsophalangeal joint pathology, *Foot Ankle Int* 29:1009–1014, 2008.

Melamed EA, Schon LC, Myerson MS, Parks BG: Two modifications of the Weil osteotomy. Analysis on sawbone models, *Foot Ankle Int* 23:400–405, 2002.

Myerson MS, Jung HG: The role of toe flexor-to-extensor transfer in correcting metatarsophalangeal joint instability of the second toe, *Foot Ankle Int* 26:675–679, 2005.

O'Kane C, Kilmartin TE: The surgical management of central metatarsalgia, *Foot Ankle Int* 23:415–419, 2002.

Trnka HJ, Nyska M, Parks BG, Myerson MS: Dorsiflexion contracture after the Weil osteotomy: Results of cadaver study and three-dimensional analysis, *Foot Ankle Int* 22:47–50, 2001.

12

CHAPTER **13**

Management of the Bunionette

SURGICAL APPROACH

The approach to surgical correction of the bunionette depends entirely on the magnitude and type of deformity. Ostectomy alone is not a good choice, because with the use of this procedure alone, the tendency is to remove too much of the metatarsal head, which causes instability of the metatarsophalangeal (MP) joint and further deviation of the first toe, with or without arthritis. Although I rarely perform an ostectomy as the definitive procedure, this operation can be considered when the fifth metatarsal head, including the plantar condyle, is painful. In such cases, an ostectomy can be performed in conjunction with a condylectomy that coutours the first metatarsal head. The removal of an excessive amount of bone, however, will lead to the development of instability of the joint, with or without arthritis, with worsening of the deformity, necessitating removal of the metatarsal head.

CHEVRON OSTEOTOMY

For deformity that involves a curvature of the *distal* metatarsal with a slightly widened intermetatarsal angle, a chevron osteotomy or one with simple translation at the neck of the metatarsal is easy to perform. With more intermetatarsal deformity, however, a proximal oblique metatarsal osteotomy is preferred. For either procedure, fixation of the metatarsal is neccessary. An interesting observation is the prolonged period required for complete radiographic healing of the osteotomy; despite the initial radiographic appearance, however, bone healing invariably occurs, and nonunion of the distal metatarsal osteotomy is rare. The fixation can be performed using a small twist-off screw, a buried or percutaneously introduced Kirschner wire (K-wire), or a bioresorbable pin. The chevron cut made in the fifth metatarsal head is technically no different from that made in the first metatarsal head for correction of a hallux valgus and bunion. For maximum bone-to-bone position, I try to ensure that the angle of the cut is no less than 60 degrees. With a smaller-angle cut, more cortical and less metaphyseal bone contact results, contributing to the risk for instability (Figures 13-1 to 13-3).

At times it is not possible to perform a uniplanar osteotomy. In patients with both lateral and plantar metatarsal head pain, a biplanar osteotomy can be performed as outlined later. For correction of recurrent deformity, particularly if arthritis is present, a metatarsal head resection is the preferred procedure (Figure 13-4). The latter procedure *cannot* be performed if any hindfoot varus is present. Such resection would simply shift the pressure slightly more proximally to the distal end of the metatarsal, producing further pain and resulting in a deformity that is far more difficult to correct. If the fifth metatarsal is painful and associated with any hindfoot varus, then the hindfoot position should be corrected and the metatarsal head left alone.

OBLIQUE FIFTH METATARSAL OSTEOTOMY

An oblique shaft metatarsal osteotomy is performed to correct a wider fourth-to-fifth intermetatarsal angle or a deformity that involves bowing with a lateral curvature to the metatarsal. The osteotomy is made in the same plane as that for correction of a modified Ludloff first metatarsal osteotomy. (In fact, I had the idea for the oblique first metatarsal osteotomy while performing this fifth metatarsal osteotomy as described by Coughlin.) The cut is made proceeding from proximal and dorsal to distal and plantar at an angle of approximately 30 degrees with respect to the metatarsal shaft. The cut should be placed according to the location of deformity, and ideally it should be as far proximal as possible to gain the maximum correction. This proximal cut is not always necessary if only a more moderate deformity is present, in which case the osteotomy can be in the midshaft of the metatarsal. As with the first metatarsal (Ludloff) osteotomy, the key to this procedure is to swivel the metatarsal around the hinge point of a K-wire, pin, or screw. After two thirds of the osteotomy has been cut, the screw is inserted, and this screw maintains control of the osteotomy. Once the screw has been inserted and the osteotomy is stabilized, the cut on the metatarsal is then completed, and correction is performed through rotation of the metatarsal around the axis of the screw, which is then tightened. The overhanging bone on the lateral and dorsal aspect of the metatarsal is then shaved down with a saw blade. This osteotomy can be used for simultaneous treatment of fifth metatarsalgia and correction of a prominent bunionette by changing the plane of the osteotomy. Normally, the saw blade cut is made exactly perpendicular to the axis of the fifth metatarsal. In the presence of metatarsalgia, however, the saw blade can be dropped slightly. For the aim to be medial and dorsal so that the metatarsal is rotated medially, the blade also is inclined dorsally. This technique is an effective means of treating metatarsalgia. Fixation of the fifth metatarsal osteotomy can be more difficult than fixation of the first, and it requires many fragment screws or K-wires. Countersinking each screw is important to avoid potentially troublesome protrusion; unless the screw(s) is buried subcutaneous pain is inevitable postoperatively, necessitating its ultimate removal (Figures 13-5 to 13-7).

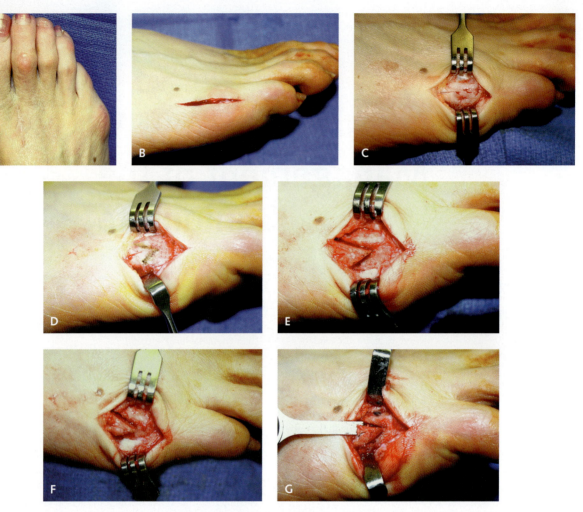

Figure 13-1 The chevron osteotomy for correction of a bunionette. **A** and **B,** The incision is longitudinal, as is the capsulotomy. **C,** First, the metatarsal head is exposed. **D,** The cut is marked out with electrocautery. **E,** A small saw blade is used to complete the cut. **F,** The metatarsal head is shifted medially by 4 to 5 mm and secured with an 11-mm twist-off screw. **G,** The lateral edge of the bone is trimmed with a saw.

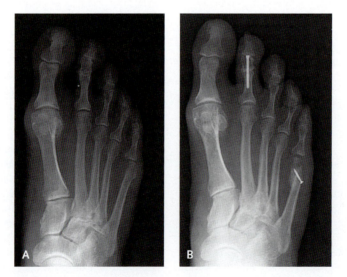

Figure 13-2 Distal metatarsal osteotomy using a twist-off screw for fixation: preoperative **(A)** and postoperative **(B)** radiographs.

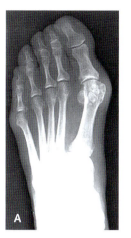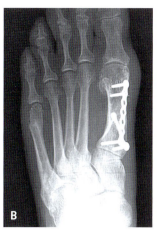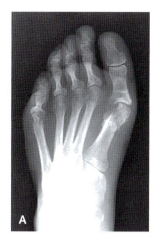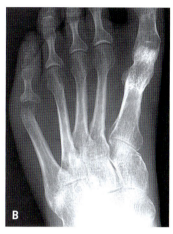

Figure 13-3 The fixation for this bunionette correction was introduced percutaneously. **A,** Preoperative radiograph. **B,** The initial internal screw fixation failed, and a K-wire was used, introduced from distal to proximal through the toe. This provided good correction; however, a superficial infection of the toe developed, which persisted. Percutaneous fixation of the fifth metatarsal osteotomy is associated with a high incidence of toe infection.

Figure 13-4 A, The patient had undergone multiple previous surgeries of the forefoot, all of which had failed. **B,** The fifth metatarsal was painful, as was the fifth metatarsophalangeal joint, so the metatarsal head was excised.

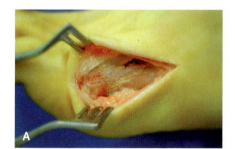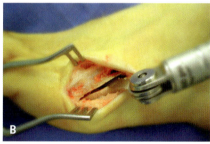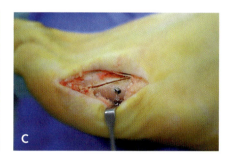

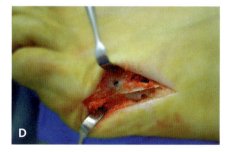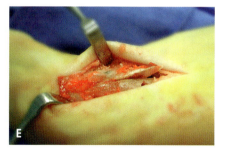

Figure 13-5 An oblique metatarsal osteotomy for correction of a bunionette associated with an abnormal metatarsal shaft angle. **A,** An incision was made along the length of the metatarsal through the capsule to expose the shaft. **B,** The osteotomy cut was made in this case with a saw blade that was slightly inclined dorsally, to simultaneously correct the fifth metatarsal angle. **C,** Note that the cut was not completed. **D,** A screw was inserted, and the distal metatarsal was rotated around the axis of the screw. **E,** The screw was then tightened, and the lateral overhanging bone was resected.

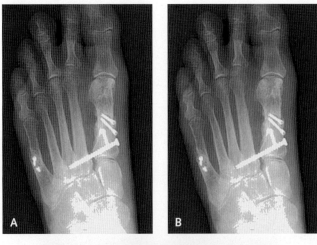

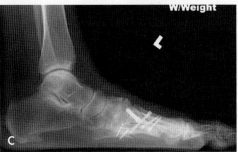

Figure 13-6 A-C, The fixation of this bunionette osteotomy was performed with two screws as outlined for the case in Figure 13-5, after the metatarsal was rotated around the axis of the first screw.

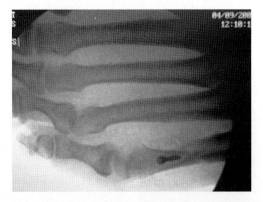

Figure 13-7 Fluoroscopic image of intraoperative correction with the first screw. The metatarsal has been cut and rotated around the axis of the screw. It usually is necessary to insert a second screw to secure the osteotomy.

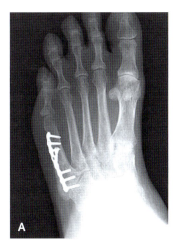
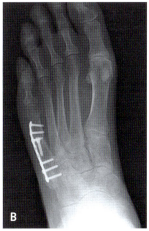

Figure 13-8 A and **B,** Failed fixation of the fifth metatarsal necessitating reoperation. The screws broke out of the bone with fracture of the metatarsal, and a small malleable plate was used for fixation.

TECHNIQUES, TIPS, AND PITFALLS

- A simple exostectomy is not ideal for correcting a bunionette. Recurrence is common, with concurrent subluxation of the fifth MP joint.

- The healing of a distal metatarsal osteotomy that is shown on a plain radiograph lags behind clinical healing, and although the radiograph may not show consolidation, the early union usually is clinically stable.

- The oblique diaphyseal osteotomy is easy to perform, provided that the fixation is stable. As with the modified Ludloff first metatarsal osteotomy, the correction is obtained by rotating the axis of the metatarsal around the screw. The use of a small bone reduction clamp is helpful to hold the metatarsal during fixation.

- For failure of exostectomy, an osteotomy can still be performed, unless a considerable amount of the fifth metatarsal head is uncovered, in which case a resection of the fifth head is preferable (Figure 13-8).

SUGGESTED READING

Coughlin MJ: Treatment of bunionette deformity with longitudinal diaphyseal osteotomy with distal soft tissue repair, *Foot Ankle* 11:195–203, 1991.

Kitaoka HB, Holiday AD Jr, Campbell DC II: Distal chevron metatarsal osteotomy for bunionette, *Foot Ankle* 12:80–85, 1991.

Vienne P, Oesselmann M, Espinosa N, et al: Modified Coughlin procedure for surgical treatment of symptomatic tailor's bunion: A prospective followup study of 33 consecutive operations, *Foot Ankle Int* 27(8):573–580, 2006.

Weitzel S, Trnka HJ, Petroutsas J: Transverse medial slide osteotomy for bunionette deformity: Long-term results, *Foot Ankle Int* 28:794–798, 2007.

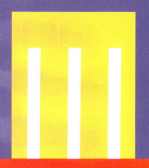

CHAPTER **14**

Surgery for the Neuropathic Foot and Ankle

Although classifying the Charcot arthropathic process as acute, subacute, or chronic is helpful from a practical standpoint, the definitions of these stages have no value because treatment will depend on the clinical severity of the deformity and the presence of bone fragmentation and periosteal new bone formation. New bone formation is apparent a month or so after onset of the acute process, often associated with marked osteopenia and bone fragmentation. Surgery at this stage may be more complicated even if the deformity is amenable to open reduction and internal fixation.

Once the process reaches the chronic phase, the midfoot typically is stable and is unlikely to deform further. However, bone prominence often is present on the plantar aspect of the midfoot, which may lead to ulceration or infection. In this context, "chronic" implies *clinically* stable, with an absence of swelling and inflammation (Figure 14-1). In these chronic arthropathies, the apex of the deformity is somewhere on the plantar foot. The "chronic" designation does not always equate with *anatomic* stability, however, because in a subgroup of midfoot arthropathies, the midfoot is quite unstable yet is not warm to touch. The deformity in such instances is very difficult to treat because of the very unstable rocker-bottom deformity of the midfoot (Figure 14-2).

Occasionally, if the first metatarsal, cuneiform, or navicular dislocates medially, the forefoot abducts and the bone prominence is directly medial. This type of deformity is easier to treat with an ostectomy than those in which bone prominences are on the lateral or plantar midfoot. The lateral rocker-bottom deformity occurs when the navicular and cuneiforms dislocate dorsally, leading to a shortening of the medial column and a laterally based prominent rocker-bottom deformity with the apex at the cuboid.

The rationale for operative treatment is to decrease the deformity, thereby minimizing the likelihood of complications, including infection and need for amputation, which otherwise may be imminent. Certainly, surgical reduction of acute dislocation makes sense, especially in patients with acute frank dislocation of the midfoot, who clearly will benefit from this more urgent operative treatment. By contrast, in patients with chronic but stable neuropathic

deformity of the midfoot, use of appropriate shoes, orthoses, and braces often can restore adequate function, so the indication for surgery is more specific: deformity that cannot be controlled by nonsurgical means, associated with recurrent ulceration and infection.

Patients can experience pain from the deformity, and although neuropathy may be thought of as being complete and not associated with any sensation, some patients experience deep, aching discomfort. Accordingly, it is appropriate to indicate surgical reconstruction with for use in such cases. Chronic deformity, recurrent ulceration, pain, and an unbraceable deformity are reasonable indications for reconstruction, but only if treatment-approach orthotics and prosthetics have failed to produce improvement or is unrealistic to begin with (Figure 14-3). There remains a "gray zone" in which the decision for performing reconstruction is more difficult if not controversial. The experienced clinician, however, gains a "feel" for the foot that helps guide decisions about the type of treatment needed. Patient factors including compliance, weight, extent of neuropathy, perfusion, skin condition, family support, opposite limb function, mobility of the ankle, and travel distance required for foot care all need to be considered in planning surgery for either the acute or the chronic stage of neuroarthropathy. The importance of these factors must not be underestimated. No matter how skillful the surgeon, the surgery will be useless if the patient lacks the means to comply with the restrictions on weight bearing and personal care requirements during rehabilitation.

CORRECTION OF NEUROPATHIC DEFORMITY OF THE MIDFOOT

During the acute phase, some absolute indications for surgery exist, including medial dislocation of the cuneiform or navicular, which will lead to skin necrosis (Figure 14-4). Initially, the associated swelling masks the bone prominence, but with resolution of swelling, a pressure sore develops or full-thickness skin loss occurs (Figure 14-5). My experience suggests that if the dislocation is diagnosed

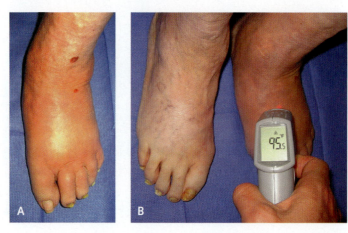

Figure 14-1 Acute neuropathic arthropathy involving the right foot. **A,** Swelling and erythema are evident. **B,** The temperature of 95° F for the midfoot is indicative of severe inflammation.

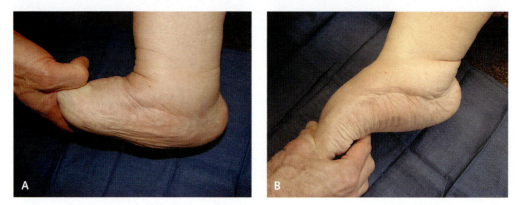

Figure 14-2 A and **B,** Midfoot subluxation in a patient with a neuroarthropathy of 5 years duration. The foot is grossly unstable in plantar flexion and dorsiflexion, but by definition this would be a "chronic" Charcot process. I prefer to consider this an unstable midfoot, rather than a chronic arthropathy.

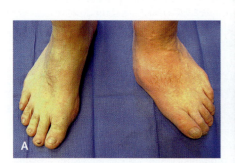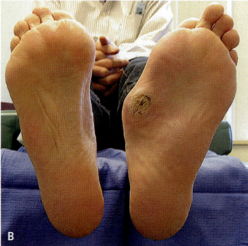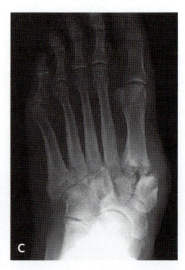

Figure 14-3 A-C, Chronic deformity of the left foot in a 69-year-old patient that had been present for 7 years. Chronic callus was present but never broke down with ulceration, and no surgery was necessary.

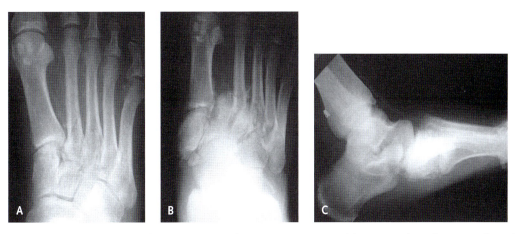

Figure 14-4 Radiographs of an acute forefoot injury. **A,** The patient was monitored for neuropathy and acute swelling of the foot, but no fracture was evident. **B** and **C,** One week later the dislocation became apparent.

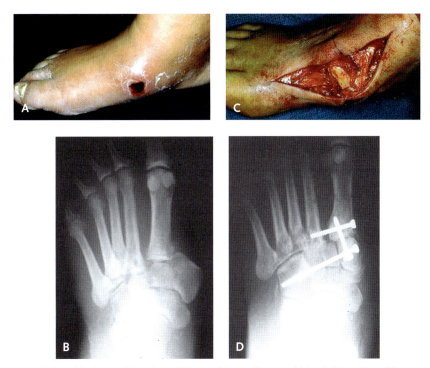

Figure 14-5 A and **B,** Acute dislocation of the medial cuneiform and lateral dislocation of the tarsometatarsal joint in a patient with neuropathy and diabetes. Eschar formation was the result of pressure of the cuneiform and the dislocation on the skin. **C,** At surgery, the cuneiform was rotated 90 degrees; the anterior tibial tendon remained attached. **D,** A primary arthrodesis of the medial column was performed.

early on in the evolution of the arthropathy, surgery will minimize the likelihood of deformity. The patient has to remain non–weight-bearing regardless of the type of treatment, and provided that the foot is not ischemic, surgery is preferable. With complete bone extrusion, operative reduction and stabilization will be necessary to prevent subsequent deformity. In patients with these acute fracture-dislocations, the issue is whether the potential morbidity of surgery outweighs the likelihood of later complications (Figure 14-6).

The key to operative treatment, however, is to take careful note of the quality of the bone. From a practical standpoint, knowing the onset of the injury is difficult, because many patients are unaware of the initial event anyway. It is preferable to use the appearance of the bone as an indicator of both the onset of the neuropathic injury and also the possibility for surgery. Performing surgery on the midfoot when the bones are crumbling as a result of osteopenia is difficult, if not frustrating, and complicated. Therefore I am more inclined to correct a subluxation or dislocation than multiple fractures around the midfoot. The traditional methods of reduction and fixation of these injuries do not work well here because they are associated with recurrence of deformity unless such techniques are combined with arthrodesis.

In the chronic stage, a complete transverse tarsal joint dislocation with dorsal dislocation of the cuneiform commonly leads to a floppy, unstable forefoot. This deformity results because the forefoot is placed into dorsiflexion by the pull of the tibialis anterior tendon while the Achilles tendon forces the hindfoot into equinus. The combination of these deformities results in a foot that is ineffective at both heel strike and toe-off, and the midfoot is at risk for ulceration.

A second deformity that frequently requires surgery in the chronic phase is the midfoot rocker-bottom deformity that is associated with supination of the forefoot. This deformity results from the heel cord pulling the foot into equinus and subsequent weight bearing on the lateral aspect of the foot.

OSTECTOMY

Ulcers may develop as a result of rubbing of anatomic bony prominences, or those produced during weight bearing in unstable joints, against shoes or other points of contact. If ulcers are intractable, ostectomy should be considered to resect the bone prominence. This procedure works well in such instances, provided that there is no associated instability of the adjacent joints. If the bone prominence is resected and the midfoot is unstable, then recurrent ulceration will occur. Ostectomy can be performed only if stability (rigidity) of the midfoot is present. Because this is a much easier and quicker procedure to recover from, with less morbidity, I prefer to perform an ostectomy, as opposed to an arthrodesis, if possible. If the ulcer fails to heal with use of a total contact cast, the ostectomy is not contraindicated. The incision has to be made carefully, however, to avoid extension of the ulcer and the possibility of infection.

Technically, the ostectomy is not difficult to perform, and the only issue is to try to minimize postoperative soft tissue problems. Rarely, I approach the ostectomy through the open ulcer. Usually, the skin has healed over the ulcer from a total contact cast program, and the incision is made off the weight-bearing surface of the foot, either medially or laterally. Large skin flaps are preserved, and full-thickness dissection using a broad periosteal elevator should be performed to reach the prominence. I use a combination of an oscillating saw, osteotomes, and a rongeur to create a contoured surface of the plantar weight-bearing foot amenable to ambulation (Figure 14-7). It is imperative not to resect too much bone, or the result will be instability, which is particularly likely on the inferior aspect of the midfoot joints. A large, solid neuropathic bone mass may be present but is uncommonly seen; resection of the undersurface of unfused midfoot joints may have the effect of worsening the deformity and secondarily exacerbating the deformity.

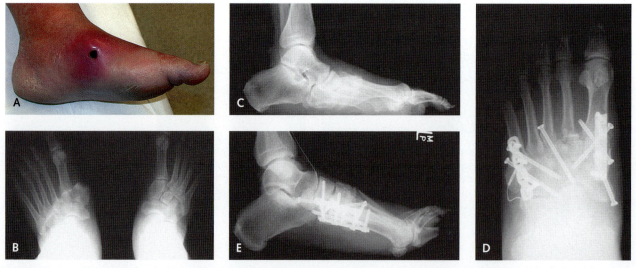

Figure 14-6 A, An acute midfoot dislocation of the left foot. **B** and **C,** Radiographic appearance. **D** and **E,** Treatment consisted of application of plantar plates and primary arthrodesis of the midfoot.

TECHNIQUES, TIPS, AND PITFALLS

- I prefer to leave large segments of the subchondral bone of the midfoot bones intact.

- If bone quality is sufficient, the medial column length can be maintained with bridge plating from the talus to the cuneiforms or first metatarsal (Figure 14-8).

- Neuropathic fracture, dislocation, or fracture-dislocation of the midfoot results in loss of medial column length secondary to comminution of an intercalary segment. Caution is indicated, because any further shortening of the medial column would cause a lateral "rocker," or adduction, of the midfoot with the apex at the calcaneocuboid joint.

- I use a burr to remove selected portions of the articular surface, rather than a chisel or an osteotome, because the ligamentous support is friable and tenuous, and with less than delicate handling, bone may literally fall out (Figure 14-9).

- Primary arthrodesis of these acute midfoot dislocations must be performed, with the joint surfaces denuded using a burr applied to subchondral bone.

- If a talo-navicular-cuneiform arthrodesis is performed, do not shorten the medial column. It may be preferable to include the calcaneocuboid joint in the arthrodesis, to avoid a lateral rocker-bottom deformity created by slight shortening of the medial column.

- If hindfoot valgus and forefoot abduction are associated with the acute midfoot Charcot arthropathy, a triple arthrodesis should be performed using lag screw fixation, but because of bone loss, plates are often necessary.

- If the navicular is fragmented and unable to be maintained as a part of the fusion mass, a naviculectomy with subsequent talocuneiform arthrodesis with similar surgical principles should be performed.

- To minimize the effect of the equinus contracture that is always present, I routinely perform a lengthening of the Achilles tendon.

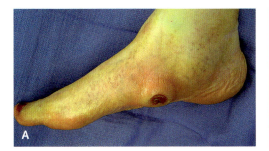
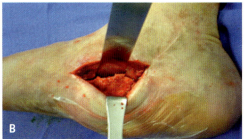
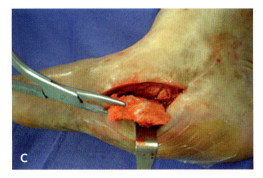

Figure 14-7 A, Ostectomy of a nonspecific plantar bone mass was performed through a medial incision off the weight-bearing surface of the foot. **B,** The flap was kept as thick as possible, and with subperiosteal dissection, the mass of bone was exposed. **C,** A curved 2-cm osteotome was used to remove the bone mass in one piece.

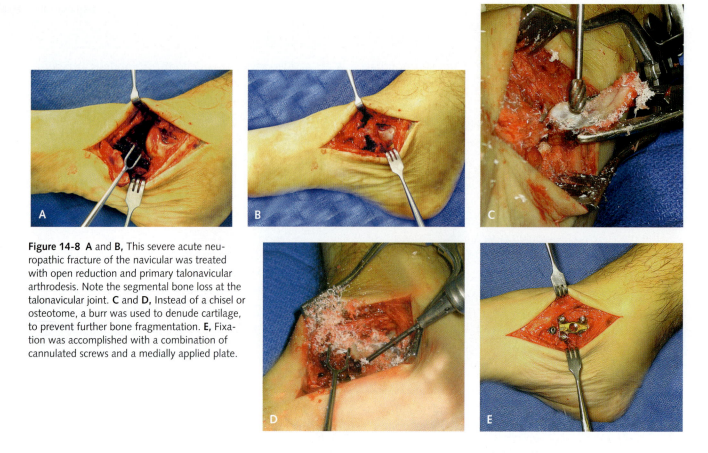

Figure 14-8 A and **B,** This severe acute neuropathic fracture of the navicular was treated with open reduction and primary talonavicular arthrodesis. Note the segmental bone loss at the talonavicular joint. **C** and **D,** Instead of a chisel or osteotome, a burr was used to denude cartilage, to prevent further bone fragmentation. **E,** Fixation was accomplished with a combination of cannulated screws and a medially applied plate.

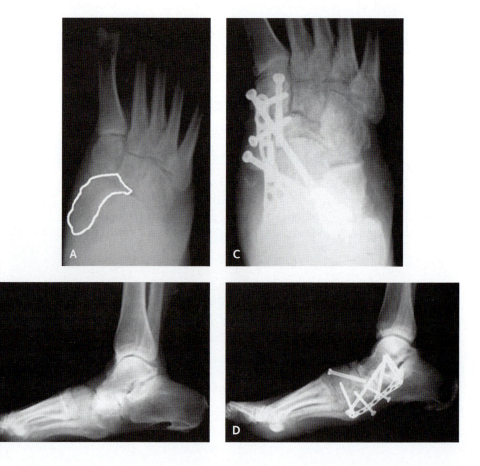

Figure 14-9 A and **B,** Chronic dislocation of the midfoot with plantar and medial subluxation of the navicular *(outlined area)* led to ulceration of the medial foot, which was refractory to all methods of nonsurgical care. The dislocation of the navicular *(outlined area)* was associated with a flatfoot and a rocker-bottom deformity. **C** and **D,** Correction was accomplished with open reduction, combined with arthrodesis of the medial column of the foot with a plantar plate.

FIXATION OPTIONS FOR THE MIDFOOT

An external fixator is used to secure and maintain reduction only when an ulcer cannot be healed before arthrodesis, and I do not routinely use an external fixation construct when the soft tissue is healed without ulceration. Occasionally, the internal fixation obtained is poor, and maintenance of the result is understandably of concern in a noncompliant patient. In such cases, I occasionally add an external fixator consisting of half-rings applied to the midfoot (Figure 14-10). I use the same half-ring external fixator for treatment of patients with open infection or ulceration with associated osteomyelitis. In the case of indolent osteomyelitis, resection of the infected bone usually is the first step in establishing a clean wound bed, which is essential for healing the associated ulcer. The dilemma

arises in the need to remove enough necrotic bone without causing destabilization of the medial column of the foot, and usually extensive ostectomy is required, followed by arthrodesis using the external fixator.

An alternative fixation technique is to use large cannulated screws, which are inserted from distal to proximal through the metatarsals. Once the reduction is complete and the midfoot alignment is obtained, the guide pins are inserted antegrade through the metatarsal at the level of the tarsometatarsal joint from proximal to distal. The midfoot is reduced, the guide pins are then redirected proximally across the midfoot, and the screws are introduced through the metatarsal heads and buried in the metatarsal shaft (Figure 14-11).

Another option for fixation is use of antegrade-inserted screws from the hindfoot through the midfoot into the forefoot. This

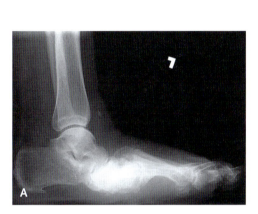
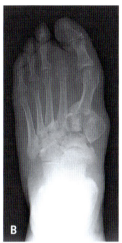
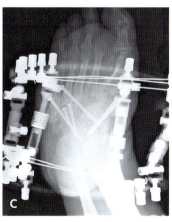
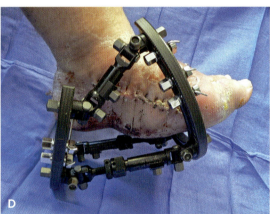
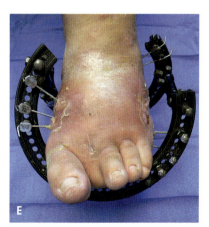
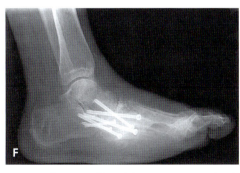
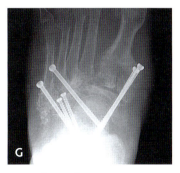

Figure 14-10 A and **B,** An acute-on-chronic midfoot dislocation associated with recurrent plantar ulceration. **C-E,** Open reduction with internal fixation using cannulated screws was performed, but the repair was not considered to be sufficient fixation for the patient, who was heavy, and two half-rings were applied to the foot. **F** and **G,** The appearance of the foot 3 years later.

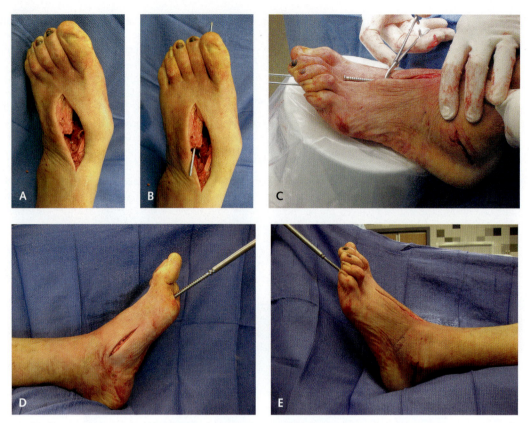

Figure 14-11 Technique of antegrade screw fixation for an acute unstable fracture-dislocation of the midfoot. **A** and **B,** After the midfoot is opened, and the joints are debrided, the guide pin is inserted directly through the metatarsal out the skin distally. As many pins as necessary are used. **C,** A screw is then laid on top of the metatarsal under fluoroscopic guidance, to allow rough estimation of the length of the screw required, because the depth gauge will not work in this location. **D** and **E,** The tarsometatarsal joints are reduced, and the guide pins are inserted antegrade across the joints. Cannulated fully threaded screws are used to secure the fixation; partially threaded screws also are used if necessary.

fixation method is particularly useful for management of a combination of midfoot and hindfoot deformity, for which a midfoot fusion is performed in conjunction with the hindfoot correction. If the midfoot is dislocated, then the entire dislocation can be reduced using screws inserted from the back of the talus into the forefoot. In Figure 14-12, a patient with neuroarthropathy and a chronic dislocation of the midfoot was treated by opening up both the medial and lateral sides of the foot simultaneously. Note that when the laminar spreader is in the midfoot, the towel can be seen through the foot laterally. The foot was manually reduced by bringing the forefoot down to the midfoot and determining that the reduction was possible. Once this was verified, a large guide pin was inserted from the anterior talus out the back of the ankle posterolaterally. The guide pin was then driven forward into the first metatarsal, and a second pin into the lateral midfoot, followed by placement of large cannulated screws from back to front (see Figure 14-12).

A similar problem is depicted in Figure 14-13: The patient had undergone numerous unsuccessful previous surgeries. Despite diabetic neuropathy, she had pain with considerable deep aching in the foot. This combination of findings presented a management dilemma because there was considerable bone loss in the midfoot and hindfoot associated with deformity. Once all the hardware was removed, I had to make the decision of either inserting a structural bone graft or shortening the foot slightly. I prefer not to use a structural graft in the midfoot of a patient with neuropathy. The failure

rate is too high, and the success rate for incorporation of these large grafts in an attempt to maintain the length of the foot is not good. I therefore shortened the hindfoot, maintaining stability through the subtalar joint, and then building up the medial column after removal of the remaining necrotic navicular. Once the medial column is shortened, then the lateral column also must be slightly shortened; otherwise a lateral rocker-bottom deformity will develop. The retrograde-antegrade guide pin and cannulated screw were inserted from the talus into the first metatarsal (see Figure 14-13)

If possible, I use the tension-banding effect of a plate applied on the plantar surface. This approach does require more stripping of the medial soft tissues and abductor hallucis muscle, but the resulting construct is stable. This procedure is particularly useful for stabilization with the medial column of the midfoot (Figure 14-14).

Dressings and sutures are removed 2 to 4 weeks after the operation. After appropriate healing of incisions has been confirmed, a non–weight-bearing, below-the-knee plaster or fiberglass cast is applied. This support is maintained with frequent cast changes for at least 2 but often 4 months. Thereafter a weight-bearing cast is applied and maintained until bridging trabeculation is observed at the surgical site. On average, 6 to 12 months of casting is required for union of arthrodesis of the midfoot. Once healing is evident, it is advisable to use a polypropylene ankle-foot orthosis for up to 1 year, which will lessen the effects of direct pressure and shear stresses encountered in normal weight bearing on the abnormal midfoot.

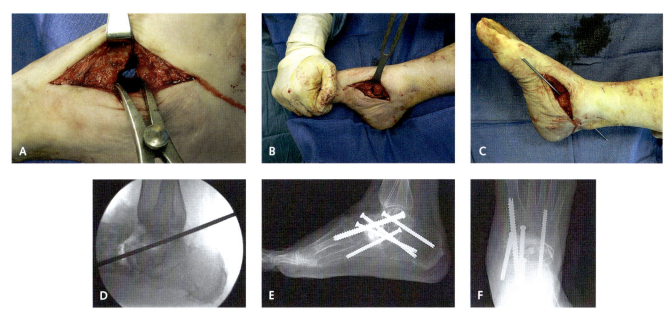

Figure 14-12 A chronic dislocation of the midfoot associated with neuropathy was treated by opening up both the medial and lateral aspects of the foot simultaneously. **A,** When the laminar spreader was in the midfoot, the towel was visible through the foot laterally. **B,** The foot was manually reduced by bringing the forefoot down to the midfoot to confirm that the reduction was possible. **C** and **D,** Once this was verified, a large guide pin was inserted from the anterior talus out the back of the ankle posterolaterally. **E** and **F,** The guide pin was then driven forward into the first metatarsal, and a second pin into the lateral midfoot, followed by insertion of large cannulated screws from back to front.

CORRECTION OF NEUROPATHIC DEFORMITY OF THE HINDFOOT AND ANKLE

In contrast with the Charcot midfoot deformity, with collapse of the hindfoot and ankle, the resultant deformity often necessitates surgery. A number of fixation options are available, and decision making in such instances depends to some extent on the magnitude and type of deformity and the individual surgeon's preference. Clearly, in the presence of sepsis, external fixation is ideal. I have found, however, that even in the presence of ulceration of the fibula, such as with a severe varus deformity of the ankle, the arthrodesis can be performed with internal fixation. For example, in the presence of the severe varus ankle, if the fibula is exposed or infected, or both, it is excised completely as part of the procedure, followed by internal fixation. In such cases I routinely mix antibiotic powder with the cancellous bone graft. Factors that indicate the need for an external fixator in management of the infection and correction of deformity include the degree of the infection and a concern for the presence of osteomyelitis.

Regardless of the type of deformity and the type of external fixator used, I prefer to close all the wounds before application of the external fixator. It is easier to close the incision before application of the frame, and closing gives a better sense of where the cross pins will be, because I prefer not to have pins going through the incision. Clearly, in the presence of infection, this part of the incision will not be closed. For example, in the presence of a severe varus deformity with exposed fibula, an incision is made over the distal fibula to perform the cheilectomy for the tibiocalcaneal arthrodesis. The incision that is extended proximally and distally is closed, but the original open wound is left open.

However, use of an external fixator obviously is necessary in the presence of sepsis, and at the opposite end and in the absence of severe deformity, cannulated screw fixation is most versatile.

It is worth noting that the goal of treatment of a Charcot hindfoot deformity is to obtain stability, and the ability to wear a shoe without risk for ulceration. Arthrodesis is a worthwhile goal, but the lack of arthrodesis does not imply failure of treatment if the foot is stable. Cannulated screw fixation is simple and allows significant deformities to be addressed. I have used a blade plate frequently to treat ankle and associated hindfoot deformities in the past with success (Figure 14-15). In the case illustrated in Figure 14-16, the patient was a 63-year-old woman with recurrent neuropathic ulceration over the head of the talus. A triple arthrodesis was performed, with cannulated screw fixation. Note that the ankle was quite deformed preoperatively, and although arthritis was present with slight valgus erosion, the ankle was stable (see Figure 14-16).

With gross instability involving the ankle or subtalar joint, use of a blade plate, locking plate, or intramedullary rod is preferable. In the 1990s I used a blade plate for most of these procedures, because control of rotation was not possible with an intramedullary rod (Figure 14-17). External fixation is necessary with patients who have neuropathic deformity, infection, and uncontrollable instability. Figure 14-18 presents an example of external fixation for a very unstable neuropathic stress fracture of the distal tibia and fibula with associated ulceration and superficial infection over the fibula. Closed reduction of the deformity was performed, and an external fixator was applied until the wound was healed and the fracture stable. In the patient in Figure 14-19, the fixator was used to augment the internal fixation of the distal tibia neuropathic fracture. This patient had very poor skin and poor perfusion to the limb, so rather than using an more extensive open reduction procedure, percutaneous fixation of the fracture was accomplished, supplemented by the external fixator. The fixator was removed at 10 weeks, and although the patient tried to remain non–weight bearing, adherence to this restriction proved impossible, and the deformity rapidly progressed. This deformity was ultimately treated

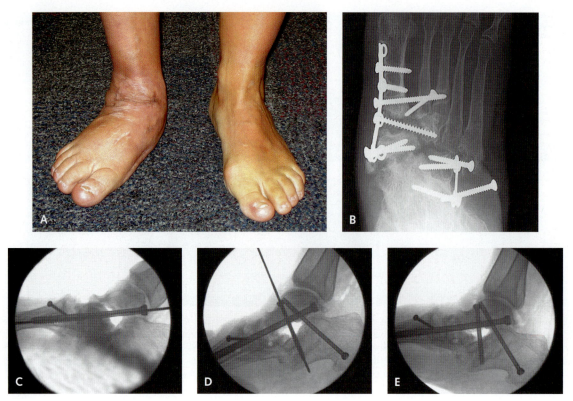

Figure 14-13 A and **B,** The patient had undergone numerous unsuccessful previous surgeries, with complications including infection. **C-E,** After removal of all of the hardware, followed by removal of the remaining necrotic navicular, the midfoot was shortened, maintaining stability through the subtalar joint and then building up the medial column. Once the medial column is shortened, the lateral column also must be slightly shortened; otherwise a lateral rocker-bottom deformity will develop. The retrograde-antegrade guide pin and cannulated screw were inserted from the talus into the first metatarsal, as shown.

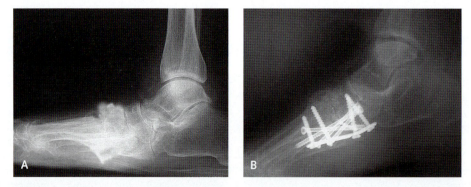

Figure 14-14 A, Chronic recurrent ulceration of the medial midfoot. **B,** Once the ulcer healed, a medial column arthrodesis was performed using screws and a plate applied to the plantar surface under the abductor hallucis.

with a closing wedge biplanar osteotomy of the distal tibia in conjunction with placement of an intramedullary rod. Note that the length of the rod is not ideal; the rod should be slightly longer in the patient with neuropathy, to prevent fracture at the tip of the rod.

The older intramedullary fixation systems did not have adequate rotational control of the limb, and supplemental screws were always required. If severe erosion was present in the calcaneus, as is frequently the case with neuropathic deformity, then it is difficult, if not impossible, to maintain control of rotation (Figure 14-20). With the advent of improved intramedullary fixation, the problem

no longer exists. Excellent compression of the ankle and or the subtalar joint is possible, using both an external and internal compression system with the nail (Phoenix nail—Biomet, Parsippany, New Jersey). Accordingly, the decision to use intramedullary fixation will depend on other factors such as the type and location of the deformity, ability of the patient to comply with non–weight bearing, and factors that include the bone quality. It is worth emphasizing that the primary goal for correction of neuropathic deformity is stability. This tenet applies whether or not surgery is performed. Although arthrodesis is desirable, the absence of arthrodesis does not in any

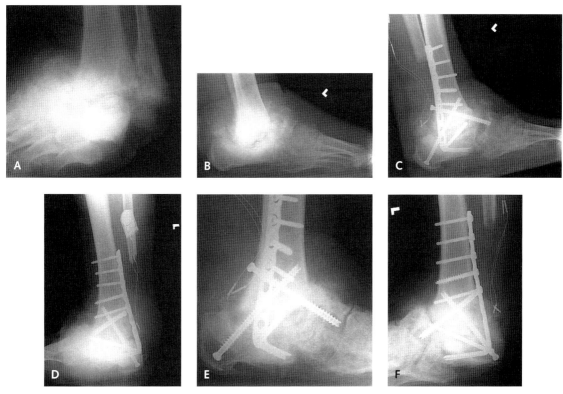

Figure 14-15 A and B, The patient had gross instability of the foot and ankle with recurrent ulceration over the fibula. C and D, Treatment consisted of a tibiocalcaneal arthrodesis with a blade plate fixation and insertion of an implantable bone stimulator. E and F, Marked bone healing is evident 4 years after the reconstruction.

way defeat the purpose of surgery, nor does it lead to failure. Under these circumstances, intramedullary fixation may be preferable for treatment of a patient who has significant deformity and a total inability to comply with restricted mobility postoperatively (Figure 14-21). One additional option for fixation of these very unstable neuropathic deformities is the use of a locking plate. There is no currently designed locking plate for fixation of the tibiocalcaneal complex, and I have used the humeral locking plate (Synthes, Westchester Pennsylvania) successfully when application of such a plate is indicated, as in Figure 14-22. In the case illustrated, a decision had to be made intraoperatively regarding the use of a structural bone graft to increase the height of the hindfoot. A laminar spreader was inserted and the hindfoot distracted and checked clinically and fluoroscopically. The foot was then manually compressed to check on the status of the skin. If bone is missing, as in this example in which the talus was fragmented, the hindfoot will widen considerably when compressed between the tibia and the calcaneus. Sufficient skin was present for closure in this foot, and the calcaneus was

aligned with respect to the tibia, and after insertion of a guide pin to maintain alignment, the locking plate was used to secure alignment.

The indication for surgery in this patient group is far easier to define. Almost all patients are treated initially with a brace of some sort to maintain the alignment of the foot under the tibia. Even gross deformities may be immobilized indefinitely in this manner, and despite the inconvenience, the brace is well tolerated. When ulceration occurs despite adequacy of bracing, surgery is indicated. Surgery is deferred until there is no evidence of clinically active infection and until swelling has decreased. If the limb is swollen, a regimen of diuretic agents, bed rest with limb elevation, and application of an Unna bandage (Carapace, Inc., Toledo, Ohio) is instituted for 48 hours before surgery. In patients with documented osteomyelitis, treatment should be initiated with culture-specific intravenous antibiotics and local wound care. Although the infection cannot always be eradicated in these patients, drainage or surrounding erythema at the time of reconstructive surgery should be minimal.

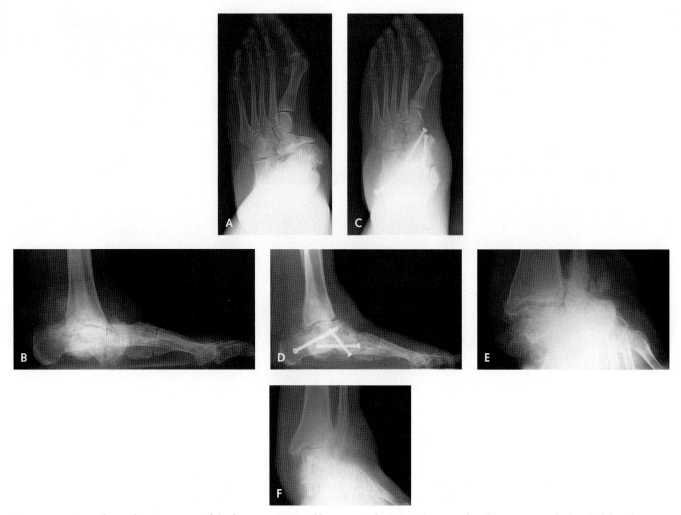

Figure 14-16 A, Radiographic appearance of the foot in a 63-year-old woman with recurrent neuropathic ulceration over the head of the talus. **B-D,** A triple arthrodesis was performed with cannulated screw fixation. **E** and **F,** Note that the ankle was quite deformed preoperatively, and although arthritis was present with slight valgus erosion, the ankle was stable.

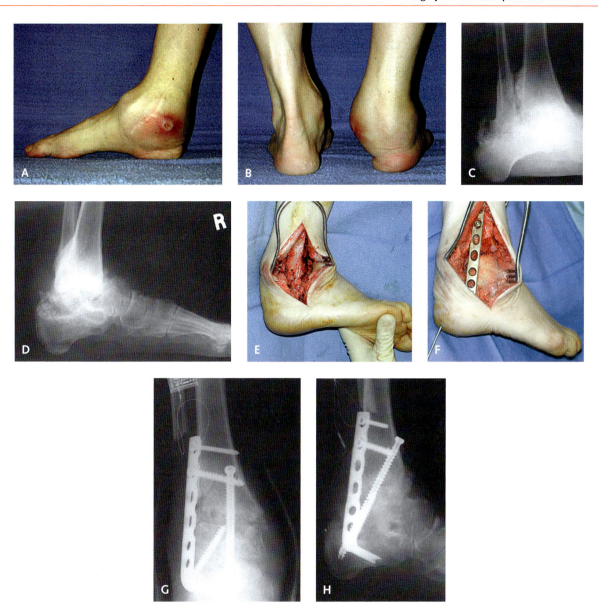

Figure 14-17 A and **B,** Severe uncontrollable neuroarthropathy associated with ulceration and hindfoot collapse. **C** and **D,** Note the profound hindfoot valgus and necrosis of the talus. **E,** When the tibiotalocalcaneal arthrodesis was planned, it was noted that once the foot was compressed between the calcaneus and the tibia, the skin did not close as a result of puckering and tension on the skin edges. For this reason, a structural bone block graft was used to increase the height of the hindfoot, facilitating distraction of the limb and skin closure.
F-H, A blade plate was used for fixation.

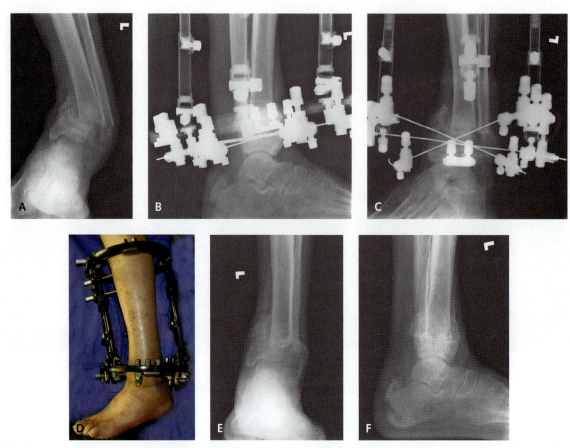

Figure 14-18 A, A very unstable neuropathic stress fracture of the distal tibia and fibula with associated ulceration and superficial infection over the fibula. **B-D,** Closed reduction of the deformity was performed and an external fixator was applied until the wound was healed. **E** and **F,** The fracture was stable when the fixator was removed.

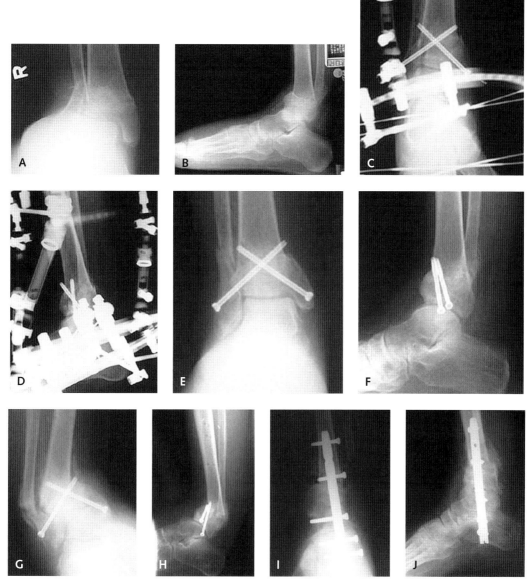

Figure 14-19 A and **B,** The patient, who had diabetic neuropathy, presented for treatment of an acute injury to the distal tibia and had been walking on the limb for 1 week. The skin condition was particularly poor, and perfusion to the limb not normal; therefore an open reduction was not performed. **C** and **D,** Fixation was provided with crossed screws, supplemented by an external fixator, which at the time seemed to be sufficient fixation, but in retrospect was not enough. **E** and **F,** The fixator was removed at 10 weeks; the alignment, although reasonable, was not perfect. **G** and **H,** Subsequently the deformity rapidly progressed. **I** and **J,** Ultimately an osteotomy of the tibia and a tibiotalocalcaneal arthrodesis were required for definitive repair.

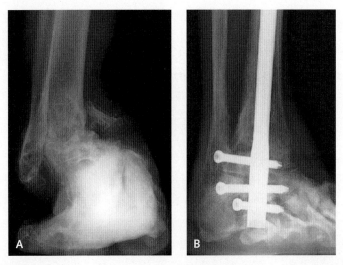

Figure 14-20 An intramedullary rod was used to correct the severe neuropathic dislocation shown in **A.** The design of this rod does not facilitate rotational control, and nonunion was present, evident in **B.**

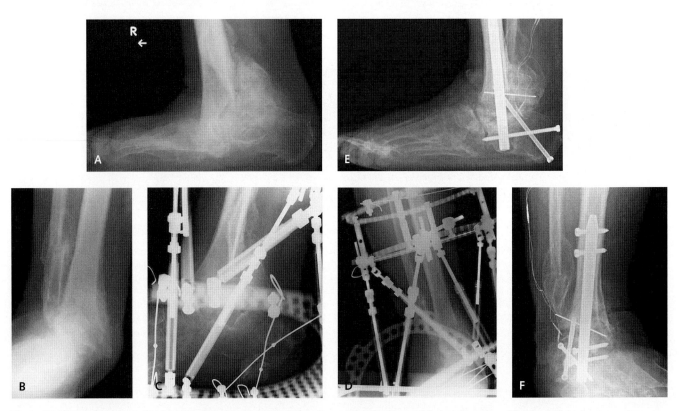

Figure 14-21 A and **B,** The patient had profound neuropathic deformity associated with medial ulceration. **C** and **D,** The initial management approach involved use of a Taylor spatial frame to effect wound healing and realignment. **E** and **F,** Once the alignment and wound healing had been obtained, the fixator was removed and intramedullary fixation was used for the tibiotalocalcaneal arthrodesis.

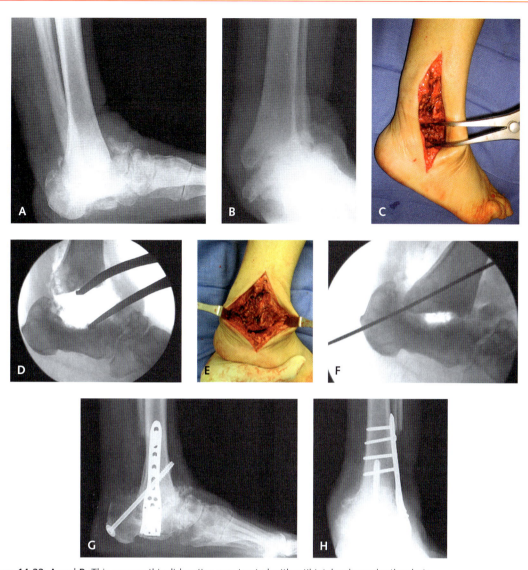

Figure 14-22 A and **B,** This neuropathic dislocation was treated with a tibiotalocalcaneal arthrodesis.
C and **D,** A laminar spreader was inserted and the hindfoot distracted and checked clinically and fluoroscopically.
E and **F,** The foot was then manually compressed to check that with the resultant hindfoot widening, the skin would still close. **G** and **H,** The calcaneus was then manually compressed and aligned with respect to the tibia, and a guide pin was inserted to maintain alignment. A locking plate was then applied for the tibiocalcaneal arthrodesis.

TECHNIQUES, TIPS, AND PITFALLS

- A curvilinear incision is made over the distal 10 cm of the fibula and is extended distally toward the sinus tarsi.

- Whenever possible, existing incisions should be used. A full-thickness skin flap is developed without regard for the sural and superficial peroneal nerves in the patient with neuropathy.

- Nerves and even the peroneal tendons are cut to prevent excessive skin retraction and dissection. The distal 10 cm of the fibula is resected after an oblique osteotomy with an oscillating saw. If the deformity is not associated with ulcer or infection, the fibula is harvested for bone graft using an acetabular reamer.

- The remnants and fragments of the talus are excised. Specifically, the fragmented body of the talus is always removed, although the head of the talus may be protected and preserved provided that it is adequately vascularized and not involved with a medial dislocation of the talonavicular joint or infection.

- The articular surface of the distal tibia is prepared by making a flat cut with an oscillating saw, and a flexible chisel is used to debride the articular cartilage on the dorsal surface of the calcaneus.

- Great care is taken to establish precise alignment of the foot under the leg. Be careful not to internally rotate the foot under the leg.

- After the deformity is reduced, it is stabilized initially with 2-mm guide pins.

- I try not to incorporate the talonavicular joint into the tibiotalocalcaneal or tibiocalcaneal arthrodesis.

- Whenever possible in the setting of neuroarthropathy, limited motion is preferable, and this applies to the talonavicular joint and to a tibiocalcaneal arthrodesis.

- With use of a lateral plate, it is placed on the lateral calcaneal subchondral bone. Care is taken to position the hindfoot in neutral, because the calcaneus tends to displace into slight valgus as compression is applied to the plate proximally.

- Allograft or autograft bone, or a combination thereof, is used; the choice is determined by the amount of bone harvested from the fibula and the size of the defect to be filled. The bone graft is then mixed with 400 mg of tobramycin and 500 mg of vancomycin powder as well as a concentrate of the aspirate from the iliac crest.

- The antibiotic–bone graft mixture is firmly packed between the bone surfaces anteriorly, in addition to the posterior aspect of the tibia and calcaneus, to facilitate an extraarticular and an intraarticular arthrodesis. The back of the tibia is debrided by raising a thick osteoperiosteal flap that extends down onto the dorsal surface of the calcaneus posteriorly. Graft is packed here as well. The wound is closed in layers using 2-0 absorbable sutures, and 3-0 nylon sutures are used for the skin incision. Any tension on the skin edges encountered during closure may be due to the change in shape of the hindfoot or to the added subcutaneous bulk of the plate, and the peroneal tendons may need to be removed.

SUGGESTED READING

Ahmad J, Pour AE, Raikin SM: The modified use of a proximal humeral locking plate for tibiotalocalcaneal arthrodesis, *Foot Ankle Int* 28: 977–983, 2007.

Assal M, Stern R: Realignment and extended fusion with use of a medial column screw for midfoot deformities secondary to diabetic neuropathy, *J Bone Joint Surg Am* 91:812–820, 2009.

Chaudhary SB, Liporace FA, Gandhi A, Donley BG: Complications of ankle fracture in patients with diabetes, *J Am Acad Orthop Surg* 16:159–170, 2008.

Jani MM, Ricci WM, Borrelli J Jr, et al: A protocol for treatment of unstable ankle fractures using transarticular fixation in patients with diabetes mellitus and loss of protective sensibility, *Foot Ankle Int* 24:838–844, 2003.

Myerson MS, Alvarez RG, Lam PW: Tibiocalcaneal arthrodesis for the management of severe ankle and hindfoot deformities, *Foot Ankle Int* 21:643–650, 2000.

Myerson MS, Henderson MR, Saxby T, Short KW: Management of midfoot diabetic neuroarthropathy, *Foot Ankle Int* 15:233–241, 1994.

Papa J, Myerson M, Girard P: Salvage, with arthrodesis, in intractable diabetic neuropathic arthropathy of the foot and ankle, *J Bone Joint Surg* 75:1056–1066, 1993.

Pinzur MS: Current concepts review: Charcot arthropathy of the foot and ankle, *Foot Ankle Int* 28:952–959, 2007.

Schon LC, Easley ME, Weinfeld SB: Charcot neuroarthropathy of the foot and ankle, *Clin Orthop Apr* :116–131, 1998.

CHAPTER **15**

Cavus Foot Correction

OVERVIEW

Correction of the cavus foot can be daunting. With adherence to some basic principles, however, the deformity usually can be well corrected and the foot dynamically balanced, with maintenance of as much motion as possible. The presurgical evaluation should ascertain the following: Where is the apex of the deformity? Is this a midfoot or a forefoot cavus? Is the forefoot in equinus? If so, is this a global equinus, or does it involve only the first or perhaps the middle metatarsal? How mobile is the first metatarsal? Is the foot rigid, or is the deformity passively correctable? Surgeons rely on the Coleman block test to determine flexibility of the hindfoot and forefoot (Figure 15-1). This test is certainly acceptable, but I also recommend manipulating the heel to see the effects of the hindfoot on the forefoot. If the heel can be reduced into heel valgus, then perhaps less correction will need to be done in the hindfoot and more in the forefoot. Finally, the most important component of the evaluation is to identify additional deforming forces on the foot. Invariably, the peroneus longus muscle is stronger than the anterior tibial muscle, and the posterior tibial muscle is stronger than the peroneus brevis muscle, with a variable degree of contracture of the gastrocnemius and soleus muscles present.

DECISION MAKING

What are the indications for arthrodesis? At times a specific indication is obvious—for example, the presence of severe ankle arthritis will necessitate an arthrodesis for correction. A varus deformity associated with ankle arthritis and global foot cavus deformity is not ideally treated with a joint replacement (Figure 15-2). A triple arthrodesis is a good procedure, provided that the foot is correctly balanced with additional osteotomy and tendon transfer. The triple arthrodesis gained a poor reputation for correction of the cavus foot, particularly that associated with Charcot-Marie-Tooth disease, correctly named hereditary sensorimotor neuropathy. These arthrodesis procedures were performed in isolation, and as might be expected, the deformity recurred. The posterior tibial tendon inserts distal to the talonavicular joint, and unless the tendon is transferred,

the medial foot deformity will gradually recur, with onset of adductovarus. Therefore, if a triple arthrodesis is thought to be the procedure of choice, it should be performed with appropriate transfer of the posterior tibial tendon, as well as additional tendon transfers as required (Figure 15-3).

Generally, I perform a combination of a calcaneal osteotomy, a first metatarsal osteotomy, and a plantar fascia release. I then add whatever else is necessary to complete the correction, which may include a resection of the base of the fifth metatarsal, an ankle ligament reconstruction, or a midfoot osteotomy (Figure 15-4). The calcaneus osteotomy is a very utilitarian procedure to correct a cavus foot and, depending on the magnitude of the deformity, is always required in one form or another (Figure 15-5).

It is rare that a triple arthrodesis needs to be performed. In fact, this arthrodesis, although not contraindicated, is associated with numerous long-term complications, particularly ankle arthritis. The mobility of the hindfoot must be preserved if possible.

Although it is possible to perform an anatomic correction of the foot initially with a triple arthrodesis, these procedures are insufficient in the long term if muscular imbalance remains. Integral to the success of any of these procedures is a corrected foot posture, a plantigrade hindfoot relative to the forefoot, and muscle balance. Even with perfectly executed surgery, if the posterior tibial muscle is overactive relative to the evertors of the hindfoot, the foot will ultimately "fail," with further adductovarus deformity. The posterior tibial muscle must therefore be transferred in many of these procedures. Frequently, a cavus deformity is associated with slight weakness of the anterior tibial muscle, and the posterior tibial tendon can be transferred as part of this corrective procedure. Usually, the transfer is to the dorsal aspect of the foot through the interosseous membrane. Occasionally, however, if the anterior tibial muscle is strong and the predominant deformity is adductovarus, then a split posterior tibial transfer can be performed, with the lateral limb being transferred into the peroneus brevis tendon. Not much of the split tendon is needed for the transfer; enough is transferred so that it can pass behind the tibia and fibula and hook into the peroneus brevis tendon with an effective suture tenodesis.

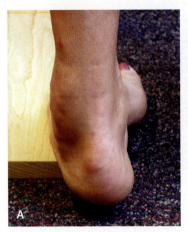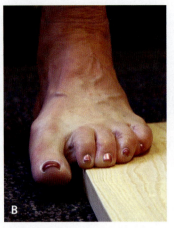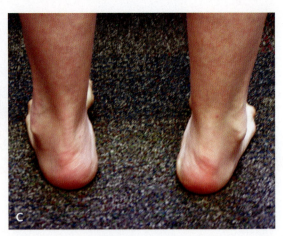

Figure 15-1 The Coleman block test is performed by placing a block under the lateral foot and allowing the first metatarsal to come to the ground. **A** and **B,** In these photographs, the foot is quite rigid, and no correction of the heel varus took place. **C,** The patient was an adolescent. The heel corrected into neutral with the test, suggesting more of a forefoot-driven varus deformity.

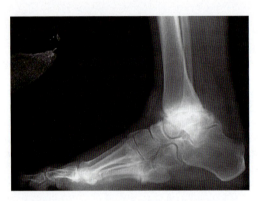

Figure 15-2 Note the severe ankle arthritis associated with the hindfoot varus and the chronic nonunion of a fifth metatarsal stress fracture. An ankle arthrodesis with a calcaneus osteotomy with resection of the base of the fifth metatarsal was selected as the treatment approach.

PLANTAR FASCIA RELEASE

The plantar fascia release is an integral part of correction of the cavus foot deformity and therefore usually is the first procedure that I perform as part of the correction. Correcting the position of the calcaneus is difficult without first releasing the plantar fascia. From a technical standpoint, although I used to make an incision directly under the arch of the foot medial to the fascia, I found this counterproductive. Although this incision was easy to perform, it always left a large hypertrophic nodular scar, almost like fibromatosis, that was difficult to soften, even with aggressive rehabilitation. Subsequently, I attempted the entire plantar fascia release from the lateral incision inferior to the calcaneal osteotomy. This approach worked fairly well, but releasing the medial bundle through this access is difficult. If there is severe cavus deformity, the medial band over the abductor fascia cannot be released. The incision does, however, provide reasonable access for the fascia release. This modification of the original Steindler procedure is performed by extending the incision for the calcaneal osteotomy slightly more distally and cutting across the fascia transversely with Metzenbaum scissors.

The easiest procedure for me is a complete fascia release through a medial longitudinal incision adjacent to the heel, which

is made slightly more distally at the junction of the dorsal and plantar skin (Figure 15-6). Unfortunately, some patients may be left with a small patch of numbness on the medial aspect of the heel pad from this incision, and the potential for this outcome must be explained to patients preoperatively. The incision is made over a 2-cm length. With the incision kept longitudinally in the axis of the foot, no problems occur with wound healing during the lengthening and flattening of the medial column; problems would occur, however, if a vertical incision were made along the axis of the tarsal canal.

The branch of the lateral plantar nerve usually is not visible and does not need to be looked for. A copious fatty tissue under the incision needs to be reflected with a large soft tissue retractor until the fascia is visualized. I then split the fascia directly off the calcaneus using scissors from a medial to lateral direction. The scissors are advanced without a cutting motion until both the medial and lateral bands are completely released.

For severe deformity, in which cavo-adductovarus is present, the fascia of the abductor hallucis tendon also must be completely released. For some of these severe deformities, the intrinsic muscles must be stripped off the calcaneus completely, in addition to the fascia release. The stripping can be done using scissors or a broad periosteal elevator from within the same medial incision. This release must be very carefully planned, because multiple incisions cannot be used for the posterior tibial tendon transfer, the abductor fascia release, and the plantar fascia release (Figure 15-7).

CALCANEUS OSTEOTOMY

The incision for the calcaneal osteotomy varies according to the type of procedure performed. If an osteotomy alone is performed, then a shorter incision is made directly inferior to the peroneal tendons. Usually, however, the calcaneal osteotomy needs to be performed with additional procedures, including repair of the peroneal tendon, reconstruction of lateral ankle instability, and a peroneus longus to brevis tendon transfer. For these cases, the incision is simply extended posteriorly along the axis of the peroneal tendons behind the fibula.

The incision is deepened through subcutaneous tissue in the plane between the peroneal tendon and the sural nerve. The nerve can be retracted either superiorly or inferiorly, depending

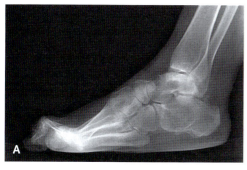

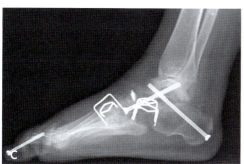

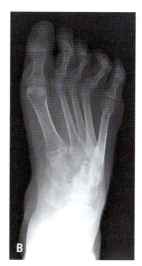

Figure 15-3 A and **B,** A very rigid cavus deformity in a 33-year-old patient with Charcot-Marie-Tooth disease. The hindfoot and forefoot were very rigid, and pain was present along the lateral foot. **C,** Correction was accomplished with a triple arthrodesis, a dorsiflexion arthrodesis of the first tarsometatarsal joint, arthrodesis procedures of the hallux and lesser toe interphalangeal joints, and transfer of the posterior tibial tendon to the dorsum of the foot.

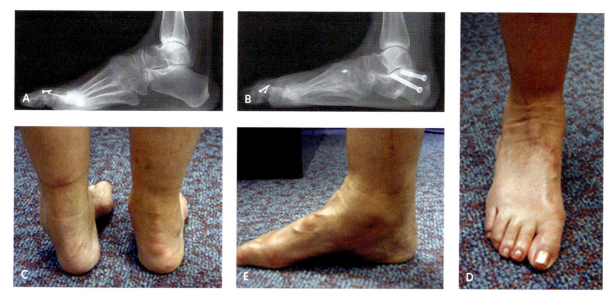

Figure 15-4 A, Bilateral flexible cavovarus deformity associated with ankle instability in a 31-year-old patient with Charcot-Marie-Tooth disease. **B-E,** Initial correction in the right foot was accomplished using a "standard reconstruction," including a triplanar calcaneus osteotomy, a first metatarsal osteotomy, a plantar fascia release, a peroneus longus-to-brevis transfer, and a transfer of the posterior tibial tendon to the dorsum of the foot, and a modified Chrisman-Snook procedure.

on its position. The periosteum needs to be elevated over a broad area, because a wedge is going to be removed. I insert a retractor to separate the soft tissues and then place two small, curved retractors on either side of the calcaneus to expose the entire lateral tuberosity. A saw, not an osteotome, should be used to make the cut; a wide, fan-shaped saw blade should be selected. The cut is first initiated perpendicular to the axis of the calcaneus at a

45-degree angle to the tuberosity. I use a punching action with the saw blade so that I can feel the medial cortex as it is perforated. Once the first cut has been made, the second cut is made at an angle to this of approximately 20 degrees, but the appropriate angle depends on the size of the wedge. It is far easier to start out with a smaller wedge and then remove more bone if the correction is not sufficient (Figure 15-8).

Figure 15-5 A, The residual effect of mild idiopathic bilateral cavus deformity in a 53-year-old woman. **B** and **C,** The deformity was corrected with a peroneus longus-to-brevis transfer, a plantar fascia release, and a calcaneus osteotomy.

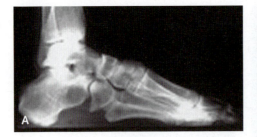
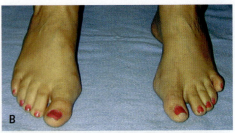
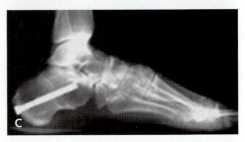

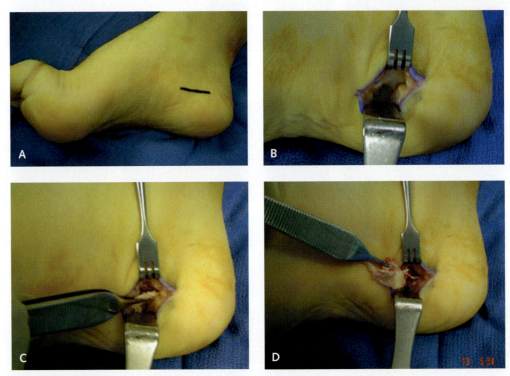

Figure 15-6 A, The plantar fascia release is performed with a short transverse incision at the junction of the dorsal and plantar skin. **B,** A retractor is used to sweep the fatty tissue toward the plantar surface, exposing the fascia. **C,** The fascia is cut with a scissors; **D,** then a segment of the fascia is excised to prevent recurrent scarring.

Once the wedge or bone has been removed, I then pull the heel into valgus. The osteotomy rarely closes down perfectly at this time, so additional perforation of the calcaneus typically is necessary to permit it to close down smoothly. This perforation to permit smooth reopposition of the cut surfaces can be accomplished by reinserting the saw blade while the osteotomy is partially closed. The cuts are then completed with multiple minor perforations (curfing). Depending on the deformity, the calcaneus is moved in two or three planes. The valgus closing wedge osteotomy constitutes the first plane. The tuberosity is then always shifted lateral to its axis under the subtalar joint, which improves the weight-bearing axis of the hindfoot. Movement in a third plane consists of a cephalic shift, which is added according to the pitch angle of the calcaneus. I try to flatten out the talocalcaneal angle, and the calcaneus–first metatarsal angle in particular flattens as the calcaneal tuberosity is moved cephalad.

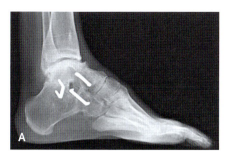
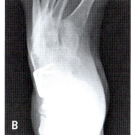
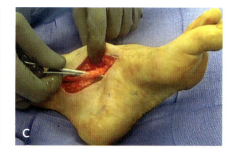
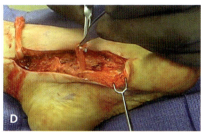
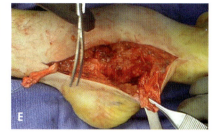
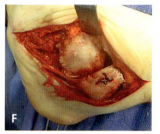
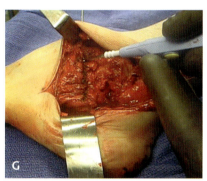

Figure 15-7 A and **B,** Very severe recurrent deformity after a failed triple arthrodesis. **C-E,** In addition to the revision of the triple arthrodesis, treatment included a transfer of the posterior tibial tendon, a plantar fascia release, and a stripping of the abductor fascia, performed from a single extensile medial incision. **F** and **G,** On the lateral aspect of the foot, the revision triple arthrodesis was performed, in addition to a modified Chrisman-Snook procedure.

I use two guide pins to hold the calcaneus in the corrected position. The first guide pin is inserted centrally into the body of the posterior tuberosity, which is then manipulated into the corrected position. While the guide pin is being held and the heel is forced into the desired position, a second guide pin is introduced for screw fixation. It is best to insert the screw from slightly posterior lateral to slightly anterior and medial to gain maximal compression. Tamping the overhanging inferior ledge of bone is unnecessary but can be done with a small bone tamp to prevent any irritation on the peroneal tendons.

PERONEUS LONGUS-TO-BREVIS TENDON TRANSFER

The peroneus longus-to-brevis tendon transfer is a useful procedure when the peroneus longus muscle is working and is flexible. Regardless of the strength of the peroneus brevis tendon, this transfer augments the weakness of the peroneus brevis muscle. Ideally, this procedure is done in younger patients and even in children to achieve maximal advantage. If the brevis tendon is scarred, torn, or absent, the longus tendon can still be transferred to the stump of the base of the brevis tendon.

The peroneus longus tendon is cut under direct vision as it passes underneath the cuboid. A stay suture is then inserted into the tendon and pulled distally to obtain the correct tension. I pull on it to achieve maximal tension; then I release it slightly and perform the tenodesis at this level of tension. The incision for the calcaneus osteotomy can be extended to perform a transfer or repair of the peroneal tendon (Figure 15-9). The sutures are inserted by burying the knot either as interrupted sutures or as a continuous locking whip suture (Figure 15-10).

FIRST METATARSAL OSTEOTOMY

As the heel is brought into valgus, increased pronation of the forefoot occurs, with an increased plantar flexion of the first metatarsal. Occasionally I perform a valgus calcaneal osteotomy without a first metatarsal osteotomy, but a decision to omit the first metatarsal cut has to be based on the specific foot deformity. In any case, the important consideration here is the balance that can be attained with the combination of the calcaneal osteotomy, the peroneus longus-to-brevis tendon transfer, and the first metatarsal osteotomy. With the peroneal transfer, the plantar flexion of the first ray is clearly weakening, and this weakening has to be considered when the osteotomy is performed to prevent overcorrection with ultimate shift of weight to the second metatarsal. Another issue is whether the forefoot cavus deformity is global or limited to one or two metatarsals. Invariably, the first metatarsal is in equinus, so this osteotomy is what I most commonly use.

An incision is made on the dorsal medial aspect of the first metatarsal extending to the metatarsal cuneiform joint. The periosteum is stripped, and the extensor hallucis longus tendon is retracted laterally. The osteotomy cut is made 1 cm distal to the articulation in metaphyseal bone. This osteotomy can be performed in two ways: In one, a closing wedge is used, which has the obvious advantage of preserving a plantar cortical hinge for stability (Figure. 15-11). In the other, a vertical osteotomy is performed; then the dorsal, proximal, and cortical rim is impacted into the metaphysis. This procedure has the advantage of correcting

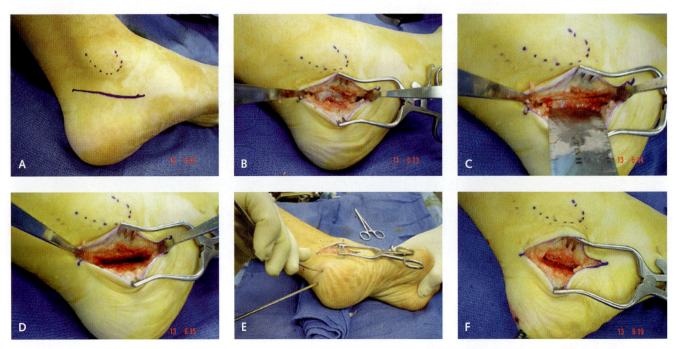

Figure 15-8 Calcaneus osteotomy procedure. **A,** The incision is placed directly above the peroneal tendons and above the level of the sural nerve. **B,** The periosteum is reflected and retractors are inserted on either side of the tuberosity. **C** and **D,** The wedge is removed using a wide saw applied with a punching action; the width of the wedge usually is approximately 5 mm but will be determined by the defect. **E** and **F,** The heel is translated laterally by approximately 5 mm, and then two guide pins are inserted, one directly through the osteotomy and the other to manipulate the heel into valgus **(E)**, followed by cannulated screw insertion **(F).**

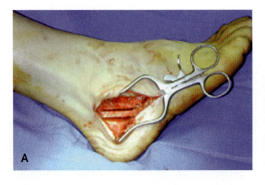

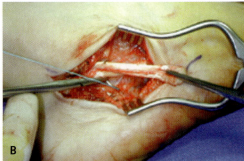

Figure 15-9 A, The calcaneus osteotomy also can be performed using the same incision as that for a peroneal tendon repair or transfer or an ankle ligament reconstruction. **B** and **C,** After the osteotomy is accomplished, a peroneus longus–to-brevis tendon transfer is performed.

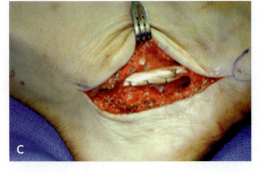

the deformity but also limits the amount of shortening of the first metatarsal (Figure 15-12).

The dorsal wedge resection osteotomy is performed with a vertical cut perpendicular to the axis of the metatarsal more proximally but is not completed, and I preserve approximately 3 mm of bone on the plantar metatarsal. The second cut is made approximately 4 mm distal to this at an angle of 15 degrees. If more bone is resected originally, overcorrection may result, with a transfer of pressure to the second metatarsal.

Once the bone wedge has been resected, the first metatarsal is pushed up dorsally, and the plantar surface of the forefoot is palpated with the foot in maximal dorsiflexion. More bone can be shaved through the osteotomy itself until an appropriate amount of the wedge has been resected. The easiest way to secure this osteotomy is with a dorsally applied two-hole plate. Once the amount of bone to be resected has been verified, the plate is applied on the proximal cortex, and then the metatarsal is pushed up into dorsiflexion. While the corrected position is maintained, the second screw is inserted, using the compression feature of the plate to compress the osteotomy (Figure 15-13). This procedure is quite stable with the method of fixation outlined, and, depending on additional

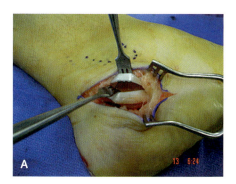

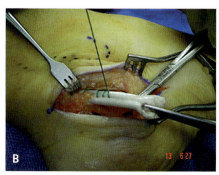

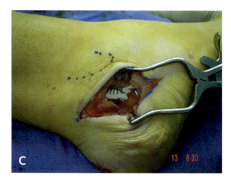

Figure 15-10 A-C, This flexible cavus foot was treated with an osteotomy of the first metatarsal and a peroneus longus-to-brevis tendon transfer.

procedures performed, patients may begin weight bearing at 2 weeks after surgery.

MIDFOOT OSTEOTOMY

The midfoot osteotomy is a complex procedure that requires careful preoperative planning. Ideally, the osteotomy is based at the apex of the deformity on the foot, which may correspond to the navicular or the cuneiforms. The osteotomy can be performed with the removal of a biplanar dorsally based wedge. It is rare that the wedge correction can be obtained with a single bone cut, and a wedge has to be removed. Because the first metatarsal declination is always more depressed than the fifth, the wedge is biplanar, with more bone removed from the dorsomedial than from the lateral midfoot (Figure 15-14).

An incision is made in the midline of the foot extending from the ankle joint distally through the midmetatarsal. This is an extensile excision, and it is imperative not to compromise the outcome by limiting the length of the incision, because skin retraction and wound dehiscence are potential risks with a shorter incision. The superficial and deep peroneal nerves are retracted laterally and medially, and a plane is developed underneath the neurovascular bundle, which is then elevated with subperiosteal dissection performed in a medial direction. It usually is necessary to cut the extensor hallucis longus brevis tendon to gain access to the dorsal aspect of the midfoot. The entire dorsal central aspect of the midfoot is now stripped using a large broad periosteal elevator. The midfoot is then marked under fluoroscopic guidance to delineate the starting point of the osteotomy.

The plane of correction depends entirely on the shape of the foot. I try to exit the osteotomy in the cuboid laterally and in the medial cuneiform medially, but this aspect of the procedure depends on how much rotation and angulation are necessary. If wedge osteotomies are performed, then both the medial and lateral limbs of the osteotomy meet at an apical point, usually over the middle cuneiform. Frequently, most of the medial cuneiform has to be resected. The base of the osteotomy is dorsal, and the cut will then be varied to some extent in accordance with the shape of the foot. As the osteotomy moves further laterally, less bone is resected, and the correction is obtained more by dorsal elevation of the lateral border of the foot with rotation than through wedge correction (Figures 15-15 to 15-17).

Planning the osteotomy with transparencies preoperatively is useful. Transparent paper is applied to a lateral view radiograph of the foot, and the position of the wedge is located. Cutouts are then made in the shape of the foot, and the planned osteotomies are marked on the transparencies. With these transparencies, the size and location of the wedge are determined. Predicting the amount of rotation or correction is difficult with these uniplanar templates, but such planning provides a good idea of the size of the dorsal or dorsomedial wedge if a midfoot osteotomy is going to be performed.

A saw is used to perform the osteotomy. If the dorsal position of the apex is in the middle lateral cuneiform joint, the medial exit point usually is at the base of the medial cuneiform. The anterior tibial tendon attachment must be reflected and retracted medially. The osteotomy cut is then shaped such that the medial limb forms one aspect of an approximately 8-mm wedge at a 15- to 20-degree angle to the dorsal plane of the midfoot. If any adduction deformity is present in addition to the cavus, then a biplanar wedge is removed. Bone is resected both dorsally and medially, and this resection removes more of the medial cuneiform itself. If a global cavus deformity of the midfoot is present, then the base of

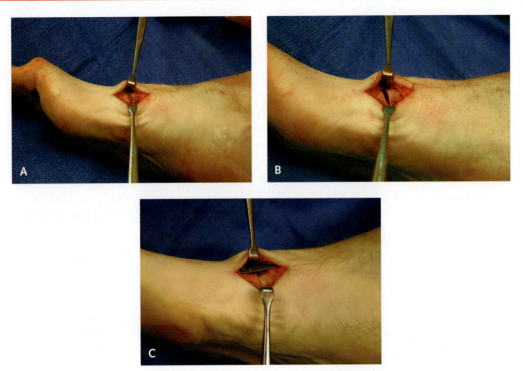

Figure 15-11 A-C, The first metatarsal osteotomy was performed with a small dorsal wedge resection and fixation with a two-hole plate. Notice that the plate does not contour well to the surface of the osteotomy.

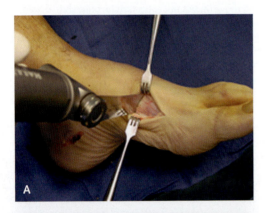

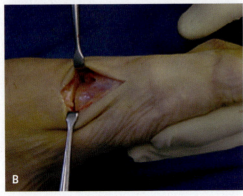

Figure 15-12 A and **B,** This first metatarsal osteotomy was performed with a vertical saw cut in the metatarsal, which was then impacted into the metaphysis to correct the declination angle.

the osteotomy dorsally extends from the center of the foot medially at much the same distance as that between the osteotomy limbs. The first lateral osteotomy cut is made extending toward the cuboid from the middle or lateral cuneiform, and then the second osteotomy cut is made at a much smaller angle so that the apex is in the cuboid without removing much of the cuboid at all. It is far easier to perform the lateral correction by dorsally translating the cuboid and then rotating it slightly to elevate the base of the fifth metatarsal.

Once the wedges have been resected, the forefoot is then dorsiflexed until good contact between the dorsal bone surfaces is achieved. The advantage of this osteotomy is that further contouring can be performed, just as with any wedge osteotomy, until sufficient bone has been removed and the forefoot position corrected relative to the hindfoot. Fixation of the osteotomy is possible with screws, a dorsal plate, or large threaded pins that are inserted percutaneously (see Figure 15-17). Using pins in this location sometimes is easier because of the plane of the osteotomy and the small bone segments between each articulation. Use of staples also is possible if adequate bone is present on both sides of the osteotomy, which is not usually the case. Frequently, I insert large pins from the medial and lateral portion of the foot, from distal to proximal, and then remove them at 6 weeks once ambulation begins. Healing of these osteotomies generally is good; however, any incomplete healing of one portion of the osteotomy does not seem to influence the outcome of the procedure.

Occasionally, the apex of the deformity is more distal at the level of the tarsometatarsal joint. Jahss described a truncated wedge arthrodesis of the tarsometatarsal joint for this type of deformity. This procedure is technically easy to perform, but arthrodesis of all of the joints is difficult to obtain. As with the wedge osteotomy

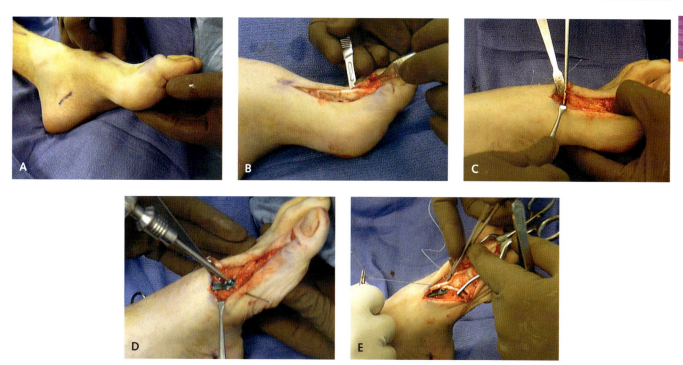

Figure 15-13 A, This cavus forefoot deformity was corrected with an arthrodesis of the hallux interphalangeal (IP) joint, a transfer of the extensor hallucis longus (EHL), and a dorsal wedge osteotomy of the first metatarsal. **B,** After the IP arthrodesis, the extensor hallucis longus (EHL) was cut distally to expose the metatarsal. **C,** The dorsal wedge was removed, and the metatarsal was levered open with an osteotome, preserving the plantar cortex. **D** and **E,** A two-hole plate was used, first to lock the metatarsal **(D)** and then to compress it distally (Orthohelix, Akron, Ohio). **E,** The EHL was then transferred through a drill hole in the metatarsal and sutured.

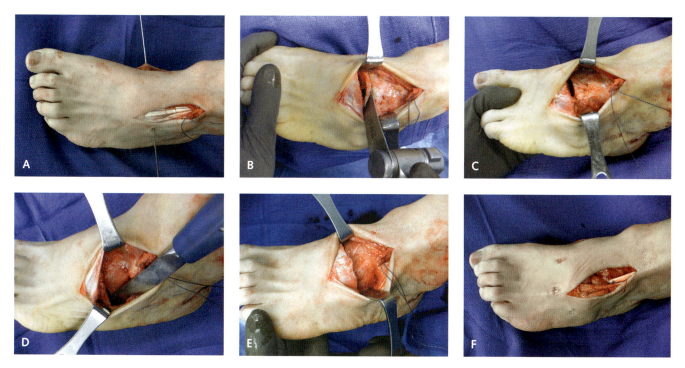

Figure 15-14 A midfoot osteotomy was performed in this patient with a complex cavus deformity and a drop foot secondary to polio. **A,** The level of the osteotomy is marked with a guide pin and checked under fluoroscopic guidance. **B** and **C,** The saw cut is made along the guide pin, and then the wedge is made with the saw and removed from the dorsomedial midfoot. **D,** The lateral foot is elevated with an osteotome. **E,** The medial foot is then closed dorsally. **F,** The posterior tibial tendon, which was transferred to correct a drop foot, is inserted directly into the osteotomy, which is then fixed with plates.

Figure 15-15 A and **B,** The apex of the cavus deformity is in the midfoot with quite severe heel varus and forefoot cavoadductus. **C,** Correction was accomplished with a midfoot derotational osteotomy with screw fixation.

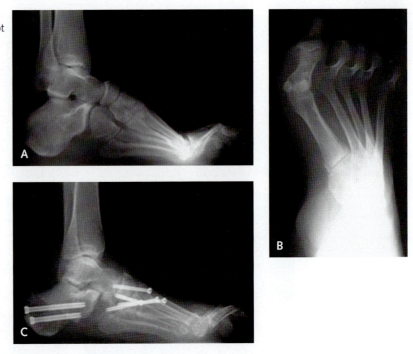

Figure 15-16 A-C, Note the typical forefoot cavus and adductus and the shape of the dorsomedial wedge removed in this foot. The forefoot was corrected at a later stage.

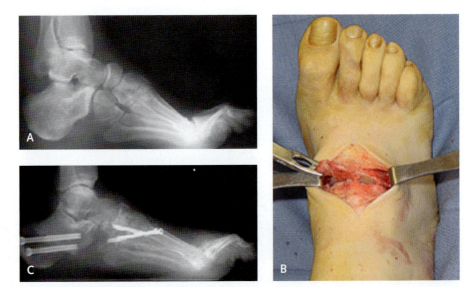

previously discussed, more bone is removed medially than laterally. In fact, it is rare that a wedge is removed from the cuboid metatarsal articulation. I do not favor this procedure because it relies on arthrodesis of the medial and middle columns of the tarsal metatarsal joint for satisfactory outcome. Furthermore, any cavus deformity is rare at the metatarsocuboid joints, and it is preferable and far easier to perform an osteotomy through the cuboid. Such an osteotomy maintains whatever motion is present in the lateral column joints. Fixation of the dorsal wedge arthrodesis from the medial and middle columns can be accomplished using staples, pins, or screws. As with the other wedge procedures, maintain-

ing the plantar aspect of the joint intact at the hinge on which to obtain some axis for the compression dorsally is useful.

CORRECTION OF FIFTH METATARSAL DEFORMITY

Correction of hindfoot deformity is essential if there is excessive stress on the fifth metatarsal (Figure 15-18). With some hindfoot deformities, resection of the fifth metatarsal will be required. In these cases, the patient exhibits tremendous callosity under the base of the fifth metatarsal and absent peroneus brevis muscle function.

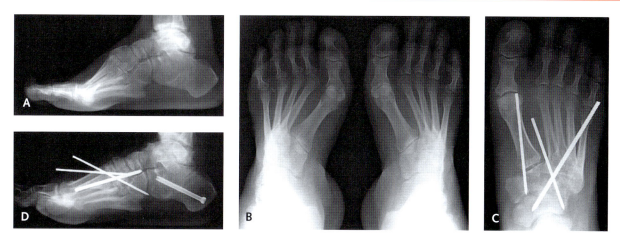

Figure 15-17 **A** and **B,** Cavoadductus deformity. **C** and **D,** Correction was accomplished with a midfoot biplanar osteotomy. Note the use of threaded Steinmann pins for fixation. Internal fixation with screws was attempted, but the plane of the midfoot was not amenable to this type of internal fixation. The pins were removed at 8 weeks, and weight bearing was begun in a boot.

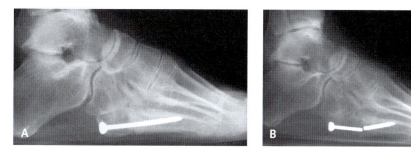

Figure 15-18 Correction of hindfoot deformity is essential following a stress fracture of the fifth metatarsal. **A,** Initially, incorrect treatment was provided for this fracture with fixation without hindfoot correction. **B,** Subsequently, the screw broke, necessitating far more extensive surgery.

These changes frequently are associated with the more severe forms of hereditary sensory motion neuropathy. Although many patients still have sensation, the deformity of fifth metatarsal can be painful. Nonetheless, to achieve better correction with a more plantigrade foot, ostectomy of the fifth metatarsal is a good procedure and can be done in conjunction with any additional necessary procedure (Figure 15-19).

The incision that is used for the calcaneal osteotomy, peroneal tendon procedure, or triple arthrodesis is extended, or an additional incision is made from the base of the fifth metatarsal distally along the course of the dorsal shaft of the metatarsal. A saw cut is made obliquely in the shaft of the fifth metatarsal in two planes so that the starting point of the osteotomy is dorsal and slightly lateral. With this orientation of the osteotomy, no bone prominence remains on the plantar lateral weight-bearing surface. The metatarsal base is grasped with a clamp, rotated on its pedicle, and then is cut sharply by detaching the short plantar ligament and the remnant of the attachment of the peroneus brevis tendon. The peroneus brevis tendon can be detached distally because it is nonfunctional. If peroneus longus-to-brevis tendon transfer is performed, however, then the longus tendon needs to be securely attached to the base of the remnant of the brevis tendon and to the fascia overlying the cuboid. At the completion of the ostectomy, the hypertrophic callus needs to be pared with a large blade. Softening the callus with a moist sponge for some time before it is cut is helpful, because this usually is extremely hard tissue.

On a lateral radiograph, if the fifth metatarsal is depressed relative to the position of the first metatarsal, then regardless of the manner in which the osteotomy or arthrodesis is performed, the fifth ray remains inferior to the plane of the cuboid and cannot be rotated sufficiently or translated dorsally to alleviate the plantar pressure (Figure 15-20). In such cases, removal of the fifth metatarsal is a very good procedure, because the peroneus brevis does not function anyway, and if eversion strength needs to be improved for hindfoot balance, then the peroneus longus can be transferred (Figure 15-21).

POSTERIOR TIBIAL TENDON TRANSFER

For a posterior tibial tendon transfer, it is essential to keep in mind the principles of correction of a cavus foot deformity. Muscle balance must be obtained. In some patients this requirement is obvious, because they have a paralytic deformity such as a footdrop in addition to the cavus deformity. I try to use whatever is available, and in particular whichever muscle is a deforming force on the foot and ankle. This applies to the EHL, the EDL, the posterior tibia tendon, the peroneus longus, and any other tendon that may be used to correct deformity (Figure 15-22). The technical details of the posterior tibial tendon transfer are described in the section on tendon transfers in Chapter 19. The principles of tendon transfers do not differ from those performed for paralytic deformity; however, the incisions must be planned more carefully when calcaneal and midfoot osteotomies are performed simultaneously (Figures 15-23 to 15-26).

Figure 15-19 A patient with Charcot-Marie-Tooth disease and neuropathy had been treated on two previous occasions for osteomyelitis at the base of the fifth metatarsal, and a decision was made to remove the metatarsal in conjunction with a hindfoot arthrodesis. **A,** The incision was made along the peroneals. **B-D,** After exposure of the base of the metatarsal, the metatarsal was cut with a large saw and removed. **E,** The peroneus brevis tendon was still attached to the soft tissues laterally, and after debridement, this tendon was used for a modified Chrisman-Snook procedure.

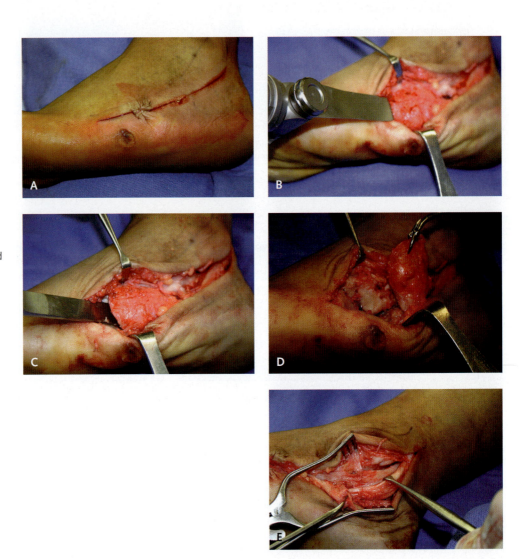

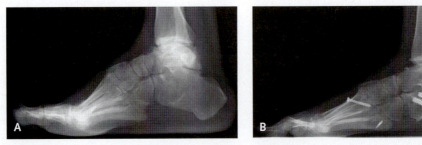

Figure 15-20 A, Severe but flexible cavus deformity was treated with calcaneal and first metatarsal osteotomies and a transfer of the posterior tibial tendon around the back of the hindfoot into the base of the fifth metatarsal, rather than with arthrodesis. **B,** Note that although the overall alignment was improved, the fifth metatarsal remained slightly inferiorly translated relative to the midfoot.

CORRECTION OF RIGID MULTIPLANAR DEFORMITY

Correction of multiplanar deformity probably is one of the more difficult orthopaedic foot and ankle procedures to perform. Not only is the structural deformity associated with bone deformity in multiple planes, but also joint contractures and muscle imbalance are other factors that must be addressed. As previously noted, the approach to correction of this type of deformity involves both structural bone alteration, in conjunction with

adequate muscle, and soft tissue balancing. Frequently, patients with this deformity have undergone multiple previous operations (commonly, a triple arthrodesis performed when the patient was an adolescent). In addition to deformity, ankle instability and ankle arthritis are also present. Throughout this chapter, I have emphasized that arthrodesis of the cavus foot is best avoided whenever possible. In clinical practice, however, such avoidance is impossible with severe multiplanar deformity, and arthrodesis is commonly performed in addition to osteotomy and ostectomy (Figures 15-27 to 15-29).

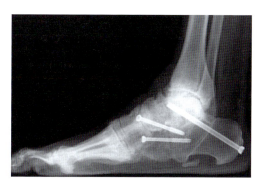

Figure 15-21 Postoperative radiographic appearance after removal of the fifth metatarsal. Although ankle arthritis was present, the joint was painless, and the foot was quite plantigrade.

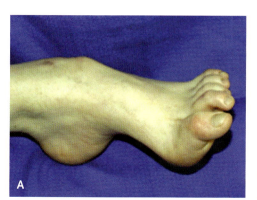
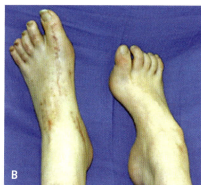
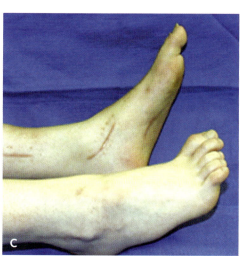
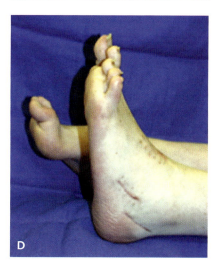

Figure 15-22 A, Bilateral severe cavo-adductus deformity, associated with footdrop on the left, in a 54-year-old patient with Charcot-Marie-Tooth disease. B-D, Correction of the dropfoot was accomplished with posterior tibial tendon transfer through the interosseous membrane into the cuboid, combined with calcaneus and first metatarsal osteotomies, and plantar fascia release. The patient eventually became completely brace-free and was able to ambulate independently.

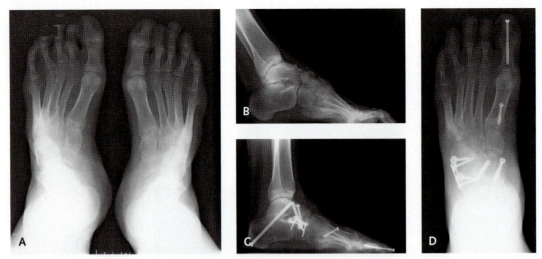

Figure 15-23 A and **B,** A rigid hindfoot deformity in a patient with Charcot-Marie-Tooth disease. **C** and **D,** Treatment consisted of a triple arthrodesis, a transfer of the posterior tibial tendon, first metatarsal osteotomy, and lesser toe interphalangeal arthrodesis.

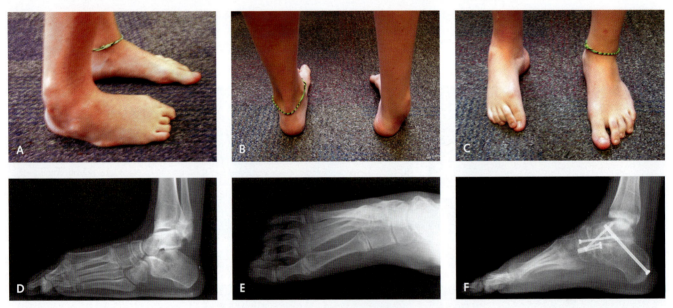

Figure 15-24 A-E, Severe equinocavovarus deformity secondary to a compartment syndrome of the foot and leg in an adolescent girl. Note the severe contracture of the posterior tibial tendon, the contractures of all of the intrinsics including the flexor hallucis brevis, and in addition to the hindfoot deformity, elevation of the first metatarsal. **F,** Treatment was accomplished with excision of the posterior tibial tendon and muscle, a triple arthrodesis, a transfer of the anterior tibial tendon to the lateral cuneiform, and a transfer of the flexor hallucis longus to the first metatarsal (a reverse Jones procedure).

15

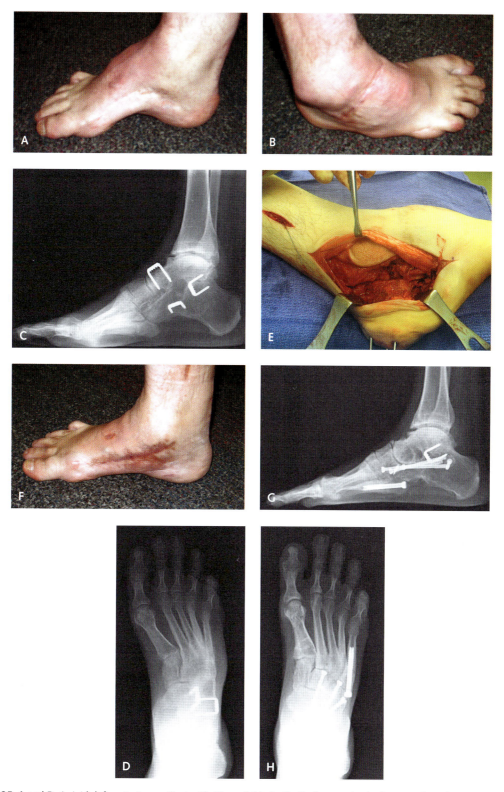

Figure 15-25 A and **B,** A rigid deformity in a patient with Charcot-Marie-Tooth disease who had previously undergone a triple arthrodesis. **C** and **D,** Note the persistent hindfoot deformity, the cavus orientation of the foot, and the stress fracture of the fifth metatarsal. Revision surgery and repair consisted of a transfer of the posterior tibial tendon, a revision of the triple arthrodesis, a modified Chrisman-Snook procedure, and open reduction–internal fixation of the base of the fifth metatarsal. **E,** The lateral incision with the extensile exposure for the revision arthrodesis and with the peroneal tendons retracted. **F-H,** The final clinical and radiographic alignment.

Figure 15-26 A-D, The clinical and radiographic appearance of the foot and ankle in a patient who had polio in childhood, after a failed triple arthrodesis complicated by avascular necrosis of the talus. **E** and **F,** Treatment consisted of a transfer of the posterior tibial tendon and a tibiotalocalcaneal arthrodesis. Note also the resection of the fifth metatarsal on the lateral radiograph **(E).**

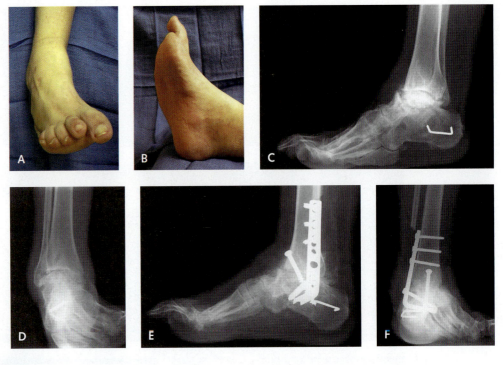

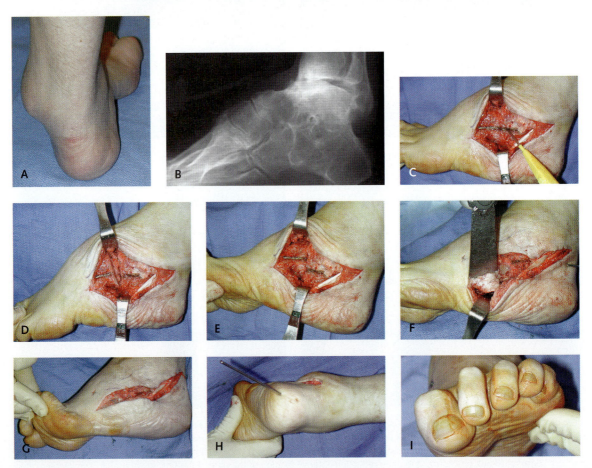

Figure 15-27 A and **B,** This severe complex multiplanar deformity developed after a failed triple arthrodesis. In addition to a transfer of the posterior tibial tendon, a revision triple arthrodesis with excision of the base of the fifth metatarsal and first metatarsal osteotomy was performed. **C,** After lateral exposure is obtained, an electrocautery marking is made horizontally over the apex of the deformity. **D,** The biplanar wedge osteotomy is made through the hindfoot. **E,** Once the cut is completed, the hindfoot is derotated, with observation of the change in the position of the cautery marking. **F,** The base of the fifth metatarsal was still prominent and was excised. **G** and **I,** The alignment of the foot was then checked in all planes before fixation; because of increased plantar flexion of the first metatarsal, a dorsiflexion osteotomy was performed.

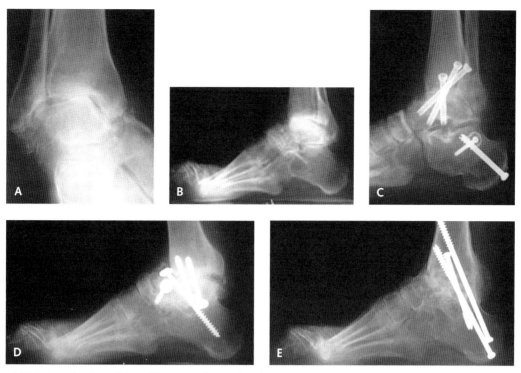

15

Figure 15-28 An arthrodesis of the ankle is a good procedure for correction of fixed ankle deformity and arthritis, and this can be performed as an isolated procedure, as shown in **A** to **C,** or as part of a tibiotalocalcaneal arthrodesis, as in **D** and **E.** Note the addition of the calcaneus osteotomy to the ankle arthrodesis. The hindfoot was not completely corrected with the tibiotalocalcaneal revision; however, the foot was quite plantigrade.

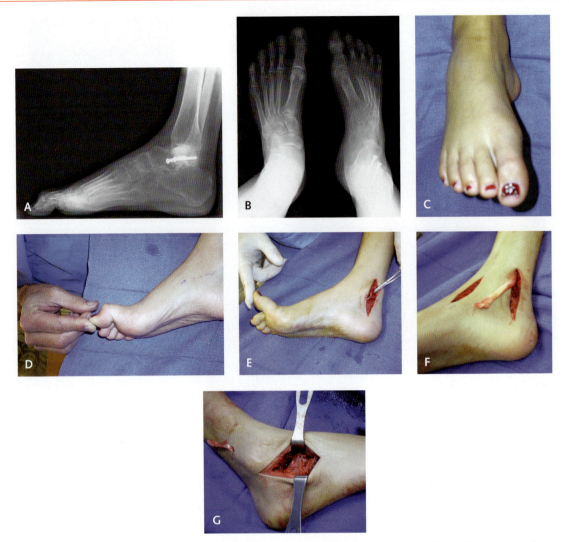

Figure 15-29 A-C, This deformity was secondary to a talus fracture associated with avascular necrosis and development of a compartment syndrome of the foot with tethering of the flexor hallucis longus (FHL). **D,** Note the contracture of the FHL with the hallux passively dorsiflexed. **E,** The FHL was first lengthened, resulting in improved dorsiflexion without hallux contracture. **F** and **G,** A transfer of the posterior tibial tendon was performed to the cuboid through the interosseous membrane and combined with a triple arthrodesis.

TECHNIQUES, TIPS, AND PITFALLS

- Avoid arthrodesis whenever possible.

- I balance the hindfoot, making sure that I slightly weaken the strong inversion and strengthen eversion. This procedure can be made with a posterior tibial tendon transfer through the interosseous membrane to correct an equinocavovarus deformity or posteriorly to augment a weak or absent peroneus brevis muscle (see Figure 15-24).

- A plantar fascia release invariably needs to be performed and should be done before a calcaneal osteotomy, because the calcaneus cannot be manipulated into valgus while the fascia is tight.

- Calcaneal osteotomy is performed in a biplanar or triplanar manner according to the pitch angle of the calcaneus. This is effected by a closing wedge osteotomy laterally, then shifting the calcaneus farther laterally, then allowing the calcaneal tuberosity to slide slightly cephalad, and improving the pitch angle if necessary.

- Always be on the lookout for an unstable ankle in the setting of a cavus foot. This varus deformity of the hindfoot creates an added load on the ankle and on the lateral aspect of the fifth metatarsal. Stress manipulation with radiographs should be performed preoperatively or intraoperatively.

- Be aware of the triad of a varus heel, ankle instability, and a stress fracture of the fifth metatarsal.

- In the setting of rigid varus deformity with hypertrophy of the base of the fifth metatarsal and thickened callosity, even with good correction of the hindfoot, the prominence under the base of the fifth metatarsal persists. This persistent prominence is due to inferior subluxation of the fifth metatarsal under the fourth metatarsal, which can only be corrected to a derotational osteotomy of the entire midfoot. Even with this osteotomy, the first metatarsal sometimes is still prominent. For this reason, in a correction of a rigid cavus deformity with a fifth metatarsal prominence, I am inclined to resect the base of the fifth metatarsal completely. Resection of the proximal third of the metatarsal recreates a smooth lateral weight-bearing surface of the foot. Generally, the peroneus brevis muscle is not functioning at all, and these rigid cavus deformities usually are corrected by arthrodesis. Therefore the function of the peroneus brevis muscle is not as relevant.

- I generally stabilize and correct the hindfoot first and stage the correction of the forefoot deformity. Multiple procedures have to be performed, particularly when the deformity is severe.

SUGGESTED READING

Aminian A, Sangeorzan BJ: The anatomy of cavus foot deformity, *Foot Ankle Clin* 13:191–198, v, 2008.

Krause FG, Wing KJ, Younger AS: Neuromuscular issues in cavovarus foot, *Foot Ankle Clin* 13:243–258, vi, 2008.

Mubarak SJ, Van Valin SE: Osteotomies of the foot for cavus deformities in children, *J Pediatr Orthop* 29:294–299, 2009.

Olney B: Treatment of the cavus foot. Deformity in the pediatric patient with Charcot-Marie-Tooth, *Foot Ankle Clin* 5:305–315, 2000.

Sammarco GJ, Taylor R: Combined calcaneal and metatarsal osteotomies for the treatment of cavus foot, *Foot Ankle Clin* 6:533–543, vii, 2001.

Ward CM, Dolan LA, Bennett DL, et al: Long-term results of reconstruction for treatment of a flexible cavovarus foot in Charcot-Marie-Tooth disease, *J Bone Joint Surg Am* 90:2631–2642, 2008.

Wulker N, Hurschler C: Cavus foot correction in adults by dorsal closing wedge osteotomy, *Foot Ankle Int* 23:344–347, 2002.

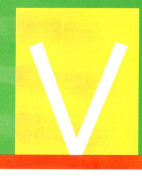

Correction of Paralytic Deformity

V

CHAPTER 16

Tendon Transfers for Management of Paralytic Deformity

OVERVIEW OF TENDON TRANSFERS

The correction of foot and ankle deformity by means of a properly performed tendon transfer can be satisfying for both the surgeon and the patient. The goal of any tendon transfer is to create a stable, functioning, and plantigrade foot. This goal applies to every tendon transfer performed for paralysis as well, because the correction of deformity, the improvement of function, and the establishment of a plantigrade foot are essential.

ANATOMY AND RELATED CONSIDERATIONS

From a simplistic perspective, any muscle (tendon) that passes anterior to the ankle joint axis functions as a dorsiflexor, and conversely, any muscle or tendon passing posterior to the axis of the ankle is a plantar flexor. This is important because the peroneal tendon and the posterior tibial tendon (PTT) are plantar flexors of the ankle, although their function is thought of primarily in terms of inversion and eversion. If a tendon lies centrally, in the axis of a joint, it exerts little influence on the motion of that joint. Conversely, the greater the distance a tendon lies from a joint axis, the greater force it exerts across the joint because of the longer lever arm. This is relevant, for example, in transfer of the PTT through the interosseous membrane. The transfer is performed subcutaneously, and the tendon is not passed inferior (deep) to the retinaculum, because this would decrease power.

The tibialis anterior muscle lies almost directly on top of the subtalar joint axis, but because it inserts on the medial cuneiform, it has an accessory function of inversion. At times, however, the tibialis anterior can become a primary invertor of the foot—for

example, in the absence of a functioning tibialis posterior muscle. The Achilles tendon lies posterior to the ankle joint axis and provides the primary plantar flexion strength for the ankle. It also normally lies slightly medial to the subtalar joint axis and therefore is a weak invertor of the subtalar joint. This effect is negated with long-standing absence of the tibialis posterior muscle, in which case the peroneal tendons then pull the heel into valgus, potentiated by the valgus force of the Achilles tendon insertion. In patients with this deformity, the position of the Achilles tendon and thus the force of the gastrocnemius muscle have to be normalized by a medial translational osteotomy of the calcaneus, in addition to any tendon transfer performed.

The PTT and the peroneal tendon form a force couple around the ankle that controls hindfoot inversion and eversion. The PTT lies posterior to the ankle joint axis and medial to the subtalar axis. It therefore plantar-flexes the ankle and inverts the hindfoot, in contrast to the peroneal tendons, which plantar flex the ankle and evert the hindfoot. Paralysis of a component of this force couple allows overpull of the antagonist, resulting in varus or valgus malalignment. Although the balance of inversion and eversion may depend on the relationship between the peroneus brevis muscle and the tibialis posterior muscle, the accessory inversion of the tibialis anterior muscle and the eversion of the peroneus longus muscle (and the gastrocnemius-soleus muscle as outlined earlier) must be considered.

In planning any tendon transfer procedure, the following factors must be considered: the relative muscle strengths and tendon excursion of every functioning muscle, no matter how weak it may appear; the positioning of the tendon to be transferred relative to the rest of the foot; the proper tensioning of a transferred tendon; and the pull-out strength necessary to secure the tendon transfer. Optimally, a tendon transfer should approximate the strength and excursion of the motor unit that it is being used to replace, but such equivalent substitution can be rarely accomplished using a single tendon. Accordingly, expecting the extensor hallucis longus (EHL) muscle to replace the tibialis anterior muscle, or the flexor digitorum longus muscle to replace the tibialis posterior muscle, is unrealistic. Such a replacement can be difficult if not impossible when an attempt is made to compensate for paralysis of the strongest muscles, such as the tibialis anterior or gastrocnemius-soleus, when multiple tendon transfers may be required.

Also, it is important to consider that most muscles will lose a grade of power when transferred, particularly if the transferred tendon is not phasic (a tendon that is primarily a flexor and is transferred to function as an extensor). As an example, a PTT transfer to the dorsum of the foot to regain dorsiflexion strength is not phasic, and muscle power is lost. By contrast, if the PTT is transferred behind the ankle to the peroneal muscles to augment eversion, it is not functioning at a mechanical disadvantage because it has been kept posterior to the ankle axis. Use of a muscle that is phasic is always preferable because less "reeducation" of the muscle is required, rehabilitation is facilitated, and less strength of the muscle is lost in the transfer. Typically, in a PTT transfer for correction of a flaccid paralysis in which the tendon is passed through the interosseous membrane to the dorsum of the foot, at least one grade of muscle strength is lost. The same applies with another, nonphasic transfer such as use of the peroneal muscle(s) to substitute for absent ankle dorsiflexion. The peroneal muscle does not need to pass through the interosseous membrane (as with the PTT transfer), however, and these muscles can be passed more directly over the fibula to the anterior foot. Although this is a nonphasic transfer, less strength is lost than when a PTT transfer is used because the change in direction of the tendon transfer is minimized.

How tight should the transferred tendon be when secured to the bone? If the tendon fixed at maximal elongation, the tendon transfer serves more as a tenodesis, although it always stretches out. If it is fixed in its relaxed state, however, it cannot generate adequate tension to pull effectively. Generally, I prefer to insert the tendon under more tension than relaxation, because some stretching out of the muscle always occurs. The converse, however, does not apply, and muscle strength can never be regained if the transferred tendon is too loose. Finally, if the tendon is transferred underneath a retinaculum, which functions as a pulley, the effective tendon excursion (range of motion) is increased. With this transfer, however, the tendon is brought closer to the ankle or subtalar axes, with consequent shortening of the lever arm and reduction in strength of the transfer unit. With a subcutaneous position of a tendon transfer, excursion is decreased, but motor strength is maximized because of the greater distance from the joint axes and the resulting greater lever arm. In general, a tendon is always transferred in a subcutaneous position. Quite apart from the biomechanical advantage outlined here, the likelihood that the tendon ultimately will get "stuck," as has been associated with transfers under the retinaculum, is greatly decreased.

Wherever possible, I perform a transfer using a tunnel with a bone-tendon-bone interference fit of the tendon. A simpler attachment of the tendon to the periosteum is never as secure. Sufficient tendon length must be present to permit its insertion

in the correct location and insertion into a bone tunnel. The options for securing the tendon in the tunnel include an interference fit with a bone peg or a screw, either metallic or bioresorbable, and use of a suture anchor. Sometimes, admittedly, I use both, which ensures excellent apposition of the tendon in the tunnel, with little tendency to pull out of the bone. The fixation of the tendon is very important, because rehabilitation with weight bearing and passive range-of-motion exercises may begin once the sutures are removed, and the strengthening and retraining that need to be initiated may start sooner. Rehabilitation is essential regardless of the type of transfer, although this is easier to accomplish if the transferred tendon is in phase with the muscle it replaced.

Timing of Procedure and Preoperative Evaluation

Recovery of muscle function may occur for up to 1 year after nerve injury. An electromyogram (EMG) may have diagnostic benefit for this determination, but repeat clinical examination during this time is more helpful. Although some muscle recovery may continue up to 2 years after injury, I generally perform a transfer for paralytic deformity at 1 year after loss of function. This timing for intervention is particularly relevant when the foot is gradually deforming because of an imbalance in muscle forces about the ankle. The longer the presence of muscle imbalance, the more likely it is that fixed deformity will occur, and bone correction is required in addition to the tendon transfer. During the recovery phase after paralytic injury, the limb must be protected to prevent progressive deformity. If a protective regimen is not followed, the reconstructive procedure becomes far more difficult, if not impossible, to accomplish. A flexible equinus deformity is far easier to correct than a fixed equinovarus deformity, which may require, in addition to the tendon transfer, hindfoot and forefoot osteotomy or arthrodesis to ensure a plantigrade foot.

In evaluation of patients for possible tendon transfer, ascertaining whether the deformity is static or progressive is important. Whenever muscle imbalance is present, deformity of the foot will eventually occur, and this deterioration will be exacerbated if the muscles used for the transfer itself are involved in the paralytic process. Correction of the foot to a plantigrade position is always possible, even in a patient with a progressive deformity such as that in Charcot-Marie-Tooth disease. If the transfer is performed in childhood, however, the initial balance of the foot subsequently will be lost if the nonfunctioning muscle then strengthens. The key to an enduring result is to create a reconstruction in which the foot is both plantigrade *and* balanced; even if further weakening of the muscles occurs, the foot generally will remain plantigrade.

Fixed deformity of either the foot or the ankle cannot be corrected by tendon transfer alone, although the transfer may be integral to the success of surgery. For example, in a patient with a rigid equinovarus deformity, a triple arthrodesis may be chosen for correction. Although this procedure may initially correct the deformity, if tibialis posterior muscle function remains in the absence of peroneal strength (or vice versa in an equinovalgus deformity), deformity will recur, and a tendon transfer should be incorporated into the treatment plan (Figure 16-1). Any fixed deformity of the hindfoot must be corrected if a tendon transfer is performed. In order to restore passive motion across the joint on which the tendon transfer acts, the joint must be in a neutral position and the foot plantigrade. Once again, it is always preferable to use muscles that are in phase.

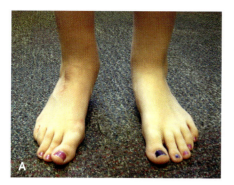 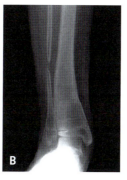 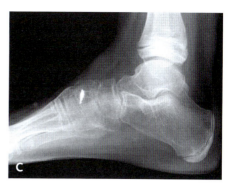

Figure 16-1 A and **B,** Overcorrection of the foot in an adolescent patient with a neuromuscular drop foot deformity associated with severe valgus deformity of the distal tibia and ankle joint. **C,** A supramalleolar closing wedge osteotomy was performed in conjunction with a posterior tibial tendon transfer to the dorsum of the foot. Although active dorsiflexion was regained, valgus deformity persisted despite the tibial osteotomy.

TECHNIQUES, TIPS, AND PITFALLS

- The transferred tendon must have adequate power and excursion. A tendon transfer should approximate both the strength and the excursion of the musculotendinous unit it is to replace. If it does not, the transfer is unlikely to provide adequate power to correct the deformity. This consideration is especially important because most tendons lose one grade of power after being transferred. A musculotendinous unit being considered for transfer should ideally have a grade of 4/5 strength or better.

- The line of pull should be direct, and acute angulation of the transferred tendon must be avoided, to maximize the effectiveness of the transferred musculotendinous unit. The force vector generated by the transfer should not be weakened by undesirable angles or turns around the foot and ankle. Such weakening is a common problem with PTT transfer through the interosseous membrane, underscoring the need to avoid acute angulation of the transfer unit. This precaution also will decrease the likelihood of the tendon's getting "stuck" from scarring or contracture.

- Tendon transfers should be fixed in a bone tunnel, to allow direct action of the tendon on the skeletal structures without a soft tissue intermediary. Tendon-to-bone healing also may be more reliable than tendon-to-tendon healing, especially in cases with underlying tenodesis or atrophy.

- A tendon transfer cannot correct fixed deformity around the foot and ankle. Correction should be done either by arthrodesis or by osteotomy before

restoration of the lost motor function. Questions then arise about when to fuse and when to perform osteotomies. A triple arthrodesis is a good procedure for correction of deformity, but for correction of neuromuscular problems, osteotomies are preferable, and a triple arthrodesis should be reserved for salvage. An arthrodesis does not guarantee that a deformity will not recur, especially if the neuromuscular condition is progressive. In these cases, tendon transfer to balance the opposing force couples is essential to prevent recurrence after arthrodesis. Similarly, tendon transfer cannot correct soft tissue contractures, which should be released or lengthened to allow adequate passive motion of the joint. An example is that of gastrocnemius-soleus muscle contracture in long-standing footdrop. When the PTT is transferred through the interosseous membrane, lengthening the Achilles tendon to provide at least 10 degrees of passive ankle dorsiflexion intraoperatively is essential.

- A potential complication of a PTT transfer is a valgus deformity of the foot. This can occur in children or adults and is difficult to predict (see Figure 16-1). Although typically the result of muscle imbalance, it is also a result from incorrect positioning of the transferred tendon. Either the transfer unit needs to be moved to a more functional position or an arthrodesis should be performed.

- Transfer of the PTT for correction of a paralytic equinus deformity should be performed very carefully in a patient with a preexisting flatfoot (Figure 16-2). Although the transfer is not contraindicated, a

TECHNIQUES, TIPS, AND PITFALLS—cont'd

subtalar arthrodesis may need to be performed simultaneously. Another option is to transfer the PTT and simultaneously move the anterior tibial tendon under the navicular to elevate the medial foot (the same concept as that in the modified Young tenosuspension procedure for correction of flatfoot deformity). The anterior tibial tendon in this instance functions only for tenodesis and can of course stretch out.

- A foot may appear to be very rigid, particularly with a cavovarus deformity, but once the PTT is transferred, the hindfoot "unwinds" (Figure 16-3). For this reason, although I may plan for an arthrodesis, until I have released the PTT and the plantar fascia, I will not

commit to the procedure, because an osteotomy may be quite sufficient.

- Planning a PTT transfer for a patient with additional deformity can be challenging. For example, in a patient with tibia vara and paralytic equinus, where should the PTT be inserted? In the case shown in Figure 16-4, the tibia vara, muscle atrophy, and slightly increased valgus of the hindfoot are the result of absence of accessory inversion function of the tibialis anterior muscle. In this instance I would select a slightly more medial insertion for the PTT transfer than at the lateral cuneiform, which is the more standard position for a PTT transfer for correction of equinus deformity.

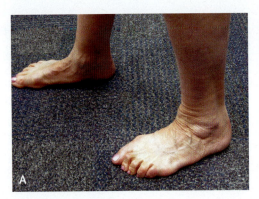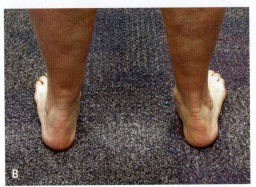

Figure 16-2 A and **B,** The patient had a peroneal nerve injury with a drop foot with a preexisting flatfoot deformity bilaterally. The dilemma in use of the posterior tibial tendon transfer in this patient lay in the recognition that this procedure would exacerbate the flatfoot deformity. In addition to the tendon transfer, therefore, a modified Young tenosuspension of the anterior tibial tendon under the navicular was performed to maintain the arch of the foot.

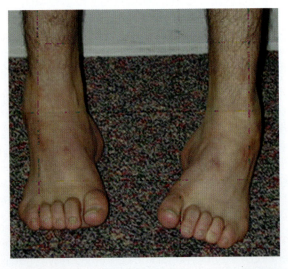

Figure 16-3 A patient with Charcot-Marie-Tooth disease appeared to have a rigid hindfoot deformity preoperatively. After the posterior tibial tendon transfer and the plantar fascia release, however, the hindfoot was quite flexible, and a calcaneus osteotomy was sufficient to obtain a plantigrade foot.

TENDON TRANSFER PROCEDURES

Posterior Tibial Tendon Transfer

I use a four-incision technique for a PTT transfer to restore ankle dorsiflexion. The operation can be done with the patient under regional or general anesthesia and positioned supine. The first incision is made medially from the level of the talonavicular joint to the medial cuneiform to harvest the PTT. The sheath is opened longitudinally, and the insertion of the tendon is exposed. An osteotome is used to remove a small osteoperiosteal flap including the attachment of the PTT to the navicular joint (Figure 16-5, *A*). If possible, an additional strip of tendon with periosteum is harvested distal to the navicular joint. The end of the tendon is then tagged with a 2-0 suture to facilitate transfer (see Figure 16-5, *B*), and the PTT sheath is split longitudinally posterior to the medial malleolus to make passage of the tendon easier (see Figure 16-5, *C*).

The second incision is made medially along the calf approximately 15 cm above the level of the ankle. This corresponds to the location of the musculotendinous junction. Dissection is carried down through the subcutaneous tissue to expose the underlying fascia, which is incised longitudinally, and the tibialis posterior muscle is then palpated while pulling on the distal tendon stump

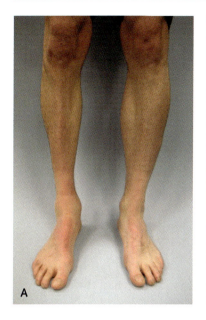

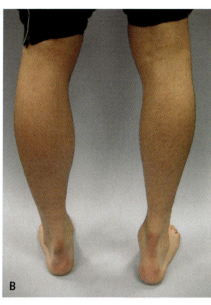

Figure 16-4 A and **B,** What is the optimal insertion site for the posterior tibial tendon in a tendon transfer in this foot? The patient has tibia vara with hindfoot valgus. Because slight valgus is already present, I would insert the tendon into the middle and not the lateral cuneiform. This has to be balanced against the existing strength of the peroneal muscles.

(see Figure 16-5, *D*). The muscle and tendon are then pulled proximally with a finger or a curved clamp. The tendon should be kept moist with a saline-soaked sponge for the remainder of the procedure. The musculotendinous junction should be maintained intact, if possible, without tearing the muscle. The less fraying that occurs, the less likely it is that scarring will develop as the tendon passes laterally.

The third incision is made on the opposite side of the leg just anterior to the fibula and slightly distal to the second incision. The incision is deepened through the subcutaneous tissue, and the superficial peroneal nerve is identified and protected. The muscles of the anterior compartment are retracted medially to expose the interosseous membrane, and a 2-cm window of the interosseous membrane is excised. Care is taken to avoid injury to the underlying neurovascular bundle, which is no longer protected by the tibialis posterior muscle belly. A blunt elevator can be used to gently push aside any soft tissue structures deep to the interosseous membrane. The PTT is "lined up" on the lateral aspect of the leg to identify the optimal angle of passage through the interosseous space (see Figure 16-5, *F*).

A large, curved clamp is then passed in a lateral direction through the interosseous window to grab the tendon or suture medially. The clamp must be held directly against the posterior surface of the tibia, to avoid neurovascular injury. The suture is grasped, and the PTT is passed from the deep posterior compartment to the anterior compartment. Optimally the tibialis posterior muscle belly should traverse the window in the interosseous membrane, rather than the tendon, to avoid adhesions.

The fourth incision is then made over the dorsum of the midfoot. Generally, it is attached somewhere between the middle and lateral cuneiforms, but the appropriate point of attachment will depend on the deformity and the strength of the remaining muscles. The soft tissues and branches of the superficial peroneal nerve are dissected and protected. The extensor tendons are then retracted and the periosteum is incised over the lateral cuneiform. A long curved clamp is passed subcutaneously from this incision to the incision over the anterolateral aspect of the leg. The suture ends are grasped, and the PTT is then passed into the incision overlying the foot. The lateral cuneiform is prepared with a gouge or trephine that

removes a plug of bone corresponding to the diameter of the tendon (Figure 16-6). The plug is removed and the tendon is advanced into the tunnel by passing the suture ends out the plantar aspect of the foot with a long straight needle. If a suture anchor is used for fixation, this should be inserted into the cancellous bone on the side of the tunnel before the tendon is inserted. While the ankle is held in 10 degrees of dorsiflexion, the transfer is tensioned almost at maximal elongation. If necessary, a percutaneous Achilles tendon lengthening should be performed to achieve this dorsiflexion (see Figure 16-6, *C*). The sutures attached to the anchor are then used to secure the tendon into the tunnel. The bone plug harvested with the gouge may then be replaced into the tunnel beside the tendon for further fixation (see Figure 16-6, *B*).

A well-padded posterior splint is applied postoperatively for 2 weeks. After suture removal, a CAM (controlled ankle motion) boot or short-leg walking cast is applied. If no lengthening of the Achilles tendon is performed, then a boot can be used instead of a cast, and active and passive exercises can begin at 2 weeks. At 6 weeks, adhesion of the tendon to the bone tunnel is adequate to discontinue immobilization. A night splint is used for 3 months postoperatively. Physical therapy is initiated at 6 weeks to retrain the PTT to become an ankle dorsiflexor. This retraining may take several months.

A modification of the PTT transfer has been proposed as a "bridle procedure," which combines a standard PTT transfer with anastomosis of the tibialis anterior muscle and an anteriorly rerouted peroneus longus muscle. The procedure is carried out in an identical fashion to that stated earlier, with the exception that when the PTT is brought into the anterior compartment, it is routed through a longitudinal slit in the anterior tibial tendon. An additional longitudinal skin incision is made posterolaterally behind the fibula to expose the peroneus longus tendon. The peroneus longus tendon is transected approximately 5 cm above the tip of the lateral malleolus. The distal limb is retrieved from under the superior and inferior peroneal retinaculum distally and subcutaneously rerouted in front of the fibula into the third incision, described previously. Here it is anastomosed to the transferred PTT, along with the tibialis anterior muscle, with nonabsorbable sutures. The proximal stump of the peroneus longus tendon is then sutured to the peroneus brevis

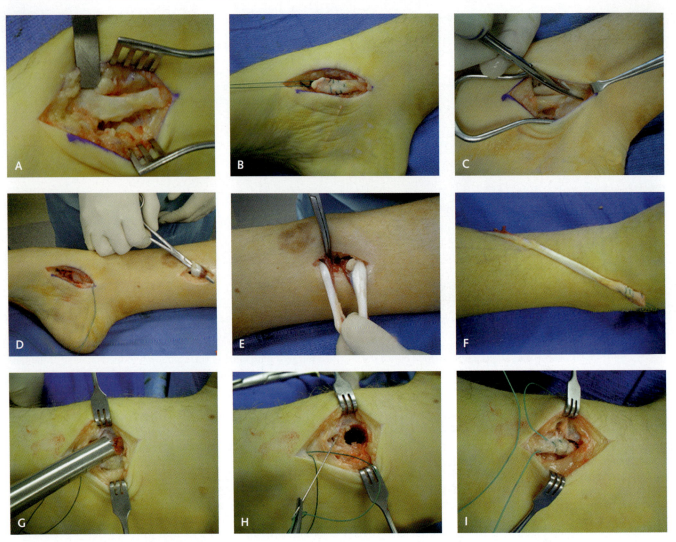

Figure 16-5 The steps in a posterior tibial tendon (PTT) transfer. **A,** The PTT is harvested from the medial foot with a small osteoperiosteal flap off the medial cuneiform. **B,** A suture is inserted into the tendon; **C,** The flexor retinaculum is then released in order to pass the tendon easily behind the ankle. **D** and **E,** The tendon is palpated in the deep compartment, the retinaculum released, and the tendon pulled through into the medial leg. **F,** The tendon is passed through the interosseous membrane and then subcutaneously to the foot. **G,** A 6-mm trephine is used to remove a plug of bone from the lateral cuneiform. **H,** The PTT is passed through the bone tunnel with a straight needle out the plantar skin. **I,** The bone plug is replaced as an interference fit against the tendon with a bone suture anchor to reinforce the insertion of the tendon.

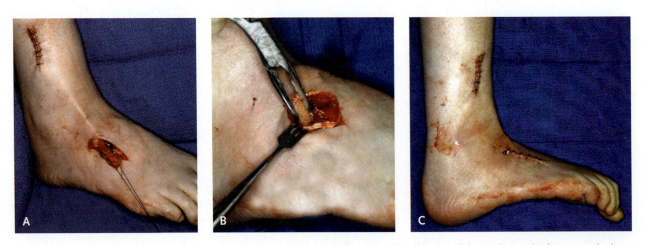

Figure 16-6 In this paralytic deformity, note the subcutaneous angle of the tendon **(A)** and the fixation of the tendon to the foot using the bone plug **(B).** The final position of the foot was in slight dorsiflexion, with marked flexion of the toes as a result of a tenodesis effect on the long flexor tendons **(C).**

tendon. I have no personal experience with this modification of the PTT transfer and have not encountered the presumptive problems with balance of the foot that purportedly are overcome with the bridle procedure.

Transfers of the Extensor Hallucis Longus and Extensor Digitorum Longus Tendons

Whenever possible, a phasic transfer should be performed for correction of deformity. With paralytic equinus, transfer of the extensor hallucis longus (EHL) or extensor digitorum longus (EDL) tendon, used either singly or in combination, is a good procedure. Traditionally, the EHL tendon has been transferred in conjunction with an arthrodesis of the hallux interphalangeal joint. This is a reasonable option when the hallux is fixed and contracted. In general, however, with Charcot-Marie-Tooth disease, the extensor hallucis brevis (EHB), along with other intrinsic muscles, is not functioning, so careful surgical planning is essential, because no active dorsiflexor of the hallux will be left if the EHL tendon is transferred. Accordingly, I use the EHL tendon transfer more frequently in patients requiring dorsiflexion in whom the PTT is not functioning. In some patients, even those who have an active PTT available for transfer, the hallux and lesser toes are fixed and contracted as a result of the use of the extrinsic extensor tendons as accessory dorsiflexors of the ankle. For these patients, transfer of the EHL and EDL tendons is a good alternative, because it simultaneously corrects deformity of the toes.

In some more isolated neuropathies, the EHL may be weak while the EDL is strong. The EDL can therefore be used to support the hallux with a transfer or tenodesis procedure (Figures 16-7 and

16-8). The EHL is, of course, very useful for transfer as an accessory dorsiflexor, to substitute for a weak tibialis anterior muscle. The tendon is inserted in the midfoot, rather than in the first metatarsal as described in the classic Jones-type transfer. Indeed, I do not like to use the EHL to elevate the first metatarsal. It is rarely strong enough, and if the first metatarsal is fixed in plantar flexion, I prefer to transfer the peroneus longus to the peroneus brevis tendon. The tendon is then passed proximally into the midfoot and positioned accordingly. Cutting the tendon distally is not necessary, nor is it ideal to insert the tendon into the metatarsal necks, as previously described; rather, the maximal mechanical advantage, which is obtained when the tendon is transferred into the base of the metatarsals or cuneiforms, should always be sought.

The use of both the EHL and the EDL tendons simultaneously is an excellent tendon transfer to correct for a footdrop deformity when the foot is in a neutral position and not in equinovarus. Generally, if the foot is in a fixed equinovarus position, the PTT transfer is preferable. If the foot is in a neutral position with the PTT and peroneals in balance, then the EHL and EDL can be used (Figure 16-9). For this procedure, I may insert the tendons on the dorsum of the foot, depending on the shape and position of the hindfoot.

Tenodesis of Extensors to Tibia (Stirrup Procedure)

Sometimes a patient does not have any available tendon to use for a transfer, and arthrodesis is neither desirable nor necessary. For these patients, the footdrop may be easily controlled during the day with an ankle-foot orthosis. Household ambulation may, however, be markedly improved with a tenodesis procedure. Tenodesis of

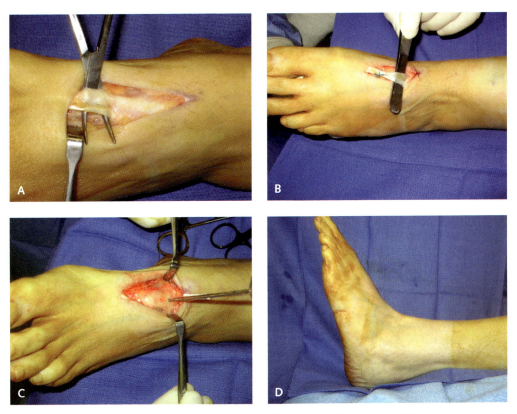

Figure 16-7 A paralytic equinus does not always "follow the rules": The extensor hallucis longus (EHL) and extensor digitorum longus (EDL) may be functioning, while the posterior tibial tendon is not functioning at all. In this case, a transfer of the EHL to the midfoot was performed. **A** and **B**, Before the transfer, tenodesis of the EHL to the EDL was performed to preserve and maintain the extension of the hallux. **C** and **D**, The EHL tendon was then transferred to the midfoot.

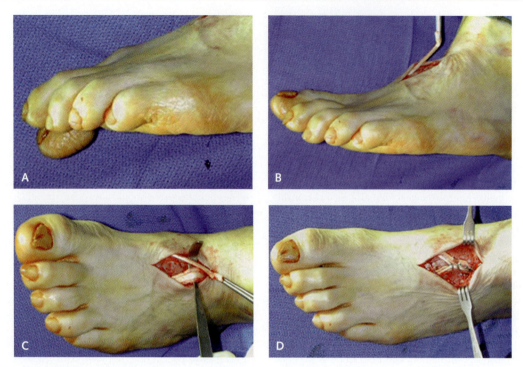

Figure 16-8 Paralysis of the extensors may be patchy. **A,** A peripheral mononeuropathy of the extensor hallucis longus (EHL) tendon in a patient with diabetes caused a drop hallux deformity. The remaining toes functioned well. **B-D,** As an alternative to transferring a functioning tendon into the hallux, a tenodesis of the EHL tendon to the extensor digitorum longus tendon under appropriate tension may be used.

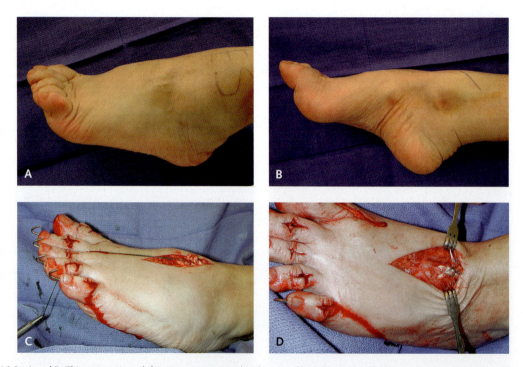

Figure 16-9   A and **B,** This cavoequinus deformity was associated with severe fixed claw toe deformities and a footdrop, but no functioning posterior or anterior tibialis muscles were available for transfer. **C** and **D,** An arthrodesis of the hallux and lesser toe interphalangeal joints was performed, and the extensor hallucis longus and extensor digitorum longus tendons were cut distally and then passed proximally. The tendons were then sutured and inserted through a trephine hole into the middle cuneiform secured by a suture anchor and the bone from the trephine tunnel.

the extensors to the tibia, also called the stirrup procedure, has been used in patients who have flaccid paralysis of all lower leg muscles, usually as a result of polio or low-level myelomeningocele. This procedure can help limit the need for use of a brace and is an alternative to pan-talar fusion (Figure 16-10). The incision is made in the distal third of the leg. The tibialis anterior, extensor hallucis longus (EHL), and extensor digitorum longus muscles are identified and placed on tension to dorsiflex the ankle 10 degrees. If this dorsiflexion is unattainable, then a percutaneous Achilles tendon lengthening is performed. For this procedure, the periosteum of the tibia where the tenodesis is planned is roughened with an osteotome to encourage tendon adhesion to the bone. The tendons are then divided and tagged with nonabsorbable sutures. The ankle is positioned in 10 degrees of dorsiflexion with the metatarsophalangeal joints held in neutral. A staple is used to affix the tendons to bone while tension on the tendon ends is maintained. The remaining sutures are then passed through a drill hole in the tibia and sutured back into the ends of the transferred tendons. Immediate weight bearing with use of a walking boot or cast is permitted. This support can be discontinued 4 weeks postoperatively. This tendon transfer unit may stretch out over 2 years but can be easily tightened again if necessary. Other tenodesis procedures may be considered, depending on the proximity and function of adjacent phasic muscles.

Correction of Equinovarus and Cavoequinovarus Deformity

Many causes for an equinovarus or cavovarus foot deformity are recognized, including Charcot-Marie-Tooth disease, trauma, compartment syndrome, and congenital or acquired defects. The overall approach to correction of these deformities is essentially the same,

with a goal of attaining a plantigrade foot. The tendon transfers for each will slightly different, but whenever the midfoot is fixed in varus, the PTT is a contributor to the deforming forces in effect, even if the tendon appears to be weak or absent. In some patients who have undergone a previous triple arthrodesis with subsequent development of further varus deformity, the PTT has to be active, even if very weak. In these patients, transfer of the PTT may not be worthwhile, particularly if the transfer is to replace a weak or absent tibialis anterior muscle. However, the PTT must be moved from its location to remove the deforming force. At this stage, with recurrent deformity, a revision of a previous triple arthrodesis usually is necessary. It is then a simple matter to see which muscles are working and which are not, and then to combine the bone correction with appropriate soft tissue balancing.

It should be possible to define the functioning muscles simply by looking at the radiograph. Good examples of this concept are presented in Figures 16-11 and 16-12. With the severe equinovarus deformity shown in Figure 16-11, it can be inferred that the tibialis anterior muscle is weak, the peroneus longus is strong, the peroneus brevis is weak, and the tibialis posterior muscle is strong. This is the starting point for planning correction of all equinovarus deformities. In this case, marked clawing of the hallux and lesser toes also is evident. These tendons can therefore be used to add to dorsiflexion strength and also to correct the dynamic deformity at the metatarsophalangeal joints. The same concept applies with the deformity shown in Figure 16-12, which was secondary to a compartment syndrome of the leg in a young woman. In this case, the elevation of the first metatarsal indicates a very strong tibialis anterior muscle and a weak or absent peroneus longus. Similarly, the tibialis posterior muscle is very scarred and contracted, and the peroneus brevis is weak or not functioning. To correct the bone deformity

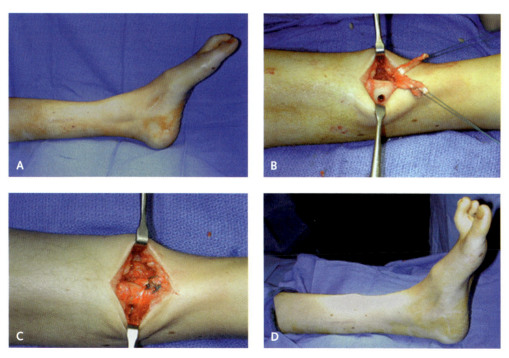

Figure 16-10 A, In a patient with flaccid paralysis with no tendons available for transfer at all, a tenodesis can be performed by attaching the tendons to the tibia. For the foot to be maintained plantigrade, the extensor tendons must be included in addition to the anterior tibial tendon. **B** and **C,** One or two drill holes are made in the tibia, and the tendons are pulled through across the tibia and then tied anteriorly. **D,** Although the foot is in neutral position, note that the hallux is below the level of the lesser toes, which could be averted with the extensor hallucis longus tendon in the tenodesis procedure.

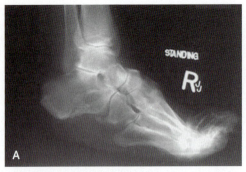

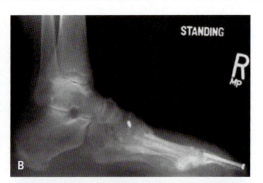

Figure 16-11 A-C, This paralytic cavoequinovarus deformity was corrected with a lengthening of the Achilles tendon; a transfer of the posterior tibial tendon and hallux and lesser toe interphalangeal fusions; an osteotomy of the first metatarsal; a transfer of the extensor hallucis longus and extensor digitorum longus tendons to the midfoot; and a transfer of the peroneus longus to the peroneus brevis tendon.

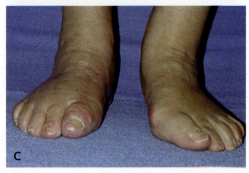

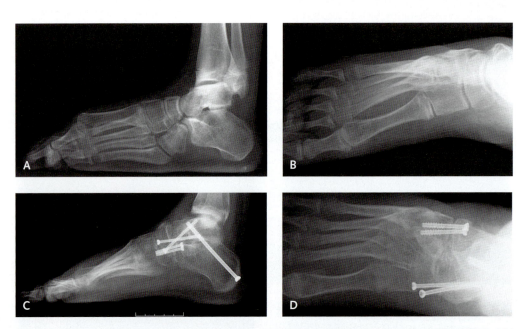

Figure 16-12 A and **B,** A compartment syndrome of the leg caused this severe hindfoot varus associated with midfoot and forefoot supination. **C** and **D,** Correction was accomplished with a transfer of the anterior tibial tendon to the lateral cuneiform, complete release with excision of the posterior tibial tendon, and a triple arthrodesis.

in this patient, a triple arthrodesis is required—this makes sense, because osteotomies are not a practical alternative to correct this rigid deformity. To correct the elevation of the first metatarsal, an osteotomy or arthrodesis may be necessary, but unless the anterior tibial tendon is moved laterally, the deformity cannot be corrected. I would start with the anterior tibial tendon transfer to the middle of the foot, in this case the lateral cuneiform. If the first ray does not come down into a neutral position, I would then consider either an opening wedge osteotomy of the medial cuneiform, or if very

unstable, an arthrodesis of the first tarsometatarsal joint. I do not particularly like the plantar flexion osteotomy of the first metatarsal, because the osteotomy is not performed at the apex of the deformity.

As I have stated repeatedly, an arthrodesis is not a good operation to correct deformity if the muscles are not simultaneously balanced. Without restoration of such blance, recurrence of the deformity is inevitable. Typical examples of recurrence in such cases are presented in Figures 16-13 to 16-15. In Figure 16-13, a

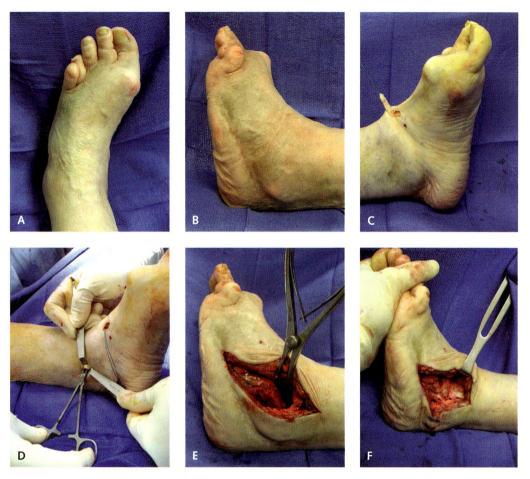

Figure 16-13 A and **B,** Severe rigid equinovarus deformity in a patient with Charcot-Marie-Tooth disease who had previously undergone a triple arthrodesis with subsequent failure. This case highlights the need for tendon balancing even with an arthrodesis. **C** and **D,** Conversion to a pan-talar arthrodesis was achieved with a transfer of the anterior and the posterior tibial tendons to the dorsum of the foot. **E** and **F,** A plantigrade position of the foot was finally obtained with a biplanar wedge resection from the ankle joint for the arthrodesis.

patient with Charcot-Marie-Tooth disease had been treated with an attempted triple arthrodesis with severe recurrent equinovarus deformity. Here again, it can be inferred that the tibialis anterior muscle is weak, the tibialis posterior is strong, and the peroneals are weak or absent. It is not easy to decide when to transfer both the PTT and the anterior tibial tendon. If only the hindfoot is in varus and the midfoot not supinated, then I transfer only the PTT. If, however, the tibialis anterior muscle is functioning, and the midfoot is fixed in supination after the PTT transfer, then I move the anterior tibial tendon more laterally (see Figure 16-13).

The patient in Figure 16-14 had been treated with a previous triple arthrodesis, also with failure as a result of persistent imbalance of the hindfoot, resulting in recurrent deformity as well as a stress fracture of the base of the fifth metatarsal. Correction was accomplished with a revision of the triple arthrodesis, fixation of the stress fracture, but most important, transfer of the posterior tibial tendon. It serves no purpose to correct a hindfoot or midfoot deformity with a triple arthrodesis if the apex of the deformity is more anteriorly located.

In Figure 16-15, the patient's cavus deformity, associated with lack of dorsiflexion, developed after a previous triple arthrodesis. The PTT was not strong enough to use for a transfer, so the EHL and EDL tendons were used to improve dorsiflexion, combined with a revision of the arthrodesis, performed at the apex of the deformity in the midfoot.

Correction of a calcaneus deformity is difficult because so few muscles function strongly enough to compensate for a weak gastrocnemius-soleus. If such deformity is associated with sensory neuropathy, ulceration will develop on the plantar heel, and treatment will require calcaneus osteotomy and transfer of the anterior tibial tendon into the calcaneus. Although the foot is not necessarily stronger postoperatively, it is more functional, and despite the need for a brace, the hindfoot is better balanced. At times, spine injury can lead to odd deformities, as demonstrated in Figure 16-16: a patient with a calcaneus deformity, a weak posterior tibial muscle and strong peroneal muscle.

Correction of Equinovalgus Deformity and Alternative Tendon Transfers

The traditional transfers for correction of paralytic equinus deformity have been discussed thus far. Some patients, however, have variations of equinus deformity for which the traditional tendon transfer is not feasible, and other tendon transfers must be used. This is particularly the case with an equinovalgus deformity, when neither the PTT nor the tibialis anterior muscle is functioning and the peroneals are strong. If no PTT function is present, then, in

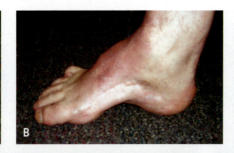

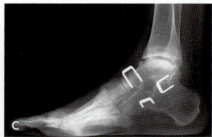

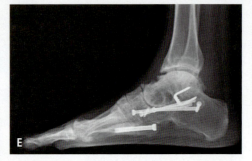

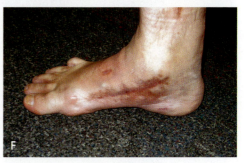

Figure 16-14 A-D, Recurrent cavovarus deformity following failed triple arthrodesis. **E** and **F,** Correction obtained with PTT transfer and revision arthrodesis.

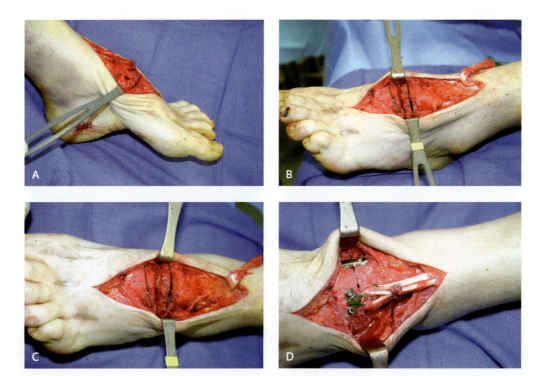

Figure 16-15 A-D, Correction of recurrent deformity after attempted hindfoot arthrodesis. The apex of the deformity was in the midfoot—hence the biplanar midfoot wedge osteotomy with arthrodesis. Both the extensor hallucis longus and the extensor digitorum longus tendons were used in a transfer to improve dorsiflexion. The tendons were fixed to the foot under the plate used for the arthrodesis.

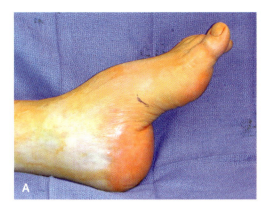
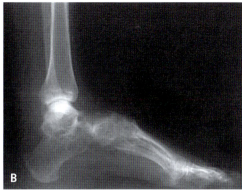
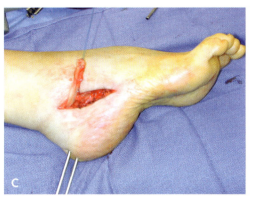

Figure 16-16 Correction of a paralytic calcaneus deformity, regardless of etiology, is difficult. **A** and **B,** The patient presented with a calcaneus deformity and poor push-off strength. The management goal was not to make her brace-free but to improve balance. **C,** A medial translational osteotomy of the calcaneus was performed with a transfer of the peroneal tendons to the calcaneus.

order of preference, I use one or both of the common digital extensors (EHL or EDL tendon), the peroneal tendon, or even the FHL tendon. The need for a peroneal transfer is not that uncommon when the tibialis posterior or other functioning muscles of dorsiflexion are absent. Both peroneal tendons are cut percutaneously on the lateral aspect of the foot, and then the peroneal retinaculum is released. The sheath is completely opened, and the peroneal tendons are transferred anterior to the fibula. The attachment is similar to that described previously for the PTT. Because no other functioning muscle is present, the tendons are always inserted in the middle of the foot into the lateral cuneiform. An osteotomy of the calcaneus (with medial translation) usually has to be performed

simultaneously to correct the hindfoot valgus, which is invariably present (Figures 16-17 to 16-19).

An interesting transfer is the use of the FHL tendon to correct equinus deformity. This is, of course, a nonphasic transfer, but the FHL tendon may be used if all else fails or if no alternative muscle is available. Many surgeons are familiar with its use to augment or substitute for a deficient gastrocnemius muscle or to augment a chronic rupture of the Achilles tendon. When the FHL tendon is used in this way, the transfer is phasic, unlike with use of the FHL tendon to substitute for a paralytic equinus deformity. It does work, although not with the same strength as that afforded by the PTT under similar circumstances.

Figure 16-17 A and **B,** Equinovalgus deformity in a patient with no functioning tibialis posterior or tibialis anterior muscle. In addition to a transfer of the extensor hallucis longus and extensor digitorum longus tendons, a peroneal transfer was planned in conjunction with a medial translational calcaneus osteotomy. **C** and **D,** The result at 1 year with active dorsiflexion **(C)** and plantar flexion **(D).**

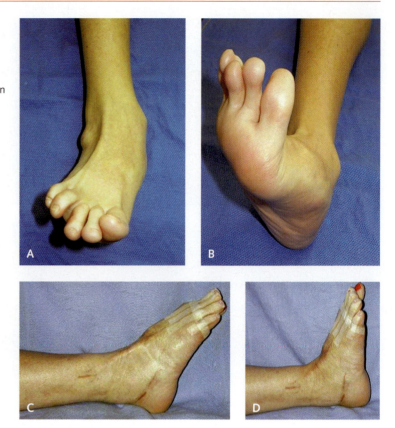

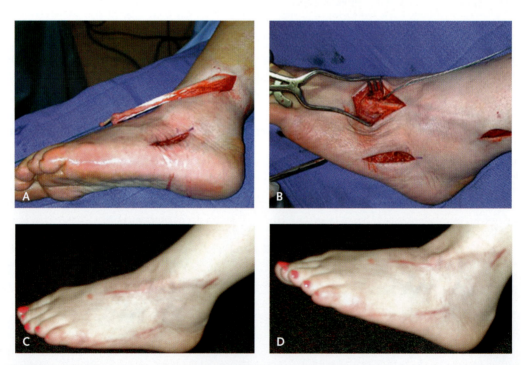

Figure 16-18 A and **B,** The patient had little functioning dorsiflexion, with a marked equinovalgus deformity of the foot. A single lateral incision was used to perform a triplanar osteotomy of the calcaneus and harvest the peroneal tendons for transfer into the middle cuneiform. **C** and **D,** Active plantar flexion and dorsiflexion 6 weeks after peroneal tendon transfer and calcaneus osteotomy.

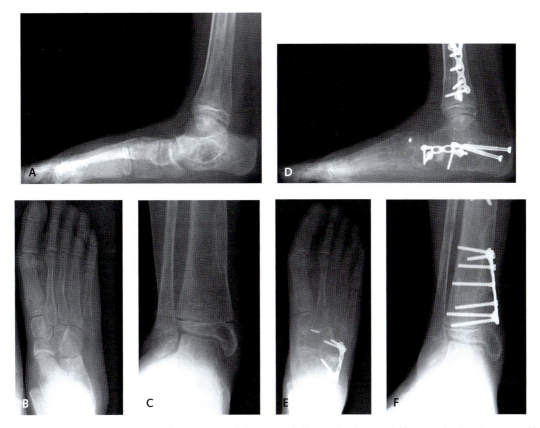

Figure 16-19 A-C, A rigid equinovalgus deformity in an adolescent with fibrous dysplasia. In addition to the footdrop caused by peroneal nerve injury, note the valgus deformity of the ankle, the hindfoot valgus, and the flatfoot. **D-F,** Correction was accomplished with a closing wedge osteotomy of the distal tibia, a calcaneus osteotomy, a lengthening arthrodesis of the calcaneocuboid joint, resection of a tarsal coalition, and a transfer of the peroneal tendons to the dorsum of the foot.

SUGGESTED READING

Hsu JD, Hoffer MM: Posterior tibial tendon transfer anteriorly through the interosseous membrane, *Clin Orthop Mar-Apr* :202–204, 1978.

Rath S, Schreuders TA, Selles RW: Early postoperative active mobilisation versus immobilisation following tibialis posterior tendon transfer for foot-drop correction in patients with Hansen's disease, *J Plast Reconstr Aesthet Surg* 63:554–560, 2010.

Rodriguez RP: The bridle procedure in the treatment of paralysis of the foot, *Foot Ankle* 13:63–69, 1992.

Vigasio A, Marcoccio I, Patelli A, et al: New tendon transfer for correction of drop-foot in common peroneal nerve palsy, *Clin Orthop Relat Res* 466:1454–1466, 2008.

Wagenaar FC, Louwerens JW: Posterior tibial tendon transfer: Results of fixation to the dorsiflexors proximal to the ankle joint, *Foot Ankle Int* 28:1128–1142, 2007.

Wenz W, Bruckner T, Akbar M: Complete tendon transfer and inverse Lambrinudi arthrodesis: Preliminary results of a new technique for the treatment of paralytic pes calcaneus, *Foot Ankle Int* 29:683–689, 2008.

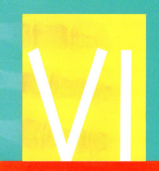

CHAPTER **17**

Correction of Flatfoot Deformity in the Child

Pes planus is a common problem, and although the condition is predominantly idiopathic, in children it may be associated with neuromuscular disease and other disorders including tarsal coalition and the accessory navicular syndrome. The discussion in this chapter is limited to the flexible flatfoot, with or without the presence of an accessory navicular. By and large, similar principles of correction apply to treatment of flexible flatfoot in the child and to management of flatfoot in the adult, with the exception that a rupture of the posterior tibial tendon is not encountered in children, in whom rigid deformities are less common as well.

The difficulty in management of the flatfoot deformity in childhood is to know for whom and when treatment is required. Children who have severe flexible flatfeet, and who are symptomatic but have not responded well to management with orthoses, will require surgery. With those children who have severe flatfoot deformity but are asymptomatic, whether to persevere with nonoperative treatment or to proceed to surgical correction becomes a difficult decision. The adolescent with severe flatfoot who has a sibling or a parent with similar deformity that was not helped by orthoses also may benefit from earlier surgery. I find it helpful to examine the child every 6 months, to get a "feel" for the severity of the deformity and to look for any progression of the deformity or symptoms. There are of course children with asymptomatic flatfoot, whose parents are anxious about the shape of the feet, but who clearly do not require any treatment at all. With the passage of time, flexible feet in pediatric patients will become more rigid; this may happen in early adolescence or young adulthood. Adaptive changes inevitably take place in the hindfoot that alter its relationship with the forefoot. In order to keep the foot plantigrade, as the hindfoot everts and the calcaneus moves into valgus, the forefoot has to supinate. The Achilles tendon moves laterally with the calcaneus, and the axis of force on the subtalar joint changes, increasing the likelihood of a contracture of the gastrocnemius-soleus. As these structural changes take place, rigidity increases, and of course, the surgical treatment alternatives become bewilderingly complex.

In the young child with a symptomatic flexible flatfoot, I hope to reduce the hindfoot into neutral with a subtalar arthroereisis, with or without a lengthening of the gastrocnemius. If the forefoot is supinated with reduction of the hindfoot deformity, then it is useful to add a plantar flexion osteotomy of the medial cuneiform to maintain the forefoot in a plantigrade position. The many variations of this basic deformity must be appreciated; in some children, for example, the heel is in far more valgus, for which a subtalar arthroereisis does not provide sufficient correction, so a medial translational osteotomy of the calcaneus is required either as an isolated procedure or in addition to the arthroereisis. As the aforementioned adaptive changes take place, gradually increasing abduction of the forefoot relative to the hindfoot occurs, and the navicular moves off the head of the talus (uncovering of the talus). In these feet, a medial translational osteotomy of the calcaneus is not sufficient for correction, and a lengthening of the lateral column of the foot is required. Perhaps the most obvious difference in management of flatfoot between children and adults is that in the former, arthroereisis and osteotomy are emphasized, and arthrodesis should be avoided. Unfortunately, arthrodesis still has to be part of the treatment algorithm, because some adolescents will have a very rigid flatfoot, not associated with a tarsal coalition. Each of these procedures is discussed next.

ARTHROEREISIS

Indications and Rationale

The goal of arthroereisis in the child is to properly orient the talus over the calcaneus; the joint is then allowed to remodel. This remodeling is expected to help prevent further problems later in life, such as degeneration or rigidity of the hindfoot. An arthroereisis implant can be considered to function as an internal orthotic device. This procedure has many advantages; most important, however, are the maintenance of motion it affords and the minimal associated morbidity. The indications for arthroereisis in the child are broad.

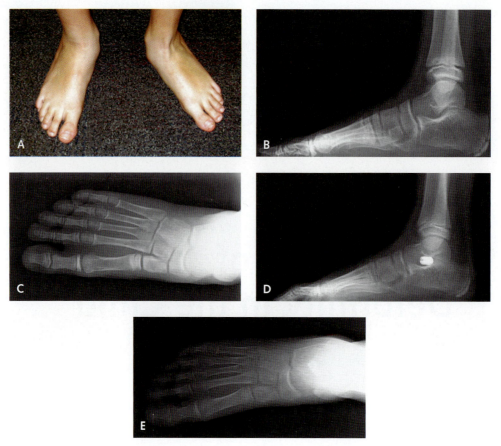

Figure 17-1 The patient was a 9-year-old girl with a painful flatfoot who was treated with an arthroereisis and percutaneous Achilles tendon lengthening. **A,** Appearance of the foot on clinical presentation. **B** and **C,** Preoperative radiographs. **D** and **E,** Postoperative result at 18 months after surgery. The implant was not painful and was left in.

Treatment results for children undergoing arthroereisis have been excellent, provided that the talonavicular joint is not significantly uncovered. The procedure seems to work very well in younger children who have predominantly heel valgus, presumably because they have more capacity for remodeling and adaptation of the forefoot (Figure 17-1). Once the talonavicular joint sags, particularly as seen on the lateral radiographic view, these feet seem to require more correction of the pronation deformity than a medial displacement calcaneal osteotomy can provide (Figure 17-2). If there is abduction deformity of the foot, with uncovering of the talonavicular joint, then neither the arthroereisis nor the medial displacement osteotomy is likely to be successful. In anecdotal reports, in the adult flatfoot, more of the talocalcaneal deformity is corrected with arthroereisis than with the abduction of the transverse tarsal joint. Most important, children are able to bear weight in a boot within days after the arthroereisis surgery.

The pediatric patient typically adapts to the arthroereisis very well, and the incidence of implant failure is low in this age-group. By contrast, in my own experience with use of arthroereisis as an adjunctive procedure in a group of carefully selected adult patients, sinus tarsi pain warranted implant retrieval in approximately half of the cases. In children, however, implant removal has been necessary in less than 10% of the cases, probably because the foot adapts as it matures.

One cause for failure of the implant regardless of the age of the patient is inadequate correction of the forefoot. When the hindfoot is restored to a neutral position with the implant, some supination

of the forefoot occurs. If the forefoot is able to compensate by increased plantar flexion of the first metatarsal, then a plantigrade foot is maintained. If the supination exceeds this adaptive ability, however, then in order to maintain the forefoot in a plantigrade position, the hindfoot has to evert during the foot flat phase of gait. This increased eversion then compresses the subtalar implant, causing pain. For this reason, an opening wedge osteotomy of the medial cuneiform is necessary if supination is excessive.

Surgical Technique

An incision is made in the sinus tarsi, approximately 1.5 cm in length. To locate the exact position for the incision, it is necessary to palpate the "soft spot" between the distal tip of the fibula and the anterior process of the calcaneus. The incision is placed inferior to the intermediate dorsal cutaneous branch of the superficial peroneal nerve and dorsal to the peroneal tendons. A guide pin that functions as a cannula for the arthroereisis dilators and sizers is inserted into the tarsal canal from lateral to medial, pushed through a puncture on the medial foot, and then clamped (Figure 17-3). The anatomy of the tarsal canal must be appreciated: The canal is shaped like an oblique cone and passes from anterolateral to posteromedial. The guide pin should therefore be inserted in the same plane as that of the tarsal canal and not directly medially. A slight resistance to the insertion of the pin can be felt as it traverses the interosseous ligament; then it is pushed through until it is protruding on the medial skin. The clamp on the guide pin prevents

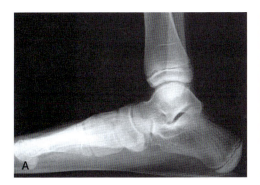 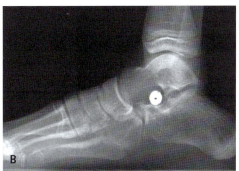

Figure 17-2 Preoperative **(A)** and postoperative **(B)** lateral radiographs of a flexible flatfoot in a 10-year-old patient. Treatment consisted of arthroereisis. No additional procedures were necessary, and the implant was left in.

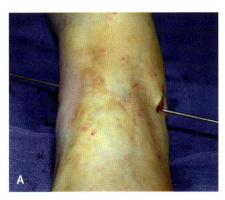 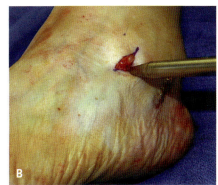

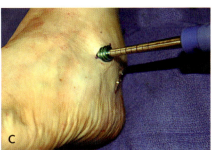

Figure 17-3 In arthroereisis, the guide pin is inserted in the same plane as that of the tarsal canal and not directly medially. The pin is placed through the tarsal canal **(A)**, followed by the dilator **(B)** and the trial arthroereisis implant **(C)**.

loss of position of the guide during repeated insertion of the sizers and trial implants.

Once the guide pin is secure, the first cannulated trial sizer is inserted to get a feel for the position, location, and size of the tarsal canal. The range of motion of the subtalar joint is carefully assessed with each incremental increase in the size of the dilator. The dorsiflexion of the foot now occurs more directly through the ankle joint, rather than in an oblique direction with a combined motion of dorsiflexion and eversion through the subtalar joint. If too large a prosthesis is inserted, motion of the subtalar joint will be limited. An important point here is that the goal of this operation is simply to limit excessive eversion of the hindfoot. If the prosthesis is too small, correction of hindfoot valgus will not be obtained, and dorsiflexion of the foot through the subtalar joint will persist. The appropriate sizer should limit abnormal subtalar joint eversion and allow for a few degrees of remaining eversion only.

The sizer is withdrawn, a trial implant is inserted, and the position of the implant is checked radiographically. The implant should rest between the middle and the posterior facets. On the

anteroposterior view of the foot, the lateral edge of the prosthesis should be 4 mm medial to the lateral edge of the talar neck. If the position of the implant is incorrect, as noted on the anteroposterior radiograph of the hindfoot, then it is easy to adjust the final position by screwing clockwise or counterclockwise in the sinus tarsi.

The range of motion of the subtalar joint is assessed. The eversion with the foot in neutral dorsiflexion should be particularly noted. As stated, the primary goal of correction is to limit excessive subtalar joint eversion. The effect of the implant on the range of motion of the ankle and the position of the forefoot is not as important as the limitation of excessive subtalar eversion. In most young children treated for a flexible flatfoot deformity, insertion of the implant is sufficient to provide appropriate correction. The forefoot should be plantigrade, and no excessive supination of the forefoot should be present after hindfoot correction. If supination is present, an opening wedge osteotomy of the medial cuneiform is an excellent procedure to correct any residual forefoot supination after correction of the hindfoot. A gastrocnemius recession also is commonly performed as required by the presence of contracture.

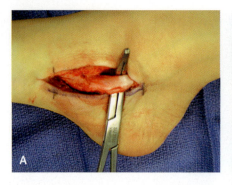

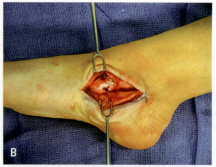

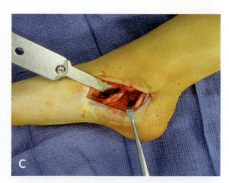

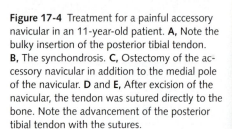

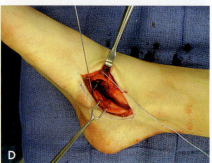

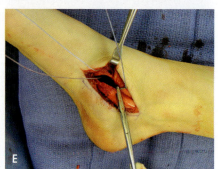

Figure 17-4 Treatment for a painful accessory navicular in an 11-year-old patient. **A,** Note the bulky insertion of the posterior tibial tendon. **B,** The synchondrosis. **C,** Ostectomy of the accessory navicular in addition to the medial pole of the navicular. **D** and **E,** After excision of the navicular, the tendon was sutured directly to the bone. Note the advancement of the posterior tibial tendon with the sutures.

CORRECTION OF THE ACCESSORY NAVICULAR SYNDROME

A painful accessory navicular bone is almost always associated with a flatfoot of variable degree. Although this condition is more prevalent among children, it also can be present in adults, with symptoms resulting from disruption of the synchondrosis. As the synchondrosis is stressed, disruption of the attachment of the accessory navicular bone and thus of the posterior tibial tendon occurs, with consequent proximal migration of the accessory navicular bone. Elongation of the posterior tibial tendon and an acquired flatfoot then occur. In the child, however, the accessory navicular bone can be painful either as a result of stress on the synchondrosis or from pressure in the shoe secondary to an uncorrected pronated flatfoot (Figure 17-4).

Various degrees of deformity and flexibility of the hindfoot are associated with the accessory navicular bone, and these also may require correction. Generally, I decide on additional surgery according to the location of deformity. Such procedures may include medial translational osteotomy of the calcaneus, lateral column lengthening, subtalar arthroereisis, medial cuneiform osteotomy, or Achilles tendon lengthening. Occasionally, if the accessory bone is large, I may use a screw for fixation of a painful os; however, trimming the excess medial bone off the navicular bone is as important as obtaining bone healing. I use screw fixation in the child or adolescent patient only if the bone fragment is large enough, with the aim of accelerating healing with bone-to-bone contact. The rationale for this operation is that because the posterior tibial tendon is not detached from the accessory bone, healing may be quicker (Figure 17-5). The only disadvantage of this procedure is the potential for continued swelling on the medial aspect of the foot. The key to success with screw fixation is generous shaving of the os navicularе as well as the medial pole of the navicular, to decrease the bulk of the bone on its medial aspect.

I use a single utilitarian incision placed medially and open the posterior tibial tendon sheath. The attachment of this tendon cannot be preserved. The location of the accessory navicular bone varies significantly, and the bone must be shelled out completely from the posterior tibial tendon. With the use of a skin hook on the accessory navicular bone, the tendon is then peeled off sharply, and the entire tendon, with the periosteal sleeve, is then preserved. Excision of the entire accessory navicular bone, including the medial pole of the normal navicula, is then necessary. The medial border of the navicular must be flush with the anterior edge of medial cuneiform and the talus so that the talonavicular cuneiform line is corrected. After the ostectomy, the tendon advancement is performed. In the child, the tendon can easily be anchored into the bone using a sharp needle inserted directly into the navicular bone, the cuneiform, or both as the capsuloligamentous tissue is advanced distally. In the older adolescent or the adult, reattaching the tendon with a bone suture anchor is easier (Figure 17-6). There should be moderate tension on the posterior tibial tendon with the foot slightly overcorrected across the midline once the tendon has been advanced. The foot is positioned in slight equinus and varus after the repair, and any additional necessary procedures are now performed. Sometimes, performing either the arthroereisis or the calcaneus osteotomy before excision and then advancing the posterior tibial tendon to get a better sense of the tension on the midfoot is easier. As with all flatfoot procedures, additional correction may be required for realignment of deformity (Figures 17-7 and 17-8).

LATERAL COLUMN LENGTHENING OF THE CALCANEUS

The indications for lengthening of the lateral column are quite specific and include a flexible foot that is amenable to correction. In this context, *correction* implies that the talonavicular joint can be covered with the procedure. The lateral column lengthening procedure does not work well if the foot is stiff. The experienced surgeon will develop a "feel" for what constitutes a stiff foot. On examination, is it possible to rotate and translate the hindfoot? How much

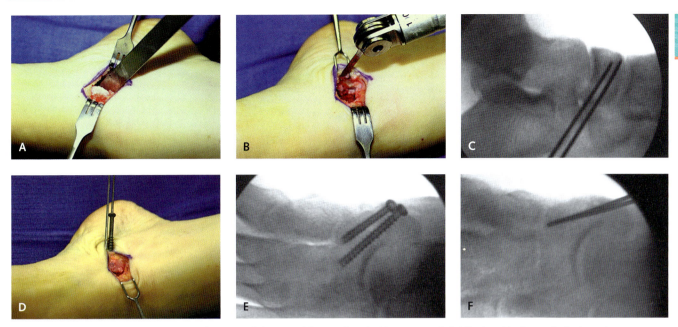

Figure 17-5 Fixation of an accessory navicular in an adolescent athlete. A short incision was used slightly dorsal to the navicular bone to expose the bone. **A,** Note the obvious separation of the os navicular. **B,** The accessory bone is cut further with a saw. **C** and **D,** Cannulated pins are then inserted and radiographs obtained to check the position of the pins relative to the os naviculare and the navicular tuberosity. **E** and **F,** Cannulated screw fixation is used to secure the fragment.

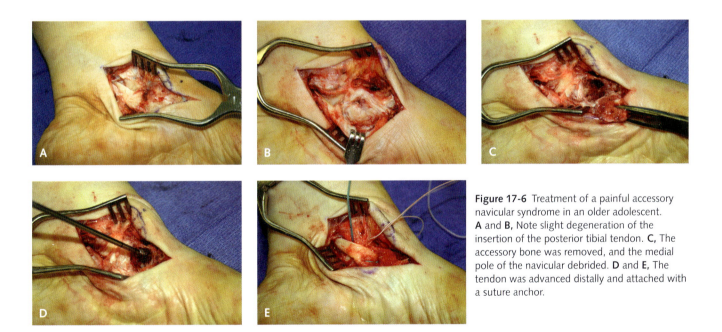

Figure 17-6 Treatment of a painful accessory navicular syndrome in an older adolescent. **A** and **B,** Note slight degeneration of the insertion of the posterior tibial tendon. **C,** The accessory bone was removed, and the medial pole of the navicular debrided. **D** and **E,** The tendon was advanced distally and attached with a suture anchor.

forefoot supination will then occur with either correct orientation of the hindfoot (Figure 17-9)?

As noted previously, the hindfoot position is first corrected with either a medial translational osteotomy of the calcaneus (to correct the heel valgus) (Figure 17-10) or a lateral column lengthening calcaneus osteotomy to correct abduction of the midfoot. A lengthening of the lateral column with an arthrodesis of the calcaneocuboid joint is not performed in childhood. The recommended

approach to lengthening of the lateral column is through a short incision over the sinus tarsi. If the incision is made too laterally over the peroneal tendons, it is harder to insert the graft and visualize the anterior subtalar joint (Figure 17-11). The osteotomy cut is made 1 cm posterior to the calcaneocuboid joint. The position of the osteotomy is marked with a guide pin and checked fluoroscopically. Osteotomy cuts are then made on either side of the guide pin and completed through the neck of the calcaneus.

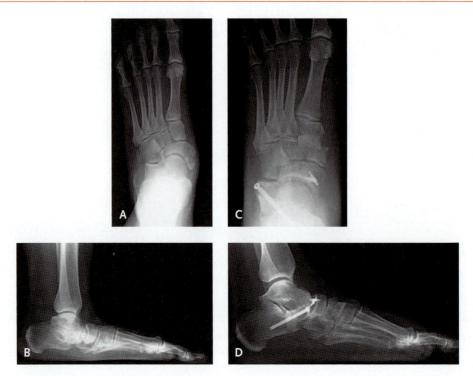

Figure 17-7 Flatfoot and accessory navicular syndrome in a 13-year-old patient. **A** and **B,** Note the marked sag of the foot on the lateral radiograph, and the abduction of the midfoot. **C** and **D,** Both deformities were corrected with excision of the accessory navicular, advancement of the tendon, and lengthening of the lateral calcaneus.

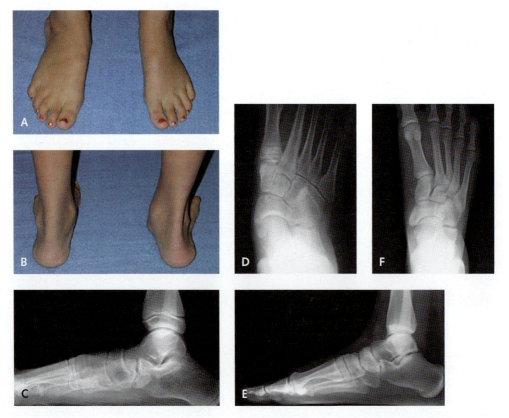

Figure 17-8 **A** and **B,** A marked flatfoot, which was very flexible, associated with an accessory navicular in a 14-year-old patient. Treatment consisted of only excision of the accessory navicular and advancement of the tendon. **E** and **F,** Correction was maintained 4 years later.

17

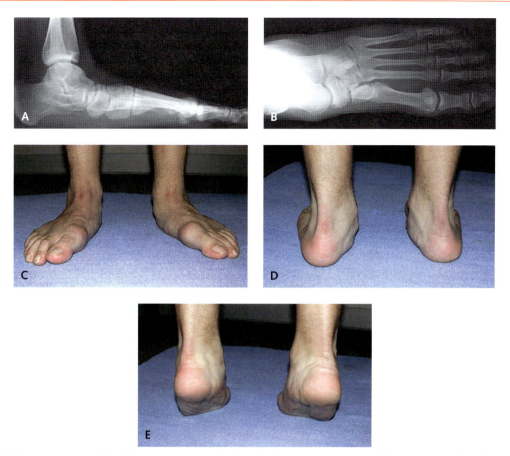

Figure 17-9 In some instances, the flatfoot may no longer be flexible despite the young age of the patient. **A** and **B,** Flatfoot with marked abduction of the midfoot in a patient 17 years of age. **C–E,** Fixed changes with elevation of the first metatarsal and fixed hindfoot valgus are already present, all in the absence of a tarsal coalition.

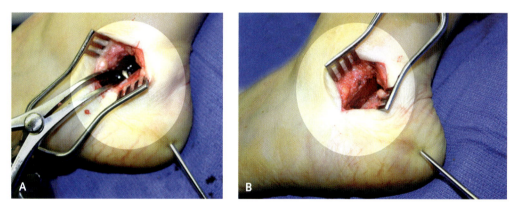

Figure 17-10 For some adolescents who have marked heel valgus only, without much midfoot abduction, a medial translational osteotomy of the calcaneus is a useful procedure. **A,** Here the osteotomy cut has been made, the laminar spreader inserted, and the guide pin placed. **B,** The calcaneus is shifted 10 mm medially.

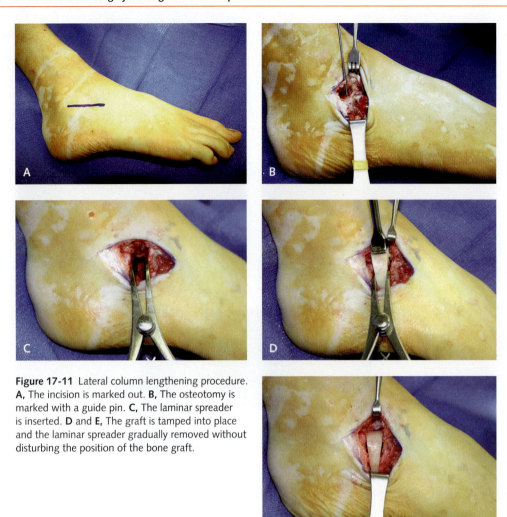

Figure 17-11 Lateral column lengthening procedure. **A,** The incision is marked out. **B,** The osteotomy is marked with a guide pin. **C,** The laminar spreader is inserted. **D** and **E,** The graft is tamped into place and the laminar spreader gradually removed without disturbing the position of the bone graft.

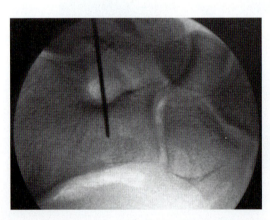

Figure 17-12 Incorrect position for insertion of the guide pin for the lateral column lengthening procedure. The pin is too far posterior.

I do not believe that the osteotomy should be made specifically between the middle and anterior facets of the subtalar joint. With this placement, the osteotomy may be too close to the posterior facet, causing impingement of the graft against the posterior facet. A common error is to make the osteotomy too far posterior

(Figure. 17-12). The osteotomy cut is opened using an osteotome and then a laminar spreader. It may be helpful to use a laminar spreader through guide pins, because the insertion of the paddles of the laminar spreader will interfere with insertion of the graft.

With the osteotomy distracted, the position of the talus relative to the navicular is checked clinically and radiographically, and once positioning is corrected, the appropriate-size graft is cut. I use an iliac crest allograft and have never experienced any problems with incorporation of the graft in children. The size of the graft in children generally is 8 to 10 mm on the lateral aspect of the graft. It is tamped into position, and then a decision is made regarding the need for fixation, which in children is not often necessary. If the repair is unstable, a screw can be used, but subsequent removal often is required if it creates a dorsal prominence. Use of a Kirschner wire (K-wire) is acceptable when it is introduced percutaneously and removed at 3 to 4 weeks. One undesirable result with lengthening is slight dorsal subluxation of the distal calcaneus, creating prominence of the anterior process of the calcaneus subcutaneously. This has not appeared to be a clinical problem other than occasional shoe irritation. One of the more common complications of this procedure is impingement of the graft in the sinus tarsi, which results when the osteotomy is made too far posteriorly (Figure 17-13).

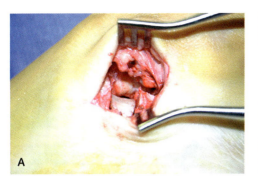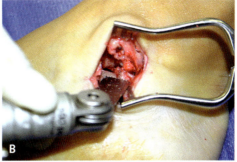

Figure 17-13 **A** and **B,** The graft has been well seated **(A),** but note the impingement between the posterior margin of the calcaneus and the posterior facet, which required ostectomy. The calcaneus moves posteriorly as well as angulating anteriorly with this type of osteotomy, which therefore cannot be made too close to the posterior facet.

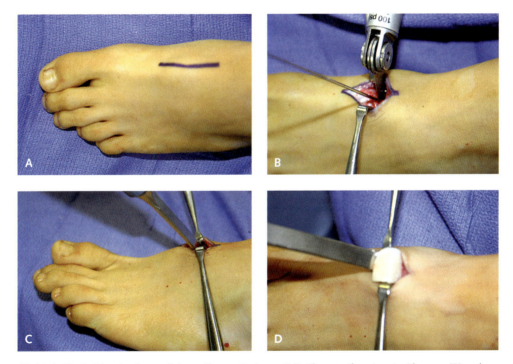

Figure 17-14 **A,** The incision for the medial cuneiform osteotomy. **B-D,** The cuneiform is cut with a saw **(B)** and opened with an osteotome **(C),** followed by tamping the graft securely into the osteotomy cut **(D).**

OPENING WEDGE OSTEOTOMY OF THE MEDIAL CUNEIFORM

The opening wedge medial cuneiform osteotomy is an excellent adjunct to many hindfoot correction procedures, including lateral column lengthening, medial translational osteotomy, excision of an accessory navicular, and placement of an arthroereisis implant. Determining the exact indications for this procedure is difficult, because the capacity of the forefoot for plantar flexion subsequent to the calcaneus osteotomy cannot be predicted. Generally, therefore, if the forefoot is supinated more than 15 degrees, I add the cuneiform osteotomy. The incision is made along the dorsal margin of the medial cuneiform between the anterior tibial tendon and the extensor hallucis longus (Figure 17-14). The extensor hallucis longus is retracted laterally, and the periosteum over the cuneiform reflected. A K-wire is inserted from dorsal to plantar in the middle of the cuneiform, and its position checked fluoroscopically. There is a tendency to make the saw cut too vertically and not along the

axis of the cuneiform. If this placement is exaggerated, the osteotomy may enter the metatarsocuneiform joint. The guide pin should therefore be directed slightly proximally, and saw cuts made on either side of the K-wire. Once the direction of the osteotomy has been obtained, the K-wire can be removed. The osteotomy should be completed up to the base of the cuneiform, and not terminate in the middle of the bone, because a fracture can occur that extends into the metatarsocuneiform joint as the osteotomy is opened. Once the cut is completed, a laminar spreader is inserted into the osteotomy, and as it is distracted, the first metatarsal is plantarflexed, correcting the metatarsal declination angle. I use a structural bone graft and wedge it into the osteotomy. The graft does not need to be wide at the base, usually measuring no more than 7 mm across at the dorsal base of the graft. It is not always easy to insert the graft while maintaining distraction with the laminar spreader, and use of a modified spreader that distracts the osteotomy by means of pins is very helpful. The osteotomy is stable once the graft is wedged into place, and fixation usually is not necessary (Figure 17-15).

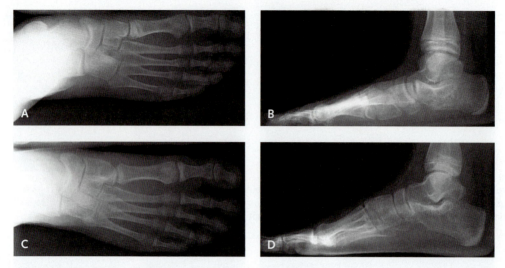

Figure 17-15 A and **B,** This very symptomatic flatfoot in a 13-year-old patient was treated with lateral column lengthening and medial cuneiform osteotomy. **C** and **D,** Radiographic appearance 4 years later.

TECHNIQUES, TIPS, AND PITFALLS

- Sinus tarsi pain may occur after arthroereisis, probably as a result of irritation from the prosthesis, impingement of the prosthesis against the posterior facet, or use of an incorrectly sized prosthesis. This pain also may occur on mild forefoot supination. For the forefoot to remain plantigrade, the hindfoot has to evert slightly, and this eversion causes jamming of the arthroereisis implant.

- If pain is present postoperatively, a boot is used for 2 to 4 weeks. If pain persists, then a corticosteroid injection is administered into the sinus tarsi.

- The implant may have to be removed for chronic pain. Removal of the implant after 1 year is not associated with a reversal of the foot structure.

- The range of motion of the hindfoot can decrease after arthroereisis, and although this decrease is not significant, it is not normal.

- A gastrocnemius recession often is necessary in a child with flatfoot.

CHAPTER **18**

Correction of Flatfoot Deformity in the Adult

Nothing in foot and ankle surgery elicits controversy as much as the "appropriate" correction of flatfoot. To some extent, this controversy has a lot to do with the many satisfactory operations that are available for correction of similar deformities. Because of the plethora of these surgical alternatives, choosing a procedure can get confusing, and at times the surgeon needs to find an operation that works well and then stick with it. This decision does, of course, depend on the severity of the deformity, the appearance of the foot, and the flexibility of the hindfoot and forefoot. Perhaps the most important aspect of decision making is the presence of flexibility in the hindfoot. Specifically, is the subtalar joint completely correctable into a neutral position? If such reduction is possible, can it be achieved without associated significant forefoot supination? (Figure 18-1). The management approach also will differ for a unilateral deformity or that associated with flatfoot since childhood that has more recently become symptomatic, perhaps unilaterally (Figure 18-2). The approach to correction of deformity is based on the flexibility of the foot; the presence of rupture of the posterior tibial tendon, the spring ligament, or the deltoid ligament; and the presence of any arthritis or secondary deformity of the midfoot.

Presented next is a very complete and thorough classification scheme for flatfoot deformity that should help with decision making regarding surgical correction.

CLASSIFICATION OF THE FLATFOOT DEFORMITY

Stage I: Tenosynovitis Without Deformity

In stage I disease, the tendon is inflamed or partially ruptured and may or may not be accompanied by systemic inflammatory disease. In either case, deformity is absent or minimal and the overall continuity of the tendon is maintained. Tendon continuity is confirmed on physical examination with an intact single-leg heel raise and good resisted foot inversion strength with the foot plantar flexed. Stage I is subdivided into three categories:

A. *Inflammatory disease:* Posterior tibial tendon (PTT) rupture that results from a systemic disease such as rheumatoid arthritis and the other inflammatory arthritides is recognized as a separate entity. In stage IA, hindfoot anatomy is maintained and the foot alignment is normal. Surgical treatment consists of tenosynovectomy.

B. *Partial PTT tear with normal hindfoot anatomy:* Care for this stage typically begins with a conservative treatment consisting of anti-inflammatory medications and immobilization in a cast, walking boot, or custom brace.

C. *Partial PTT tear with hindfoot valgus:* Presence of a slight (deviation of 5 degrees or less) deformity distinguishes stage IC from stage II disease. Although care begins with conservative treatment, this stage may represent a more incipient rupture, and the foot should be monitored closely. Surgical treatment consists of a tenosynovectomy and a medial translational osteotomy of the calcaneus.

Stage II: Ruptured Partial Tibial Tendon and Flexible Flatfoot

Stage II disease is defined by presence of PTT tendon rupture, as evidenced on physical examination by a clinically apparent flatfoot, weakness with inversion of the plantar-flexed foot, and inability to perform a single-leg heel raise. Stage II disease is subdivided into five categories on the basis of the most salient feature present. Because some patients exhibit several of the following features, some degree of overlap may exist.

A. *Hindfoot valgus:* In stage IIA, once the heel is reduced from valgus to neutral, there is a varying degree of residual forefoot supination. Treatment options include a flexor digitorum longus (FDL) tendon–to–PTT transfer combined with either a subtalar arthroereisis implant to limit subtalar eversion or a medial displacement calcaneal osteotomy ("calcaneal slide") to reduce hindfoot valgus.

B. *Flexible forefoot supination:* In stage IIB, reducing the hindfoot from valgus to neutral results in forefoot supination because of gastrocnemius muscle contracture (Figure 18-3). However, the forefoot deformity is flexible; if the ankle is plantar flexed to relax the gastrocnemius muscle, the forefoot supination is corrected (Figure 18-4). Recommendations for this stage would be similar to those for stage IIA, but with the addition of an Achilles tendon lengthening or a gastrocnemius muscle recession, depending on the cause of equinus.

C. *Fixed forefoot supination:* In stage IIC, as a consequence of long-standing hindfoot valgus, adaptive changes have occurred in the frontal plane of the forefoot. Thus, although

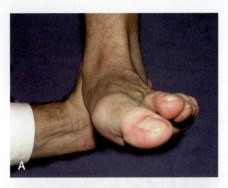

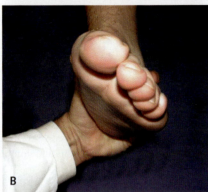

Figure 18-1 A, In this flatfoot, the heel is cupped in the resting position, reflecting the extent of the valgus deformity. **B,** The heel is then reduced to the neutral position, to determine whether the hindfoot is reducible but also to observe the position of the forefoot, which in this case is markedly supinated.

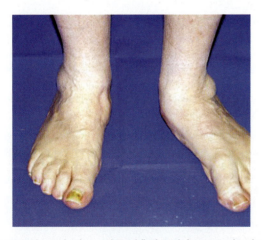

Figure 18-2 This is clearly a unilateral flatfoot deformity and in the adult is most likely due to a rupture of the posterior tibial tendon. Is the foot easily reducible? Where is the apex of the deformity? (See Figure 18-3.)

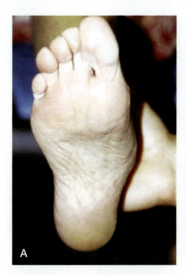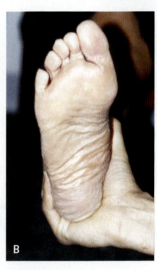

Figure 18-3 A, The hindfoot is in valgus, with moderate abduction of the forefoot at rest. **B,** The foot is very flexible and can be completely restored to a neutral position by holding the heel in neutral.

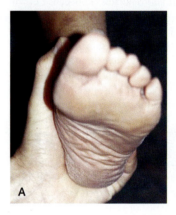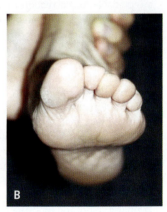

Figure 18-4 A, In this case, slight forefoot supination is apparent with the heel reduced to neutral. **B,** This forefoot supination disappears when the forefoot is held in equinus, thereby ruling out an effect of the Achilles tendon or the gastrocnemius muscle in producing contracture in the foot.

the hindfoot deformity is supple and reducible to neutral, the forefoot deformity becomes fixed once the heel is held in a reduced position. In other words, when the ankle is plantar flexed while the hindfoot is held in reduction, the forefoot remains supinated. The operative treatment recommendation for stage IIC is to angulate the medial ray plantarward to rectify the fixed forefoot supination and restore a plantigrade foot (in addition to the treatment for stage IIA or IIB

disease). Correction typically is accomplished with a dorsal opening wedge osteotomy of the medial cuneiform with insertion of an allograft bone wedge.

D. *Forefoot abduction:* This may occur at the transverse tarsal joint (most commonly) or at the first tarsometatarsal (TMT) joint. The first TMT joint instability can be either a primary deformity or a result of TMT joint arthritis. The simplest way to make this distinction is through examination of the lateral view radiograph for a gap at the plantar joint surface, which is present with primary deformity. Primary deformity of the first TMT joint also may result in secondary hindfoot deformity, including rupture of the PTT. Surgical treatment consists of an FDL tendon transfer combined with a lateral column lengthening procedure such as a modified Evans procedure. This is accomplished with a lateral opening wedge osteotomy of the calcaneus 1.5 cm posterior to the calcaneocuboid joint with insertion of allograft bone.

E. *Medial ray instability:* As in stage IIC (fixed forefoot supination), the stage IIE foot retains forefoot supination with reduction of the valgus heel to neutral. This supination persists even with ankle plantar flexion, as a result of instability of the medial column, and may arise from any component structure of the medial column. It may occur at the talonavicular, naviculocuneiform, or medial cuneiform–first metatarsal joint, or a combination thereof. This situation is similar to that in stage IIA; after the heel is corrected to neutral, however, the unstable medial ray will tend to dorsiflex; this dorsiflexion causes the foot to collapse to pronation, leading to painful subtalar joint impingement. Generally, the treatment used is the same as for stage IID disease. The addition of medial column arthrodesis (naviculocuneiform or TMT) could be considered. This arthrodesis usually is unnecessary for most patients, however, because medial column stability commonly is restored after lateral column lengthening with the addition of an opening wedge osteotomy of the medial cuneiform.

Stage III: Rigid Hindfoot Valgus

Stage III disease generally is associated with a more advanced course of tendon rupture and deformity and typically is characterized by rigid hindfoot valgus. Forefoot deformity also may be present and usually consists of rigid forefoot abduction.

A. *Hindfoot valgus:* Treatment usually consists of triple arthrodesis.

B. *Forefoot abduction:* Treatment also consists of triple arthrodesis, but in certain cases lateral column lengthening with a bone block arthrodesis of the calcaneocuboid joint also may be required to fully adduct the forefoot back to neutral.

Stage IV: Ankle Valgus

Stage IV disease occurs after chronic tendon rupture and is associated with deltoid ligament rupture and medial ankle instability, leading to ankle (tibiotalar) joint valgus deformity. It can occur in the setting of previous triple arthrodesis. Several variants of this condition have been seen. It may or may not be associated with ankle instability and arthritis and a flexible or rigid hindfoot.

A. *Flexible ankle valgus:* In this setting, reconstructing ankle deformity with medial-sided ankle procedures is appropriate. This condition is relatively rare.

B. *Rigid ankle valgus:* This is the more common presentation of stage IV disease. In stage IVA, the ankle valgus deformity is mostly rigid and is almost irreducible. Nonoperative treatment consists of use of an ankle orthosis such as a custom Baldwin or Arizona brace, and operative treatment is with ankle arthrodesis (in the setting of previous triple arthrodesis), pan-talar arthrodesis, tibiotalocalcaneal arthrodesis, or talectomy with tibiocalcaneal arthrodesis.

SURGICAL PROCEDURES FOR CORRECTION OF FLATFOOT

Tenosynovectomy

A tenosynovectomy is indicated in patients who have inflammatory changes in the PTT but do not have deformity. Usually tenosynovectomy is necessary early in the course of the disease process as the tendon is beginning to tear. In some patients, however, an inflammatory tenosynovitis may be associated with a seronegative spondyloarthropathy. I am more inclined to perform earlier surgery in

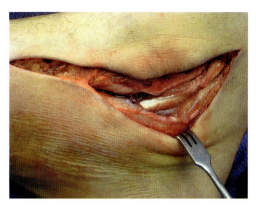

Figure 18-5 Inflammatory changes in the tendon in a patient who had psoriasis with multiple additional symptoms, including pain of 2 months duration in the posteromedial ankle.

these patients, because infiltrative tenosynovitis will eventually cause rupture of the tendon (Figure 18-5). A tenosynovectomy is indicated after failure of nonoperative care, whatever that happens to consist of. The nonoperative regimen generally consists of a period of immobilization in either a boot or a cast, followed by use of some sort of brace or orthosis. In addition, a decision has to be made whether to correct any (mild) deformity of the hindfoot along with the tenosynovectomy.

If, as is probable, tenosynovitis represents the early stage of rupture of the PTT, then some hindfoot deformity also is likely to be present. This deformity usually consists of valgus of the heel, slight pronation at the midfoot, and contracture of the gastrocnemius-soleus muscle. In patients with such deformity, therefore, the performance of a medial translational osteotomy of the calcaneus, along with the tenosynovectomy, may be prudent. Certainly, adding this procedure would be a good idea if minor fissuring indicative of early rupture was present in association with the tenosynovitis. This additional surgery usually is not necessary, however, when the tenosynovitis is associated with a seronegative inflammatory disorder. In patients with such disorders, the tenosynovitis develops as part of a spondyloarthropathy and enthesopathy, and deformity occurs much later, after complete rupture of the tendon. The goals of the tenosynovectomy are to decrease pain and to remove any of the inflammatory tissue that may hasten the rupture. Then the foot should be rested until healing takes place.

To begin the tenosynovectomy, an incision is made posteromedially along the length of the tendon, and the retinaculum is opened completely (Figure 18-6). Occasionally, the tenosynovitis is a result of a stricture or stenosis of the retinaculum immediately behind the medial malleolus. This stricture creates an hourglass shape to the tendon, with obvious deformity and inflammatory change visible in the tendon. Once the retinaculum has been opened, the tendon is inspected. The inflammatory change is not always that obvious and frequently is on the posterior surface of the tendon and tendon sheath. The tendon must then be rotated to inspect the posterior surface. I find that skin hooks are the easiest way to do this, by flipping the tendon around to inspect the posterior surface. The inflammatory tissue is then removed from the tendon sheath and the tendon itself; either dissection scissors or a knife blade is used in this procedure. Rubbing the tendon vigorously with a sponge also facilitates removal of this inflammatory tissue. Finally, the tendon should be inspected for any tears, which, as stated, usually are on the posterior surface (Figure 18-7). If a tear is identified, it is repaired with a running suture of monofilament absorbable suture. I use a 2-0 suture and bury the knot and then run

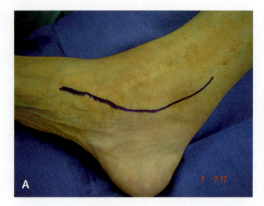
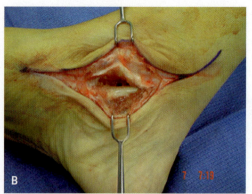
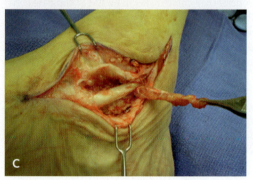

Figure 18-6 A, The incision is made along the course of the posterior ankle. **B,** The tendon sheath is then opened. **C,** Note the extensive tenosynovitis along the length of the tendon, evident in **B.** Involved tissue was removed by sharp dissection.

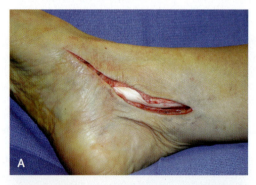
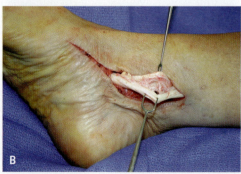

Figure 18-7 A 44-year-old athletic patient presented with postero-medial ankle pain of 6 month duration. **A,** Opening the tendon sheath revealed hypertrophic and proliferative tenosynovitis. **B,** On further exploration, the tendon was noted to be torn longitudinally and was repaired. No associated deformity whatsoever was present. In order to protect the tendon during the healing process, a medial translational osteotomy of the calcaneus was performed simultaneously.

the suture along the length of the tendon, imbricating the tendon along the way as the repair is performed. I do not repair the flexor retinaculum, because the tendon will not subluxate provided that the foot is immobilized for a few weeks after surgery. It is always a good idea to support the tendon if there is a tear, which is simultaneously repaired; in such instances, either an arthroereisis or a calcaneus osteotomy can be performed. Weight bearing can be started as tolerated in a boot, and gentle passive range-of-motion exercises can start after 2 weeks, followed by non–weight-bearing exercise, including swimming and cycling.

Medial Translational Osteotomy of the Calcaneus

Correction of the flexible flatfoot deformity, with or without an associated tear of the PTT, begins with the lateral approach, including calcaneus osteotomy. Once the osteotomy has been completed, the incision is closed, and the patient is turned from the lateral to the supine position for the tendon transfer and PTT correction.

This osteotomy is an extremely utilitarian procedure, and I use the medial translation osteotomy for correction of multiple types of deformities whenever hindfoot valgus is present and when the medial aspect of the foot needs to be supported. Restructuring the medial column of the foot, leaving the hindfoot in valgus, does not correct the hindfoot deformity. The rationale for the medial translation is not only the movement of the calcaneal tuberosity medially, with corresponding improvement of the mechanical tripod of the heel with respect to the forefoot, but also the medialization of the insertion of the Achilles tendon relative to the axis of the subtalar joint.

Many clinical and biomechanical studies have supported this osteotomy, with its positive impact on both the foot and the ankle. The osteotomy can be used to improve the mechanics of the tibiotalar joint because medial translation will increase the contact pressure on the medial aspect of the tibiotalar joint when valgus

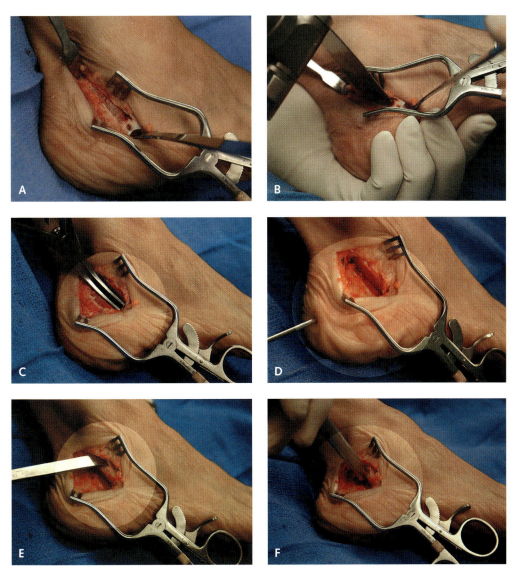

Figure 18-8 The steps in a medial translational osteotomy. **A,** The incision is marked out just inferior to the peroneal tendons, the sural nerve is retracted inferiorly and the tendons superiorly, and the periosteum is reflected as Hohman retractors are used to expose the calcaneus. **B,** A saw blade is used to cut the calcaneus while the opposite hand holds the foot to appreciate the sense of the saw blade as it perforates the medial calcaneus. **C,** A laminar spreader is inserted lengthwise to prevent crushing of the bone. **D,** The calcaneus is then shifted medially by 10 mm, and a cannulated guide pin is inserted followed by a 6.5-mm cannulated threaded screw. **E** and **F,** The dorsal periosteum is elevated, and the overhanging bone is tamped down to smooth out the ledge of bone, which may impinge on the skin.

deformity is present in the ankle. The osteotomy also can be added to a triple arthrodesis to improve the mechanical support of the ankle in a stage IV rupture of the PTT in conjunction with reconstruction of the deltoid ligament. This is an extremely reliable operation, and nonunion is not a problem. With internal fixation, the tuberosity can be shifted at least 12 mm without any concern for instability or nonunion. Overcorrection into slight varus can occur, albeit rarely.

An incision is made two fingerbreadths below the tip of the fibula in line with the peroneal tendon (Figure 18-8). The incision is deepened into subcutaneous tissue, and immediately the sural nerve and lesser saphenous vein must be identified and retracted. A retractor is inserted into the tissue, and then once the nerve is retracted, the incision is deepened onto periosteum, which is reflected to expose the calcaneus. I try to perform the osteotomy as close as possible to the axis of the subtalar joint. After subperiosteal dissection, two curved soft tissue retractors are inserted on the dorsal and inferior aspect of the tuberosity. The inferior retractor is pushed between the calcaneus and the plantar fascia and serves as a retractor of the soft tissues during the osteotomy. The cut is made perpendicular to the axis of the tuberosity at a 45-degree angle with respect to the calcaneal pitch angle. An osteotome should *not* be used, because more control is afforded by the use of a wide saw blade. A punching action of the saw is used for the osteotomy, to permit the perforation through the medial aspect of the tuberosity to be felt. A smooth laminar spreader with no teeth is inserted into the osteotomy site to distract the calcaneus, and the medial

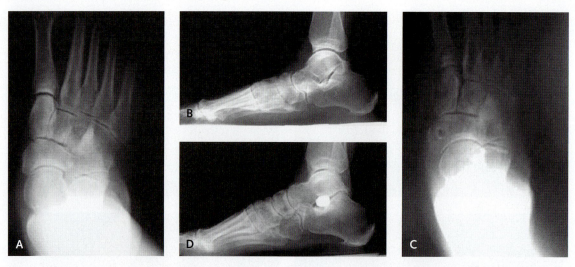

Figure 18-9 A and B An interesting combination of slight abduction of the transverse tarsal joint, moderate heel valgus, and mild forefoot supination with the heel reduced. **C** and **D,** In addition to the FDL tendon transfer, a subtalar arthroereisis was performed to support the partially ruptured posterior tibial tendon (PTT). A medial translational osteotomy of the calcaneus may have been a good alternative to the arthroereisis, but in view of the extent of uncovering of the talonavicular joint, the latter was thought to be preferable. It is possible to perform the calcaneus osteotomy, and then, if the heel remains in valgus or the forefoot abduction persists, the arthroereisis can be added.

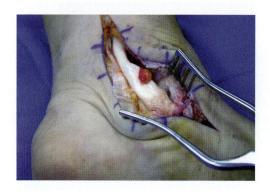

Figure 18-10 The tendon was markedly stenosed behind the malleolus and was partially torn. Note also the granulations behind the tendon, indicative of a tear of the deltoid ligament.

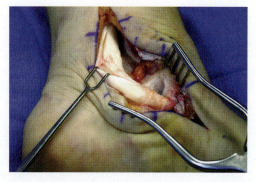

Figure 18-11 In addition to the obvious tears of the posterior tibial tendon, note the granulation over the deltoid ligament as well as the defect in the talonavicular capsule.

periosteum is separated. The medial translation is then facilitated, but cephalic translation is avoided. Once the calcaneus is held in the desired position, which is approximately 10 to 12 mm of medial shift, it is fixed with one 6.5-mm cannulated screw introduced from inferolateral to anteromedial to enter the harder sustentacular bone. Compressing the overhanging lateral ledge of bone is important because presence of a ridge can cause irritation on the soft tissues and sural nerve. This is a stable osteotomy, and weight bearing can start after 10 days, either in a cast or in a boot, depending on the additional procedures performed.

Flexor Digitorum Longus Tendon Transfer

The indications for FDL tendon transfer are a flexible flatfoot and a reducible subtalar joint with or without forefoot supination. Obesity does not appear to be a contraindication to this procedure, and provided that the foot is flexible, the addition of a calcaneal osteotomy to the FDL tendon transfer will support the foot. Occasionally, if I am concerned about the ability of the tendon transfer and the osteotomy to support the foot completely, I may add a subtalar arthroereisis to support the subtalar joint. This is particularly helpful in patients who have an increase in the talar declination but have good coverage of the talonavicular joint (Figure 18-9).

To begin the FDL tendon transfer, an incision is made medially starting behind the medial malleolus and extending distally toward the medial cuneiform. This incision is deepened to the flexor retinaculum, and the PTT sheath is opened. Frequently, the PTT rupture is partial and longitudinal, and it fissures in the posterior aspect of the tendon and is visible once the tendon is rotated and rolled backward. In addition to tears of the tendon, the entire capsule-ligament complex must be inspected for any defect, tear, or rupture that could involve the deltoid ligament, the talonavicular capsule, or the spring ligament. Each of these much be addressed in addition to the tendon transfer (Figures 18-10 to 18-14). I have at times left behind the ruptured posterior tendon, in an effort to increase the strength medially. This makes perfect sense provided

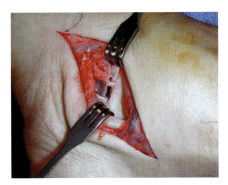

Figure 18-12   Note the tear in the spring ligament. The posterior tibial tendon, which had a minor tear, has been retracted posteriorly.

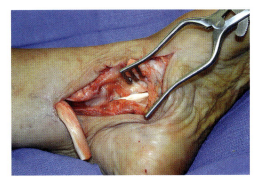

Figure 18-13   The posterior tibial tendon tear, which was significant, was more distally located, and the tendon was cut distally. Note, however, the mild inflammation of the deltoid ligament.

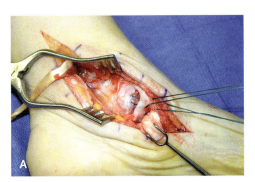

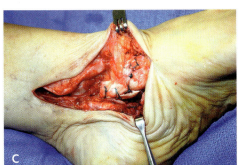

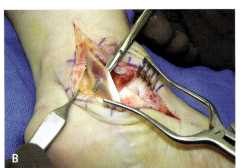

Figure 18-14 A, The posterior tibial tendon (PTT) has been resected, and the stump of the tendon retracted distally with the skin hook. The flexor digitorum longus (FDL) tendon has been cut distally in the foot for the transfer and retracted posteriorly. **B,** Note the significant tear in the talonavicular capsule with sutures inserted to begin the repair before tendon transfer. **C,** The FDL has been transferred and sutured to the stump of the PTT tendon.

that the tendon does not generate pain as a result of the persistent scarring and inflammation from the tear. Another potential problem with leaving the PTT behind is the swelling and thickening of the foot that accompanies this treatment. It also is difficult to correctly tension the FDL transfer if the PTT is left behind at its resting tension, because the PTT is not shortened (Figure 18-15). If a side-to-side tenodesis is done more distally, increased thickening, bulk, and scarring will be present. Accurately restoring the balance between the transferred FDL tendon and the adjacent redundant PTT with this method is impossible. The FDL tendon normally is transferred with considerable tension in the knowledge that it will stretch out in time. If I plan to leave the tendon, following debridement, the degenerated tendon is split off and then the tendon is tubularized with a running absorbable suture (Figure 18-16). In general I do resect the distal tendon, and other than the distal 2 to 3 cm, the torn portion of the PTT is excised. If, however, there is considerable insertional tendinopathy and the distal tendon is torn, it is completely cut from its attachment to the navicular. If the posterior tibial muscle is still functioning and has some mobility and

excursion to it, then a proximal tenodesis can be performed. The entire excursion of the posterior tibial muscle is approximately 1 cm, so with fissuring and elongation of the tendon, the muscle does not function well. If, at the completion of the flexor tendon transfer, excursion of the PTT is noted, then a side-to-side tenodesis of the PTT to the FDL tendon is performed, proximal to the medial malleolus. I excise the central segment of the PTT, leaving a distal stump of 2 cm to facilitate the attachment of the FDL tendon for transfer. The proximal stump is cut at the level of the medial malleolus.

Once the PTT has been prepared, the FDL tendon is harvested. The sheath for the FDL tendon lies immediately posterior to the PTT, and the sheath is opened with a knife and is then split longitudinally with scissors. No effort is made to preserve the flexor sheath, because the FDL tendon moves into the sheath of the PTT and the sheath of the FDL tendon is split proximally far enough that the tendon is mobile. The plane of dissection for harvesting the FDL tendon is important and should be extended between the abductor fascia and the medial border of the foot. A retractor is inserted between the abductor fascia and the undersurface of the

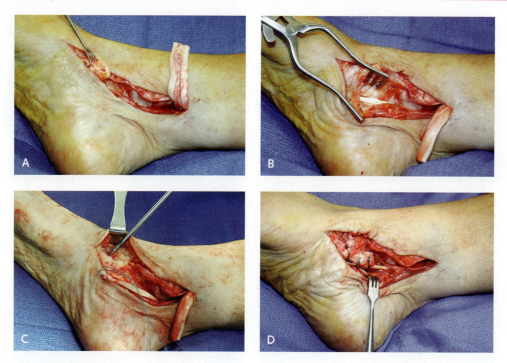

Figure 18-15 The steps in the flexor digitorum longus (FDL) tendon transfer for posterior tibial tendon (PTT) rupture. **A,** The severely torn PTT tendon is cut, leaving a 2-cm stump distally. **B,** The sheath of the FDL tendon is opened. **C,** The FDL tendon is cut under direct vision distally, and a 4.5-mm drill hole is made in the navicular. **D,** The FDL tendon is passed through the drill hole from plantar to dorsal and then sutured to the underside of the stump of the PTT.

medial cuneiform, and then, by gradually putting this on stretch, the dissection is facilitated under direct vision.

The sheath of the FDL tendon must be released up to the junction of the flexor hallucis longus (FHL) tendon at the master knot of Henry, and the tendon is cut under direct vision with scissors. No effort is made to perform a side-to-side tenodesis to the FHL tendon. Sufficient cross-connection functions between the two tendons, and deficit of toe function is not noticed by the patient. A suture is inserted into the tip of the FDL tendon, and the tendon is then passed from plantar to dorsal through a 4.5-mm drill hole. This drill hole is made after subperiosteal dissection on the dorsal medial pole of the navicular bone; it is important to keep the drill from getting too close to the medial pole of the navicular bone or to the talonavicular and navicular cuneiform joint. If inadvertent fracture of the medial pole of the navicular bone occurs intraoperatively, the tendon can then be attached with a biointerference screw or a screw with a spiked ligament washer directly into the navicular bone. The use of the drill hole, however, does facilitate early rehabilitation because of the strength of the bone-tendon-bone fixation. Once the drill hole is made, the suction tip is introduced from dorsal to plantar, and the suture on the FDL tendon is withdrawn into the suction tip and pulled through the hole from which the tendon can be pulled up dorsally.

The tendon is now tightened maximally to get an idea of where the foot is positioned with maximal tension on the tendon. The tendon must not be overtightened, because overtightening also may tend to cause subluxation of the FDL tendon out of the PTT groove. If the tendon can possibly subluxate, then the retinaculum must be repaired loosely to prevent stenosis and friction with the potential for abrasion of the FDL tendon. The extent to which the tendon is tightened for the repair depends in part on the weight of the patient

and the deformity. The heavier the patient and the more extensive the deformity, the tighter I make the repair. The tendon should not be at what would be considered a physiologic tension, in which the tendon would be somewhere between maximum relaxation and maximum tension. The foot should be positioned medially in inversion beyond the midline, because the tendon always stretches out, and the foot will assume a more neutral position over time.

Before the sutures are inserted for the FDL tendon repair, the deltoid ligament, talonavicular capsule, and spring ligament must again be inspected, and if a repair on the soft tissue is needed, it should be performed before the FDL tendon is tensioned. Usually a 1- to 2-cm strand of FDL tendon passes through the navicular bone, and this can be used to suture the tendon back down onto the stump of the PTT on both the lower and the dorsal surfaces of the tendon.

At the completion of the FDL tendon transfer, the excursion of the tibialis posterior muscle is again checked with a clamp on the tip of the tendon, and provided that a 1-cm excursion is present with a yield point on the pulling of the muscle, a proximal tenodesis is performed. The PTT is grasped and pulled as far distally as possible, and then the repair is performed just distal to the musculotendinous junction to the FDL tendon with a running locking stitch using 0-0 nonabsorbable suture.

Rehabilitation after this procedure depends on the extent of additional operations performed. After a straightforward medial translational osteotomy of the calcaneus and flexor tendon transfer, patients can start bearing weight at 2 weeks in a removable walker boot. Exercise, excluding swimming, can be initiated at this time. If, however, a ligament repair is performed (e.g., talonavicular capsule, spring ligament, or deltoid ligament), then the rehabilitation is prolonged,

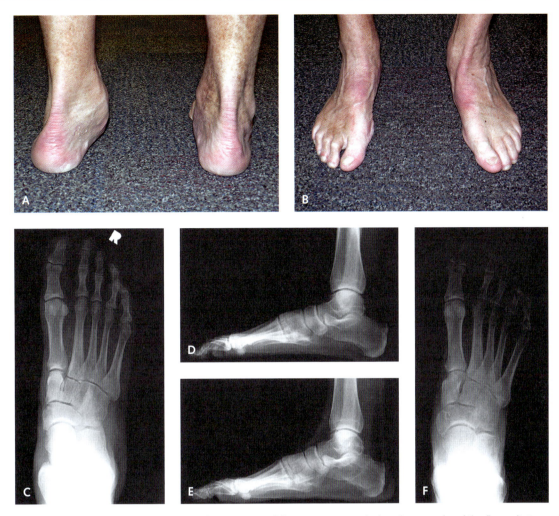

Figure 18-16 A and **B,** Clinical appearance 4 years after resection of the torn posterior tibial tendon, transfer of the flexor digitorum longus tendon, and medial translational osteotomy of the calcaneus. Note the correction of heel valgus as well as the arch height on the right foot. **C** and **D,** Preoperative radiographs. **E** and **F,** Postoperative radiographs. The calcaneal screw has been removed.

and weight bearing is initiated at 6 weeks to permit full healing of the soft tissues. When a ligament repair has been performed, the patient should continue wearing the boot for up to 9 weeks and then use a soft brace to support the ankle with walking activities and exercise.

Subtalar Arthroereisis

The indications for a subtalar arthroereisis in the adult are different from those in the child, because the surgeon has numerous alternative repair procedures from which to choose. The subtalar implant procedure is useful as an approach to the heel that remains in valgus after medial translational osteotomy and for any other type of flexible hindfoot correction when the talonavicular joint has subluxated but an arthrodesis is to be avoided. The arthroereisis is not a good or sufficient procedure when the talonavicular joint is markedly uncovered, a condition best treated with lateral column lengthening. Sag of the talus, with an increase in the talocalcaneal angle, and heel valgus, however, are conditions that are most amenable to correction with this procedure.

The technique for insertion of the implant is identical to that described previously for use in the child. Generally, I plan to remove the implant between 6 and 12 months, although this removal occasionally is not necessary because the patient is symptom-free. The adult patient is, however, warned about the potential for pain after the arthroereisis, because even when this repair is performed under ideal circumstances, the incidence of pain necessitating removal is greater than 50%. In addition to the static correction provided by the arthroereisis, the mechanical support from the prosthesis has a beneficial effect while soft tissue healing is taking place. An arthroereisis can be used as an adjunct to other hindfoot and midfoot procedures such as tarsometatarsal arthrodesis (Figure 18-17).

Spring Ligament and Capsuloligamentous Repair

Rupture of the spring ligament may occur as an isolated injury unassociated with a tear of the PTT, or it may be torn as an attritional process, the result of a tear of the PTT, both of which will cause a flatfoot deformity. Repair of the spring ligament is not easy, because it is a thick, strong ligament and does not support sutures well. If sutures are to be used, they need to be extremely stout, on the order of No. 2 nonabsorbable suture material. I do not excise a vertical ellipse from the talonavicular joint to shorten this as a routine part of the repair process, unless a defect is visible in the capsule. If a defect in the talonavicular capsule is significant,

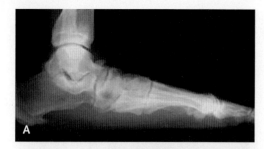

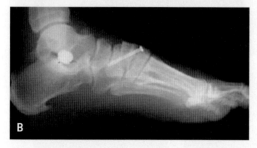

Figure 18-17 A, A tarsometatarsal arthrodesis was performed as part of a modified Lapidus procedure. **B,** At the completion of the procedure, it was noted that the hindfoot was in more valgus than anticipated, and a subtalar implant was inserted.

then this joint usually is unstable, and the transverse tarsal joint is abducted. This abduction will necessitate a lateral column lengthening procedure to correct the alignment. If severe instability is associated with complete disruption of the spring ligament and talonavicular complex, then an arthrodesis of the talonavicular joint may have to be performed. Generally, once the lateral column lengthening has been performed, then an FDL tendon transfer is sufficient to stabilize the medial column and is added for dynamic correction.

The other option for correction of an unstable spring ligament and talonavicular capsule is the use of a heavy suture anchor inserted into the pole of the navicular tuberosity. Sutures are used to imbricate the talonavicular capsule. This is done in a U-shaped suture line after the capsuloligamentous tissue is pulled down onto the navicular bone (Figure 18-18).

Insertional Posterior Tibial Tendinopathy and Excision of the Accessory Navicular in the Adult

A painful accessory navicular in the adult is not uncommonly associated with sudden development of an acquired flatfoot and pain on the medial insertion of the PTT. Unlike with rupture of the tendon as outlined previously, the tendon can easily be palpated on resisted inversion, although the foot remains weak. Pain is located at the insertion of the tendon, and the mass of the accessory navicular also is palpable. The principle of correction for an accessory navicular is different from that for a noninsertional rupture of the PTT. If the pain is present specifically at the insertion of the tendon without much thickening and tendinopathy, then excision of the bone is required, with advancement of the tendon into the navicular. A transfer of the FDL tendon may be necessary in these patients if considerable tendinopathy is present, necessitating excision of the distal PTT. Excising the medial pole of the navicular is important because the navicular will be prominent even after excision of the accessory bone. In the adult, however, unlike in the child, the tendon cannot be attached through

Kirschner wire (K-wire) holes made in the navicular bone, and a suture anchor is ideally used.

Lateral Column Lengthening

The indication for a lateral column lengthening is greater than 40% uncovering of the talonavicular joint. The lengthening can be performed through either the calcaneocuboid joint or the neck of the calcaneus. The lengthening through the joint is preferable in older patients and in those with osteopenia, or if a little more rigidity of the hindfoot is present (Figure 18-19). As a rule, if an arthrodesis is required in the older adult, it will be a triple arthrodesis, but in some instances in which the foot is still reasonably flexible, a lengthening procedure can be considered. Such a procedure would be used in patients who have a flexible hindfoot, with abduction across the transverse tarsal joint and with 40% or greater uncovering of the talonavicular joint and osteopenia. A problem in elderly patients or those with osteopenia is the potential for crushing of the cancellous bone in the neck of the calcaneus during the lengthening. If crushing occurs, then the graft collapses, with involution into the cancellous surface.

Patients with arthritis of the calcaneocuboid joint also benefit from arthrodesis. This procedure is not as common, because isolated arthritis of the calcaneocuboid joint is not common, and arthritis usually implies a rigid hindfoot, for which a triple arthrodesis would need to be performed. In this group of patients with severe rigid deformity, however, a triple arthrodesis can be performed with the addition of a lateral column lengthening procedure with insertion of a structural graft into the calcaneocuboid joint. In my experience, the incidence of arthritis after lengthening osteotomy is minimal and does not warrant the increased risk for performing an arthrodesis of the calcaneocuboid joint. The risk for nonunion of this joint is high despite advances in internal fixation techniques, and malunion seems to be much more of a problem than with osteotomy.

The incision for the lateral column lengthening osteotomy is made along the dorsal surface of the peroneal tendons, extending from the tip of the fibula to the calcaneocuboid joint. The incision should be slightly more dorsal than lateral, because visualizing the neck of the calcaneus from the dorsolateral rather than the lateral direction is easier. Once the incision is deepened onto the periosteum, the peroneal tendons are reflected inferiorly and are retracted through the rest of the procedure. The periosteum on the dorsal surface of the neck must be completely elevated, and the anterior aspect of the subtalar joint must be visualized.

With adequate soft tissue retraction, the neck of the calcaneus is cut with a saw, perpendicular to the axis of the calcaneus and approximately 1 cm proximal to the articular surface of the calcaneocuboid joint. A saw cut is made through both cortices, and the calcaneus is loosened. Inserting a small osteotome to free up the medial cortex is the easiest method. I originally thought that keeping the medial cortex intact might be desirable, but this restriction does not allow significant lengthening of the calcaneus. A lamina spreader is now inserted into the calcaneus or a pin distractor used (Figure 18-20). The foot must be examined while the lamina spreader is inserted under distraction. The spreader should be inserted along the thicker cortical rim of the osteotomy to prevent crushing of the central bone. A radiograph is obtained while the lamina spreader is in place to ensure correct coverage of the talonavicular joint. Usually the calcaneus has been opened approximately 10 to 12 mm. A graft is now fashioned, and I use a structural allograft, either from the iliac crest or from a femoral head. The graft is now cut to shape and inserted. This step is difficult because the lamina spreader gets in the way. Although specially designed lamina spreaders are available

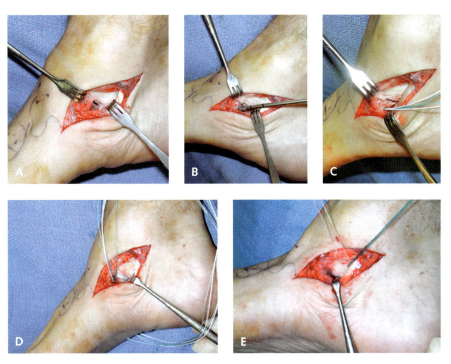

Figure 18-18 The patient sustained a rupture of the spring ligament with an acquired flatfoot deformity. **A,** The posterior tibial tendon was completely intact. Note the defect in the spring ligament, which extends up into the inferior aspect of the talonavicular capsule. **B,** The edge of the navicular was debrided down to bleeding bone, and the suture anchor was inserted. **C-E,** These were then inserted as a U-suture to pull the flap down toward the navicular. A medial translational osteotomy of the calcaneus was performed simultaneously.

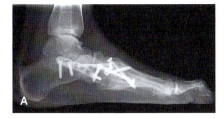

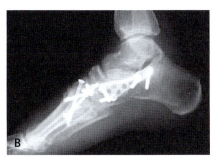

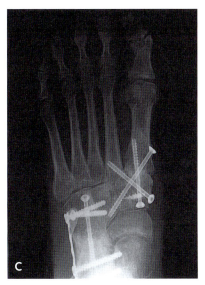

Figure 18-19 A-C, The patient was a 46-year-old woman with approximately 50% uncovering of the talonavicular joint, but a little more rigidity than I would have preferred for a lengthening through the calcaneus. The bone block lengthening was therefore performed through the calcaneocuboid joint. Further deformity and arthritis of the first metatarsocuneiform joint resulted, and an arthrodesis was performed, adding plantar flexion to the first ray.

for this purpose, the graft must be inserted dorsolaterally without abutting the lamina spreader, which blocks its insertion. If the lamina spreader is inserted more inferiorly, however, it is in soft bone, which increases the risk for crushing. The graft is tamped into place and must be checked dorsally. The graft tends to be visible from the lateral aspect but not entirely from the dorsal aspect, and some dorsal migration of the graft may occur with abutment up against the anterior aspect of the subtalar joint. This less-than-optimal positioning will cause a painful impingement. Generally, the graft is secured with a fully threaded 4-mm cancellous screw, which is introduced from the anterolateral tip of the calcaneus at the calcaneocuboid joint. If the overhanging bone, which may cause impingement at the anterior aspect of the posterior facet, is still present, it should be trimmed down with a saw. Ideally, the foot should be examined fluoroscopically and then rotated through all planes of motion for examination to ensure correct position of the graft before closure

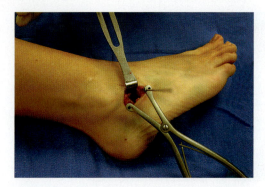

Figure 18-20 As an alternative to a regular laminar spreader, the distractor with pins is quite useful, because the paddles of the spreader are present to interfere with the bone graft.

(Figures 18-21 and 18-22). In some circumstances, lengthening of the lateral column is not sufficient. It is important to recognize that the mechanism for improvement with this osteotomy is by virtue of an angular correction laterally to adduct the forefoot. A slight increase in plantar flexion may be obtained as well, but this would be a secondary effect. The lengthening of the lateral column will not correct marked heel valgus. Of interest, the deformities associated with a flatfoot seem to be different. If the forefoot is abducted, there is not that much heel valgus, and vice versa. Although addition of a medial calcaneus osteotomy is not necessary as a routine procedure, at times this modification is useful (Figure 18-23).

Medial Cuneiform Osteotomy

Although the hindfoot is flexible and the talonavicular joint and the subtalar joints are reducible, when the heel is brought into a neutral position, a fixed forefoot supination often is present. In some patients, this deviation is exacerbated as a result of the gastrocnemius muscle contracture. Also, forefoot supination, which is marked with the heel in the neutral position, may reduce as the foot is plantar flexed. In these patients, hindfoot reconstruction is possible in conjunction with a gastrocnemius muscle recession without any need to address the medial column instability.

On the other hand, if the forefoot supination persists or is excessive, then it must be corrected. A number of procedures can be used for treatment, all of which rely on structural correction rather than dynamic support on the medial aspect of the foot. The structural changes must take place at the first TMT joint, the medial cuneiform, or the navicular cuneiform joint. To some extent, the location depends on the extent of instability present on the lateral weight-bearing radiograph. If the instability is excessive with a gap on the plantar surface, then an arthrodesis of this joint must be considered. This is usually the case with the TMT joint and not the navicular cuneiform joint. I do not focus as much on the navicular cuneiform joint unless arthritis is present. Furthermore, even though instability may be apparent in the medial column, invariably the instability is in the talonavicular joint, and I do not think that arthrodesis is warranted in a flexible flatfoot. In such cases, I prefer to perform an opening wedge osteotomy of the medial cuneiform. With this osteotomy, the medial column stabilizes, and even though instability may have been present on stress film intraoperatively, this will be corrected by increasing plantar flexion and thereby tightening the windlass mechanism.

An arthrodesis of the first TMT joint may be performed if instability or arthritis is present at that joint, but I generally prefer an opening wedge osteotomy of the medial cuneiform joint for correction. The incision is made over the dorsal aspect of the foot immediately medial to the extensor hallucis longus tendon and lateral to the anterior tibial tendon. This interval is used directly onto the dorsal aspect of the cuneiform, which is exposed with subperiosteal dissection. If an incision has been used for a PTT reconstruction, this can be extended distally, although the more dorsally located incision is easier to use.

A guide pin is inserted from dorsal to plantar through the cuneiform and aimed slightly proximally. The position is checked laterally to ensure that the middle of the cuneiform has been reached. Saw cuts are now made on either side of the guide pin, and as each cut is made, the guide pin can then be removed. The osteotomy cut is made vertically, but the plantar cortex of the medial cuneiform joint should be preserved. The cut generally is in line in the same plane as the second metatarsal cuneiform joint. Rarely, the cut may enter into the edge of this joint. Once the cut is complete, a lamina spreader is inserted dorsally after the cut has been pried open with an osteotome. The graft size used here is not as large as that for the lateral column lengthening. Usually, a 6-mm graft is sufficient. This is a triangular or trapezoidal graft that should be wider dorsally than on the plantar surface in both planes. Insertion of the graft is difficult with the lamina spreader in place. Either the lamina spreader needs to be opened maximally to facilitate insertion of the graft, or the graft needs to be between the margins of the lamina spreader, which can then be removed. This ought to forcibly plantar flex the first metatarsal by dorsiflexing the hallux during this maneuver of graft insertion. The graft should be tamped down flush with the margin of the cuneiform and then checked fluoroscopically. This "press-fit" bone graft is generally stable, and, although rare, if fixation is necessary, I use one threaded 4-mm cancellous screw from the dorsal surface at the level of the metatarsal cuneiform joint aiming proximally (Figure 18-24).

Arthrodesis Procedures

The indication for isolated arthrodesis (in contrast with a double or triple arthrodesis) is not always clear. In a case from my own experience, although I did not anticipate the need to perform a talonavicular arthrodesis, the necessity for the procedure became evident when gross instability of the talonavicular joint was observed intraoperatively. Furthermore, with some feet in which the talonavicular joint is very abducted and found to be grossly loose on examination, the natural inclination is to avoid an arthrodesis and to use a lateral column lengthening procedure in an attempt to reduce the joint. As a consequence of rupture of either the spring ligament or the talonavicular capsule (or both), however, the joint may be so unstable that the talonavicular arthrodesis becomes a good choice of procedure. This procedure generally reduces the hindfoot deformity; in some flexible deformities for which the apex is at the talonavicular joint, however, heel valgus persists (Figure 18-25). For these patients, the talonavicular arthrodesis generally is performed in conjunction with a medial osteotomy translation of the calcaneus. Addition of a tendon transfer to the arthrodesis not necessary, but it is essential to ensure that the medial column is adequately plantar flexed.

Even less clear than with the talonavicular arthrodesis is when to perform a subtalar arthrodesis. Occasionally, in a heavier patient, the deformity is predominantly in the talonavicular joint, with marked heel valgus and an increase in the talocalcaneal angle on the lateral radiograph. With this type of patient, the subtalar arthrodesis may provide more definitive correction, but here I would add a tendon transfer to support the medial arch of the foot, because the arthrodesis normally will not provide adequate correction. The role

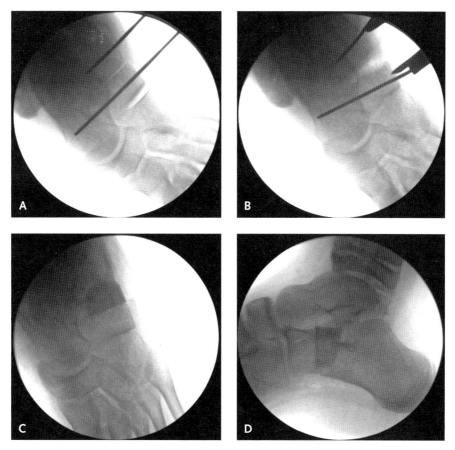

Figure 18-21 The lateral column-lengthing calcaneus osteotomy. **A,** The guide pins were inserted fluoroscopically, leaving room for the osteotomy. **B,** Using a pin distractor, the gradual covering of the talus by the navicular was noted under fluoroscopic guidance. **C** and **D,** Insertion of the graft. The osteotomy has been performed slightly too far proximally, and is abutting on the posterior facet. The graft was removed, and narrowed slightly, and further impacted into the osteotomy.

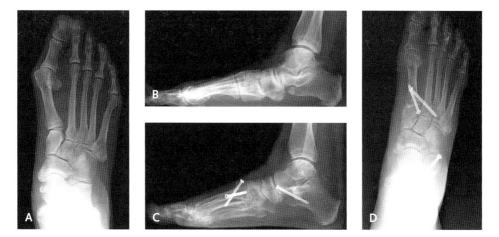

Figure 18-22 A and **B,** The patient was a 56-year-old woman who experienced sudden onset of pain at the insertion of the posterior tibial tendon associated with a flatfoot deformity. Abnormalities included an accessory navicular, uncovering of the talonavicular joint, and hallux valgus. **C** and **D,** Correction was accomplished with a lengthening osteotomy of the calcaneus, reattachment of the posterior tibial tendon into the navicular, and a modified Lapidus procedure.

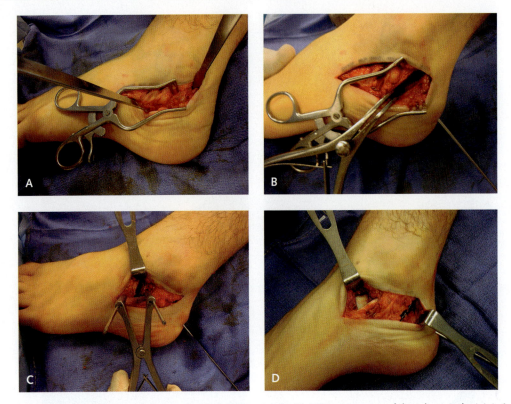

Figure 18-23 A combined deformity of severe heel valgus associated with 50% uncovering of the talonavicular joint. **A,** The procedure commenced with an extensile incision exposing the calcaneus. **B,** The medial osteotomy of the calcaneus was first performed, noting the laminar spreader in place. **C,** Once the tuberosity was stable, the lateral column lengthening was performed using a pin distractor. **D,** Postoperative appearance of both osteotomies. It is important not to overcorrect with either of these osteotomies, because their combined effect is magnified.

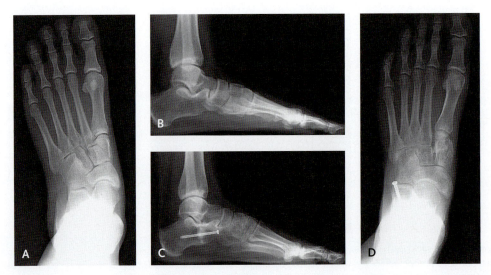

Figure 18-24 **A** and **B,** Flexible flatfoot deformity in a 27-year-old man with bilateral flat feet. **C** and **D,** The lateral column lengthening was first performed, and the supination of the forefoot was corrected with osteotomy of the cuneiform.

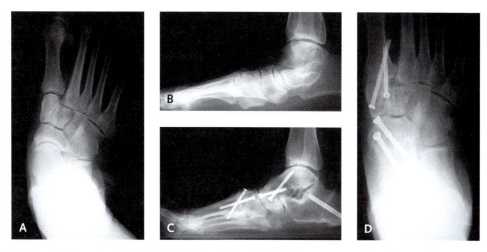

Figure 18-25 A and **B,** A marked flexible flatfoot deformity, including 55% uncovering of the talonavicular joint, and arthritis with instability of the first metatarsocuneiform joint in a 33-year-old man. **C** and **D,** The correction commenced with the talonavicular arthrodesis, but the heel remained in valgus, necessitating the calcaneus osteotomy in addition to the planned arthrodesis of the first tarsometatarsal joint.

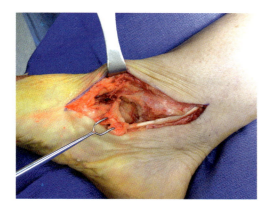

Figure 18-26 The patient was a 54-year-old woman who presented with posteromedial ankle pain and a rupture of the posterior tibial tendon that was absent. Note the inflamed flexor digitorum longus tendon and the degeneration of the deltoid.

of the triple arthrodesis is quite clear in managing rigid deformity and is discussed elsewhere.

Management of the Deltoid Ligament Tear (Stage IV Posterior Tibial Tendon Rupture)

A standardized repair of a ruptured deltoid ligament for a degenerative tear associated with a stage IV flatfoot does not work. Many variations of this repair have been attempted, including end-to-end repair, a "vest-over-pants" repair, and advancement of the ligament up into the medial malleolus. With all of these repairs, the ligament tends to stretch out after a while because of the inherent degenerative nature of the local tissue. From a mechanical standpoint, this condition is vastly different from a lateral ankle ligament reconstruction, for which an anatomic repair (Broström repair) works well. Histopathologically, the deltoid ligament is different, and when associated with degeneration, this simply stretches out again, possibly compounded by the mechanical deformity and the

preexisting changes associated with the rupture of the PTT. The typical changes in the medial ankle are shown in Figure 18-26.

The reconstruction of the deltoid ligament is performed using a hamstring allograft; From a technical perspective, this reconstruction is similar to that for the lateral ankle ligament. Autogenous tissue may be used, but I would refrain from using the local tissue because even the remaining stump of the PTT failed when I tried to use it. The hamstring allograft is attached with an interference screw system. An incision is made medially extending along the course of the ruptured PTT from 4 cm proximal to the malleolus toward the navicular joint. Adjunctive procedures, which may include a triple arthrodesis, a medial calcaneal osteotomy, or an FDL tendon transfer, are performed as required. A 4.5-mm drill hole is made directly into the medial malleolus, and the tendon graft is then secured with an interference screw (Figure 18-27). The dorsal limb of the graft is inserted into the talus using a blind-end tunnel technique. Rather than a talar blind-end tunnel, a through-and-through tunnel is used in the calcaneus, to maximize tension on the tendon graft. Ideally the exit point on the lateral side of the foot should be in the calcaneus, because pulling the graft through on the lateral side of the talus, which is protected and covered by the overhanging fibula posterolaterally, is difficult. The drill hole is made in the posterior tuberosity of the calcaneus with a cannulated guide pin with a sleeve for the drill bit used to protect the soft tissues. The suture is attached to the tendon, which is measured so that no more than 2 cm of tendon passes through the tunnel. If the tendon is longer, sufficient tension on the lateral aspect of the calcaneus cannot be generated when the tendon is pulled on. The suture is passed through the calcaneus with a straight needle and is pulled out laterally, avoiding the sural nerve. While tension is being applied to the tendon, the foot is positioned in neutral dorsiflexion, and stability on forced passive eversion or valgus stress on the ankle is assessed. The interference screw is inserted in a standard fashion, and a larger-diameter screw is used to secure the calcaneus depending on the quality of the bone (Figures 18-28 and 18-29).

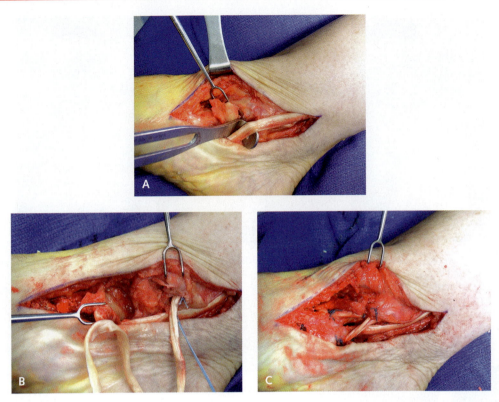

Figure 18-27 Treatment for a flexible stage IV rupture of the posterior tibial tendon and deltoid ligament. **A,** Note the torn deltoid and the inflamed flexor digitorum longus (FDL). **B,** A forked hamstring allograft was used. The proximal end was inserted into the medial malleolus with an interference screw. **C,** The distal end of the graft was then split and the dorsal end inserted into the talus, and the plantar limb of the graft into the calcaneus. A calcaneal osteotomy with transfer of the FDL tendon was then performed.

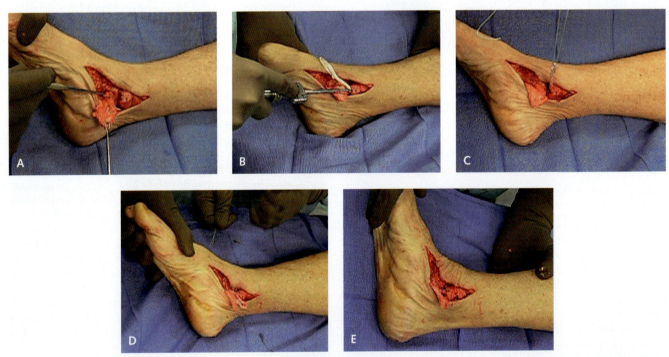

Figure 18-28 Chronic medial ankle instability was corrected with a forked hamstring allograft procedure. **A,** The defect in the ankle is apparent in this intraoperative photograph. **B,** The drill hole in the malleolus was made with a 4.5-mm drill bit. The graft is inserted into the medial malleolus with an interference screw. **C,** The graft is then split into two short tendon grafts distally. **D,** The talar graft is inserted obliquely into the body of the talus with a blind-end tunnel technique, and into the calcaneus with a through-and-through technique. **E,** Appearance at completion of the graft procedure.

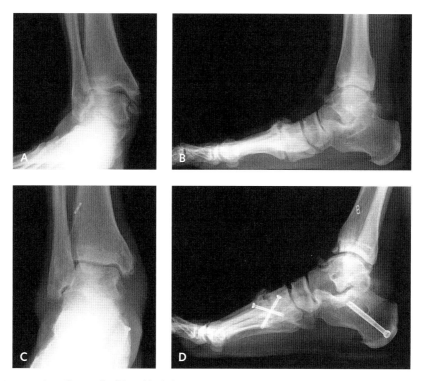

Figure 18-29 A and **B,** Chronic flexible ankle deformity associated with a deltoid tear and first metatarsocuneiform arthritis and instability. A forked hamstring allograft was used for the reconstruction, in addition to a calcaneus osteotomy and arthrodesis of the first tarsometatarsal joint. The graft was inserted into the medial malleolus using a fiber wire attached to an anchor "TightRope" (Arthrex, Inc., Naples, Florida). **C** and **D,** Good correction was maintained at 3 years after surgery.

TECHNIQUES, TIPS, AND PITFALLS

Calcaneus Osteotomy and Flexor Digitorum Longus Transfer

● The principle of the calcaneal osteotomy is to shift the tuberosity medially, thereby altering the axis of pull of the Achilles tendon on the hindfoot. As the tuberosity shifts medially, the Achilles tendon is now slightly medial to the axis of the subtalar joint. Plantar flexion is then facilitated in a neutral position, and the valgus deformity of the heel is not augmented. As long as the osteotomy includes the tuberosity, it probably does not make a difference in how close to the axis of the subtalar joint the osteotomy is performed. I have seen problems occur when the osteotomy is made too far posteriorly when it does not include enough of the tuberosity of the calcaneus. Any postoperative pain is largely the result of an uneven step-off on the back of the calcaneal tuberosity.

● The average amount of medial shift used in this procedure is 1 cm, but the amount can be varied according to the size of the patient and the magnitude of the deformity. In patients with more significant heel valgus and a larger heel, which will tolerate more medialization, I will then shift the calcaneus up to 14 mm. The diameter of the calcaneus at the level of the osteotomy is approximately 30 mm; therefore a shift of 15 mm is easily tolerated, and fixation is not compromised.

● Tamping down the overhanging ledge of bone on the dorsal ridge of the calcaneal osteotomy is important. The effects of this overhanging ridge can be determined by palpation of the bone through the skin. This can be uncomfortable and may need revision if this is not adequately smoothed down at the time of surgery.

● Neuritis does not seem to be a problem after the osteotomy, provided that the surgeon looks for the nerve and retracts it if it is visible. Usually, however, the nerve is not visible during the operative procedure.

● Overcorrection from this osteotomy is rare but can occur. If the heel seems to be in slight varus postoperatively, this is probably not arising from overtightening of the tendon transfer medially. I have had to reverse the osteotomy for two patients, and although this reversal does bring the heel back to a better position, the heel is slightly shorter and wider.

● What should be done when the PTT is intact with minor fissuring but has good excursion? Often, the more minor tears are associated with additional disease on the medial side of the capsuloligamentous complex. Rarely, the tendon is left intact if it appears to be completely healthy. Be careful with this approach, because minor fissuring and tearing do lead to functional elongation with a decrease in function.

● I prefer not to leave the PTT intact when I am doing an FDL tendon transfer. Even if the tendon has moderate tears only, I cut out a central portion approximately 6 cm in diameter. Leaving a distal 2-cm stump facilitates the attachment of the flexor tendon; the proximal stump can then be used for the tenodesis to the FDL tendon.

● A proximal tenodesis is performed only when a healthy tibialis posterior muscle is present, with confirmation of good excursion. Performing a tenodesis of any sort to the PTT is not recommended if the PTT is diseased because this would inhibit the function of the healthy FDL tendon transfer.

● Looking for additional disease in the capsuloligamentous complex is important. Changes may range from a defect in the deltoid ligament to fissuring and elongation of the talonavicular capsule to a complete rupture of the spring ligament. At times a flexible flatfoot associated with a normal PTT and complete disruption of the medial capsuloligamentous complex, requiring repair, may be present.

● How tight should the transferred FDL tendon be made? I have done this procedure using different tensions in the belief that the tendon with the muscle should be attached at resting tension to function adequately. At present, however, I am not sure that this is correct. In the patients in whom I have tightened the tendon maximally, the foot does not stay inverted, and gradually some elongation occurs with settling out of the hindfoot and the arch. Nowadays, I tighten the FDL tendon transfer so that when the sutures are inserted, the forefoot is approximately 10 degrees beyond the midline.

● Preserving a pulley for the FDL tendon is unnecessary. Open up the sheath between the FDL and PTT and reroute this accordingly. Subluxation does not occur.

● When cutting the FDL, visualize the tendon in the arch of the foot. A plexus of veins is adjacent to the master knot of Henry, and if it begins to bleed, maintaining visualization of the tendon during dissection is difficult.

- Distal tenodesis between the stump of the FDL and the FHL tendons seems unnecessary. Weakness is not perceived by the patient and is barely discernible even on careful examination.

Lateral Column Lengthening

- The key to the lateral column lengthening procedure is to avoid crushing of the calcaneus. Crushing can be prevented by carefully inserting the lamina spreader on the dorsolateral aspect of the calcaneus right at the junction of the neck and avoiding the soft cancellous bone.

- Once the graft is inserted, removal of the laminar spreader is not always easy. Ideally, if the incision is more dorsal and less lateral, then the graft can be inserted and directed vertically, and removal of the laminar spreader from the lateral side of the incision is easier.

- The graft should be trapezoidal and wider laterally and dorsally. The greatest change in the position of the joint of the graft, however, should be directly lateral.

- Be careful of the position of the graft once insertion is complete. Obtaining a good lateral radiographic image of the foot intraoperatively is important. A possible complication is pain from impingement between a slightly dorsally subluxated graft and the anterior aspect of the subtalar joint. This problem occurs when the most lateral aspect of the graft appears to be in perfect position, whereas the more medial graft is dorsally subluxated. The posterior facet must be visible at completion of graft insertion.

- The combination of the lateral column lengthening and an opening wedge osteotomy of the medial cuneiform is extremely useful for correction of a flexible flatfoot that is associated with a fixed forefoot supination.

- The purpose of the lateral column lengthening is to correct the coverage angle of the talonavicular joint.

Rarely, the heel remains in valgus despite the lateral column lengthening, and the medial translation of osteotomy of the calcaneus can be performed simultaneously.

- Failure of the lateral column lengthening occurs as a result of bone impingement in the sinus tarsi when the graft is extruded. This extrusion may not, however, occur postoperatively and is a result of incorrect placement of the graft intraoperatively. Graft placement must be checked visually to ensure that no impingement is present up against the undersurface of the posterior facet.

- If the lamina spreader crushes the graft or crushes the calcaneus, the graft will sink into the center of the neck of the calcaneus and will not provide structural support. The bone graft should rest on the cortical rim and should not sink into the center of the calcaneus. If there is a tendency for crushing of the center of the calcaneus with the lamina spreader, the calcaneus will need to be held open in a slightly distracted position with a plate. An H plate is ideal for this repair. In this instance, a structural graft is not as important, because the plate maintains the position of the calcaneus.

- Before the cut is made on the calcaneus, inserting a guide pin transversely across the neck of the calcaneus is helpful to ensure the correct position. The cut tends to be too close to the calcaneocuboid joint, and the guide pin should be adjusted until the planned cut is approximately 10 to 12 mm proximal to the articular surface.

- The lateral column lengthening may be performed at the calcaneocuboid joint. As previously noted, this approach is not my preference, because most of these lengthening procedures can be performed through the neck of the calcaneus without the loss of motion that commonly results with lengthening at the calcaneocuboid joint. Nonetheless, this remains a reasonable alternative for correction in the appropriate patient.

SUGGESTED READING

Bluman EM, Myerson MS: Stage IV posterior tibial tendon rupture, *Foot Ankle Clin* 12:341–362, 2007:viii.

Bluman EM, Title CI, Myerson MS: Posterior tibial tendon rupture: A refined classification system, *Foot Ankle Clin* 12:233–249, 2007:v.

Bohay DR, Anderson JG: Stage IV posterior tibial tendon insufficiency: The tilted ankle, *Foot Ankle Clin* 8:619–634, 2003.

Greisberg J, Hansen ST Jr, Sangeorzan B: Deformity and degeneration in the hindfoot and midfoot joints of the adult acquired flatfoot, *Foot Ankle Int* 24:530–534, 2003.

Kadakia AR, Haddad SL: Hindfoot arthrodesis for the adult acquired flat foot, *Foot Ankle Int* 8:569–594, 2003.

Kann JN, Myerson MS: Intraoperative pathology of the posterior tibial tendon, *Foot Ankle Clin* 2:343–355, 1997.

Myerson MS: Adult acquired flatfoot deformity: Treatment of dysfunction of the posterior tibial tendon insufficiency, *Instr Course Lect* 46:393–405, 1997.

Myerson MS: Adult acquired flatfoot deformity. Treatment of dysfunction of the posterior tibial tendon [abstract], *J Bone Joint Surg Am* 78A:780–792, 1996.

Myerson MS, Corrigan J: Treatment of posterior tibial tendon dysfunction with flexor digitorum longus tendon transfer and calcaneal osteotomy, *Orthopedics* 19:383–388, 1996.

Myerson MS, Corrigan J, Thompson F, Schon LC: Tendon transfer combined with calcaneal osteotomy for treatment of posterior tibial tendon insufficiency: A radiological investigation, *Foot Ankle Int* 16:712–718, 1995.

Neufeld SK, Myerson MS: Complications of surgical treatments for adult flatfoot deformities, *Foot Ankle Clin* 6:179–191, 2001.

Pinney SJ, Van Bergeyk A: Controversies in surgical reconstruction of acquired adult flat foot deformity, *Foot Ankle Clin* 8:595–604, 2003.

Toolan BC: The treatment of failed reconstruction for adult acquired flat foot deformity, *Foot Ankle Clin* 8:647–654, 2003.

Trnka HJ, Easley ME, Myerson MS: The role of calcaneal osteotomies for correction of adult flatfoot, *Clin Orthop Aug* :950–64, 1999.

Zaret DI, Myerson MS: Arthroereisis of the subtalar joint, *Foot Ankle Clin* 8:605–617, 2003.

CHAPTER 19

Complications of Treatment of Flatfoot

Errors in management of flatfoot fall into two broad categories: errors of decision making and technical errors related to surgery. Complications resulting from such errors often can be effectively managed with appropriate revision surgery. Other complications may occur as part of the natural history of the disease process, including arthritis and deformity. This chapter considers some of the more commonly encountered complications in this clinical setting, with a range of examples using the staging system for acquired flatfoot in adults, as described in the previous chapter.

TENOSYNOVITIS

A common error in the management of the flexible flatfoot is failure to recognize the presence of tenosynovitis in patients who have a seronegative spondyloarthropathy. This condition is not necessarily associated with a flatfoot deformity, but if it is not treated with a tenosynovectomy, the tendon will be progressively infiltrated until rupture and deformity occur. In the older patient with tenosynovitis associated with a mild flatfoot deformity, or no flatfoot, one issue is whether or not an osteotomy of the calcaneus should be performed with the tenosynovectomy.

HOW TO MANAGE THE FAILED TENDON TRANSFER

It is important to establish why a tendon transfer procedure failed. Was the selected tendon transfer not strong enough for the specific foot deformity? Is the patient obese? Did preoperative assessment fail to detect some stiffness of the hindfoot? Is there additional deformity of the medial column? Should an osteotomy of the calcaneus have been performed, and if so, with lengthening or medial translation?

Figure 19-1 presents an example of failure of a previous flexor digitorum longus (FDL) tendon transfer. The patient was a 54-year-old active woman weighing 76 kg. The hindfoot was quite flexible, and with the heel reduced to neutral there was a fixed forefoot supination deformity of 20 degrees. No active inversion was noted, and pain was present along the medial border of the foot and ankle, in addition to sinus tarsi pain, the result of subfibular impingement. Traditionally, if the FDL has already been used in a tendon transfer, little is left to function as an invertor. The lateral side of the foot can be weakened with a peroneus brevis-to-longus transfer, which

would have the added benefit of plantar-flexing the first ray. The lateral radiograph (see Figure 19-1, *A*) shows a break in the foot at both the talonavicular (TN) and naviculocuneiform (NC) joints. Certainly a fusion of the NC joint could be added to the procedure without loss of too much function, but this procedure would not address the weakness and lateral foot pain. The patient had already undergone a successful triple arthrodesis on the opposite foot for management of a very rigid flatfoot deformity and wanted to avoid another arthrodesis. In this patient, uncovering of the TN joint was not so extensive as to necessitate a lengthening of the lateral column, whether by osteotomy or by arthrodesis. I do not like to use a subtalar implant in the adult, and although this would be a reasonable indication, this procedure still does not address the muscle imbalance. I therefore selected the anterior tibial tendon (ATT) for transfer, modifying the original Young procedure.

For this modified procedure, the navicular is exposed, and a thick osteoperiosteal flap is raised from the center of the navicular and retracted inferiorly (see Figure 19-1, *C*). This flap can include the remnant of the posterior tibial tendon (PTT) as well. A ridge with an overhang of approximately 5 mm is then prepared under the navicular with a curette or chisel, to function as a ledge for the transferred ATT. The retinaculum of the ATT is opened and released proximal to the ankle joint under direct vision. The ATT is then pulled below the navicular into the prepared slot (see Figure 19-1, *D*) and sutured either using the osteoperiosteal flap or by adding a suture anchor into the body of the navicular. If an anchor is used, fluoroscopic guidance is recommended to ensure that it is in the navicular and not protruding into the joint. The remnant of the PTT can now be cut, sacrificed, or repaired, depending on the status of the tendon (see Figure 19-1, *E*). In this patient, after these procedures there was slightly more forefoot supination than I would accept, and plantar flexion of the medial column was obtained with an opening wedge osteotomy of the medial cuneiform. The postoperative radiographs showed excellent restoration of the height of the arch of the foot, as well as coverage of the TN joint (see Figure 19-1, *F* and *G*).

A similar example of the same problem is shown in Figure 19-2. The patient was a 61-year-old man who had been treated with a previous calcaneus osteotomy and a transfer of the flexor hallucis longus. The hindfoot was quite flexible, and the heel was in moderate valgus. On observation of the heel from posterior, the calcaneus osteotomy did not appear to have accomplished much.

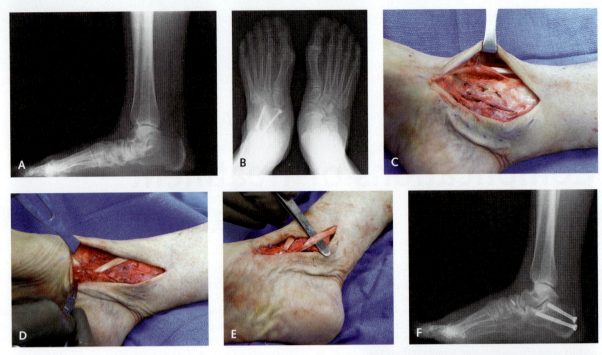

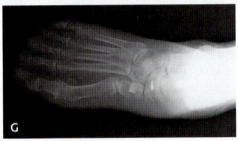

Figure 19-1 A and **B,** A 54-year-old woman with an active lifestyle had undergone a previous tendon transfer to correct a flexible flatfoot. The hindfoot remained flexible. **C,** The navicular was exposed, and a thick osteoperiosteal flap elevated from the center of the navicular and retracted inferiorly. **D** and **E,** The anterior tibial tendon was then pulled below the navicular into the prepared slot **(D),** and sutured with an anchor into the body of the navicular **(E). F** and **G,** The postoperative radiographs show excellent restoration of the height of the arch of the foot as well as coverage of the talonavicular joint 3 years after surgery.

Figure 19-2 A and **B,** A 61-year-old patient had been treated with a prior calcaneus osteotomy and a transfer of the flexor hallucis longus for correction of deformity. The hindfoot remained quite flexible, and the heel was in moderate valgus. **C** and **D,** Revision surgery was accomplished with the modified Young procedure, transferring the anterior tibial tendon under the navicular to support the medial arch of the foot.

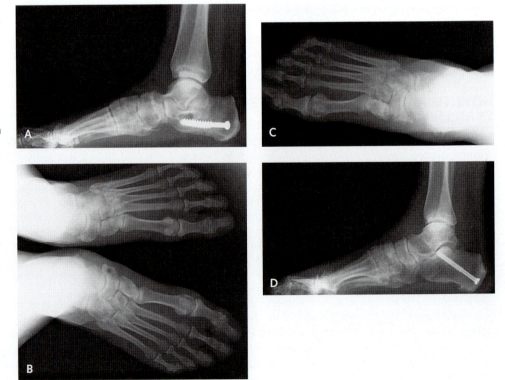

The elements of surgical decision making were similar to those in the case shown in Figure 19-1, in which an arthrodesis was an option; however, maintaining flexibility seemed preferable in that very active patient. The ATT was transferred under the navicular, and the calcaneus osteotomy was repeated. It was not necessary to include an osteotomy of the medial cuneiform. An important point is that the ATT is not detached from its insertion and is levered inferiorly under a prepared osteoperiosteal flap in the edge of the navicular. The extent of bone resected in this process can be appreciated on the anteroposterior radiographic view (see Figure 19-2, C), in which the medial pole of the navicular has been removed to create the ridge under which to attach the ATT. It is important to leave no sharp edges on the ridge on the proximal navicular, because consequent damage to the ATT can lead to its rupture—a complication that has occurred in one of my own patients. When the rupture occurred, the patient noticed a sudden change in the foot at 8 weeks after surgery, and the ATT was no longer palpable dorsomedially. The rupture was repaired by reattaching the ATT to the dorsal central aspect of the navicular using a suture anchor.

Although errors in decision making and technique are inevitable, some of these are entirely avoidable. In the case illustrated in Figure 19-3, a 47-year-old woman was treated with a transfer of the FDL for correction of a flatfoot deformity. At 9 months after the surgery she presented with considerable pain in the anterior ankle, and on an anteroposterior radiograph of the foot, marked loss of the TN joint space was readily apparent. The diagnosis of rheumatoid arthritis was confirmed with a positive rheumatoid factor titer, and a TN arthrodesis was used for correction.

A simple error in technique is illustrated in Figure 19-4: In the case depicted, an opening wedge osteotomy was performed in conjunction with a transfer of the FDL tendon and a calcaneus osteotomy. The incorrect insertion of the bone wedge into the cuneiform, which fractured into the first metatarsocuneiform (MC) joint (see Figure 19-4), is evident. This technical error can be avoided by inserting a guide pin in the cuneiform from dorsal to plantar and obtaining a lateral view radiograph to ensure the correct orientation of the osteotomy. The cuneiform inclines obliquely,

and the osteotomy is not perpendicular to the axis of the foot but must be oriented to the axis of the cuneiform. The osteotomy cut also must be completed with the saw and not end in the cuneiform, because use of an osteotome to complete the cut may result in fracture extending out into the MC joint, which probably happened in this case. Although arthritis did not develop in this patient over 3 years of follow-up, the potential for this complication nonetheless remains worrisome. The "hump" evident in the midfoot was the result of the incorrect axis of the osteotomy, which unfortunately caused abutment and symptoms in shoes.

What is the optimal approach to treatment of the extremely flexible flatfoot? Is it always possible to avoid arthrodesis? In Figure 19-5, illustrating the case of a 44-year-old man with a unilateral flexible flatfoot, significant uncovering of the TN joint is apparent. The lateral radiographic view showed quite a lot of sag at the TN joint as well, with a fairly marked alteration in the talocalcaneal angle. In such cases, I have found that despite addition of a lateral column–lengthening procedure, instability may persist at the TN joint, increasing the likelihood of subsequent failure. Accordingly, although it is therefore always preferable to perform a tendon transfer with osteotomies, a TN arthrodesis is a good, reliable procedure and was performed in this patient with a successful result. The postoperative improvement in the talocalcaneal angle can be readily appreciated on the lateral view, even on a non–weight-bearing radiograph (see Figure 19-5, D).

Perhaps a similar result could be achieved with a lengthening arthrodesis through the calcaneocuboid (CC) joint, but this too has not been my experience, and persistent abduction of the forefoot may be present (Figure 19-6). An arthrodesis of the CC joint preserves more medial column motion, and although it still locks up inversion and eversion, it is nevertheless preferable to the TN arthrodesis under similar circumstances. It is, however, associated with some risk for nonunion of the CC joint, although this is far less common than with the TN joint. The case illustrated in Figure 19-6 involved a number of errors, including perhaps that related to decision making—the extensive correction required was too much to expect from this procedure. Persistent abduction of the foot was present, insufficient lengthening was achieved, and a nonunion of the joint further complicated the outcome, which was resolved with a triple arthrodesis.

Another, similar dilemma is illustrated in Figure 19-7. In this case, the patient was a 57-year-old man with bilateral flexible flatfoot. Indeed, because of the extreme flexibility the use of

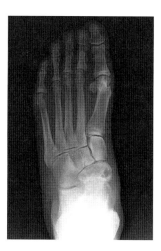

Figure 19-3 A patient who had been treated with a transfer of the flexor digitorum longus tendon for correction of a flatfoot deformity now presented with talonavicular pain. After appropriate investigation, the patient was found to have rheumatoid arthritis, which was the cause of the pain. A tendon transfer will not work no matter how flexible the foot if arthritis is present, particularly that associated with a rheumatologic process.

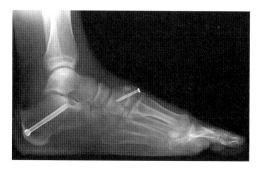

Figure 19-4 A fracture of the cuneiform occurred during performance of an osteotomy on this foot. Although the alignment of the foot is good, the fracture could potentially cause painful arthritis. The responsible technical error was an incorrectly made osteotomy cut, which was not completed to the plantar surface of the cuneiform, so that when the cuneiform was distracted, it fractured into the first tarsometatarsal joint.

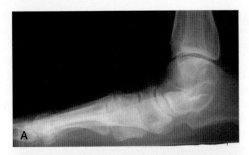

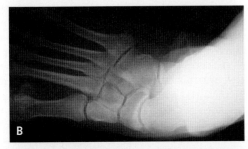

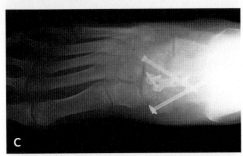

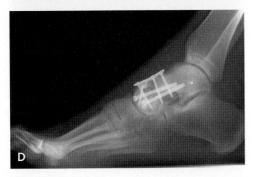

Figure 19-5 A and **B,** This was an extremely flexible deformity with marked uncovering of the talonavicular (TN) joint and a collapse pattern on the lateral radiographic view. **C** and **D,** A talonavicular arthrodesis was selected for correction. Although lengthening of the lateral column might have worked, I have found the latter procedure to be less reliable in the presence of significant TN instability.

osteotomies to perform the correction was appealing. Nevertheless, perhaps because of just a sense of when things are more likely to go wrong, derived from experience, I selected a triple arthrodesis for correction. In realigning the foot intraoperatively, it was apparent that correction of the TN coverage was possible only if a lengthening of the lateral column was simultaneously performed. The triple arthrodesis was therefore accomplished with a bone block graft in the CC joint (see Figure 19-7).

Complications of arthrodesis of the CC joint are quite common, including nonunion, as well as under- and overcorrection. It is far more difficult to manage a nonunion of the CC joint since there

is necrosis of bone, impaired vascularity, and increasing deformity. This is well illustrated in Figure 19-8 in a patient who was treated for a flexible flatfoot with a lateral column lengthening, a transfer of the FDL, and a medial cuneiform osteotomy. Subsequent nonunion of the CC joint, persistent abduction of the foot with uncovering of the TN joint, and erosive changes about the CC joint with avascular bone were resolved with additional structural bone grafting, bone stimulation with bone morphogenic protein, and repeat fixation (see Figure 19-8, *C* and *D*). It seems to get harder, not easier, to revise the CC joint nonunion. Perhaps this tendency has to do with the local anatomy and the patient, but most often, the problem is just poor bone with surrounding sclerosis. This is exemplified in Figure 19-9, in a patient for whom four surgeries were performed to obtain an arthrodesis. The first procedure was performed with a lengthening of the CC joint with arthrodesis and a medial translational osteotomy of the calcaneus (see Figure 19-9, *A* and *B*). A nonunion resulted, and the bone grafting was repeated with different fixation (see Figure 19-9, *C* and *D*). Although the initial appearance was satisfactory, another nonunion ensued and was treated with repeat bone grafting and placement of implantable bone stimulator, which also failed to effect healing (see Figure 19-9, *E*). Ultimately, healing was obtained with repeat grafting with use of a different method of fixation and bone stimulation with bone morphogenic protein (see Figure 19-9, *F* and *G*).

In certain circumstances, it is reasonable to avoid an arthrodesis for correction of flexible flatfoot. I made a mistake in retrospect in the case illustrated in Figure 19-10. The patient was a 69-year-old man with a very flexible unilateral flatfoot, with an obvious rupture of the PTT. There was associated arthritis as well as instability of the first tarsometatarsal (TMT) joint, necessitating an arthrodesis. Given the requirement for an arthrodesis of the first TMT joint, I wanted to avoid having to perform a triple arthrodesis, so I chose to lengthen the lateral column with an osteotomy and bone graft (see Figure 19-10). Although the initial result was excellent, with improved alignment (see Figure 19-10, *C* and *D*), the osteotomy did not heal, and a nonunion resulted, followed by collapse of the hindfoot and recurrent flatfoot deformity. I did not think that revision of the nonunion would be easy, in view of the sclerosis and collapse at the margins of the nonunion. I therefore decided to convert this to a triple arthrodesis with bone graft. At this stage, the midfoot arthrodesis had healed, and the difficulty was how to address the nonunion of the calcaneus and simultaneously obtain an arthrodesis of the hindfoot. When the revision was performed, very little bone was available to work with within the distal neck of the calcaneus, and even less once the CC joint was denuded. Cancellous bone graft was used in the nonunion defect, supplemented by an implantable bone stimulator, and fixation across the nonunion and the CC joint was achieved simultaneously, with quite a successful outcome (see Figure 19-10, *F* and *G*). Perhaps the error in this case was not to go straight to the arthrodesis to begin with. Obviously, the experienced surgeon will be reluctant to perform an arthrodesis of the midfoot in addition to a triple arthrodesis, because the open joint might be expected to undergo stress with eventual development of arthritis. This does not often happen, however, and these extended triple arthrodesis procedures (including either naviculocuneiform or tarsometatarsal joints) are at times necessary.

Such a case is illustrated in Figure 19-11. The patient was a 66-year-old woman with a rigid flatfoot deformity, with marked instability of the first TMT joint, as well as slight sag at the NC joint. In view of the rigidity of the foot, a triple arthrodesis was clearly necessary, but then so was a first TMT arthrodesis, which

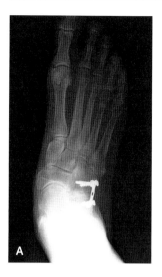
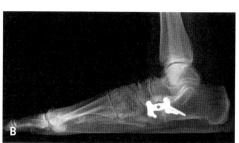

Figure 19-6 Persistent abduction of the foot after an attempted arthrodesis through the calcaneocuboid joint. A and B, Insufficient lengthening resulted in a nonunion of the joint, further complicating the outcome, which was resolved with a triple arthrodesis.

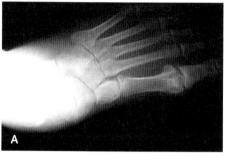
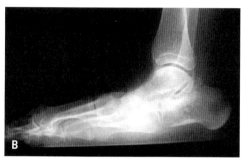
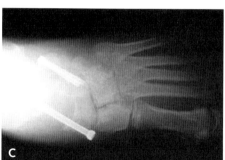
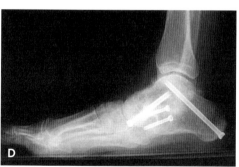

Figure 19-7 A and B, Rigid flatfoot deformity and moderate uncovering of the TN joint in a 47-year-old woman. C and D, Although a triple arthrodesis was performed, it was necessary to either shorten the medial column or lengthen the lateral column. These procedures were performed simultaneously with insertion of a bone block graft in the calcaneocuboid joint.

was performed simultaneously with good realignment. At 3 years after surgery, the foot remained aligned without development of arthritis in the NC joint (see Figure 19-11, C and D). A similar example is presented in Figure 19-12, in which the patient was a 62-year-old man with a rigid hindfoot deformity, dislocation of the TN joint, and a moderate hallux valgus deformity with painful arthritis of the first TMT joint. Note also the changes of the fibula on the anteroposterior view of the ankle, indicative of chronic stress (see Figure 19-12, C). This was addressed with a triple arthrodesis and a modified Lapidus procedure simultaneously with success (see Figure 19-12, D and E). It is therefore evident that when necessary, an extended medial column arthrodesis should be performed in conjunction with a triple arthrodesis if indicated. The procedure should not be avoided merely to prevent added stiffness of the foot.

A slightly different problem with a flexible flatfoot arises in the older adult with a painful accessory navicular, usually associated with insertional PTT tendinopathy. The foot is often still fairly flexible, and pain is typically present at the insertion of the PTT.

Should one correct this with excision of the accessory navicular, and advancement of the PTT, or excise the painful PTT and perform a tendon transfer. Structural deformity frequently is associated with the flatfoot, so that regardless of what is performed medially, something has to be done in addition to correct the deformity, much along that outlined for treatment of the adult flatfoot. This approach was taken in the 51-year-old patient whose case is illustrated in Figure 19-13, who presented with a painful flatfoot associated with recent onset of pain at the insertion of the PTT. Given the pain at the insertion of the PTT with some recent avulsion of the tendon and gradual retraction of the accessory navicular, I elected to excise the accessory navicular, and reattach the PTT with an anchor to the navicular. A subtalar arthroereisis was performed to correct the alignment of the calcaneus (see Figure 19-13, C). The initial alignment was satisfactory, although certainly not excellent. Over the course of the next year, however, the patient complained of pain in the sinus tarsi, and the implant was removed (see Figure 19-13, D). This too did not alleviate her pain, and eventually a subtalar

Figure 19-8 A and **B,** Nonunion of the calcaneocuboid (CC) joint, persistent abduction of the foot with uncovering of the talonavicular joint, and erosive changes about the CC joint with avascular bone followed treatment for a flexible flatfoot with a lateral column lengthening, a transfer of the flexor digitorum longus, and a medial cuneiform osteotomy. **C** and **D,** Correction with resolution of pathologic changes was accomplished with additional structural bone grafting, bone stimulation with bone morphogenic protein, and repeat fixation. (Case courtesy Dr. John Campbell.)

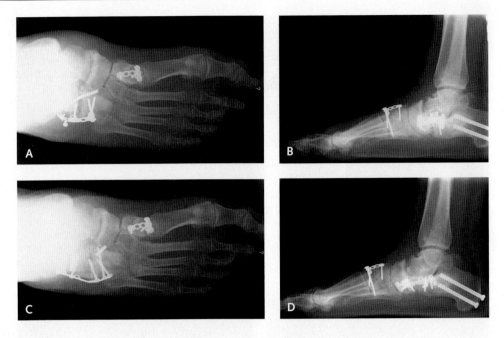

Figure 19-9 A and **B,** A flexible flatfoot deformity in a 39-year-old woman was corrected with a lengthening of the calcaneocuboid joint with arthrodesis and a medial translational osteotomy of the calcaneus. **C** and **D,** A nonunion resulted, and the bone graft procedure was repeated with use of different fixation. **E,** Although the initial appearance was satisfactory, another nonunion ensued and was treated with repeat bone grafting and placement of an implantable bone stimulator, which also failed to produce healing. **F** and **G,** Ultimately, healing was obtained with repeat grafting, changing the screw fixation, and adding bone morphogenic protein. (Case courtesy Dr. Clifford Jeng.)

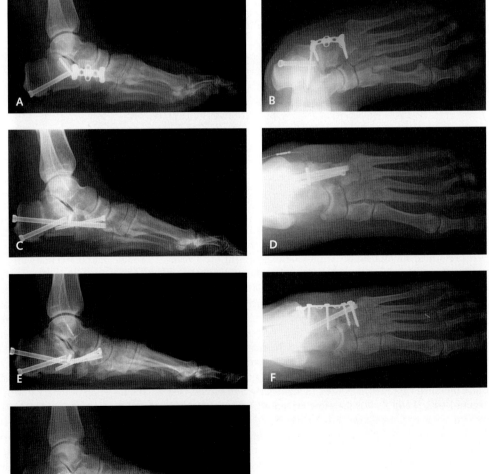

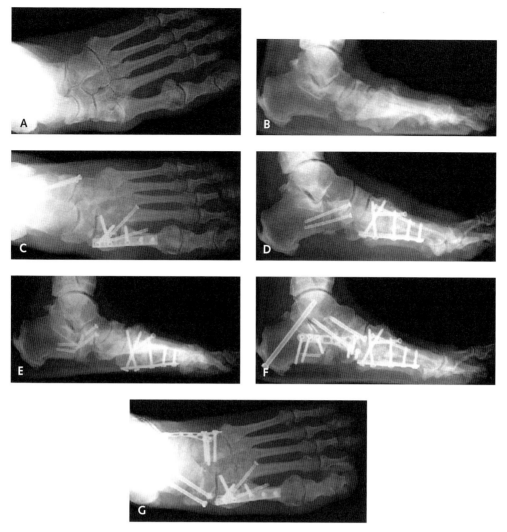

Figure 19-10 A and **B,** A unilateral flexible flatfoot with arthritis as well as instability of the first tarsometatarsal (TMT) joint in a 69-year-old man. **C** and **D,** This was treated with lengthening of the lateral column with an osteotomy and bone graft and arthrodesis of the first TMT joint. **E,** At 3 months, a nonunion was noted with collapse of the hindfoot and recurrent flatfoot deformity. **F** and **G,** A triple arthrodesis with bone graft across the nonunion as well as the calcaneocuboid (CC) joint was performed. At this stage, the midfoot arthrodesis had healed, and the difficulty was how to address the nonunion of the calcaneus and simultaneously obtain an arthrodesis of the hindfoot. When the revision was performed, there was very little bone to work with within the distal neck of the calcaneus, and this was worsened once the CC joint was denuded. Cancellous bone graft was used in the nonunion, supplemented by placement of an implantable bone stimulator, with fixation across the nonunion and the CC joint simultaneously, with quite a successful outcome.

arthrodesis was performed (see Figure 19-13, *E*). Although the subtalar pain had been addressed, the hindfoot was not corrected, and persistent midfoot supination was present with pain under the fifth metatarsal and cuboid, ultimately treated with a triple arthrodesis (see Figure 19-13, *F*). Although the pain resolved, I did not think that the alignment was correct. What went wrong here? First, the subtalar implant does not work well in the adult. It certainly aids in realigning the hindfoot; however, the rate of removal of the implant as a consequence of pain in the adult has been approximately 50% in my experience. It is always difficult to go straight to a triple arthrodesis in a foot like this, and perhaps an isolated subtalar arthrodesis with excision of the PTT and a transfer of the FDL tendon would have been a better alternative.

Perhaps the use of the implant is warranted nonetheless in the adult as a temporary adjunct to maintain correction of the flexible

flatfoot (Figure 19-14). However, unless the forefoot is perfectly plantigrade, and in particular, if there is any forefoot supination, then as the foot moves into foot flat in weight bearing, in order to maintain the forefoot plantigrade, the hindfoot has to evert, causing compression of the subtalar implant with consequent pain. An additional osteotomy of the medial cuneiform was used in this patient in an effort to increase the plantar flexion of the medial forefoot, thereby decreasing the force on the hindfoot in foot flat. The arthroereisis can lift up the talus and improve the talar declination, but it cannot correct the abducted forefoot. My advice is to use this procedure sparingly in the adult, but to have it available as a surgical alternative.

With the adult flatfoot, an association with rupture of the PTT causing a unilateral flatfoot deformity is the first thing that comes to mind. Perhaps the flatfoot was congenital, however, with

Figure 19-11 A and **B,** A rigid flatfoot deformity with instability of the first tarsometatarsal (TMT) joint, as well as slight sag at the naviculocuneiform joint, in a 66-year-old woman. **C,** A triple arthrodesis and a first TMT arthrodesis were performed. **D,** Radiographic appearance at 3 years after surgery.

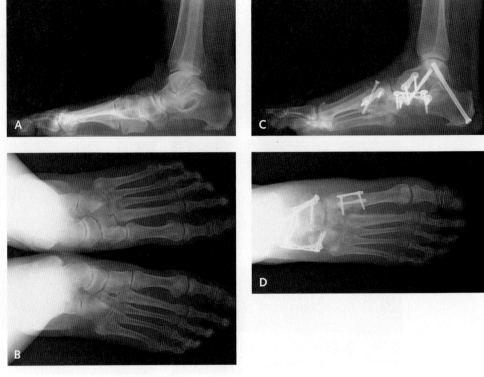

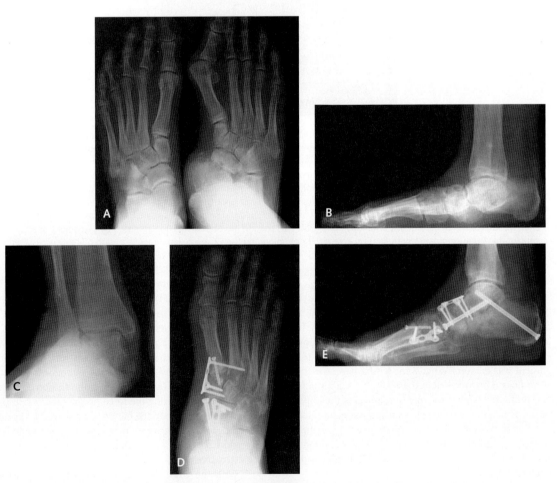

Figure 19-12 A-C, Rigid hindfoot deformity, dislocation of the talonavicular (TN) joint, and a moderate hallux valgus deformity with painful arthritis of the first tarsometatarsal joint in a 62-year-old man. **D** and **E,** Correction was accomplished with a modified triple arthrodesis and a modified Lapidus procedure.

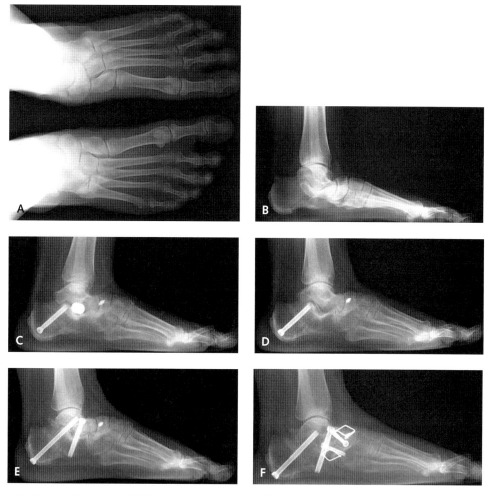

Figure 19-13 **A** and **B**, A painful flatfoot associated with pain of recent onset at the insertion of the posterior tibial tendon (PTT) in a 51-year-old patient. **C**, The accessory navicular was removed, and the PTT reattached with an anchor, combined with a subtalar arthroereisis. **D**, The patient had persistent pain in the sinus tarsi, and the implant was removed at 1 year. **E**, This did not alleviate pain, and 3 months later a subtalar arthrodesis was performed. **F**, Despite arthrodesis, the hindfoot problems were not corrected, and pain under the fifth metatarsal and cuboid ultimately necessitated a triple arthrodesis.

many years of flexible flatfoot eventuating in a deformity that was more pronounced and symptomatic on one side. It is important to consider the effect of midfoot deformity on the hindfoot. This is a common cause of the adult flatfoot, which should not be considered as an isolated arthritic process but should be regarded as a global problem of the hindfoot and midfoot. Treatment for the arthritis that does not attempt to correct the hindfoot deformity is not adequate treatment. This is well illustrated in Figure 19-15, in the case of a 65-year-old patient referred for management of severe plantar midfoot and hindfoot pain after unsuccessful surgery. Her postoperative radiographs (Figure 19-15, *A-C*) show a persistent rocker-bottom deformity, lateral overload under the cuboid, and abduction of the foot, in addition to nonunions. Comparison with the opposite foot (see Figure 19-15, *D*) serves to highlight the midfoot rocker-bottom deformity, as well as the hindfoot collapse. The equinus deformity of the previously operated foot is evident, with severe compromise of the calcaneus pitch angle and similar degree of abnormality in the talar declination angle. The challenge with this type of deformity is to correct not only the midfoot rocker-bottom and abduction deformities but also to treat the persistent arthritis, the nonunion, and the hindfoot deformity. This complex correction can be accomplished only with a triple arthrodesis, extended to the

midfoot. The CC joint is the apex of this deformity, so the correction must hinge on this axis.

An extensile lateral incision was used, from the tip of the fibula to the mid-metatarsal, and the CC joint was levered open. Once all the joints were debrided and prepared, the cuboid was levered dorsally and then temporarily pinned. This approach contrasts with that in most triple arthrodesis procedures, in which either the TN or the subtalar joint is the hinge on which the hindfoot deformity is corrected. Personally, I normally prefer to begin the arthrodesis at the TN joint and find that reduction of the subtalar joint follows. It is only with severe subtalar joint deformity that reduction of the latter must be accomplished first, followed by derotation of the TN joint. The effect of these manipulations on the alignment of the TN joint must then be ascertained. To correct the medial foot alignment, if the subtalar joint is fixed first, the navicular has to be adducted and translated slightly inferiorly to the talus. In Figure 19-15, the foot has an excellent clinical appearance, but the radiograph appears a little odd, because the axis of the TN joint is not perfect. Nonetheless, the result was excellent, as is evident on even a non–weight-bearing radiograph (see Figure 19-15, *E* and *F*). The lesson here is the necessity for correction of not only the presenting problem—in this patient, painful tarsometatarsal arthritis—but also

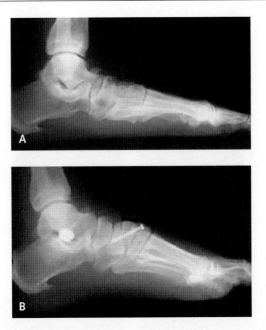

Figure 19-14 A and **B,** A subtalar arthroereisis implant was used as an adjunctive treatment for this flexible deformity, previously corrected with a transfer of the flexor digitorum longus and an osteotomy of the medial cuneiform.

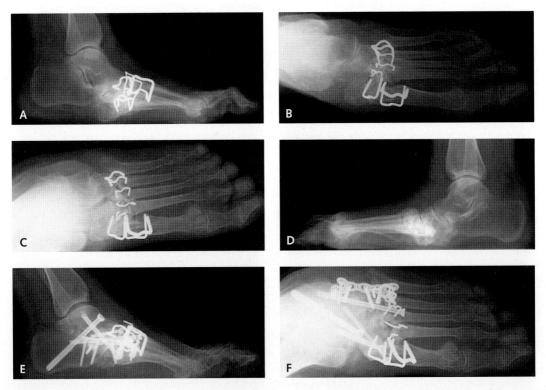

Figure 19-15 A-C, A 65-year-old patient was referred for management of severe plantar midfoot and hindfoot pain following attempted tarsometatarsal arthrodesis. This was complicated by a persistent rocker-bottom deformity, lateral overload under the cuboid, abduction of the forefoot, and nonunion of the tarsometatarsal joints. **D,** The opposite foot is shown for comparison. **E** and **F,** Correction was accomplished with a triple arthrodesis with a revision of the midfoot arthrodesis.

the potential cause of the problem—here, the hindfoot deformity. As illustrated in Figure 19-16, the patient presented with painful arthritis of the first TMT joint. If the focus of correction was only on the painful TMT joint, the foot would remain flat and abducted, and pain would continue. The hindfoot as well as the midfoot must be corrected, even though the problem is perceived as isolated to the midfoot.

Perhaps the most challenging problem in management of flatfoot, and the one associated with the most frequent complications, is the grade IV deformity. Rupture of the deltoid ligament associated with a flatfoot, whether rigid or flexible, and with or without associated arthritis of the ankle, represents a difficult problem. Clearly, a fusion of the ankle, with or without the hindfoot included, would address important components of the deformity—but most surgeons would find it difficult to consider an arthrodesis if the hindfoot is flexible and the ankle is unstable, but without arthritis. When the magnitude of this problem was recognized in the 1990s, the potential for failure of repair of the deltoid was not appreciated. In the example presented in Figure 19-17, the foot was flexible, and a rupture of the PTT was present; a tendon transfer was performed in addition to a medial translational osteotomy of the calcaneus. The deltoid was found to be completely ruptured, with the ankle joint exposed, and the medial malleolus was debrided and an anchor inserted, followed by advancement of the deltoid into the medial malleolus. Failure

occurred by 4 months, with recurrence of valgus deformity. It was apparent even then that the remnant of the deltoid was not sufficient mechanically to support the valgus forces on the ankle. Perhaps it is the quality of the tissue, as well as the additional deformity, that leads to failure. Regardless, simple repair, advancement, or reinforcement of the existing deltoid does not seem to work for correction of this deformity.

So what is the role for some sort of deltoid reconstruction? I have tried different variations of a deltoid reconstruction using a graft or even a tendon transfer with one of the peroneals, but outcome with these older approaches too has been unpredictable. In the case illustrated in Figure 19-18, a 72-year-old patient had previously undergone a triple arthrodesis, followed 5 years later by onset of lateral ankle pain resulting from subfibular impingement. At that time, the ankle was easily reducible. A hamstring tendon graft reconstruction was performed, with good intraoperative restoration of ankle stability. The triple arthrodesis was revised, and the forefoot was plantigrade at the time of this reconstruction, but complete failure with recurrent valgus as well as ankle arthritis was evident at 6 months after surgery. Why the failure? It is possible that the reconstruction must be performed anatomically, restoring the deltoid ligament and including both the superficial and deep components, along with establishing complete muscle balance of the foot and a plantigrade forefoot.

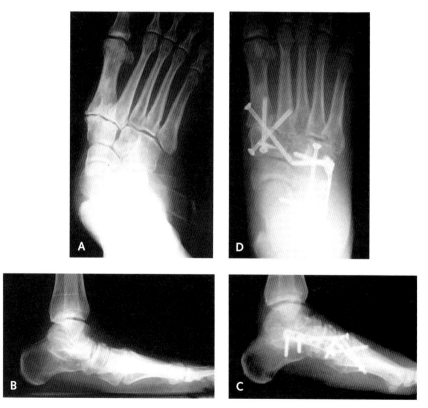

Figure 19-16 A and **B,** A painful first tarsometatarsal joint in a 41-year-old man. **C** and **D,** Treatment consisted of a lateral column lengthening and a modified Lapidus procedure.

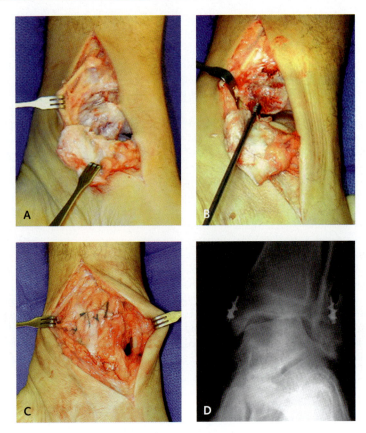

Figure 19-17 Correction of a flexible flatfoot and a flexible ankle not associated with any arthritis in a 68-year-old patient. **A,** Note the complete deltoid rupture, with the ankle joint exposed. **B** and **C,** The medial malleolus was debrided and a suture anchor inserted, followed by advancement of the deltoid into the medial malleolus. **D,** Radiograph of the ankle at 4 months after surgery demonstrates recurrent valgus deformity.

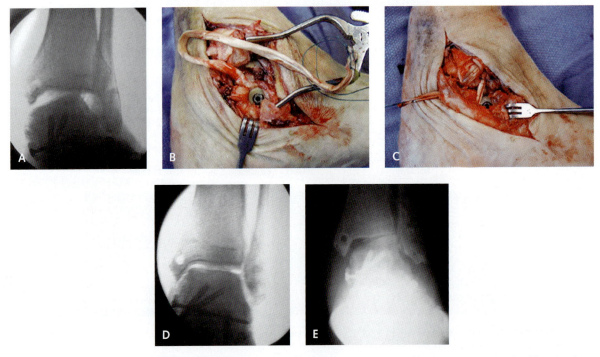

Figure 19-18 A, A 72-year-old who had previously undergone a triple arthrodesis, followed 5 years later by lateral ankle pain, the result of subfibular impingement with a reducible ankle. **B-D,** A hamstring tendon graft reconstruction was performed, with good intraoperative restoration of ankle stability. **E,** Revision of the triple arthrodesis was performed, and the forefoot was plantigrade at the time of the reconstruction, but complete failure with recurrent valgus as well as ankle arthritis was evident 6 months later.

CHAPTER **20**

Management of Tarsal Tunnel Syndrome

A tarsal tunnel release is performed for intractable refractory pain, burning, tingling, and numbness on the plantar and medial aspect of the foot. These symptoms can be associated with aching in the foot or leg, cramping, and vague sensations of soreness, fatigue, and burning, with or without activities. The common recognized causes of tarsal tunnel syndrome include hyperpronation of the foot, a valgus hindfoot, stress or pressure on the tibial nerve from a mass effect, varicosities, and trauma; in many patients, however, no identifiable cause for their symptoms can be found.

Before starting an operation for tarsal tunnel release, I routinely perform electrophysiologic testing. Although a normal test result does not contraindicate the performance of surgery, having confirmation of the clinical condition from an electromyogram (EMG) and nerve conduction studies is certainly useful. The problem arises when the patient has vague symptoms suggestive of a tarsal tunnel syndrome but not confirmed on EMG. The results of tarsal tunnel release are not that predictable; probably approximately 80% of well-selected patients improve satisfactorily. Therefore it is imperative to approach this condition with caution, and certainly to avoid operating on the patient with chronic pain or recurrent tarsal tunnel syndrome. In the latter condition, improvement is extremely difficult to obtain. Patients who have been previously operated on through a short incision over the tarsal canal and who continue to have more distal symptoms may constitute an exception: Perhaps the repeat surgery is indicated in this group of patients, for whom an inadequate release was initially performed.

The approach to tarsal tunnel release must include an incision that extends distally over the abductor hallucis muscle. The most frequent error in performing a tarsal tunnel release is to ignore the compression that occurs deep to the abductor hallucis muscle. The more proximal portion of the tibial nerve under the laciniate ligament (the flexor reticulum) is rarely the source of compression other than in patients who have lesions, masses, or varicosities in the tarsal tunnel immediately behind the medial malleolus.

The incision is deepened through subcutaneous tissue, and in the more proximal area of the tarsal tunnel the flexor retinaculum is perforated and opened proximally. Rarely, an entrapment is found in the more proximal aspect of the tarsal tunnel behind the malleolus. The flexor retinaculum (the laciniate ligament) is inspected and released slightly more distally to the level of the medial malleolus, and the nerve is inspected (Figures 20-1 and 20-2). A neurolysis is unnecessary for the success of the tibial nerve release and is not recommended. The less the nerve itself is irritated, the lower the risk for epineurial scarring.

The key to the operation is in the identification of the bifurcation of the nerve into the medial and lateral plantar nerves. The nerve is traced distally after release of the laciniate ligament, and then the abductor hallucis muscle is gently pulled distally. Using a retractor is the best way to identify the deep fascia directly underneath the abductor muscle. Once the fascia is identified, the lateral plantar nerve is released by completely splitting the deep fascia under direct vision while retracting the abductor muscle distally. After the dorsal, more proximal aspect of the fascia is released, retraction is performed in the reverse direction: The abductor muscle is identified distally at the inferior margin of the muscle and then is pulled proximally. In this way, definitive release of the entire deep fascia is accomplished. Occasionally, the superficial fascia on the abductor muscle is thick, and it also needs to be released, to allow the abductor muscle to be pulled in both directions.

Once the deep fascia of the underlying abductor muscle has been released, a decision can be made about whether to extend the incision more distally, if, for example, additional entrapment of the lateral plantar nerve or the first branch of the lateral plantar nerve, in conjunction with the heel pain syndrome, is present. The medial plantar nerve is released in a similar fashion, again under direct vision as it courses deep to the abductor hallucis muscle but slightly more anteriorly. The abductor muscle is pulled plantarward, the fascia is identified, and the split is made immediately below the flexor digitorum longus tendon. Palpation with the tip of the scissors distally is needed to ensure that the retinaculum has been completely released.

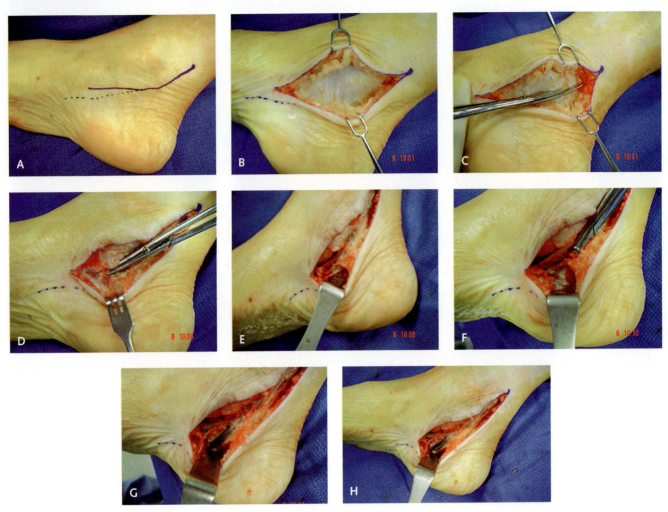

Figure 20-1 Release of the tarsal tunnel. **A,** The incision for extensile release of the tarsal tunnel. The *dotted line* represents an alternative extensile approach to the plantar aspect of the foot for a more complete nerve release. **B** and **C,** The retinaculum is exposed **(B)** and is released with a sharp scissors **(C). D,** A hemostat is then passed under the deep retinaculum into the medial plantar canal tunnel. **E,** The medial plantar nerve is completely released. **F,** The abductor fascia is exposed by pulling down on the abductor muscle with a large retractor. **G** and **H,** The lateral plantar nerve is released completely.

Any bleeding should be controlled before skin closure. I have found that this incision is prone to inflammation and dehiscence unless the foot is immobilized for a short time. I use nylon sutures in the skin and immobilize the ankle in a splint or short nonarticulated boot for 2 weeks until the sutures are removed and then allow full weight bearing as tolerated in a boot. Physical therapy and rehabilitation are important to the recovery process after this procedure and should be initiated as soon as tolerated.

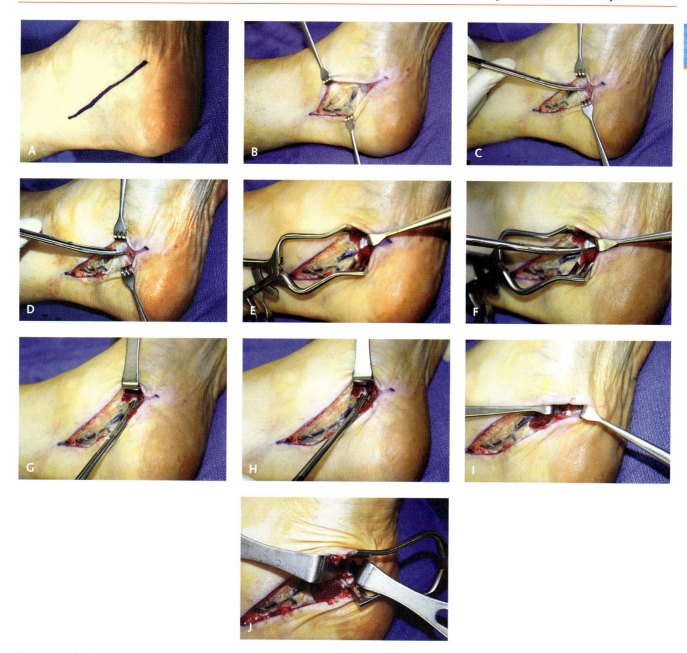

Figure 20-2 Tarsal tunnel release in a patient with nerve symptoms only. **A,** The incision is more vertical than in Figure 20-1. **B,** Note the bulging appearance of the neurovascular bundle after release of the flexor retinaculum. **C,** The distal retinaculum is split to expose the branching of the medial and lateral plantar nerves. The abductor hallucis muscle belly is abnormally large, which in this patient may have been the cause of the nerve entrapment. **D** and **E,** The muscle is swept off the deep fascia **(D)** and is released with scissors to free the lateral plantar nerve under the muscle **(E). F-H,** The muscle is then pulled forward, and the deeper course of the lateral plantar nerve is released under direct vision. **I** and **J,** In this patient, the plantar fascia was exposed and release as well.

SUGGESTED READING

Gondring WH, Shields B, Wenger S: An outcomes analysis of surgical treatment of tarsal tunnel syndrome, *Foot Ankle Int* 24:545–550, 2003.

Lau JT, Daniels TR: Effects of tarsal tunnel release and stabilization procedures on tibial nerve tension in a surgically created pes planus foot, *Foot Ankle Int* 19:770–777, 1998.

Lau JT, Daniels TR: Tarsal tunnel syndrome: A review of the literature, *Foot Ankle Int* 20:201–209, 1999.

Raikin SM, Minnich JM: Failed tarsal tunnel syndrome surgery, *Foot Ankle Clin* 8:159–174, 2003.

Sammarco GJ, Chang L: Outcome of surgical treatment of tarsal tunnel syndrome, *Foot Ankle Int* 24:125–131, 2003.

Skalley TC, Schon LC, Hinton RY, Myerson MS: Clinical results following revision tibial nerve release, *Foot Ankle Int* 15:360–367, 1994.

CHAPTER **21**

Management of Nerve Entrapment Syndromes

NEURECTOMY AND NERVE BURIAL

I must state at the outset that I have not obtained good results over the decades with nerve surgery, regardless of the type and extent. Revision nerve surgery is worse, with unpredictable results, especially in patients with chronic pain syndromes, who are very difficult to treat. Moreover, I have seen numerous patients actually harmed by repeat nerve surgery performed with the best expectations. Accordingly, the need for caution in recommending nerve surgery for management of foot and ankle pain cannot be overemphasized.

An isolated neuroma of the sural nerve may be treated surgically in the appropriate patient. By this I mean a patient who does not have chronic pain and who has localized discomfort only, from pressure over the traumatized nerve. In general, the outcome with neurectomy and nerve burial seems to be better in patients in whom the nerve was scarred or cut as a result of previous surgery than in patients who present with isolated nerve pain after an injury. In the latter group of patients, the affected foot frequently is sensitive to pressure, light touch, compression, and nerve irritation. Many of these patients with chronic pain syndromes initially are treated with topical anesthetic medications and oral neuroleptic agents, and surgery often is undertaken as a last resort. In such cases, inadequacy of pharmacologic management or of the attempted surgical correction may be the beginning of a chronic pain syndrome, with never-ending problems. I therefore rarely perform these procedures unless absolutely necessary.

Neurectomy and nerve burial may be performed in conjunction with additional procedures for correction of midfoot or hindfoot deformity, the most common of which is a subtalar arthrodesis after a calcaneus fracture, when a sural neurectomy is performed. The incision varies according to the presence of previous incisions, the location of the neuroma, and the type of additional operation performed. From a vertical incision made posterior to the peroneal tendon sheath, the nerve is identified and inspected. The nerve must be traced from proximal to distal—that is, from the healthy to the abnormal portion of the nerve. Identifying a discrete neuroma is difficult because it usually is encased in scar. The neuroma frequently is a consequence of previous surgery and is not mobile, particularly if it is located under the earlier incision. The sural nerve should be traced more distally until either the scar or a definite neuroma is identified. The nerve is dissected further distally, and if no further continuity with the main body of the nerve is observed, it is transected, including the neuroma.

The nerve is now clamped and the tip of the nerve is cauterized either using the electrocautery or with phenol. More proximally, the nerve is passed with a clamp and a 4-0 suture deep to the peroneal tendons or musculature, depending on the level in the leg. Simple resection of the neuroma is never sufficient. Burial in a muscle may work, but the recurrence rate seems to be high, and burying the nerve in bone is preferable. The key is to obtain sufficient length on the exposed nerve so that with movement of the leg and contracture of the peroneal muscles, there is no tension on the nerve.

Burying the nerve in bone is difficult, because the nerve does not easily stay in position. Two small 2.5-mm unicortical drill holes are made through the fibula perpendicular to each other and about 1 cm apart. The nerve is positioned at one end of the bone tunnel, and the suction is applied to the other drill hole to draw the nerve deep into the hole in the fibula. This drill hole technique seems to be the most effective means of burying the nerve inside the fibula. Once the nerve has been passed into the fibular hole, the epineurium can be sutured onto the periosteum. The ankle should be taken through full dorsiflexion and plantar flexion to ensure that there is no traction on the nerve and that the nerve is freely mobile in the posterior aspect of the limb and encased in the fibula itself (Figure 21-1).

Occasionally, after certain types of injuries, including crush injuries, a neurectomy may not be necessary, and a nerve release after removal of the ligament or tendon may be sufficient (Figures 21-2 to 21-5). This approach commonly is applicable, for example, in the dorsum of the foot, where the deep peroneal nerve is irritated by the extensor hallucis brevis tendon and an osteophyte from the base of the first or second metatarsal usually is a result of arthritis. Removal of the osteophytes, with release of the extensor hallucis brevis tendon, is sufficient to treat this nerve irritation. Less commonly seen nerve compression syndromes in the foot may involve, for example, the medial calcaneal branch of the tibial nerve or the first interspace branch of the medial plantar nerve. I have performed neurolysis in such cases with some success, but I rarely resort to surgery for these conditions.

MANAGEMENT OF INTERDIGITAL NEUROMA

For the management of all primary and most revision neuromas, I use a dorsal approach. This incision is centered over the affected web space if a single web space neuroma is excised. If both the

237

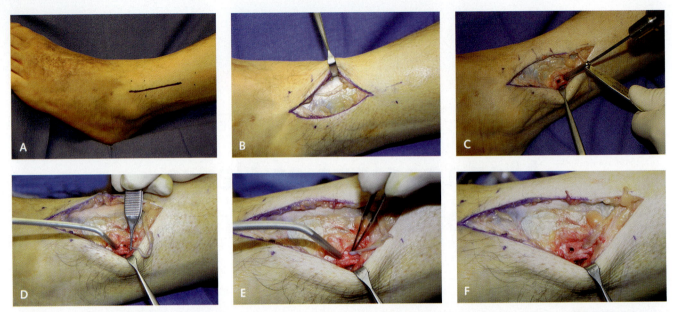

Figure 21-1 The steps in resection of a superficial peroneal nerve with burial into the fibula. The patient had sustained a severe crushing injury to the foot with consequent posttraumatic scarring of the nerve. **A,** The vertical incision. **B,** Note the thinned-out appearance of the nerve just distal to the anterior fascia. **C,** Two unicortical drill holes are made in the fibula at a 45-degree angle to each other with a 2.9-mm drill. **D** and **E,** The nerve is then placed at the edge of one of the drill holes, and the sucker tip is placed at the second hole. **F,** The nerve is sucked into the hole, allowing it to be buried without tension.

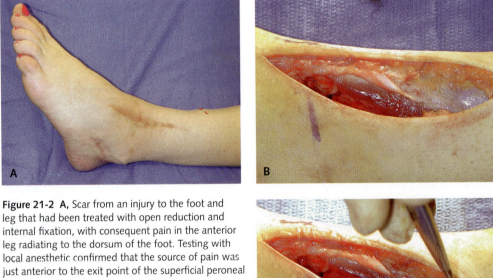

Figure 21-2 A, Scar from an injury to the foot and leg that had been treated with open reduction and internal fixation, with consequent pain in the anterior leg radiating to the dorsum of the foot. Testing with local anesthetic confirmed that the source of pain was just anterior to the exit point of the superficial peroneal nerve from the deep fascia. **B,** Extensive scarring of the fascia over the superficial peroneal nerve is evident. **C,** Appearance after release and neurolysis. The patient did not improve after revision surgery, and pain continued in the same location. No further surgery was provided.

second and third web space nerves are to be excised, then the incision is centered over the third metatarsal. Removing both web space neuromas through a single incision is easy; use of two incisions is not recommended because it will lead to unnecessary retraction, scarring, and the potential for wound compromise. The decision regarding whether the surgical approach will include one or both web spaces clearly depends on the clinical evaluation.

Neither magnetic resonance imaging (MRI) nor ultrasound studies are useful in the management of primary neuroma excision. Although ultrasound examination certainly can be used in difficult cases to differentiate scar from nerve enlargement in revision procedures, I have not found any role at all for it in the primary case. If the nature of the clinical findings is in doubt, sequential administration of 1 mL of lidocaine in potentially affected web spaces usually is

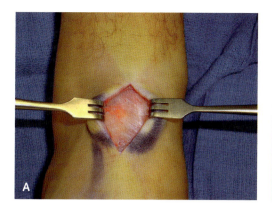

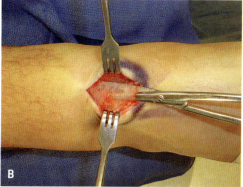

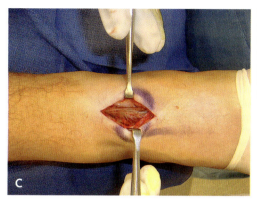

Figure 21-3 The patient experienced sharp pain with radiation over the dorsum of the first web space when wearing shoes. **A,** An osteophyte was present over the first tarsometatarsal joint compressing the deep peroneal nerve. **B** and **C,** The patient was successfully treated with release of the retinaculum and removal of the osteophyte without arthrodesis.

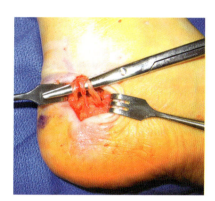

Figure 21-4 The patient was a middle-distance runner who complained of burning pain on the medial heel refractory to shoe changes and topical anesthetic agents. A neurolysis of the calcaneal nerve branches was performed with good relief of pain.

diagnostic. If the extent of the nerve involvement is still uncertain, I excise the nerve in the most symptomatic web space and then release the deep metatarsal ligaments in the adjacent web space; if on inspection this nerve also appears enlarged, it is excised as well. The only problem with excision of both the second and third web space nerves is the development of considerable numbness in the third toe, extending slightly proximal to the toe and potentially also including the third metatarsal fat pad. Although successful treatment of interdigital neuritis by release of the deep transverse metatarsal ligament, performed as either an open or an endoscopic procedure, has been reported, I have not had positive results with this operation. In fact, some years ago I started a prospective randomized study on nerve excision and release of the deep transverse metatarsal ligament. The study was abandoned when most of the patients for whom the release of the deep transverse metatarsal

ligament was performed were already returning with more symptoms and requiring further treatment.

The *standard dorsal neurectomy* is performed through a dorsal longitudinal incision 3 cm long. I do not use a short incision and prefer to expose and identify the entire nerve. A lamina spreader is inserted between the lesser metatarsals and placed on stretch, and the soft tissue is released off the dorsal surface of the deep transverse metatarsal ligament (Figure 21-6). A curved incision is now inserted from distal to proximal directly across the deep transverse metatarsal ligament, and the ligament is split. I prefer not to use a cutting motion with the scissors, to prevent any inadvertent injury to the nerve that lies immediately below it. Once the ligament is split, it is easy to hook the nerve with a curved hemostat clamp, pull the nerve up into the web space, and then trace it distally to the bifurcation. The nerve is clamped distally and cut distal to the bifurcation. The nerve is elevated out of the web space, and then the small plantar cutaneous branches of the main interdigital nerve also are cut to prevent recurrent neuroma formation. The nerve is then traced as far proximally as possible, lifted out from between the interosseous musculature, and cut as far proximally as possible. I have recently begun to bury the nerve in the interosseous muscle, and found that this improves the rate of success.

The approach to *revision neurectomy* is slightly different, although as noted, I generally use a dorsal incision even for revision. This is by far the least traumatic approach, and a scar is avoided on the plantar surface of the foot. Although the nerve is always identifiable, finding the nerve with the dorsal approach can take longer because the nerve stump frequently is stuck to the undersurface of the metatarsal, the volar plate, and the soft tissue. This dorsal approach should always be used in a revision when a previously attempted neurectomy has been performed through a short incision. Frequently, in these cases, the nerve lies under the scarred deep transverse metatarsal ligament in the center of the web space,

and this procedure is easy to perform. Unfortunately, results of revision neurectomy, whether performed through a dorsal or plantar approach, are not uniformly good. In fact, any revision should be approached with caution because excellent results are uncommon. A plantar incision can be made either transversely or longitudinally, and both types of incision have proponents. I use a plantar foot incision only when a plantar incision has already been used for a previous procedure and exquisite sensitivity is present in the skin, associated with Tinel's sign, as opposed to the more typical nerve pain that is in the web space. If a plantar incision is to be used, I prefer to make it transverse, rather than longitudinal, because the latter placement carries a greater risk of causing irritation adjacent to the metatarsal heads. Problems with the plantar incision include the potential for wound healing problems, scarring, and then difficulties with skin and orthotic management. With weight bearing, during toe-off, the fat pad is pulled forward and the incision has to be at least 1 cm proximal to the weight-bearing surface of the metatarsal.

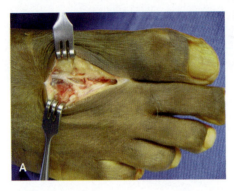

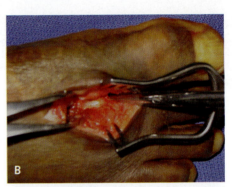

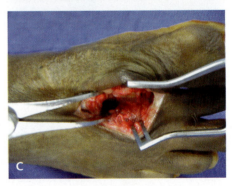

Figure 21-5 A first web neuroma involving the common plantar digital nerve developed after a crush injury to the forefoot. **A,** After exposure of the dorsal web space, the branches of the deep peroneal nerve were identified. **B,** A laminar spreader was inserted into the web space, and the deep transverse metatarsal ligament was identified and cut. **C,** The nerve was identified, and because it was noted to be intact after release of the deep metatarsal ligament, a neurectomy was not performed.

Figure 21-6 **A** and **B,** The standard approach to web space neurectomy includes an extensile web space incision, insertion of a laminar spreader between the metatarsals, and insertion of a scissors under the deep transverse metatarsal ligament, which is cut, exposing the nerve.

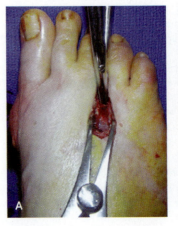

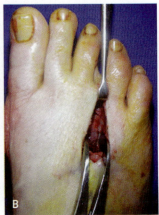

A revision neurectomy is performed as stated through a dorsal incision, and the deep transverse metatarsal ligament, which is always reconstituted, is again split. The lamina spreader is used, and the nerve has to be found more proximally. Sometimes, using a curved hemostat is easier; the instrument is swept underneath the metatarsal or deep to the interosseous muscle and tendon to try to find the nerve more proximally, where it is still normal. Once the nerve has been identified, it can be traced distally to where the stump neuroma is identified and removed. I try to identify any cross connections that may be present between the recurrent neuroma and the normal interdigital nerve in the adjacent web space (Figures 21-7 and 21-8).

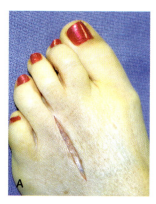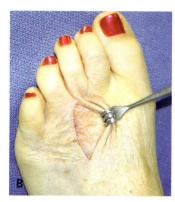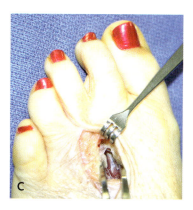

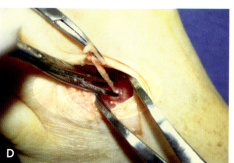

Figure 21-7 A, Because the surgical approach included both the second and third interdigital nerves, the incision was centered over the third web space. **B** and **C,** Skin retraction **(B)** and insertion of a laminar spreader into the second web space permit good visualization of the third web space **(C). D,** The nerve is then resected and buried with a suture into the interosseous muscle.

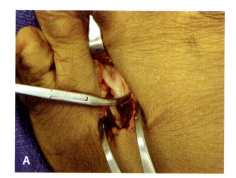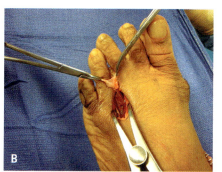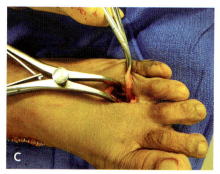

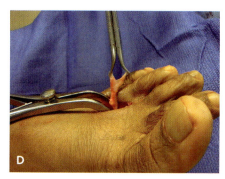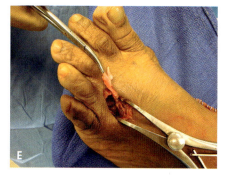

Figure 21-8 A, The neuroma is identified in a standard manner with a laminar spreader in the web space and a retractor distally pulling on the soft tissues between the toes. **B,** The bifurcation of the nerve into the two digital branches is identified, and the nerve is clamped. **C** and **D,** The nerve is then elevated distally, and each branch is cut separately. **E,** The nerve is retracted proximally, ensuring that all plantar cutaneous branches are dissected off the main nerve, and then is cut proximally between the interosseous muscles.

If a plantar incision is used, a tourniquet is applied, and the incision is made transversely and carried as far proximally as possible. The nerve is not easily identifiable and lies in the web space in fatty tissue between the flexor tendons. If the flexor tendon is indeed identified, then the dissection is too deep. Usually, once the retinaculum is incised, the fatty tissue pouches outward, and the nerve must be identified in this tissue. I find it helpful to identify all of the nerves before excising the pathologic structure. If a revision is being performed from a previous plantar incision, then an extensile approach to the plantar aspect of the foot is used to trace the interdigital nerve back to the more common trunk of the lateral plantar nerve. Neurectomy is performed in standard fashion, and here it is probably preferable to apply phenol to the tip of the stump of the cut nerve, which can then be buried in the musculature without any tension.

SUGGESTED READING

Stamatis E, Myerson MS: Treatment of recurrence of symptoms after excision of an interdigital neuroma, *J Bone Joint Surg Br* 86:48–53, 2004.

CHAPTER **22**

The Use of Bulk Fresh Allografts in Ankle Reconstruction

OSTEOARTICULAR FRESH ALLOGRAFT ANKLE REPLACEMENT

A role for use of bulk fresh allografts in ankle surgery has been well established. Although the enthusiasm for large fresh allograft osteoarticular ankle replacement has diminished over the past several years, this technique remains an effective approach to reconstruction in the appropriate patient. Furthermore, the options for treating sizable cystic lesions in either the distal tibia or the talus are very limited without the use of fresh osteoarticular grafts. In general, the smaller the size of the graft used, the less likely it is that failure will occur, whether from necrosis, collapse, graft fracture, or development of arthritis. The evidence to date suggests some critical volume of graft material or immunogenic load that the ankle can tolerate before rejection or failure occurs. In my own clinical experience in numerous patients, large bulk osteoarticular replacement grafts of the ankle have lasted more than 8 years with no complications. Such cases, however, constitute the exception rather than the rule, because a majority of these grafts have failed over time. The decision to use a fresh graft in reconstruction for a massive osteochondral lesion is far easier, because few realistic alternatives are available, and the results with this procedure have been excellent over the years.

The osteoarticular replacement procedure is indicated for patients with end-stage arthritis and for whom either an arthrodesis or total ankle replacement is not ideal. Considerations in selection of suitable candidates for this procedure include the patient's age, activity level, weight, and desire for continued mobility of the ankle. The most significant aspect of surgical planning involves assessing the potential for failure. Certainly, a *primary* ankle arthrodesis has a recognized success rate, from a technical standpoint, that should be greater than 95%. If an ankle arthrodesis becomes necessary after failure of an osteoarticular allograft replacement, clearly this success rate is lower, with failure attributed to graft collapse, sclerosis,

or avascular necrosis. The other options after failure are to repeat the graft procedure or to perform a total ankle replacement. These procedures are much easier, provided that the appropriate criteria for an ankle replacement are met. Accordingly, committing to an osteoarticular replacement procedure is a difficult clinical decision, because the failure rate over the past several years has been approximately 60%. I therefore limit use of the graft procedure to patients who have met most of the criteria for an ankle replacement but who prefer a more "physiologic" approach. Undoubtedly the worst candidate for grafting procedures is a patient who is young and active and has limited motion of the ankle to begin with, the result of posttraumatic arthritis.

Tissue typing is not necessary for this procedure. The most important aspect of planning this surgical procedure is correct sizing of the graft, because it must fit perfectly. If the graft is a few millimeters too small, the ankle will still function well, because the "fit" occurs between the articular surfaces of the tibia and the talus. If the graft is too large, however, it will not fit at all, and although the tibia can be cut laterally, the talus will abut against the malleoli.

The incision is identical to that for total ankle replacement: an anterior central midline incision over the ankle. Once the joint has been exposed and denuded of all juxtarticular osteophytes, the anterior aspect of the distal tibia is resected so that the plafond can be completely visualized. This clear view helps with planning the tibial cut correctly. Although the cuts on the tibia can be made freehand, use of a cutting block for the tibial cut is easier and permits better precision. The sizing of the cutting block is important, and 7 mm of distal tibia is removed. Judging the position of the cutting block relative to the lateral aspect of the ankle, which is not cut, is unimportant. The position of the block must be verified carefully by fluoroscopic examination, and minor adjustments must be made until the block is positioned to remove approximately 7 mm of the distal tibial surface.

243

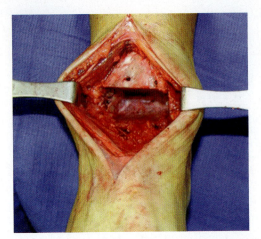

Figure 22-1 The appearance of the ankle after removal of the distal tibia. Except for the preservation of the fibula, the cut on the tibia and medial malleolus is similar to that used for the Agility Total Ankle Replacement System (DePuy Orthopaedics, Inc., Warsaw, Indiana).

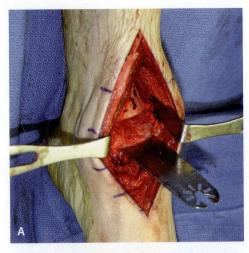

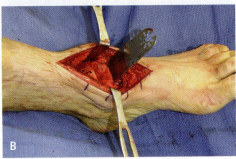

Figure 22-2 The talus is partially cut to a depth of approximately 5 mm (**A**), and a free saw blade is inserted into the bone cut (**B**), which is then checked fluoroscopically for correct placement. The talar graft is sized according to the bone resected and is cut freehand.

In cutting the tibia, it is important to protect the articular surface of the fibula and the medial malleolus. Sometimes the fibular articular surface is abnormal because of articular wear or deformity, such as shortening or external rotation. I do not normally disturb the fibula, although clearly for some cases, an osteotomy of the fibula may be required to restore length and correct rotational deformity simultaneously. The bone is then carefully pried off the tibia, and the remaining lateral tibia is then removed in segments with a small osteotome until the entire joint is visible (Figure 22-1). The talar cut is made freehand, with removal of approximately 5 mm of bone in the center of the dome of the talus (Figure 22-2). The tibial graft is then sized, and the cutting block is applied to the tibia under fluoroscopic guidance so that an identically sized matching graft can be harvested (Figure 22-3). At times, it is easier to remove a larger-size graft from the distal tibia and then shave this to a perfect cut once the size match is confirmed on the patient. The tibial graft rarely fits perfectly because of the anatomic constraints of the anterior and posterior ankle and the position of the fibula posterolaterally. The graft is then slotted into place, and minor adjustments to the diameter and depth of the graft can be made with a saw to ensure a perfect fit.

The cut on the talar allograft is made freehand, again to the size of the ankle. Cutting sufficient talus to prevent fracture is important. The position of the graft must now be checked fluoroscopically. The talus needs to be centered, under the tibia, and the graft tends to position itself perfectly with forced passive dorsiflexion of the ankle as the talus finds its resting position under the tibial articular surface. The tibial graft is then secured with the two 4-mm screws, and the talus can be fixed with a bioresorbable pin, which is inserted through the anterior aspect of the articular surface of the talus (Figure 22-4). Alternatively, if more talus is cut from the graft, then some of the neck of the talus may be present, through which screws can be inserted.

Weight bearing is not permitted for 3 months, although range-of-motion exercises are commenced as soon as they can be tolerated, and once the incision is healed, water activities with fins are encouraged.

In my own experience, the medium-term results with use of these grafts for osteoarticular joint replacement have not been gratifying. To date, over a period of approximately 10 years, the failure rate has slowly crept up to approximately 60%. Included in this large "failure" category are patients who experience marked reduction in symptoms but exhibit so-called radiographic failure, with evidence of fracture, graft nonunion or collapse, or changes consistent with arthritis. Nonetheless, with longer-term (7 year) follow-up evaluation, some patients have done extremely well (Figures 22-5 and 22-6). Of interest, many patients have noted a significant decrease in pain and have maintained range of motion despite the presence of cartilage failure and arthritis (Figure 22-7). The reason for the lack of symptoms in these patients is not well understood. Various modes of failure have been identified, including early fracture or fragmentation of the graft and late development of arthritis (Figures 22-8 and 22-9). Failure of incorporation of the graft also has been observed but is rare.

OTHER USES OF BULK FRESH ALLOGRAFTS IN THE ANKLE

The treatment of large cystic lesions of the distal tibia and talus is difficult. Some type of bone grafting procedure is necessary, and this can be accomplished using cancellous autograft or allograft supplemented by a chondral resurfacing of some sort. Results with these procedures have not been very successful, however, and cancellous bone grafting on its own does not have much success. Another, more effective option is to perform the cancellous grafting and then cover the bone with a periosteal or scaffold graft with host autologous cells incorporated into the graft. This cannot be performed as a closed procedure, and although

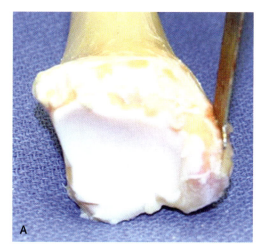
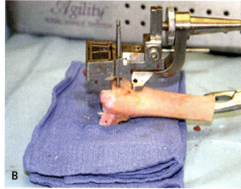

Figure 22-3 A, The graft is carefully preserved during the operation and then is cleaned of all soft tissue before the bone cuts are made. **B,** The tibia is cut through the cutting block of the Agility Ankle Replacement System (DePuy Orthopaedics, Inc., Warsaw, Indiana).

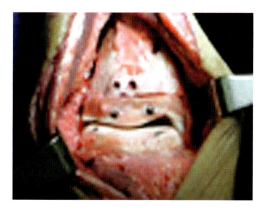

Figure 22-4 Note the good overall alignment of the grafts in the joint.

the first stage may be performed arthroscopically to harvest the cells and debride the lesion, the second stage must be performed with open technique in order to fill these massive defects. My preference is to perform this restoration as a single-stage open procedure using arthrotomy or osteotomy as needed. Regardless of approach, it is difficult to shape the graft correctly so that a precise fit is obtained.

After removal of the necrotic avascular bone and cartilage debris, I cut the margins of the lesion so that it will accept a graft of the correct size and shape. Once the host defect has been pre-pared, I fill the defect with bone wax. The wax is then removed, with the overall shape of the mold maintained as much as possible, and then is used to model the cut of the donor graft. These grafts can be used on the medial talar dome, the central or lateral talar dome, or the distal tibia. Once the graft is inserted, the natural concavity and convexity of the ankle are used to compress the graft into position with flexion and extension of the ankle. Fixation of the graft is not always necessary for large central defects of the talus. Marginal grafts should be fixed with a bioresorbable pin (Figures 22-10 to 22-14).

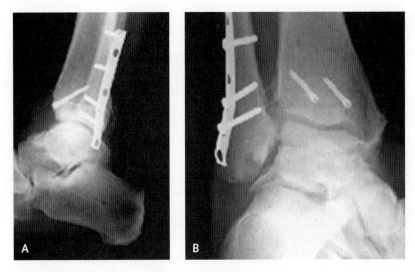

Figure 22-5 A and **B,** Radiographs of the ankle of a 49-year-old patient 5 years after an osteoarticular allograft for the treatment of posttraumatic arthritis.

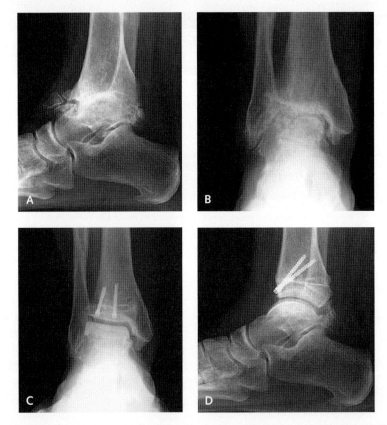

Figure 22-6 A and **B,** The patient presented with post-traumatic arthritis and demonstrated excellent range of motion of the ankle despite the impingement present anteriorly. **C** and **D,** At 7 years after the osteoarticular allograft, the joint was well preserved, with no evidence of arthritis.

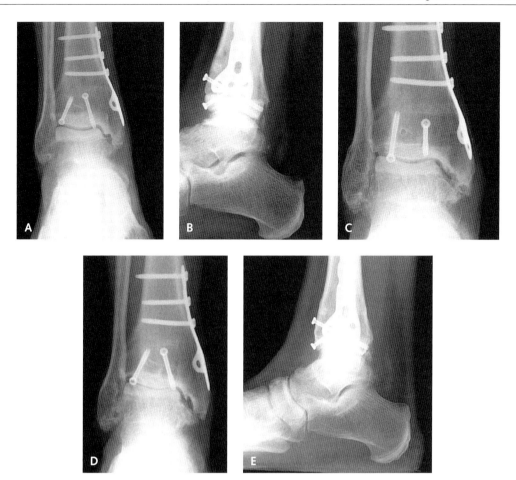

Figure 22-7 Radiographic appearance of an osteoarticular graft: **A** and **B,** at 2 years after replacement; **C** and **D,** at 6 years. **E,** Note the decrease in the joint space and the cartilage wear. The patient remained asymptomatic.

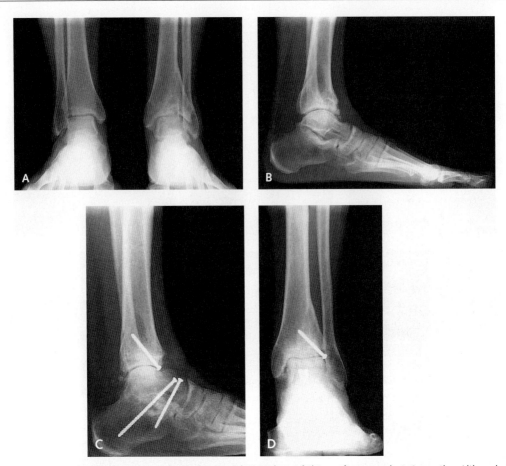

Figure 22-8 A and **B,** Preoperative radiographs. **C** and **D,** Failure of this graft occurred at 6 months. Although the radiographs show some maintenance of the joint space, healing of the graft, and good alignment, the patient was very symptomatic with limited range of motion and underwent ankle replacement 2 years later.

22

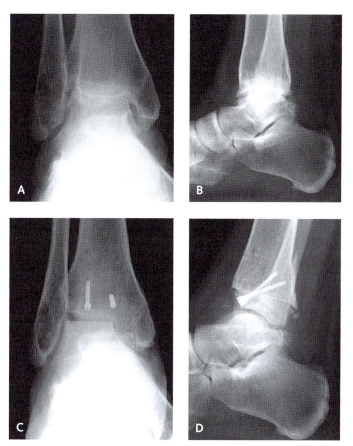

Figure 22-9 A and **B,** The patient was a 43-year-old woman who presented with posttraumatic arthritis of the ankle, normal alignment, and no instability. **C** and **D,** Radiographs at 4 months after a graft procedure. Note the lack of congruity of the graft to the host ankle and the overall inadequate match in shape. Anterior collapse of the tibial graft occurred 3 months later, with consequent arthritis. Graft replacement surgery was performed, but 9 months later, anterior collapse of the tibial graft recurred, with development of arthritis.

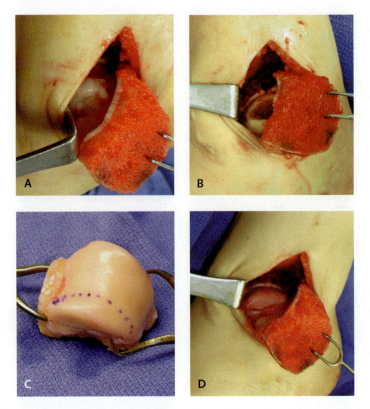

Figure 22-10 The osteochondral lesion in this case involved the entire medial dome of the talus. **A,** The medial malleolar osteotomy was performed. **B** and **C,** Debridement of the lesion and then preparation of the defect with a small saw and chisel **(B)** were accomplished next, followed by marking of the size of the graft **(C). D,** The graft fitted well into the recipient bed and was fixed with an absorbable pin.

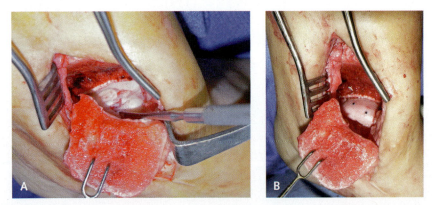

Figure 22-11 A, A lesion in the ankle of a 17-year-old boy that involved the entire medial dome of the talus at its margin and included the medial wall of the talus. **B,** Note the very good fit of the graft with two bioresorbable pins in place.

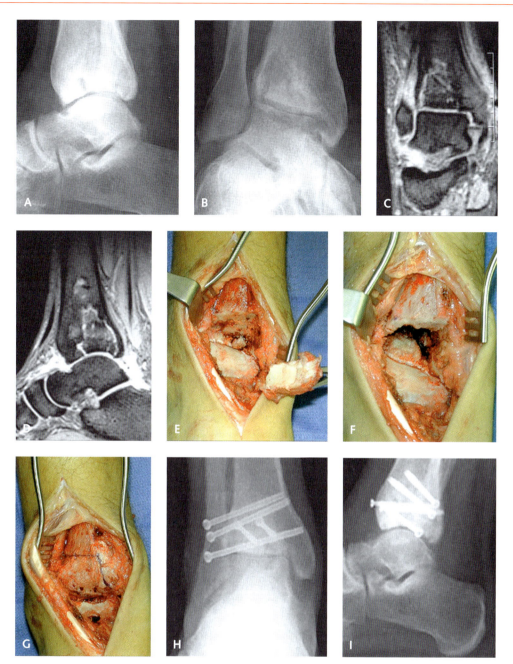

Figure 22-12 Osteonecrosis of the distal tibia developed after traumatic injury in a 34-year-old patient. **A-D,** Note the extensive necrosis and articular defect on the radiographs (**A** and **B**) and the magnetic resonance images (**C** and **D**). **E** and **F,** After anterior arthrotomy, an osteotomy of the distal tibia was performed, removing a wedge-shaped piece of the anterior articular margin **(E),** and exposing the defect **(F). G,** A fresh osteoarticular distal tibia graft was inserted to match the defect, and the tibial window was replaced and fixed with screws, as shown. **H** and **I,** Radiographic appearance at 3 years.

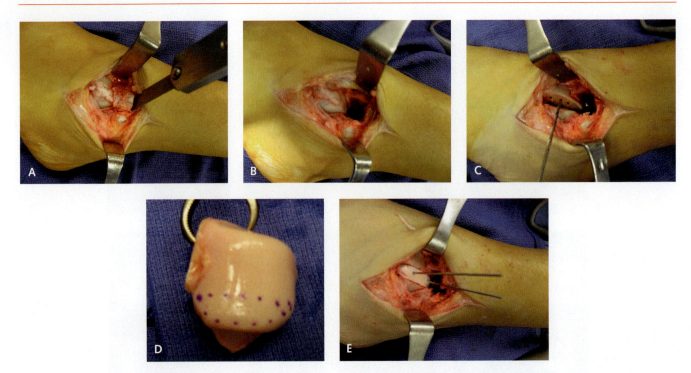

Figure 22-13 A, This large osteochondral lesion in the ankle of a 21-year-old woman is in an unusual location and involves the entire medial dome from front to back, but with the medial wall left intact. **B** and **C,** An osteotomy of the distal tibia was performed to create a window for insertion of the graft. The talus was cut with a chisel, and then the margins were trimmed with a saw to create smooth edges. **D** and **E,** The graft was then marked out using a negative mold of a bone wax impression to shape the size of the talus graft.

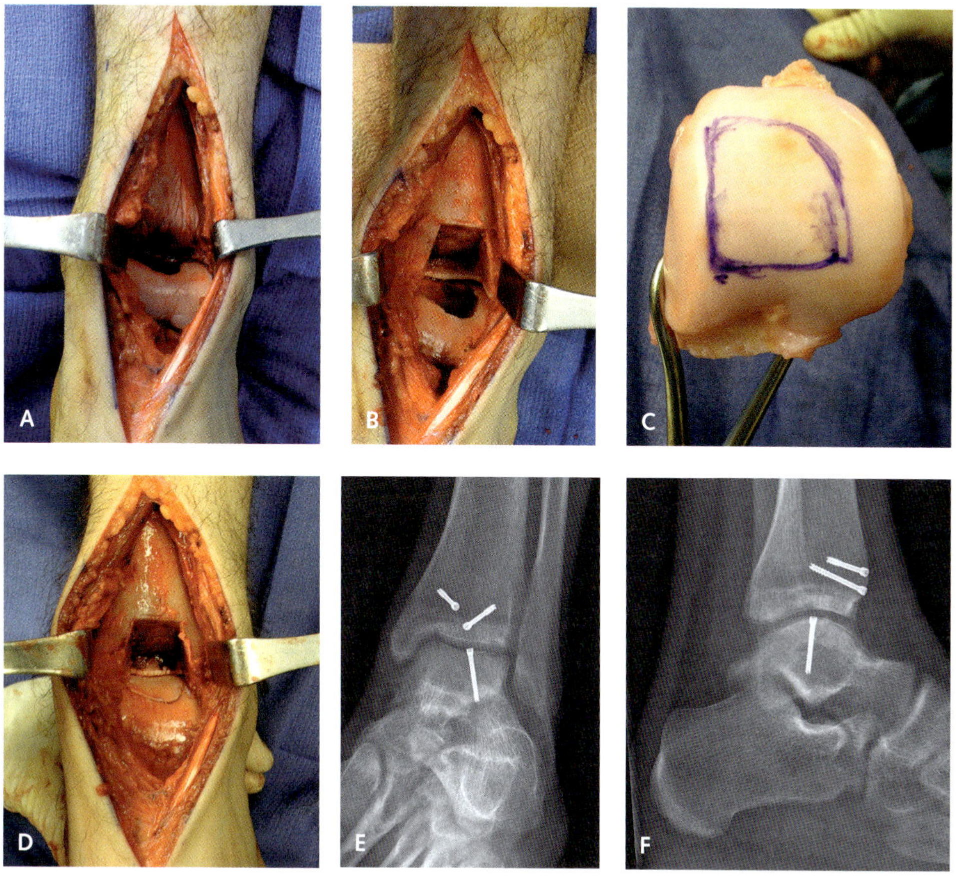

Figure 22-14 A, This large central defect of the talus included approximately 60% of the dorsal surface of the talar dome. **B,** The tibial window was made with a saw, and then a fracture created at the articular surface to expose the lesion fully. **C,** The defect was filled with bone wax to make a positive mold for the shape of the donor graft. **D,** The graft fitted extremely well and with plantar flexion and dorsiflexion of the ankle was compressed firmly into the recipient bed. **E** and **F,** Radiographs at 2 years after grafting.

CHAPTER **23**

Reconstruction of Malunited Ankle Fractures

DECISION MAKING AND RECONSTRUCTION

The premise for reconstruction of a malunited ankle fracture is joint preservation. Frequently, the joint may appear to be irreparable, with articular wear and erosive changes on the medial or lateral plafond. Even with these more advanced changes, however, restoring the alignment of the ankle is worthwhile. Most of these cases involve a malunion or a nonunion, or both, of the fibula. Occasionally, the medial malleolus or the posterior tibia also is involved in this malunited fracture, necessitating simultaneous correction. Lateral weight-bearing radiographs and a computed tomography (CT) scan of the ankle are helpful to plan the reconstruction. The CT scan is not necessary but does aid in determining the required degree of rotation of the fibula. It is always worth the effort to attempt a reconstruction of the malunited ankle fracture. If this fails, an arthrodesis and joint replacement are still options. The results with osteotomy of the fibula or the tibia, or both, are excellent even in ankles with considerable deformity and arthritis (Figures 23-1 and 23-2). In some situations, a reconstruction simply cannot be performed for technical reasons, and an arthrodesis is the best alternative. An important point in this context, however, is that an arthrodesis is not the only treatment option after severe trauma (Figure 23-3).

Débridement: Arthroscopy or Arthrotomy?

A decision needs to be made whether arthroscopic debridement of the joint is to be performed simultaneously. Arthroscopic evaluation of the joint is very helpful in these cases to document and stage the extent of ankle arthritis. In particular, arthroscopy is indicated for evaluation of a suspected posterior and inaccessible chondral defect that would not be visible with anterolateral arthrotomy. The hypertrophic tissue between the medial malleolus and the talus must be excised from the medial gutter for the reposition of the talus. Surprisingly small amounts of tissue in the medial gutter can actually block the correct medial shift of the talus back into the mortise (Figure 23-4). Fibular malunion generally is associated with a lateral translational deformity of the talus with an increase in the medial clear space, and the medial joint recess must be debrided, under visualization afforded by either arthrotomy or arthroscopy.

For this procedure, a vertical incision is made medial to the anterior tibial tendon directly over the anterior notch of the medial ankle over a 2-cm length. The incision is deepened through the joint. Then the capsule is incised, and the hypertrophic synovium, capsule, and scar are excised completely from the medial gutter. The insertion of a rongeur is useful; it should be turned around 180 degrees to ensure that the medial gutter is completely free and that the talus is mobile. The medial gutter will again be checked subsequently for correction of the fibula malunion as the talus is pushed over medially.

Fibular and Medial Malleolus Deformity and Osteotomy

The fibula is commonly shortened and externally rotated in a malunion, although only one of these may be present, determining the type of osteotomy and bone graft. Ideally, it should not be necessary to strip the entire syndesmosis in order to lengthen the fibula. In cases in which the syndesmosis must be included in the procedure, such as arthrodesis requiring creation of a tibia pro fibula, then the syndesmosis should be taken down completely (Figures 23-5 and 23-6). If the fibula is externally rotated and not shortened, then a derotational osteotomy can be performed without lengthening, thereby preserving the syndesmosis (Figure 23-7).

An extensile excision is made laterally directly over the fibula, frequently corresponding to the original incision. Existing hardware is removed. The key to this operation is to obtain the correct length and rotation of the distal fibula. These parameters are easy to judge by virtue of the bimalleolar axis, which should be measured out and planned preoperatively by comparison with the contralateral normal ankle. Correction of the external rotation, which usually is present, is not as easy. If healing of the fibula is complete, then an osteotomy has to be performed. This should be done at a level that permits application of adequate fixation distally.

The plane of the fibular osteotomy can be either exactly transverse or oblique. The advantage of a transverse osteotomy is that adequate lengthening of the fibula is far easier to obtain with this type of osteotomy. This is particularly the case if the fibula is short and needs to be lengthened with a laminar spreader. If a transverse osteotomy in the fibula is made, structural interpositional bone graft should be used, provided, of course, that shortening of the fibula is present. Occasionally, external rotation of the fibula is present without shortening, and an internal rotational osteotomy is performed without lengthening (see Figure 23-7).

The alternative is to lengthen the fibula with an oblique osteotomy and to slide the fibula more distally. The better bone contact may obviate the need for an interpositional bone graft, as seen in Figure 23-8. In this case, the long oblique malunion of the fibula facilitated an oblique osteotomy with the lengthening, and no bone graft was required. Owing to the ankle valgus deformity and early arthritis, however, a simultaneous osteotomy of the tibia was performed to realign the weight-bearing forces on the ankle. With either type of osteotomy, the syndesmosis needs to be taken down to facilitate the actual lengthening. The tissues surrounding the fibula are stripped, the periosteum is completely elevated, and then the fibula is mobilized on its distal pedicle. If a transverse osteotomy is made, a laminar spreader is inserted in the osteotomy site, the fibula is distracted, and provisional fixation is obtained from the fibula into both the talus and the distal tibia to lock the fibula at the correct length. In the case of a long oblique malunion, bone graft is not usually required, and provided that stable fixation of the fibula and syndesmosis is obtained, the ankle alignment can be markedly improved (Figure 23-9).

The position of the fibula is then checked fluoroscopically. Axial lengthening is easier to obtain without internal rotation, but some rotation usually is required. For control of the length and rotation, a bone reduction clamp should be applied to the distal fibula while it is lengthened with the laminar spreader. Then the clamp should be internally rotated to facilitate insertion of the guide pins into the fibula to hold it in position. If an oblique osteotomy is preferred, the plane of the osteotomy should be made over

a length of approximately 2 cm, with the cut beginning proximal lateral, then going to distal and medial, and ending proximal to the joint. The fibula is stripped of soft tissues in the same manner, and then the plate is applied to the distal fibula. With the plate in position, a screw is then inserted into the fibula, proximal to the plate, and then a laminar spreader is positioned between this screw and either the plate or one of the more distal screws to facilitate the lengthening. Internal rotation is performed in a similar manner with a bone reduction clamp, and then the fibula needs to be held in position with guide pins. As noted, this type of lengthening does not always require a structural or interpositional bone graft. Nonetheless, the plane of the osteotomy is such that once the distal fibula is internally rotated, apposition of the osteotomy site is not perfect, and some form of cancellous grafting may be required.

One variant of malunion of the fibula is associated with compression of the lateral plafond and valgus tilting of the ankle mortise. As outlined previously, such cases may be amenable to management by osteotomy of the fibula in addition to a closing wedge osteotomy of the medial tibia to realign the ankle. Another option is to perform an opening wedge osteotomy of the distal lateral tibia (a plafond-plasty) to achieve a plantigrade ankle. The deformity typically is the result of a crushing-type injury to the lateral ankle and plafond, and regardless of the realignment and fixation of the fibula, if the lateral plafond remains depressed, deformity and arthritis will be

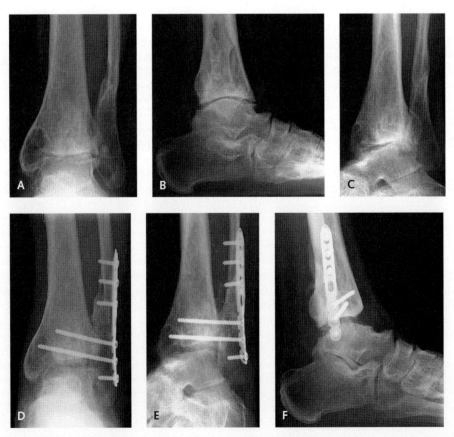

Figure 23-1 A-C, This ankle fracture malunion was associated with considerable shortening and external rotation of the fibula in addition to ankle arthritis. An arthroscopic debridement of the joint and removal of the hypertrophic tissue in the medial gutter was followed by a lengthening of the fibula and syndesmosis stabilization. **D-F,** Note the marked improvement in the alignment of the ankle as well as the apparent joint space.

23

the result. Through a lateral incision, the fibula is exposed and the osteotomy is performed if necessary. It is easier to expose the lateral tibia if the syndesmosis is taken down completely and the fibula rotated on its distal soft tissue pedicle. Once the osteotomy of the fibula is complete, under fluoroscopic guidance, the osteotomy of the tibia is made approximately 1 cm proximal to the joint line but not completed medially. The osteotomy cut should terminate at approximately two thirds of the width of the tibia and then should be opened gradually by plastic deformation of the distal lateral tibia. The defect is then filled with cancellous bone graft. Depending on the magnitude of the defect, the graft can be cancellous or structural, in which case a triangular graft is used (Figures 23-10 and 23-11).

The medial malleolus generally is involved as part of a more global ankle problem, and it is unusual to find an isolated problem on the medial aspect of the ankle. Malunion can occur of course and must be treated along with any additional deformity (Figure 23-12). A nonunion of the medial malleolus is far less common and if not treated will result in arthritis of the medial ankle with joint failure (Figures 23-13 and 23-14). Realignment and stabilization of the syndesmosis for management of chronic ankle joint pain are necessary if it can be demonstrated that the syndesmosis is the source of pain. Often after ankle fracture, patients report vague ankle soreness, and it is not easy to determine the source of the problem. If the ankle appears to be normal on imaging, I obtain a

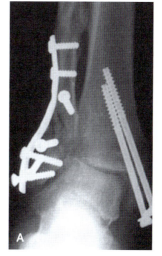
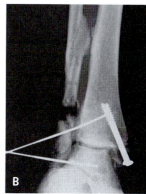

Figure 23-2 A, Despite severe deformity and joint incongruency associated with nonunion and malunion of fractures of the fibula and the medial malleolus and erosion of the lateral tibial plafond, the reconstruction is worth attempting. **B,** Note the overall improvement in the alignment of the ankle with revision of the medial malleolus fixation and lengthening of the fibula.

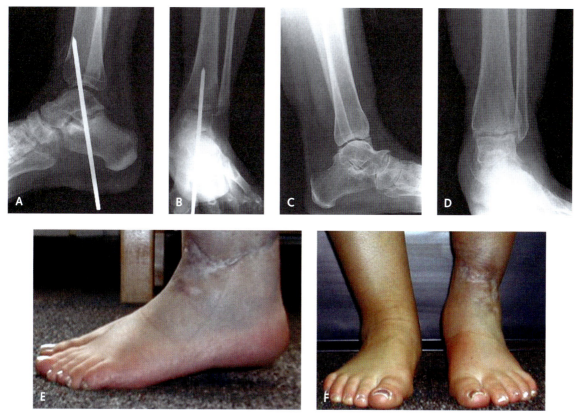

Figure 23-3 A and **B,** The patient was a 25-year-old woman who presented 6 weeks after an ankle open fracture-dislocation, which was treated with removal of the malleoli and insertion of a large retrograde pin for stabilization, resulting in development of an osteomyelitis of the calcaneus. After debridement, the ankle appeared stable, and other than periodic brace use, no additional treatment was provided. **C-F,** Five years later the ankle was stable, albeit somewhat arthritic, with restricted motion and a fixed equinus deformity.

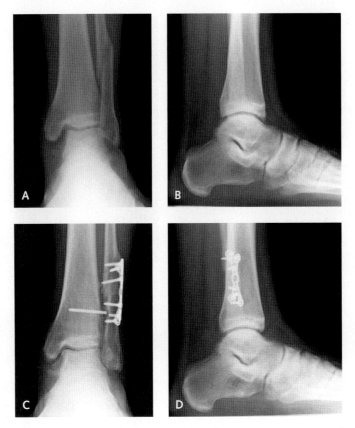

Figure 23-4 A 37-year-old patient presented for treatment after nonoperative management of an ankle injury. **A** and **B,** Note the shortening and external rotation of the fibula, the loss of the lateral talofibular alignment, and the increase in the medial joint clear space. **C** and **D,** Treatment consisted of arthroscopic debridement of the medial joint, arthroscopic cheilectomy and removal of bone debris and hypertrophic scar, and lengthening of the fibula. The overall ankle structure and in particular the distal talofibular alignment have been restored.

CT scan that includes both fibulas, to determine if rotation of the fibula or slight shortening is the problem. Sometimes the fibula is well aligned, and the pain originates in the syndesmosis. This pain can be localized with selective joint and syndesmosis injection. Depending on the magnitude of the associated deformity, as well as the bone quality, I often include the syndesmosis in the fixation and occasionally attempt an arthrodesis of the syndesmosis. If an arthrodesis is not performed, then at the very least, multiple screws will be used from the fibula across into the tibia to provide more rigid and stable fixation. After failed syndesmosis fixation, it is helpful to use larger screws and distribute the load across the fibula with a plate functioning as a washer (Figures 23-15 to 23-17).

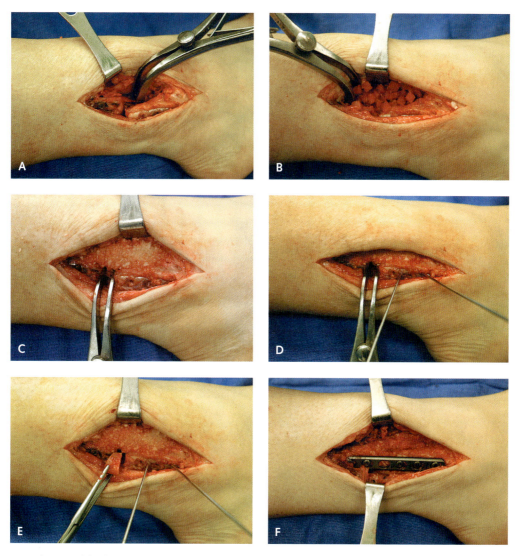

Figure 23-5 Lengthening of the fibula without internal rotation. **A,** The osteotomy is made transversely, and the syndesmosis is separated with a laminar spreader. **B** and **C,** In this case, a syndesmosis arthrodesis was performed and a cancellous graft was inserted before the lengthening procedure. **D-F,** Once the fibula was out to length, guide pins were inserted distally to lock it in place; then the graft was inserted and a plate applied.

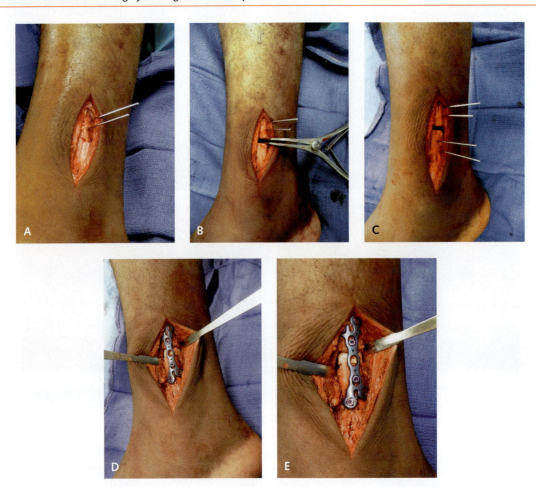

Figure 23-6 Treatment for a short and internally rotated fibula. **A,** Before osteotomy, pins were inserted more proximally to prevent proximal shift of the fibula. **B,** Once the length was corrected with a laminar spreader, multiple pins were inserted to maintain the length. **C-E,** Then the bone graft was inserted and a custom fibula-contoured plate (Orthohelix, Akron, Ohio) was applied.

23

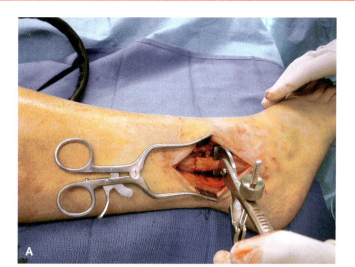

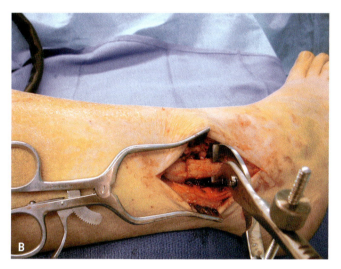

Figure 23-7 A and **B,** The fibula in this case was not short but was externally rotated. A derotational osteotomy was therefore performed, using a bone reduction clamp, after a transverse osteotomy.

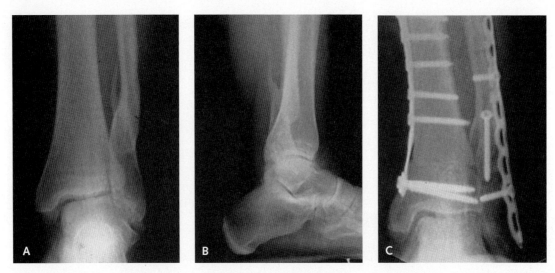

Figure 23-8 **A** and **B,** The long oblique malunion of the fibula facilitated an oblique osteotomy with the lengthening, and no bone graft was required. **C,** Owing to the ankle valgus deformity and early arthritis, however, a simultaneous closing wedge medial osteotomy of the tibia was performed to realign the weight-bearing forces on the ankle.

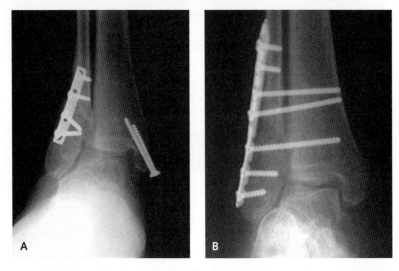

Figure 23-9 **A,** This fibula malunion was associated with marked shortening, external rotation, and nonunion, as well as valgus tilting of the ankle. **B,** Treatment consisted of a lengthening osteotomy with bone grafting and stabilization of the syndesmosis without arthrodesis.

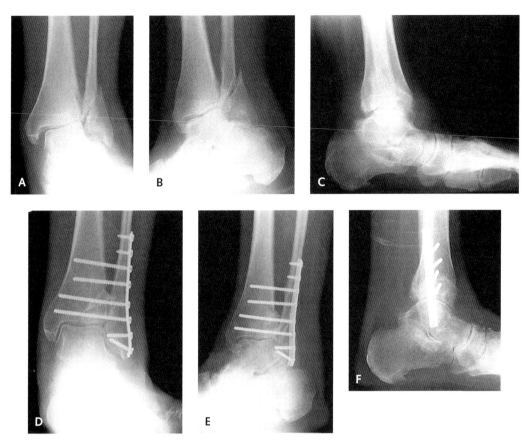

Figure 23-10 A-C, A fibula osteotomy would not be sufficient to correct the tibial alignment in this chronic 3-month-old malunion and nonunion of the distal fibula associated with compression of the lateral tibial plafond. **D-F,** A lengthening osteotomy of the fibula was performed through the plane of the fracture without bone graft, but the key to this procedure was the opening wedge osteotomy of the lateral tibia (a plafond-plasty).

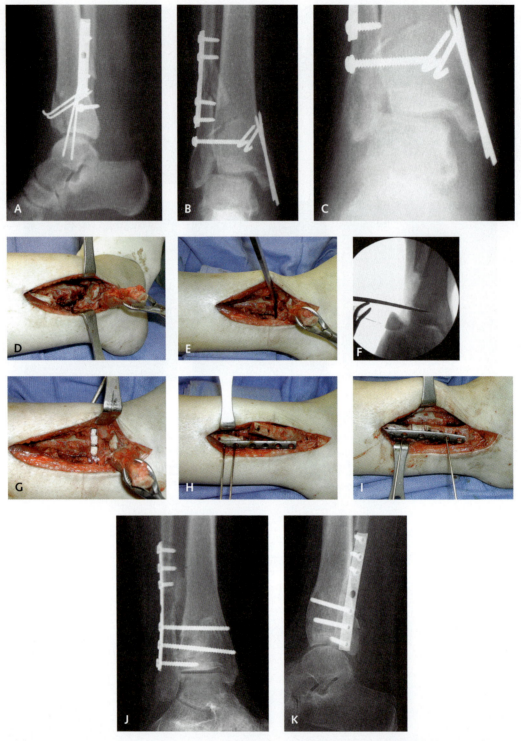

Figure 23-11 A and **B,** Infected malunion and nonunion of the distal tibia and a nonunion of the fibula in an 18-year-old patient. The tissue at the loose Kirschner wires in the anterior tibia was the location of infection. **C,** On the enlarged view of the malunion, the lateral tibia is seen to be compressed superiorly. The hardware was removed and antibiotic therapy used for 6 weeks, followed by reconstruction. **D,** The fibula was opened through the nonunion. **E** and **F,** Then an osteotomy was made through the lateral plafond of the tibia under fluoroscopic guidance. **G,** The tibia was gently levered open and filled with cancellous bone graft. **H** and **I,** The lengthening of the fibula was then performed, with plate fixation and structural grafting. **J** and **K,** The radiographic appearance
4 years later.

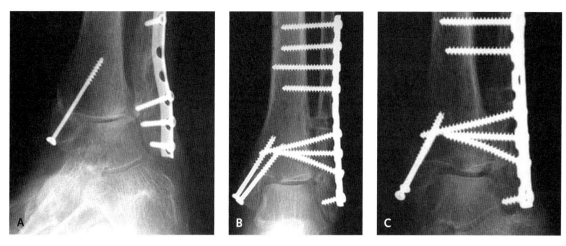

Figure 23-12 A, The patient was a 61-year-old woman who was referred for an ankle replacement at 1 year after bimalleolar ankle fracture with malunion. Range of motion was excellent, and despite a severe malalignment of the medial malleolus, as well as the fibula, reconstruction was considered to be appropriate. An osteotomy of the medial malleolus was performed with lengthening of the fibula. **B** and **C,** Because of questionable bone quality on the lateral aspect, the syndesmosis was included in the fibula fixation.

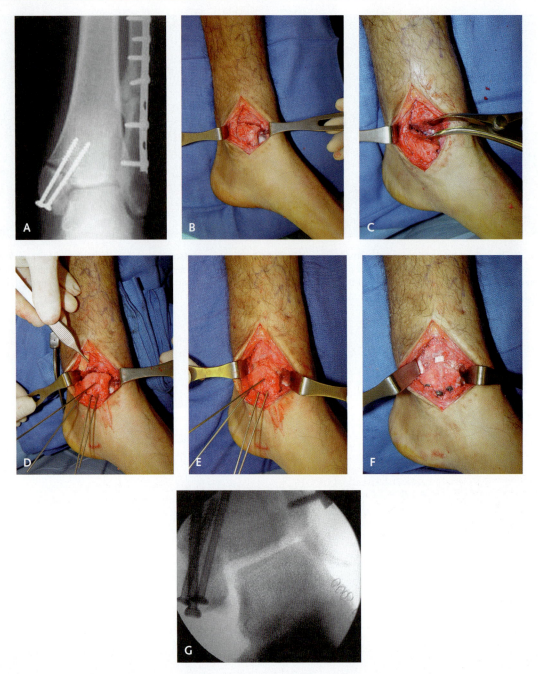

Figure 23-13 Treatment for a nonunion of a fracture of the medial malleolus in a 19-year-old patient. **A,** The fibula was healed despite the radiographic appearance. **B** and **C,** The malleolus was exposed, both sides of the malleolus were perforated with a 2-mm drill, and cancellous bone harvested from the calcaneus was inserted. **D-G,** Temporary Kirschner wire fixation was obtained, followed by definitive screw fixation.

23

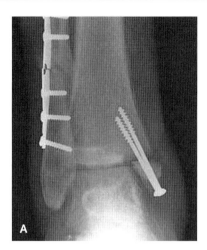
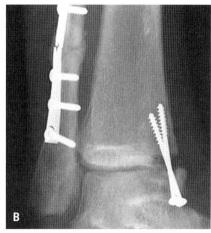

Figure 23-14 A and **B,** A nonunion with comminution of the medial malleolus, associated with severe medial compartment arthritis. The joint was not considered to be salvageable, and an arthrodesis was performed.

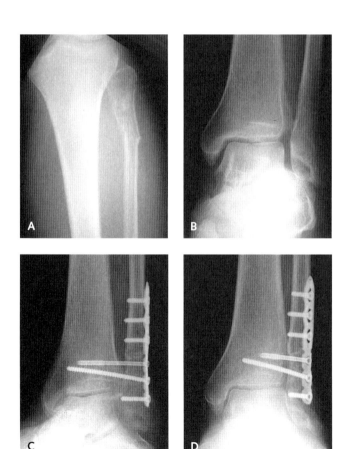

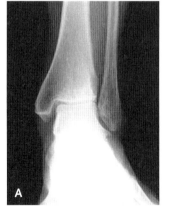
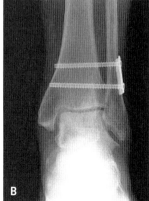

Figure 23-15 The patient sustained a high fibula fracture, which was managed with bracing in a boot that permitted functional mobilization. **A,** The fracture healed, but 9 months later, persistent anterolateral ankle pain was present. **B,** Note the slight widening of the distal syndesmosis. **C** and **D,** Treatment consisted of syndesmosis débridement and plate fixation.

Figure 23-16 The patient sustained an ankle sprain 2 years previously and never quite recovered despite immobilization and therapy. **A,** Note the slight widening of the syndesmosis. **B,** Repair was accomplished with debridement and application of a compression plate and screws.

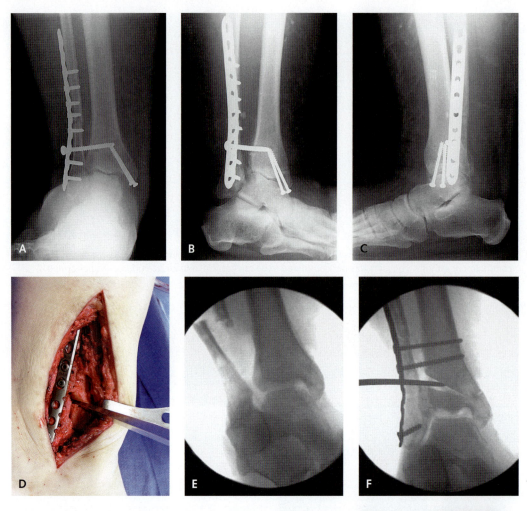

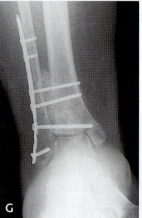

Figure 23-17 A-C, The patient was a 61-year-old woman who had sustained this fracture 9 months earlier. Two previous attempts at fixation of the syndesmsosis had failed. Note the widened syndesmosis, the nonunion of the fibula, and the valgus inclination of the ankle joint. **D-F,** Treatment consisted of fibula osteotomy through the nonunion and an opening wedge osteotomy of the lateral tibia, in conjunction with syndesmosis arthrodesis. **G,** Radiographic appearance 3 years later.

TECHNIQUES, TIPS, AND PITFALLS

- Correction of malunion is worth the effort despite marked deformity. The ankle seems to be forgiving with respect to deformity in some patients, and corrective osteotomy provides pain relief despite the appearance of arthritis.

- The length of the fibula and its rotation must be restored. Internal rotation usually is necessary to correct malunion of the fibula.

- Rarely, if the deformity is significant, then a slight medial closing wedge osteotomy of the tibia may be performed, in addition to the lengthening osteotomy of the fibula.

- If a malunion of the medial malleolus is present, it needs to be addressed specifically. Thus, in addition to the fibular osteotomy, either an ostectomy or an osteotomy of the medial malleolus may be necessary. The ostectomy usually detaches the superficial deltoid ligament, which can be reattached through K-wire holes in the malleolus. Rarely will the deep deltoid ligament be disrupted with this ostectomy.

- If the deformity of the medial joint cannot be corrected, the lateral aspect of the ankle should be corrected, particularly if a nonunion is present.

- Some injuries necessitate an osteotomy of the medial malleolus, the fibula, or even the anterior distal tibia. These osteotomies are covered in the approaches to the ankle in the section on osteochondral injury. Of relevance here, a window can be removed from the distal tibia to perform the bone grafting in patients who have avascular necrosis of a segment of the distal tibia. The window can be made in a number of ways, preserving the articular surface or incorporating the articular segment into the window. The window is made large enough, however, that the bone can be replaced with screws.

SUGGESTED READING

Borrelli J Jr, Leduc S, Gregush R, Ricci WM: Tricortical bone grafts for treatment of malaligned tibias and fibulas, *Clin Orthop Relat Res* 467:1056–1063, 2009:Epub Jan 15, 2009.

Chu A, Weiner L: Distal fibula malunions, *J Am Acad Orthop Surg* 17:220–230, 2009.

Perera A, Myerson M: Surgical techniques for the reconstruction of malunited ankle fractures, *Foot Ankle Clin* 13:737–751, 2008.

Stamatis ED, Cooper PS, Myerson MS: Supramalleolar osteotomy for the treatment of distal tibial angular deformities and arthritis of the ankle joint, *Foot Ankle Int* 24:754–764, 2003.

Stamatis ED, Myerson MS: Supramalleolar osteotomy: Indications and technique, *Foot Ankle Clin* 8:317–333, 2003.

CHAPTER **24**

Total Ankle Replacement

OVERVIEW

This chapter outlines the indications for ankle replacement in the ideal patient, as well as in those patients for whom this procedure poses a higher risk for failure. Descriptions of the different prostheses I use for ankle replacement, as well as techniques and tips for each type of implant device, also are presented. The step-by-step process is not reviewed for each procedure, although critical techniques for specific implants are highlighted.

Who is the ideal candidate for an ankle replacement? What should the surgeon tell a patient who presents with ankle arthritis, and how should decision making proceed in this setting? Selection of the treatment approach should not be the surgeon's decision alone. For an ideal patient with good alignment, good bone support, and reasonable range of motion, with no contraindication to joint replacement, what is the best surgical advice? What are the advantages of ankle replacement over arthrodesis? Is the functional improvement with ankle replacement so much greater than arthrodesis that it warrants performing the procedure despite its much higher complication rate? Many patients recognize the potential problems with ankle arthrodesis, the inherent stiffness, the limitation to certain activities, and in particular the likelihood of adjacent joint arthritis developing in the future. Within this group of patients, however, some prefer not to deal with potential for failure of an ankle replacement and want more predictability in the outcome and therefore select the arthrodesis. I outline all of the potential advantages and disadvantages, as well as the possibility of complications for each procedure; selection of the most appropriate procedure then becomes a joint decision that the patient and I make together.

An important consideration in surgical planning is the preoperative range of motion of the ankle. One of the most critical factors affecting the postoperative range of motion is a preexisting contracture, which is often the case with posttraumatic arthritis. The soft tissue envelope around the posttraumatic and arthritic ankle joint usually is quite scarred, at times significantly so. Contractures developing over long-term periods of immobilization further adversely affect the ankle joint mobility. In such cases, it is more difficult to obtain a satisfactory range of motion even intraoperatively, despite aggressive soft tissue release. A patient with severe ankylosis may never achieve an acceptable range of motion regardless of how the procedure is performed. For such patients, arthrodesis may

not be perceived as disabling (in comparison with those in whom the clinical presentation includes a reasonable range of motion but some degree of preoperative pain) (Figure 24-1). It is important to identify the true range of motion of the ankle joint, which can be clinically deceptive because "motion" may actually represent mobility of the transverse tarsal joints (Figure 24-2). I routinely obtain dynamic lateral plantar flexion and dorsiflexion radiographic views of the ankle during the preoperative evaluation to identify the exact location of sagittal plane motion.

The alignment of the foot and ankle is an important determinant of suitability for replacement surgery. There are limits to correction of a varus or valgus deformity, which I generally set at approximately 20 degrees for varus and 10 degrees for valgus. As discussed later in the section on managing associated deformity, if the deltoid ligament is torn, the likelihood of obtaining a well-aligned ankle is significantly decreased (Figures 24-3 and 24-4). Tibia varus or valgus deformity should be addressed before ankle replacement, particularly if the knee is affected, in which case the knee must be first corrected (Figure 24-5).

Bone quality is an important consideration, and if severe osteopenia is present, the likelihood of subsidence of the prosthesis is increased. The risk increases if avascular necrosis is present. The talar component is more likely to subside than the tibial component, particularly if osteopenia or avascular necrosis is present. To circumvent this problem of poor-quality bone, selection of a prosthesis with a long stem is a good option. This is combined with a subtalar arthrodesis, providing a very stable platform for the prosthesis (Figure 24-6).

Preoperative instability of the ankle is very important to ascertain, and treatment should be planned accordingly. Certain deformities seem trivial but should be approached with caution. An unstable ankle typically is thought to be associated with a lack of lateral ligamentous support. Such instability is problematic only if not identified intraoperatively, because a ligament reconstruction is always possible to restore stability. If the deltoid is torn, however, restoration of medial stability will be unpredictable. Another pattern of instability that is difficult to treat is anterior subluxation of the talus under the tibia (Figure 24-7). This displacement may resolve with correct positioning of the prosthesis and correct tensioning with a larger polyethylene ("poly") insert, but the outcome is not predictable, and anterior subluxation should be approached surgically with caution.

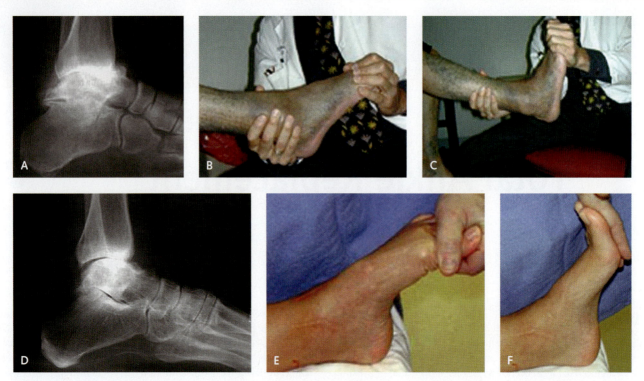

Figure 24-1 The range of motion of the ankle is important in surgical decision making and may have no correlation with the radiographic appearance. **A-C,** In this example, a patient with hemachromatosis had severe ankle arthritis but retained excellent range of motion. **D-F,** By contrast, a patient with posttraumatic arthritis may have no ankle motion at all despite only moderate arthritis as indicated by radiographically evident changes, as in this case. This patient may be a better candidate for an ankle arthrodesis than another patient with excellent motion but with far more extensive radiographic changes, for whom a replacement is preferable.

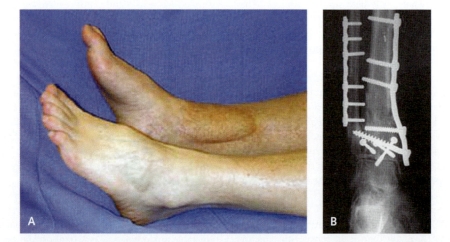

Figure 24-2 A and **B,** The patient developed ankle arthritis after treatment of a pilon fracture requiring plate fixation and a free flap. He was not a good candidate for replacement. Minimal motion was present in the ankle, and the flap could not be safely elevated. The hardware would need to be removed, which would add to the soft tissue dissection. Even if this patient had good anterior skin, it would still be necessary to remove the hardware as a staged procedure and perform the replacement months later, once the skin bridge was less likely to fail.

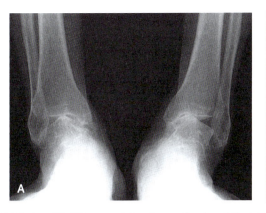
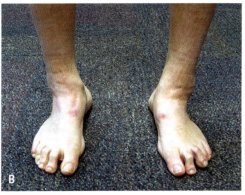

Figure 24-3 **A** and **B,** This varus deformity was fixed, and the joint was not passively reducible. At 25 degrees of varus angulation that was irreducable, this is excessive, and a joint replacement was not contemplated.

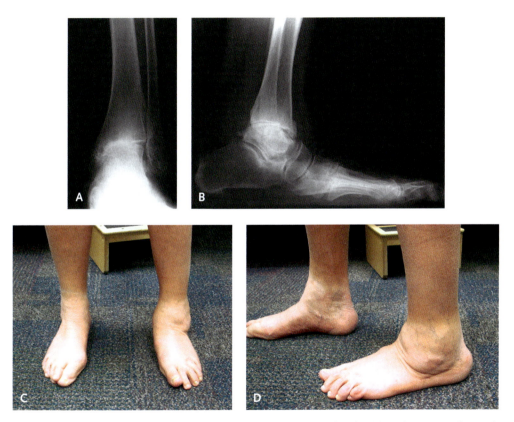

Figure 24-4 **A** and **B,** This varus deformity is not excessive and could be be treated with ankle replacement. Of note, the marked compensatory deformity of the foot must be corrected simultaneously, to avoid recurrent ankle deformity. **C** and **D,** Note the medial translation of the foot under the tibia; despite the varus ankle deformity, the hindfoot is in valgus and the midfoot is unstable. If the ankle varus deformity is corrected, greater valgus deformity of the foot will result.

Combined surgeries are commonly performed for associated deformity and arthritis. I recommend simultaneous hindfoot arthrodesis. The talonavicular arthrodesis is straightforward, because the incision is simply extended slightly distally. A lateral incision can be used for an isolated subtalar arthrodesis or a subtalar and calcaneocuboid arthrodesis (Figure 24-8). The fixation of these joints can be difficult, but correctly positioned screws or plates are used without interfering with the prosthesis. This consideration is of particular importance in patients with rheumatoid arthritis. Repeated bouts of immobilization lead to increased osteopenia with the potential for implant subsidence or fracture. Simultaneous joint replacement–arthrodesis has its advantages (Figure 24-9). If hardware is present

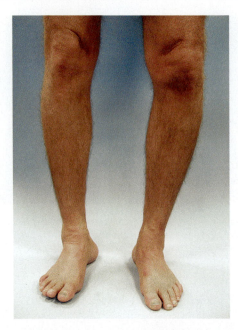

Figure 24-5 Joint replacement should be staged if there is tibia vara. The tibial osteotomy can, however, be performed simultaneously with the ankle replacement.

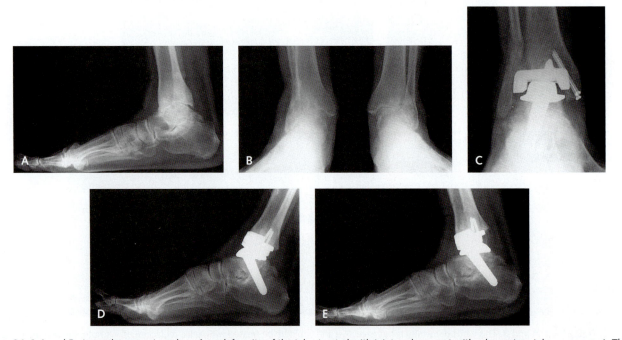

Figure 24-6 A and **B,** Avascular necrosis and a valgus deformity of the talus treated with joint replacement with a long-stem talar component. The stress fracture of the fibula was the result of the valgus deformity. The replacement was performed in combination with a subtalar arthrodesis, and a long-stem talar component was used to overcome the poor bone quality and distribute the load into the calcaneus. **C-E,** Excellent range of motion of the ankle and a stable implant at 3 years after surgery.

in the tibia or talus, it obviously has to be removed if it interferes with correct positioning of either the tibial or the talar component. Of note, however, removal of hardware may create a stress riser, particularly in the medial malleolus (see Figure 24-9). Screws that strip on attempted removal constitute more of a problem: additional bone has to be removed to core out the screw with a screw removal device. Screws in the medial malleolus may interfere with insertion of the tibial component, and they should not be removed intraoperatively, regardless of the type of prosthesis, unless the malleolus is reinforced with temporary Kirschner wires (K-wires).

Text Continued on 281

24

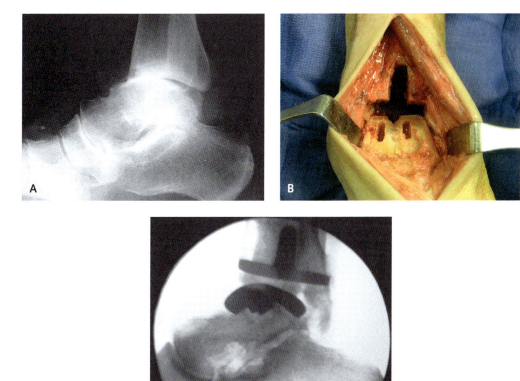

Figure 24-7 A, Anterior subluxation of the ankle was noted preoperatively in a 70-year-old patient with ankle arthritis. **B** and **C,** At the time of surgery, the joint was well prepared for the Mobility prosthesis (DePuy Orthopaedics, Inc., Warsaw, Indiana), and the cuts made for the talar component were correctly centered on the talus, yet subluxation persisted. This was addressed by appropriate tensioning with the poly insert, and correct axial alignment returned 6 months after joint replacement.

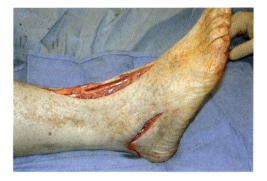

Figure 24-8 A subtalar arthrodesis was performed simultaneously with the joint replacement through a separate lateral incision. It is important to maintain as large a skin bridge as possible.

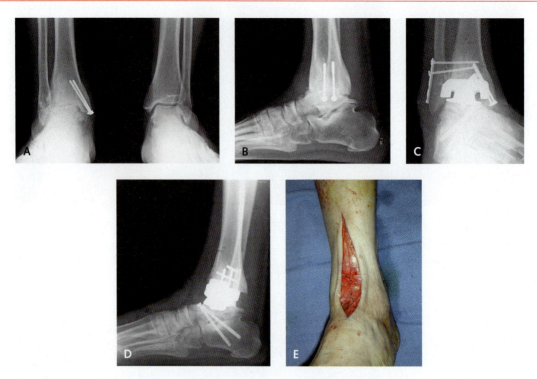

Figure 24-9 A and **B,** Ankle replacement for management of intractable posttraumatic arthritis. Note the medial malleolar screws. The screws were left in place, and the replacement was performed with a simultaneous subtalar arthrodesis.

TECHNIQUES, TIPS, AND PITFALLS

Replacement With All Implants

- After the skin incision the extensor retinaculum is carefully incised to create two flaps, which are *not* retracted during dissection until the tibial periosteum is reflected. The central aspect of the incision directly over the ankle is at the most risk for subsequent wound dehiscence, and very gentle retraction is necessary. Use finger retraction, and do not pull on the skin with an instrument. Simultaneous retraction of both sides of the incision should be avoided.

- For all implant systems, it is necessary to be able to change the size of the prosthesis at the final stage of the surgery. This is particularly the case if the range of motion is compromised, and under these circumstances, I down-size the prosthesis in the hope of improving the range of motion. Select the smaller prosthesis only if it adequately covers the cortical rims of talus and distal tibia and provides sufficient clearance. If the prosthesis has been correctly sized and matches the tibia and the talus, then it is preferable to recut the bone, which can be removed from either the talus or the tibia, depending on the available bone.

If the plan is to remove more bone from the talus, then the amount to be removed should be projected by fluoroscopic imaging, to ensure that the posterior subtalar joint is not compromised. Any further cuts on the talus must therefore be made with the ankle fully dorsiflexed.

- Do not overstuff the joint, which will lead to stiffness, pain, and ultimate joint failure. If considering a lengthening of the Achilles tendon, review whether this is in fact necessary; it may be far simpler and ultimately more reliable to shave 2 mm off the tibial cut and decrease the tension on the joint.

- The retinaculum over the anterior tibial tendon must be carefully repaired if the tendon is exposed. In the event of a wound dehiscence, provided the tendon is not exposed, the management of the wound is not difficult. The anterior incision must protect the sheath of the anterior tibial tendon and should be made slightly lateral to the tendon. If the retinaculum tears, inserting a suture in it early is preferable to repairing the retinaculum after surgery to maintain the tendon

TECHNIQUES, TIPS, AND PITFALLS—cont'd

in the sheath. The retinaculum must be closed to prevent bowstringing of the tendon and to minimize the potential for disaster if a wound dehiscence occurs postoperatively (see Figure 24-9, *E*).

- A synovectomy and debridement of these osteophytes will facilitate improved exposure, including a sense of the position and plane of the ankle joint. Performing an extensive ostectomy or cheilectomy of the anterior distal tibia to improve visualization of the joints is always helpful, regardless of the implant used. A problem may arise with exposure of the distal fibula at the talofibular articulation. This is not easy to visualize and is best done slowly, with movement of the ankle until the joint is easily visible.

- When the posterior tibial cut is made in cases of posttraumatic arthritis, removal of the posterior lip of the tibia is difficult. The tibia can be prominent posteroinferiorly, and the flexor hallucis and peroneal tendons may be scarred down to the underlying bone. Do not rip out the bone with a rongeur, but slowly remove the hypertrophic osteophytes with a pituitary rongeur. When making the tibial bone cut, pay attention to the posterior soft tissues, in particular the posterior tibial tendon and the flexor hallucis longus tendon, with the cut on the posterior aspect of the tibia. The posterior tibial tendon frequently is visualized with the medial malleolar cut (when the medial malleolus is cut as with an Agililty replacement), and it should therefore not be surprising that posterior tibial tendon symptoms may develop postoperatively. When the posterior tibial cut is made in cases of posttraumatic arthritis, it is difficult to remove the posterior lip of the tibia, and the flexor hallucis and peroneal tendons may be scarred down to the underlying bone. Do not rip out the bone with a rongeur, but slowly remove the hypertrophic osteophytes.

- A fracture of either malleolus must be recognized and fixed intraoperatively. Fracture of the medial malleolus creates more of a problem and usually is caused by a combination of osteopenia, previous stress on the medial malleolus (such as with a varus deformity), difficulty with sizing or positioning of the tibial component, or inadvertent manipulation of the ankle. If a fracture does occur intraoperatively, it should always be secured with internal fixation, because the malleoli are required for the stability of the prosthesis. Fracture of the medial malleolus creates more of a problem and usually is caused by carelessness with sizing or positioning of the tibial component or inadvertent manipulation of the ankle. Perhaps the most common error causing fracture of the medial malleolus is making an oblique (not vertical) cut of the medial malleolus, when the swing of the blade cuts deeper into the malleolus posteriorly.

- Once the trial components are inserted, it should just be possible to separate the components by a few millimeters from each other with maximal pulling on the ankle. This criterion ensures the correct tension.

- Initial splinting of the ankle joint in maximum dorsiflexion is essential to avoid creating an equinus contracture, because the dorsiflexion is difficult to regain later on. I do not like using the traditional splints—these are applied presumably with the foot in dorsiflexion; subsequently, however, because of the bulk of the dressing, the foot may be found to have drifted into equinus. A circumferential cast may be used but will need to be split in the recovery room.

- Early initiation of range-of-motion exercises is recommended. A fracture boot locked in extension should be used to immobilize the joint during the periods when exercise is not performed. Control of postoperative swelling minimizes patient discomfort and increases ability to perform the necessary exercises. Early weight bearing is permitted with the Salto prosthesis, and once the incisions are fully healed, the patient is permitted to begin swimming and walking in a pool. Progressive resistance exercises are gradually added to the postoperative rehabilitation regimen.

- Patient weight should be taken into consideration by the expected size of implant to be used and the body mass index. A large muscular man with a large joint who requires a large implant would be expected to have fewer complications with subsidence and wear than those typical for an obese patient of the same weight with a small ankle requiring a smaller implant. In general, the exact-size prosthesis should be inserted; in some instances, however, it may be best to "err" in one direction or another with regard to size. For example, in patients with severe ankle ankylosis secondary to trauma, an acceptable range of motion may not be attainable; this limitation can be minimized to some extent by downsizing the prosthesis.

Continued

TECHNIQUES, TIPS, AND PITFALLS—cont'd

Agility Ankle Replacement

- Accurate positioning including correct external rotation of the talar component is important. This is based on the anatomic external rotation of the talus and is particularly relevant for the Agility ankle replacement (i.e., the Agility LP Total Ankle Replacement System—DePuy Orthopaedics, Inc., Warsaw, Indiana). The rotation of the component should be checked visually and under fluoroscopic imaging, and the alignment can be changed if necessary (Figures 24-10 to 24-12).

- External rotation of the fibula can be a problem. This is present after trauma or associated with a congenital equinovarus deformity or a cavus foot. Unlike other prostheses, the Agility prosthesis rests on the fibula and accordingly distributes the load on the ankle. If the fibula is markedly externally rotated, it lies posterior to the tibia, and will be cut when the osteotomy for the tibial component is made. In these circumstances, it is necessary to perform an osteotomy of the fibula before the syndesmosis arthrodesis. An alternative is to completely free up the fibula, then pin it in a reduced, more anterior location, insert the prosthesis, and the fix the fibula with a plate for the arthrodesis (Figure 24-13).

- The most unique characteristic of the Agility prosthesis is that it takes advantage of successful arthrodesis of the distal tibiofibular syndesmosis. This converts a three-bone joint to a two-bone joint, which theoretically should simplify the mechanical loads about the ankle joint. It is easier to expose and debride the syndesmosis before planning the bone cuts. Once the fibula has been loosened, the syndesmosis exposure is facilitated by the insertion of a laminar spreader just proximal to the joint, and the debridement can be extended more distally to the ankle joint (Figure 24-14). A common error is to debride a portion of the anterior fibula and to ignore the posterolateral inclination of the distal fibula. This is a particular problem with posttraumatic arthritis, in which the margin of the anterior aspect of the talofibular joint is poorly defined. I start with an ostectomy of the anterior and lateral distal tibia using a chisel, followed by a thorough decortication. All soft tissue and loose bone that may impede syndesmosis arthrodesis must be removed. The biggest problem here is failure to adequately debride the fibula out of concern for a fracture of the fibula—a potential problem that can be ignored because a plate is routinely applied to the fibula for syndesmosis fusion (see Figure 24-14, B).

- In most previous reports on the use of the Agility prosthesis, the technique has been described with the use of an external fixator to distract the joint and align the ankle under the correct tension. I no longer use distraction and have found that it distorts the correct tension of the joint. The correct alignment of the cutting block for the tibia is important, but once the tibia has been correctly cut, the talus is cut free hand, to remove 4 mm of the talar dome. The foot must be in neutral dorsiflexion for making the talar cut. If the foot is in plantar flexion, the cut may enter the posterior talus and subtalar joint.

- The bone cuts for implantation of the tibial component require resection of the inner one third of both the medial malleolus and the fibula. Before making these cuts, be sure that nothing will block the saw (e.g., previously inserted hardware). Leaving hardware in whenever possible is preferable, to prevent fracture. Hardware removal in the medial malleolus presents a particular problem because it creates a stress riser, which is prone to intraoperative fracture. If there is concern about the viability of the medial malleolus, insert a temporary guide pin into the malleolus before making the bone cuts, to help prevent fracture. The screws that can give the worst problem are those in the anterior tibia that are either buried or stripped. They block the correct bone cut, and worse, when an attempt is made to remove them, the small chunk of bone that often comes out with the screw leaves a bone void. I always prefer to err on the side of taking less bone. If I am not certain about the plane of the cuts on the malleoli, I use a smaller cutting block; the margins of the bone cuts can be increased later on, if necessary.

- The correct positioning of the cutting block is the most important phase of the joint replacement. It should not be performed visually, and it must be done with careful fluoroscopic monitoring to ensure optimal alignment. With the ankle viewed from the anteroposterior position, both malleoli are not visualized in correct orientation simultaneously, and the ankle needs to be rotated around under fluoroscopic imaging to ensure perfect alignment of the cutting block.

- Pay attention to the position of the posteromedial soft tissue structures, in particular the posterior tibial tendon with the medial malleolar cut and the flexor hallucis longus tendon with the cut on the posterior

24

aspect of the tibia. The posterior tibial tendon may lie more posteriorly than medially and can be visualized when the medial malleolar cut is made.

- A common error that leads to fracture of the medial malleolus is making an oblique (not vertical) cut of the medial malleolus, so that when the tibial component is inserted, the posterior margin of the component abuts the obliquely cut medial malleolus. This incorrect cut is caused by slight external rotation of the cutting block.

Mobility Ankle Replacement

- Performing an extensive ostectomy or cheilectomy of the anterior distal tibia to improve visualization of the joints is always helpful regardless of the implant used. The Mobility ankle replacement (Mobility Total Ankle System—DePuy Orthopaedics, Inc.) is illustrated here (Figure 24-15). Removal of the osteophytes at the neck of the talus as well as the anterior tibia helps visualize the joint, and in particular the plane of the plafond for correct bone resection (see Figure 24-15, *B* and *C*).

- Proximal displacement of the cutting block results in resection of more tibia, impingement of the gutters, and likelihood of subsidence into softer metaphyseal bone.

- The "tibia follows the talus" with respect to sizing. To determine the correct tibial implant, the tibia must be sized from posterior to anterior. The sizer should be perfectly lined up over the talus, equidistant at 1 mm on either side of the talus. The sizer does not determine the talar size, because the talus can be bigger or smaller than the tibial component. It is more important that the tibial component cover the tibial surface from back to front than from side to side.

- The bone cut on the tibia varies depending on the "slack" of the joint. After the tibial cut is done, the white spacer ("lollipop") should fit comfortably, to ensure that everything will fit. It is always best to undercut the tibia and then adjust it as necessary later.

- Resect more anterior talus osteophytes than seems necessary, because this will save time in the end and make anterior chamfer burring much easier.

- If the tibial window is slightly medial or lateral, a thin wafer of bone can be cut and transferred to the other side of the window to medialize or lateralize the tibial component if an error has been made.

- When doing talar center guide, make sure there is a bump behind the ankle, to avoid creating an unwanted anterior drawer when the central pin is placed in the talus (Figures 24-16 and 24-17).

- For correction of the anterior subluxated talus, the talar center pin can be shifted anteriorly slightly to relocate the talus under the center of the tibial component.

- When the drill bits are being drilled into the talus guide, that the ankle *must* be dorsiflexed to neutral. This is the most critical step in the procedure. The two pins in the talus will guide everything from here on. With the initial tibial cut, the "tibia follows the talus" by placing the tibial base plate centered over the talus. The ankle joint should be held at 90 degrees, and care should be taken to establish the correct rotation on the talus. In most cases, the handle of the centering guide should line up with the second ray. There should be equal distance between talus exposed medial and lateral to the talar guide—approximately 1 mm. It is better to undersize than to oversize the talus, because talar component impingement on the malleoli will lead to pain and potential fracture. Once the drill hole is made through the guide hole the drill should stay parallel to either the medial or the lateral border of the talus. This is another critical step. If the guide pins are inserted in internal or external rotation, correct this placement now, because there is no turning back later. All talar cuts are made referencing the position of the pins (Figures 24-18 and 24-19).

- Check the lateral fluoroscopic image to ensure the talar center pin is indeed centered. Especially avoid a placement too far posterior, because then the cuts will remove excessive anterior talar neck.

- If after applying the posterior flat cutting guide there is no bone to resect with the saw, the block typically has been placed a bit too far posteriorly. With the "tuning fork," I always use the C-arm to confirm central placement in the anterior-posterior direction. The operator may suspect that the central pin was incorrectly placed during use of the barrel drill to do the superior and posterior grove drill. A look down the barrel should show approximately half of the barrel filled with bone. That is almost always the case on the top surface of the talus. If no bone is seen through the posterior barrel, the block is too far posterior. If the

Continued

TECHNIQUES, TIPS, AND PITFALLS—cont'd

barrel is completely filled with bone, the block is too far anterior. It is difficult to change the block position at this point and maintain stability, again emphasizing the importance of getting the initial central pin placement correct.

- The "footprint" for talar sizes 1 to 4 is the same, and 5 and 6 footprints are the same. Size 1 to size 4 talar components are therefore interchangeable in this respect, without the need for any additional cuts. If initial templating indicates the need for somewhere between a 4 and a 5, the decision is more difficult; as a rule, it probably is best to go smaller, unless the tibia clearly requires a 5 or 6.

- It is acceptable to mismatch sizes. In up to 30% of cases in my experience, the tibial component used is one size bigger. Also, the talar component quite often lies 1 or 2 mm medial or lateral to the tibia, for as-yet undetermined reasons. As noted earlier, I do not use radiographic confirmation at any point. If the bone is of really good quality, upsizing components is not essential but of course may be necesssary in patients with rheumatoid arthritis.

- The talar component does not have to be the same size as the tibial component. If mismatched sizes will be used, the poly insert should be of the same size as that of the talar component.

Salto Talaris Ankle Replacement (Figure 24-20)
- Unlike with the other implants discussed here, with the Salto Talaris ankle replacement (Salto Ankle Prosthesis—Tornier, Edina, Minnesota), the anterior tibial cheilectomy must fully expose the tibial articular surface, because the plafond marks the point from which the tibial resection is measured.

- The purpose of the locking pins in the tibial alignment guide is to accomplish just that—to hold the guide in a firm position relative to the ankle. The medial pin may not align well with the tibia and actually can be situated anywhere on the tibia. If the guide is shifted, then the distal cutting block is adjusted eventually. If the tibia has a difficult anterior configuration, the pin can be inserted laterally.

- The tibial alignment guide must not be completely flush on the distal tibia, leaving 2 mm of clearance for translation of the cutting block guide proximally for adjusting the resection level. The guide must, however, be flush with the surface of the plafond, aided by removal of all anterior osteophytes.

- The foot must be plantigrade for correct use of the alignment guide. As with other implant systems, soft tissue correction should be done before the bone cuts are made.

- The recommended distal tibial resection thickness is 9 mm, which will permit downsizing to an 8-mm insert.

- Use of an 8-mm resection level is recommended for loose joints in an effort to preserve bone, even though this can be made up with a larger poly insert thickness.

- As with all implants, sizing of the prosthesis is important, although not critical at this stage, because the size of the tibial implant can be changed. The edge of the of the medial malleolus and the lateral edge of the syndesmosis mark the lines for selection of the implant size

- Use half-pins in the tibial cutting guide to protect the malleoli during the tibial resection.

- Before making the tibial cut, insert a free saw blade and verify the angulation of the tibial cut, which can still be adjusted

- As with the Mobility implant, a bump should always be present underneath the distal tibia to raise the heel off the table, to prevent anterior translation of the foot under the tibia.

- Anterior translation of the talus will lead to anterior insertion of the talar component, and the foot must be in neutral to allow placement of the talar cutting guide pin in the correct location. If the foot is dorsiflexed, the talar dome resection will be too anterior, and if the foot is plantar flexed, the talar dome resection will be too posterior. This is a malleolus-sparing implant, and the narrow saw blade should be used to cut the talus and protect the malleoli. Verify the position of the talar cutting pins fluoroscopically to ensure that they are correctly oriented. As with the Mobility replacement, it is useful to remove all anterior osteophytes on the neck of the talus before the talus champfer cuts are made. Make sure that the chamfer guide is sitting flush on the talus. Use a laminar spreader and check this positioning fluoroscopically.

- A critical step in this procedure is the correct position of the lateral chamfer cut. Remember that the sizes 1 to 3 have a constant width of the talar implant laterally, and the variability is on the medial side of the implant.

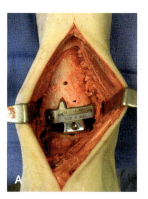
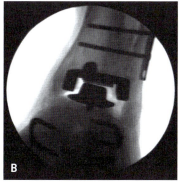
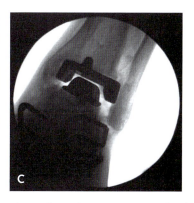

Figure 24-10 A, The external rotation of both the tibia and the talus in this case of an agility replacement was considered to be inaccurate. Both were excessively externally rotated. **B** and **C,** The slot for the fin of the tibial component and also the cuts for the medial malleolus and fibula were recut free hand, and the components were slightly internally rotated to a correct alignment.

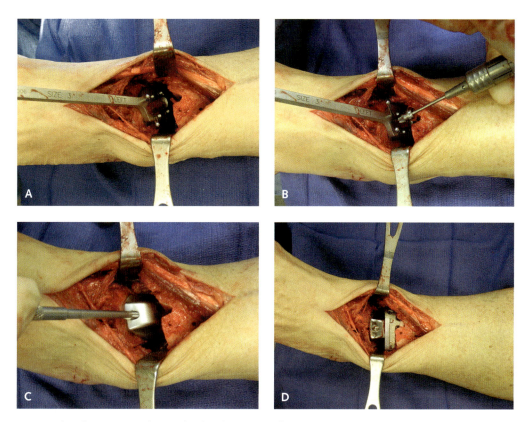

Figure 24-11 A, The talar cutting guide must be placed symmetrically on the talus, with an equal amount of bone on either side of the guide. **B,** The cutting burr is used to prepare the slot for the talar fin, and the trial talus must fit flush on the surface. **C** and **D,** The slot can be recut if necessary, or filled with cancellous graft if the fit is not correct. Cancellous bone graft was added to the anterior and lateral tibia once the final implant was inserted.

CORRECTION OF DEFORMITY

One should reconstruct the ankle joint by placing the prosthesis parallel to the ground. Adequate soft tissue balancing and complete ankle and hindfoot alignment are therefore critical. To what extent has the foot compensated for ankle deformity? For example, in a patient with a *varus* ankle, the hindfoot attempts to compensate by increasing valgus. With reduction of the ankle into a neutral position, does the hindfoot remain in valgus or is it reduced to a plantigrade position? Patients with significant mechanical malalignment of the knee or tibia should be considered for reconstructive procedures of these deformities *before* a total ankle replacement. I do, however, consider performing a supramalleolar osteotomy at the same time as ankle replacement when necessary (Figures 24-21 and 24-22). Most additional procedures below the ankle joint can be performed simultaneously with the ankle replacement, or as a staged procedure. As a generalization, preservation of foot flexibility, as opposed to any hindfoot arthrodesis, is always preferable. If staged procedures are indicated, the interval between such a procedure and the ankle replacement should be reduced, to avoid

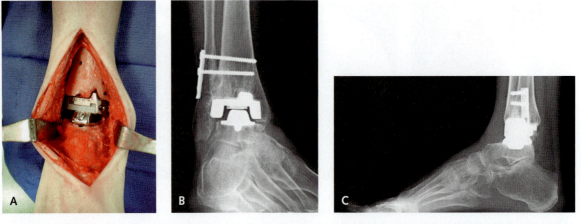

Figure 24-12 A-C, The rotational alignment of the components did not appear to be correct, although the foot was correctly aligned under the leg, as verified radiographically.

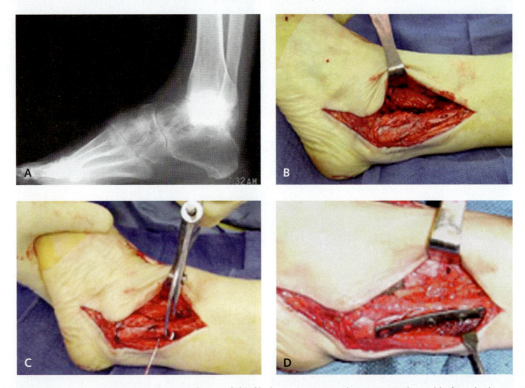

Figure 24-13 A-C, Severe traumatic posterior translation of the fibula was recognized preoperatively, and before the bone cuts were made, two incisions were made **(A),** the syndesmosis was exposed **(B),** and the fibula was pulled forward with a bone reduction clamp **(C)** and pinned in a corrected anterior position. **D,** Once the implants were in place, the fibula was plated over the cannulated guide pins.

osteopenia, which may jeopardize future implant support. There are, however, reasons to perform the surgery simultaneously, in particular, to prevent the fibrosis of the soft tissues that follows staged procedures. I perform a talonavicular or a subtalar arthrodesis at the same time as for the ankle replacement, but if a triple arthrodesis is required for correction of deformity, it is performed as a staged procedure approximately 6 months before the ankle replacement.

Planning the strategy for the correction of a *varus* ankle deformity probably is the most difficult part of any ankle joint replacement. A wide spectrum of deformity exists, ranging from a slightly deformed ankle joint with minimal soft tissue contracture to a severely deformed cavovarus foot and ankle with lateral ligament and peroneus brevis muscle insufficiency, which should not be corrected with ankle replacement. Depending on the severity and the nature of the deformity, the preoperative evaluation must ascertain the presence of the following: the contracted deltoid ligament, the contracted posterior tibial muscle, lateral ankle ligament insufficiency, motor deficit of the peroneus brevis muscle, focal bone loss on the medial aspect of the distal tibial articular surface, the varus heel, the plantar flexed first metatarsal, and a medially displaced Achilles tendon. Inserting the prostheses parallel to the ground is imperative, and adequate soft tissue balancing and complete ankle and hindfoot alignment are important before insertion of the prosthesis. The cut of the talus must be rectangular, rather than triangular, because the latter cut leads to an oblique cut of the talus and recurrent deformity.

Correcting varus deformity that is associated with bone loss on the medial distal tibial plafond is easier, because the perpendicular positioning of the cutting block relative to the limb axis always removes slightly more bone from the lateral than from the medial distal tibia. This additional resection, however, is not adequate to realign the ankle. With many chronic varus deformities, the medial malleolus and the medial distal tibia are dysplastic. Regardless of the prosthesis used, there will be no contact between the medial malleolus and the tibial component, and therefore insufficient support will be present medially, leading to varus joint tilt and failure. In such instances, a distal medial opening wedge supramalleolar osteotomy is performed, preferably before the joint replacement as a staged procedure. This reorients the alignment of the medial malleolus from an oblique to a more vertical position, a more favorable configuration for accepting the prosthesis (Figure 24-23). When the varus deformity is intra-articular, it is not generally necessary to plan additional procedures, because the tibial bone cut will correct the orientation of the joint (Figure 24-24).

In commencing with the joint replacement for correction of a varus ankle deformity, the deep deltoid is initially released, and then while a valgus force is applied to the ankle, the other portions are palpated and sequentially released. Correction of this problem usually requires opening the joint, initially cleaning out the gutters to bring the foot and talus to neutral. If a neutral position cannot be achieved after the gutters are cleaned out and there is no other mechanical blockage, then frequently, the deltoid ligament must be lengthened. The deep portion can be severed from inside out with an osteotome, but the superficial portion usually must be approached through a separate incision. The posterior tibial tendon is lifted out of its groove, and the superficial portion of the deltoid is "pie crusted" to achieve the desired length. This procedure also can be done at the termination of the procedure if it appears that the components have been put in too tight or if there is an apparent contracture of the superficial deltoid. After an adequate medial release, the lateral ligaments usually are loose, the ligaments are redundant, or the ankle is unstable, and a ligament reconstruction must be performed (which is done only after the prosthesis is inserted). The lateral gutter osteophytes must be debrided to allow rotation of the talar body in the mortise. Once the realignment is complete and the ankle is stable, a decision is made regarding the necessity for a calcaneus osteotomy (Figure 24-25).

The easiest method for lateral ligament reconstruction is to use half of the peroneus brevis tendon, which is passed under the fibular plate and over one of the screws. The tendon is pulled around the screw, and then the plate is compressed against the tendon, which is then sutured onto itself (Figure 24-26). An alternative method is to use half of the peroneus brevis in a modified Evans procedure, passing the tendon through a drill hole in the fibula to exit posteriorly and then sutured to the periosteum (Figure 24-27).

A *valgus* ankle deformity is potentially associated with combinations of a contracted lateral ligament, deltoid ligament

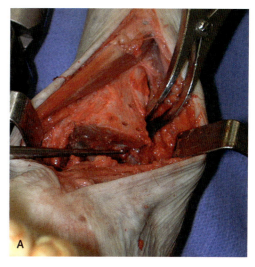

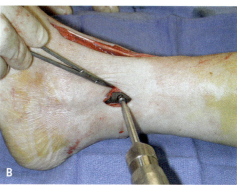

Figure 24-14 A, The syndesmosis is prepared by inserting a laminar spreader into the joint, followed by very thorough and aggressive debridement. **B,** After insertion of the implant, the syndesmosis is compressed with the application of a 2- or 3-hole plate. Plating essentially provides a large washer effect for compression of the fibula and can be extended if a fracture is present.

insufficiency, a valgus heel, a laterally displaced Achilles tendon that acts as a hindfoot evertor, a shortened and deformed fibula due to chronic impingement, and spring ligament and posterior tibial tendon rupture. Correction of a valgus deformity must be undertaken with caution (Figures 24-28 to 24-30). Unlike with the varus deformity, a ruptured deltoid and a valgus ankle are far less predictable to treat; a laminar spreader should be inserted into the lateral joint space to balance the talar cut. With severe valgus deformity, a joint replacement should not be performed because the deltoid ligament is completely torn, severely stretched, and irreparable. Joint replacement may be considered after flatfoot correction and a deltoid reconstruction, but I recommend waiting at least 1 year to ensure that the deltoid reconstruction has been successful. If the deformity is more minor, with heel valgus and foot deformity without a deltoid tear, then joint replacement is a very reasonable alternative (Figure 24-31).

In a very lax ankle, the initial tibial cut should be minimal to allow adequate tensioning of the ligaments. The Mobility system has polyethylene insert components ranging in thickness from 3 to 11 mm, in 2-mm increments, that can be used even in primary cases to achieve additional medial stability. The forefoot is important in all deformity work, and in valgus, the forefoot frequently is hypersupinated. Proper alignment of the forefoot often is necessary, by fusion

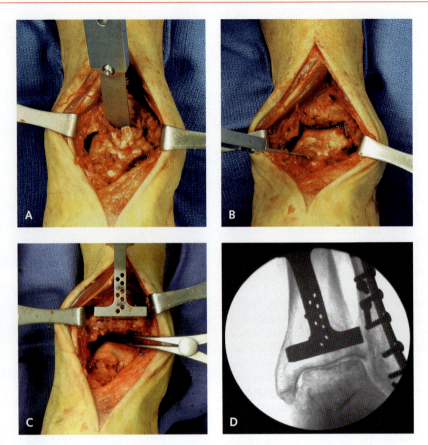

Figure 24-15 A, A chisel is used to perform an extensive ostectomy of the anterior distal tibia in preparation for this Mobility replacement. **B,** The osteophytes at the neck of the talus are removed. **C** and **D,** This helps to visualize the joint, and in particular the plane of the plafond, for correct bone resection.

of the first metatarsal cuneiform joint or stabilization of any other joints in cases involving gross instability. After the ankle prosthesis has been inserted, the forefoot stabilized, and equinus contracture corrected, only then should the case be considered completed.

ADDITIONAL PROCEDURES

When a subtalar arthrodesis is required, I use long small screws inserted from the dorsal aspect of the tarsal neck directed in multiple projections into the calcaneus (Figure 24-32). Large screws should not be inserted into the talus from bottom to top, because the direction of the screws is unpredictable. Insertion of the correct length of screw also is difficult, because it may abut the undersurface of the talar component, causing displacement. The head of the screw must

not abut the anterior edge of the talar component, because movement of the screw can lift it up off the talus.

Conversion of ankle arthrodesis to a prosthesis is technically possible but is a complex procedure. Regardless of what has been described in the literature to date, this is a salvage procedure performed as an alternative to amputation. Candidates for this procedure should have severe pain in the hindfoot, with no possibility of conversion to a pan-talar arthrodesis. If the ankle fusion has been successful, as an isolated procedure and subtalar and or transverse tarsal joint arthritis is the preferable if not the required procedure. The ideal patient for this procedure is someone who presents with a painful nonunion of the arthrodesis, with avascular sclerotic bone margins, and for whom a revision arthrodesis poses further potential for failure (Figure 24-33).

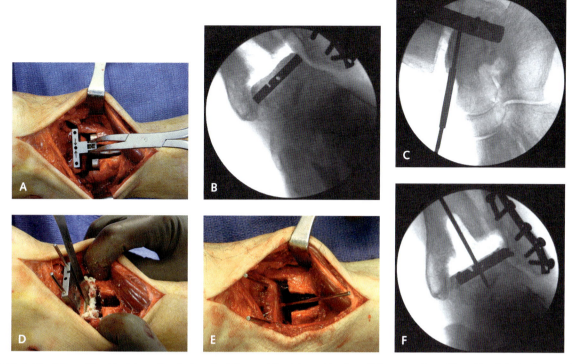

Figure 24-16 A, The talar cutting block is well seated on the talus, and the talar guide pins will line up well on either side of the body. **B** and **C,** Fluoroscopy is useful to confirm correct alignment of the talar cutting block. **D,** The bone removal from the body may be quite minimal, with only a millimeter or two shaved off. **E** and **F,** The central guide pin is correctly located in the center of the talus. This is a critical step in positioning the prosthesis.

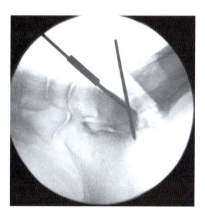

Figure 24-17 The central guide pin is not seated correctly in the talus. It is too far posterior, and the talus has subluxated forward while the guide was centered. This must be changed so that the pin enters the center of the talar body.

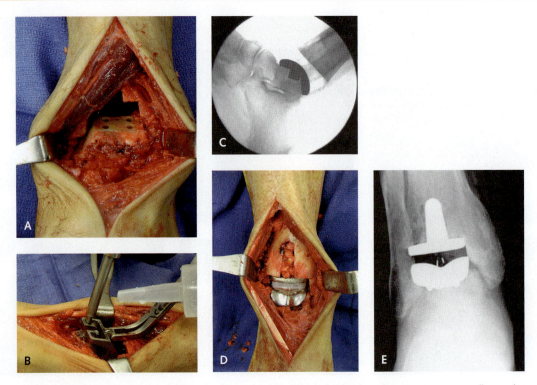

Figure 24-18 The important steps of the Mobility replacement. **A,** The guides holes for the talar component are well seated symmetrically. **B,** The burr shaping for the anterior talus must be done with the cutting block firmly seated on the talus. **C,** It is useful to obtain a radiograph of the talar trial seated before proceeding with the permanent implant, in case adjustments need to be made. **D** and **E,** Note the use of bone graft anterior to the stem and good alignment of the tibia over the talar component.

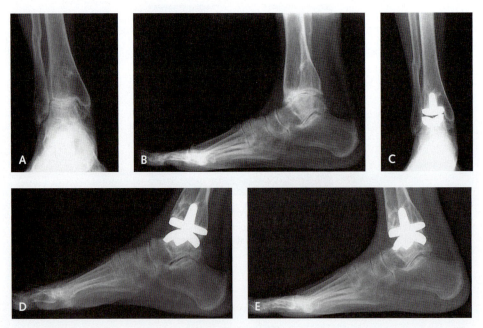

Figure 24-19 A and **B,** Replacement using the Mobility ankle implant is a malleolus-preserving procedure. **C-E,** Despite the presence of osteophytes in the medial gutter, it is not necessary to debride the osteophytes unless deformity is present, blocking correction.

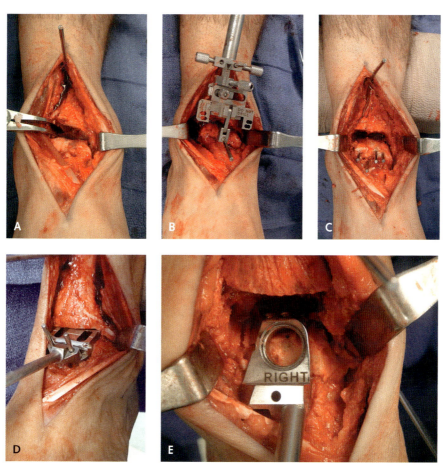

Figure 24-20 The steps of the Salto prosthesis replacement. **A,** The undersurface of the tibial plafond must be visible after cheilectomy to allow accurate positioning of the tibial cutting block. This is easiest to assess with a laminar spreader in the joint. **B,** The rotation of the component is determined by the talar alignment pin, which is a very important step. **C,** In a small talus, three and sometimes only two pins can be inserted for the talus cut. **D,** Here, the talus is pushed too anterior, and either there is no bump under the distal leg, pushing the heel forward, or the anterior margin of the talar cut is incorrect. **E,** The talus centering cut is critical because it aligns the mediolateral position for the talar component.

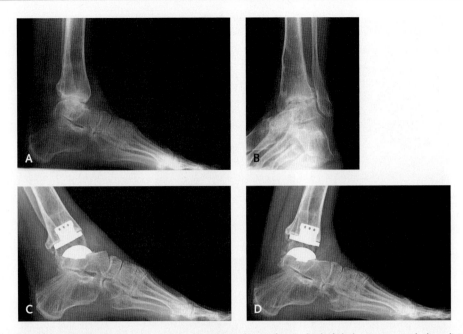

Figure 24-21 A and **B,** The patient presented with ankle arthritis after multiple failed surgeries, including distraction arthroplasty. **C** and **D,** Replacement with a Salto Talaris prosthesis resulted in good alignment and range of motion.

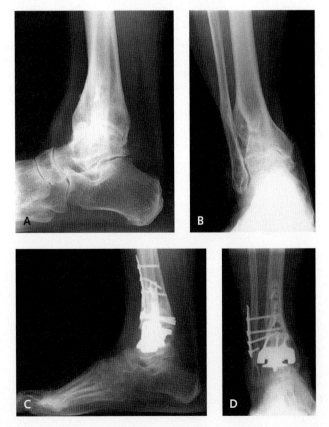

Figure 24-22 A and **B,** The patient presented with multiplanar deformity of the tibia and ankle arthritis. **C** and **D,** A dome supramalleolar osteotomy of the tibia was performed, and once the alignment was corrected, the ankle replacement was simultaneously performed.

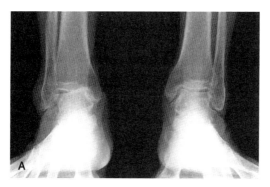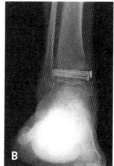

Figure 24-23 The patient was treated for varus ankle arthritis and instability with a staged medial opening wedge tibial osteotomy (a medial plafond-plasty). **A,** Obliquity of the medial malleolus is evident on the preoperative radiograph. **B,** The correct orientation of the malleolus can be seen on the postoperative radiograph.

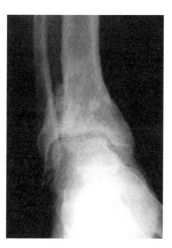

Figure 24-24 This ankle varus deformity was associated with erosive medial plafond deformity and a prominent lateral ridge of the distal tibia. The joint replacement was easier because the deformity was intra-articular and not associated with changes in the foot.

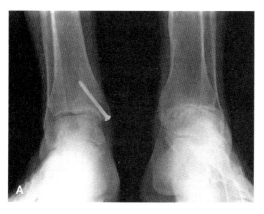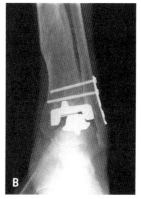

Figure 24-25 **A** and **B,** This varus deformity was corrected with deltoid release, removal of osteophytes in the lateral gutter, calcaneus osteotomy, and a modified Evans procedure.

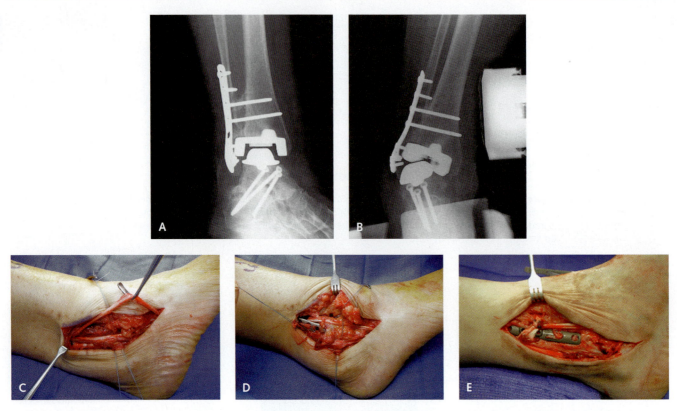

Figure 24-26 A, The patient underwent a successful joint replacement with a combined subtalar arthrodesis. **B,** An unstable ankle developed as a consequence of injury. **C** and **D,** Correction was accomplished with a modified Evans procedure using the anterior half of the peroneus brevis tendon, passed beneath the fibular plate under tension. **E,** The tendon was then looped anterior to the plate to be tied back onto itself.

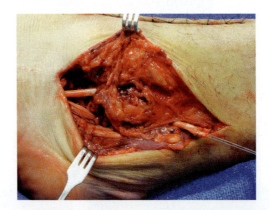

Figure 24-27 After a Mobility replacement, the patient was noted to have lateral ankle instability. This was corrected with a modified Evans procedure performed through a drill hole in the fibula, with suturing of the tendon onto the surrounding periosteum.

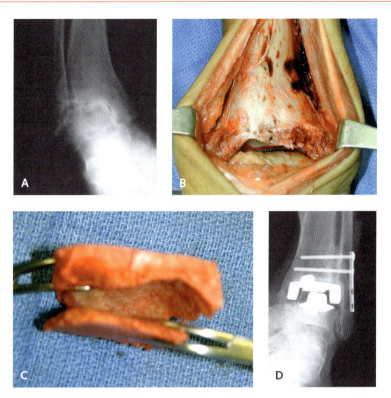

Figure 24-28 A, This varus deformity was mostly intraarticular, and although lateral instability was present requiring correction, this type of varus deformity is not a contraindication to replacement. **B** and **C,** Intraoperative erosion is evident in the medial tibial plafond (**B**) and in the resected bone, where both the talar and the tibial cuts are symmetrical (**C**). **D,** Note the good alignment of the prosthesis.

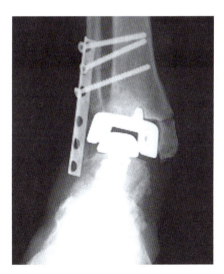

Figure 24-29 Treatment for ankle arthritis with medial joint instability in a 72-year-old patient initially was successful. At 7 months after replacement, however, a stress fracture of the medial malleolus occurred, leading to multiple subsequent complications. Too much stress remained on the medial ankle, which caused the fracture, despite what appeared to be a plantigrade foot.

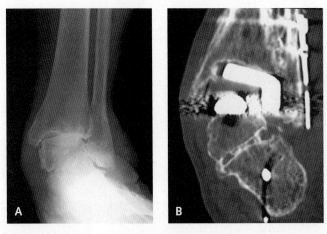

Figure 24-30 A, The patient was treated for ankle arthritis with valgus deformity. **B,** The initial alignment of the foot and ankle was excellent, but over the ensuing 2 years, recurrent valgus deformity developed, as seen on the computed tomography scan.

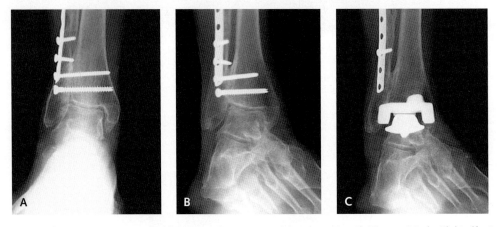

Figure 24-31 A, The patient was 67-year-old woman who was treated for traumatic arthritis associated with hindfoot valgus and slight valgus deformity of the ankle. **B** and **C,** No osteotomy was required, and the alignment was obtained with ligament balancing and correct tension on the prosthesis using a slightly thicker poly insert.

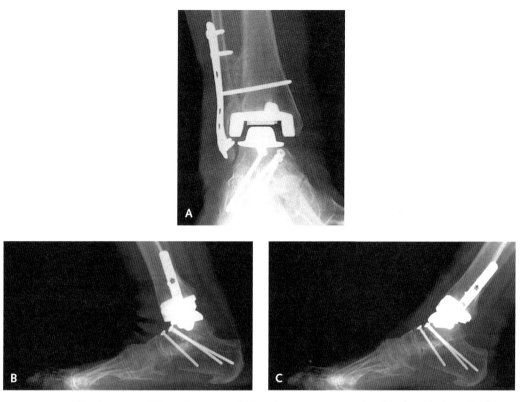

Figure 24-32 A-C, Note the alignment of the replacement, which in this patient was combined with a subtalar arthrodesis using small screw fixation.

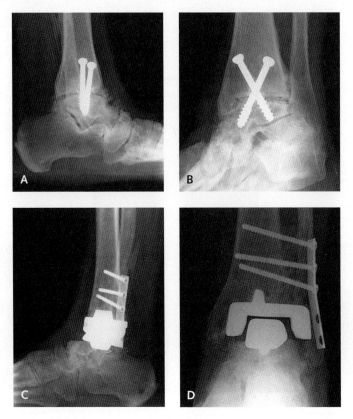

Figure 24-33 **A** and **B,** Painful nonunion of an ankle arthrodesis in a 66-year-old patient. **C** and **D,** The arthrodesis was successfully converted to an ankle replacement.

SUGGESTED READING

Cerrato R, Myerson MS: Total ankle replacement: The Agility LP prosthesis, *Foot Ankle Clin* 13:485–494, 2008.

Coetzee JC: Management of varus or valgus ankle deformity with ankle replacement, *Foot Ankle Clin* 13:509–520, 2008.

Easley ME, Vertullo CJ, Urban WC, Nunley JA: Total ankle arthroplasty, *J Am Acad Orthop Surg* 10:157–167, 2002.

Haddad SL, Coetzee JC, Estok R, et al: Intermediate and long-term outcomes of total ankle arthroplasty and ankle arthrodesis. A systematic review of the literature, *J Bone Joint Surg Am* 89:1899–1905, 2007.

Hobson SA, Karantana A, Dhar S: Total ankle replacement in patients with significant pre-operative deformity of the hindfoot, *J Bone Joint Surg Br* 91:481–486, 2009.

Leszko F, Komistek RD, Mahfouz MR, et al: In vivo kinematics of the Salto total ankle prosthesis, *Foot Ankle Int* 29:1117–1125, 2008.

Mroczek KJ, Myerson MS: Perioperative complications of total ankle arthroplasty, *Foot Ankle Int* 24:17–22, 2003.

Myerson MS, Won HY: Primary and revision total ankle replacement using custom-designed prostheses, *Foot Ankle Clin* 13:521–538, 2008:x.

Myerson MS, Miller SD: Salvage after complications of total ankle arthroplasty, *Foot Ankle Clin* 7:191–206, 2002.

Stamatis ED, Myerson MS: How to avoid specific complications of total ankle replacement, *Foot Ankle Clin* 7:765–789, 2002.

Wood PL, Sutton C, Mishra V, Suneja R: A randomised, controlled trial of two mobile-bearing total ankle replacements [Published erratum appears in *J Bone Joint Surg Br* 91:700, 2009], *J Bone Joint Surg Br* 91:69–74, 2009.

Wood PL, Clough TM, Smith R: The present state of ankle arthroplasty, *Foot Ankle Surg* 14:115–119, 2008:Epub Jul 7, 2008.

CHAPTER **25**

Revision Total Ankle Replacement

OVERVIEW

Over the past decade, a resurgence of interest in total ankle replacement (TAR) has emerged, largely as a consequence of an improved understanding of ankle kinematics, better implant designs, and advances in surgical techniques producing better results and long-term outcomes. As a result, the implants in current use have experienced greater popularity. The longevity of these arthroplasties, regardless of design, is as yet unpredictable, with unknown long-term survivorship. Quite apart from the short-term failures, which mostly are related to wound healing, it is the longer-term potential for complications that is of greatest concern. In view of the potential for failure of a primary joint replacement related to poor bone quality (as a result of either osteopenia or avascular necrosis), as well as the intermediate- and longer-term complications such as osteolysis, subsidence, and loosening, careful consideration of the available salvage options is essential.

Failure of ankle replacements may be the result of patient, implant, or surgical factors, or a combination thereof. Poor selection of patients stemming from lack of attention to physiologic (comorbid conditions, obesity), psychological, and lifestyle factors (occupational and recreational) can jeopardize the outcome. Outcomes can be affected by surgical decisions or technique dictating implant choice, sizing, placement, and alignment; balancing of varus and valgus deformity; and adequately addressing coexisting hindfoot arthritis and deformities. Other uncontrollable factors such as soft tissue complications, wound breakdown, deep infections, and intraoperative technical failures, and fractures of bone or components also can cause failure.

Avoiding complications to begin with is always preferable than having to manage them after failed surgery. Optimizing outcomes begins with patient selection. The factors that I take into consideration are the patient's activity level, lifestyle, and interest in exercise. The limb alignment, the quality of the bone, and the presence of adjacent joint arthritis are important. I may exclude patients who smoke and those in whom the surgery poses too high a risk, including those with peripheral vascular disease, diabetes, peripheral neuropathy, and skin conditions that preclude use of the appropriate surgical approach. Problems with wound healing may occur with increased frequency in patients who smoke and older patients with peripheral vascular disease. Bone quality is important as well, particularly in those patients with periarticular osteopenia, who have

a higher risk for subsidence. Avascular necrosis of the talus does not preclude TAR, particularly with partial involvement of the joint. Even with severe avascular necrosis, an arthroplasty using a custom long-stem talus component may be considered. The larger or heavier patient should be very carefully selected, even if sedentary, and if osteopenia is present I do not perform arthroplasty.

MANAGEMENT OF FRACTURES

The medial malleolus is at risk for fracture regardless of the type of implant used, but more so with the Agility prosthesis, for which a vertical cut is made in the malleolus. For malleolus-sparing procedures, the risk for fracture is nevertheless still present, and in any patient with osteopenia, I protect the malleolus with prophylactic pinning. I insert two Kirschner wires (K-wires), and if there appears to be higher risk for malleolar fracture, I use cannulated screws over the guide pins. The medial malleolus is at particular risk for fracture in the patient who has sustained a previous fracture, and in whom the screws are still present and are in the path of the prosthesis (Figure 25-1). If the implant can be inserted with the screws left in, this is preferable, but if hardware removal is necessary, then multiple guide pins or K-wires should be inserted to protect the malleolus.

The largest-sized prosthesis available that will fit adequately should always be used, but care should be taken not to encroach on the medial malleolus. All tibial components are designed as a press fit—they should be reasonably tight-fitting, but not at the expense of risking fracture. It is important to be flexible regarding the size of the components and to change the size during the procedure as needed. For the Agility prosthesis, cutting additional bone from the medial malleolus should be avoided when possible; no more than 25% of the malleolus should be removed. A common error leading to fracture of the medial malleolus is making an oblique (not vertical) cut of the medial malleolus, such that when the tibial component is inserted, the posterior margin of the component abuts the obliquely cut medial malleolus.

If fractured, the medial malleolus must be fixed using small cannulated screws or a tension band during the same procedure. The replacement is at tremendous risk for subsequent disaster unless the malleolar fracture is treated accurately. It is essential to make sure that there is no deformity of the foot causing subsequent stress of the malleolus, which would be the source of a delayed malleolar fracture. This pathogenic mechanism is more common with

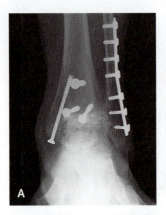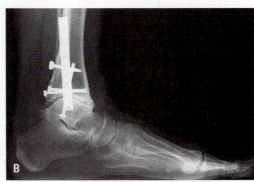

Figure 25-1 A and **B,** In ankle replacement surgery, nothing is more challenging than posterior screws blocking the path of the tibial component. I therefore prefer to stage this procedure, to ensure that the hardware is removed with no complications, and then proceed with the joint replacement at a subsequent date. (Because it is often fraught with unexpected problems, hardware removal can be a humbling experience.)

a valgus foot deformity, with stress on the deltoid and medial malleolus. It may be necessary to sacrifice some range of motion for the need for stability and to immobilize the ankle postoperatively. Screw fixation should be used as a preventive measure in patients with severe osteopenia, and a fracture that occurs intraoperatively should always be repaired with screws (Figures 25-2 and 25-3).

In general, I am not as concerned for the fractured fibula, because these fractures are easy to fix. Once again, if a fracture occurs, it must be surgically stabilized and the anatomy restored. Fractures may occur inadvertently with the cut on the tibia, regardless of the type of prosthesis (Figure 25-4). Severe valgus instability with lateral shift and tilt of the talus may result. Although all implant procedures carry a risk of fracture, the risk is higher with use of the Agility prosthesis, which emphasizes the enhanced stability of the tibial component by syndesmotic fusion. A point to remember is that the fibula lies far posteriorly relative to the tibia and is at risk for fracture when the tibial cut is made. Another source of fracture with the Agility prosthesis is overcompression of the fibula during syndesmotic screw fixation. This too presents a potentially serious problem: overcompressing the fibula can cause valgus failure of the prosthesis. Because a plate is routinely used on the fibula to enhance syndesmosis fusion, the complication of fibula fracture is not as important, but the alignment of the fibula must be maintained.

MANAGEMENT OF WOUND HEALING PROBLEMS

The soft tissues surrounding the ankle joint are not well vascularized and are relatively thin and tenuous. No deep subcutaneous tissue or muscle is present surrounding the ankle, and there is little to locally cover the components in the event of wound dehiscence. The blood supply to the extremity must be monitored with measurement of the ankle-brachial index in the elderly if pulses are questionable. Patients with rheumatoid arthritis, particularly those on immunosuppressant medications or prednisone, lose subcutaneous fat, and their thin fragile skin is more prone to wound complications.

Perhaps the most important preventive measure is to avoid any retraction and tension on the skin margins during surgery. The incision should be long enough to allow for optimal exposure without excessive retraction. I do not retract the skin edges until the periosteum is reflected, and I do not perform any simultaneous medial and lateral retraction at the same skin level. In fact, if visualization is inadequate with simple finger retraction, a slightly longer incision probably is necessary. Exactly what constitutes too much retraction of the skin to cause wound breakdown is not known, but blood flow must be maintained. The anterior tibial tendon should not be exposed at all, and if retinaculum over the anterior tibial tendon is not preserved with the incision, it must be repaired.

A minor dehiscence of the incision is not uncommon postoperatively. The very best treatment of this complication is use of simple topical antibiotic agents, dressing changes, and topical care of the skin (Figure 25-5). If a superficial dehiscence occurs, it is treated with daily changes of wet-to-dry saline dressings. I like to use a wound vacuum-assisted closure (VAC) device whenever there is drainage with breakdown of the incision. Deeper wound breakdowns are treated with silver sulfadiazine (Silvadene) dressings. If an eschar develops over an area of the incision, it is best left alone. The wound is not debrided and is kept as dry as possible (see Figure 25-5, *C-F*). The size of the eschar does not seem to be of any consequence, and over time and in the absence of infection, these dry eschars demonstrate quite a remarkable potential for healing. With more extensive wound dehiscence and exposure of the anterior tibial tendon, the use of a wound VAC device works well; in this setting, formal debridement of the wound and tendon is not necessary, because the VAC device may promote granulation and complete coverage of the tendon, without increased risk of infection. If deeper breakdown does occur, and the component is potentially exposed, coverage with a free flap usually is required to prevent infection and failure of the joint replacement. Removal of the prosthesis should not be necessary if coverage is adequate. I have no experience with acute infection of the joint; if this occurs, however, exchange of the polyethylene ("poly") insert plus irrigation as is performed for other joints would be prudent.

More advanced infection should be treated with removal of the components, insertion of an antibiotic spacer, and administration of intravenous antibiotics. Although antibiotic beads can be made to fill the gap, a solid cement spacer acts to keep the joint space open, distracted at the correct soft tissue tension, and more stable. I permit patients to walk on the ankle as soon as the skin incision has

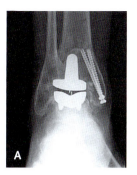
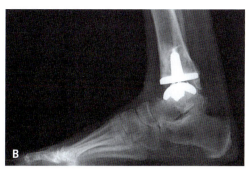
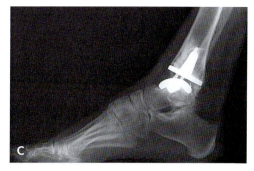

Figure 25-2 A-C, A greater degree of osteopenia was found intraoperatively than had been expected. Accordingly, two cannulated screws were inserted before the tibial osteotomy cut was made.

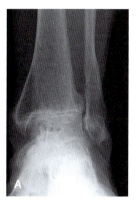
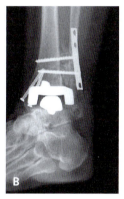
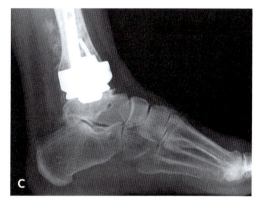

Figure 25-3 A-C, A fracture occurred intraoperatively when the tibial bone was being removed. The osteotomy had been performed, and as the bone was being removed, the malleolus cracked. Even though the fracture was not displaced, cannulated screws were inserted to maintain stability.

healed after treatment of infection, without concern for any further bone loss or subsidence. After 6 weeks, an aspiration of the joint is performed, and if results of aspirate culture are negative, 4 weeks later the prosthesis is reimplanted. Before the surgery, I take a biopsy specimen of the synovium, and if the cell count is greater than 6 white blood cells per high-power field, the joint is debrided and another antibiotic cement spacer is inserted until the joint is proved to be infection-free. It is curious how well some patients tolerate the cement spacer. One of my patients who underwent an ankle replacement 5 years earlier developed a deep infection shortly after surgery performed through a lateral incision. The prosthesis was removed, and an antibiotic-impregnated cement spacer was inserted. During his subsequent follow-up care, the patient commented that this was the best that his ankle had felt in years, and he did not desire any further treatment. At the 5-year follow-up evaluation, no evidence of subsidence or erosion of bone was found, and the patient retained approximately 15 degrees of motion (Figure 25-6).

CYST FORMATION

The early detection of loosening and subsidence is not easy, requiring a high index of suspicion, thorough history and examination, and various investigations to confirm the type of loosening. The typical history in patients with loosening of prosthetic components is one of pain on starting up with activities that is relieved shortly thereafter once "warm-up," has been achieved. If the patient

presents with pain and difficulty with ambulation, the decision to investigate the cause further, usually with computed tomography (CT) scan, may be more readily made. The situation is very different, however, if the patient presents with an asymptomatic cyst. These cysts can be massive and presumably arise in response to irritation from polyethylene wear debris, secondary to abnormal joint mechanics and typically worsening over time.

If the patient presents with an asymptomatic cyst on the plain radiograph, obtaining a CT scan is helpful, but the surgeon must be prepared to perform a revision if the size of the cyst is progressively enlarging (Figure 25-7). The CT findings are always far worse than expected, and as noted, these cysts can be quite massive.

"Expansile" osteolysis resulting from polyethylene wear debris tends to progress, with consequent destabilization of the implant, leading to loosening and, ultimately, periprosthetic fracture. So, despite the total lack of symptoms in some patients, I try to encourage them to understand the cause, with its implications for the need for a timely revision to prevent catastrophic mechanical failure and to preserve and supplement the remaining bone support. A real therapeutic dilemma arises if the patient is asymptomatic, with good range of motion, and plain radiographs and CT scans show an apparently stable prosthesis but large osteolytic cysts. It is hard to convince a patient to undergo a revision when the joint is entirely asymptomatic. Serial investigations and close follow-up examination may be acceptable to help the patient decide when a revision or bone grafting is needed.

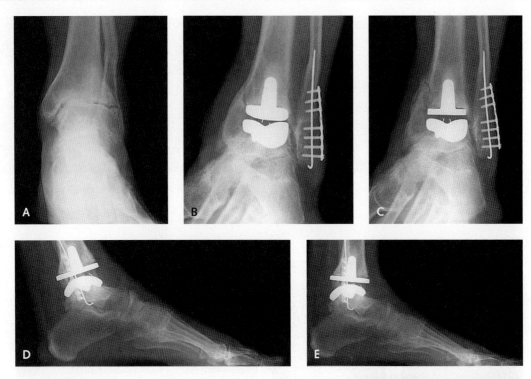

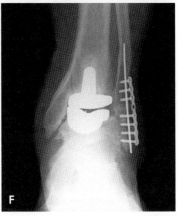

Figure 25-4 A-C, Fracture of the medial malleolus occurred 7 months after Mobility ankle replacement. The alignment of the foot was good, and no significant edge loading of the medial malleolus was apparent. Because the alignment was good and no displacement was present, immobilization without fixation constituted appropriate treatment. **D-F,** Good range of motion of the ankle was evident on a lateral radiograph obtained 2 years later without deformity.

These large asymptomatic cysts are worrisome. I do not know what the natural history is of these cysts, but it is reasonable to assume that they are progressive and will ultimately perforate the tibial or talar cortex, making revision more complicated. No studies quantifying the rate and exact likelihood of bone defect progression have been performed. Many prosthesis designs are difficult to evaluate radiologically, particularly on the talar component side, because here it is not possible to see if there is any structural loss of bone support underneath. For example, in the Salto, STAR, and Hintegra systems, the talar component covers the body of the talus, which can "hide" what is going on underneath it, thereby masking bone necrosis. Earlier signs such as periprosthetic radiolucent lines also should be looked for on serial follow-up radiographs. CT scans are very helpful to evaluate for cystic defects or loosening.

Once a decision for surgical management of the cysts has been made, it generally is necessary to revise the prosthesis, or at the very least, the "poly" liner. Generally, there is some minor abnormality with alignment causing the abnormal poly insert wear. The cysts often are far deeper than is apparent on plain radiographs, and a large curette is used to remove the lining of the cyst without perforating the bone. I pack the cyst with a mixture of cancellous allograft chips and an iliac crest aspirate concentrate. The cancellous graft is packed in firmly, particularly when the bone loss is at the margin of the tibial component (Figure 25-8). It probably is not enough to simply fill the cyst with bone graft. This approach ignores the underlying pathology and the cause of the problem. If an assumption of abnormal poly wear is, is it enough to just change the poly insert, or is a change in the prosthesis necessary? This is well illustrated in Figure 25-9 in a patient who underwent an ankle replacement 8 years previously and presented with asymptomatic cyst formation in the medial malleolus. Because the joint was asymptomatic, I made the error of assuming that it would be easier just to bone-graft the cyst, thereby preventing fracture of the malleolus. Despite an acceptable radiographic appearance at 1 year, cystic degeneration subsequently recurred, necessitating revision of the prosthesis and bone grafting.

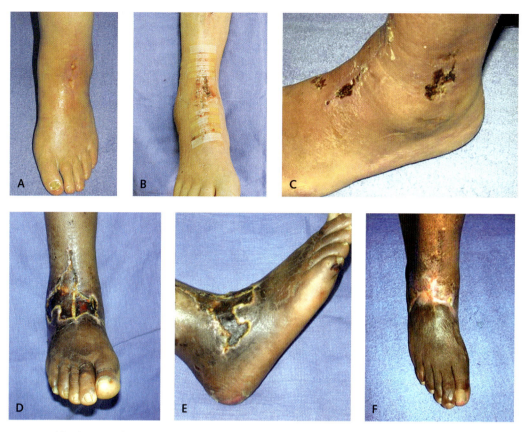

Figure 25-5 Wound healing complications are common after ankle replacement procedures. **A** and **B,** Minor dehiscence is not a concern. **C,** Eschars should be left intact, kept dry, and left to granulate in from below. **D-F,** Even a very large eschar will eventually fill in well without infection, in the absence of peripheral vascular disease. In the case shown, the patient had rheumatoid arthritis, probably with mild vasculitis, and it took 7 months for the eschar to heal. The ankle replacement was performed 4 months after a triple arthrodesis.

COMPONENT SUBSIDENCE, REVISION, AND CUSTOM REPLACEMENT

One particular problem with all of the available prostheses and implants is the potential for subsidence of either the talar or the tibial component. Talar component subsidence was more of a problem with the earlier models of the Agility prosthesis and was encountered in particular in patients who were not suitable candidates for the procedure because of poor bone quality, an increased body mass index, or a high activity level. An incorrect cut on the talar body also can increase the likelihood of subsidence. Although larger standard prostheses are available for all implant systems, their effectiveness depends on proportionate size of the ankle relative to the patient. One problem that arises in clinical practice is management of ankle problems in obese shorter patients with small ankles in keeping with overall smaller bony anatomy. Accordingly, I use a body mass index less than 35 as the cutoff criterion for a standard ankle replacement, and if the patient meets other criteria for replacement, then use of a custom prosthesis is considered with a long talar stem as the *primary* prosthesis.

With talar subsidence, for instance, the supportive talar body is crushed, and the component is pushed inferiorly into the talus. This was a particular problem with the older versions of the Agility prosthesis but has been most effectively addressed with the newer LP prosthesis, which covers the major portion of the surface of the talar dome. In fact, although several years have passed since this latter implant came into use at my institution, talar subsidence

has not been a problem. When subsidence occurs, regardless of the prosthesis, the previous supportive rim of cortical bone also becomes the source of impingement, limiting range of motion. Although the overhanging bone in the medial and lateral gutter can be debrided and decompressed, the structurally compromised base is vulnerable to further subsidence and eventually fracture of the remaining talus. This debridement can be performed as either an open or an arthroscopic procedure; in the long term, however, simply decompressing the impinging bone may not be mechanically sound. Although revision of the talar component, bone grafting, and use of a standard component may be possible, the same loads are present, and failure may recur. Performing arthroscopic or open debridement of the talar gutters has its proponents, but I do not think that this makes sense (Figure 25-10). If the cause of the problem is indeed heterotopic bone formation, then debridement is a reasonable procedure. If the bone has built up as a result of subsidence, however, in all likelihood the talar component has compacted the bone and will not further subside to allow the joint debridement to succeed. This consideration applies in particular with those implants for which coverage of the surface area of the talus is incomplete.

Depending on the pathology, the implants may be already loose, or they may still be well fixed. The latter scenario may present considerable technical difficulties—specifically, fractures and further bone problems may occur with attempts to pry the components loose. Removal of well-fixed components must be done meticulously, working at the interface with small, thin osteotomes to preserve as much bone as possible (Figure 25-11). Any overlying exostosis, debris, or granulation and scarred synovial tissue must be removed to aid visualization. If it is possible, I generally first remove the poly implant to give more working space. With respect to the Agility replacement system, removal of the older versions of the poly insert may be difficult, because it is bottom-loaded and will not slide out anteriorly until the edge rails are completely disengaged (see Figure 25-11). If scarring is significant and the joint cannot be distracted, the poly insert needs to be cut in segments with a reciprocating saw and removed piecemeal in large sections. Although destructive, this technique is the most efficient

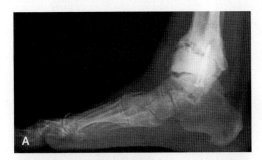

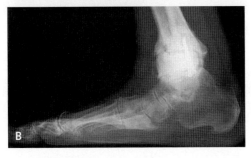

Figure 25-6 An ankle replacement performed in a 71-year-old man was complicated by a deep infection developing shortly after surgery. The prosthesis was removed, and an antibiotic-impregnated cement spacer was inserted. During subsequent follow-up care, the patient commented that this was the best that his ankle had felt in years, and he did not desire any further treatment. **A** and **B,** At 5 years, no subsidence or erosion of bone is evident, and the patient has retained approximately 15 degrees of motion.

way of disrupting the edge-locking section of the older Agility poly tibial component (Figure 25-12). The poly insert generally is easiest to remove once the talar component has been removed. With the additional available room under the tibial component, an osteotome can be inserted under the poly insert to lever it out. If the joint still seems too tight for removal of the poly insert, then a laminar spreader can be inserted under the medial or lateral column of the tibial component, gaining more room to lever it out.

An option for treating subsidence or revision is with a similar device, one of a larger size, or use of a custom-designed prosthesis. Of course, a custom prosthesis is not necessary for all of these revision cases even when severe subsidence is present. It is far simpler just to insert a larger Agility prosthesis component, regardless of the type of prosthesis used initially. This prosthesis is larger than other commonly used prostheses and may adequately "fill" any bone void. Revisions using standard primary components can still be successful for management of contained defects, which can be bone grafted, and smaller central segmental defects can be supported with structural graft. As an alternative to structural or cancellous bone graft, bone cement can sometimes be used, adding to early stability—for example, at the keel section of the tibial component to restrict rotational and translational motion.

I do not have any experience using cement to stabilize subsidence of the tibial component. This is a plausible alternative, particularly in the patient who has osteopenia, is frail, and requires more immediate mobility and ambulation. However, there is always the risk for cement failure with further bone resorption, setting the stage for an even more difficult reconstruction. Another alternative is to remove any necrotic or avascular talus and then seat the revised implant directly on the posterior facet of the calcaneus, while simultaneously performing a subtalar arthrodesis (Figure 25-13).

The most useful indication for a custom prosthesis is after a failed ankle replacement, particularly in the setting of mechanical failure resulting from severe osteolysis, loosening, and subsidence. Loss of bone in the talus can make the procedure with either primary or revision surgery too difficult with a standard implant, because the amount of supportive bone is insufficient, making it difficult to achieve stability and fixation with a standard component. This restriction applies in patients with osteopenia, avascular necrosis, or loss of bone in the talus. A long-stem custom implant would transfer the load to the calcaneus, providing stability while bone graft incorporation and implant interface bony ingrowth occur (Figure 25-14). As noted, it typically is the talar component

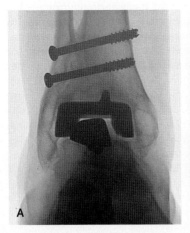

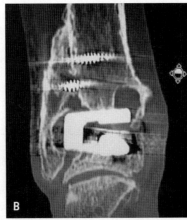

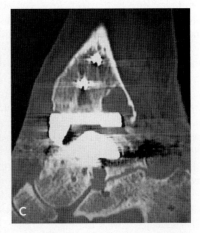

Figure 25-7 A, The patient underwent ankle replacement 8 years earlier and was entirely asymptomatic. **B** and **C,** The appearance of the cysts on a computed tomography scan was far worse than that on the plain radiograph.

that subsides, and in many cases, the well-fixed tibial implant from the original primary arthroplasty may be retained while the talar side is revised and the polyethylene insert is exchanged.

The tibial component also may subside, with valgus or anterior deformation. In the case illustrated in Figure 25-15, the patient underwent the ankle replacement 5 years previously, when the joint became symptomatic. Radiographs showed an obvious nonunion of the syndesmosis and lateral subsidence of the tibial component with valgus deformity. Revision was accomplished using a larger prosthesis, with cancellous bone grafting behind the prosthesis. The graft was mixed with an iliac crest aspirate, and bone morphogenic protein was applied to the anterior surface of the tibia. Only limited weight bearing was permitted for 2 months after cancellous impaction grafting. Improved alignment of the components was noted 2 years after revision. Revision of a tibial component that has subsided is not easy, because it is essential to maintain the position of the tibial component while back-filling with bone graft. The other option is to use a larger implant, which has more of a press fit, and then use bone graft behind the prosthesis. A useful technique is to place laminar spreaders under the tibial component to compress the implant and then confirm position with fluoroscopy (Figure 25-16).

The custom stem of the talar and tibial components can be fabricated to the required angle, diameter, and length relative to the calcaneus. The body section also can be enhanced to the desired thickness and inclination to act as augmentation for the anticipated bone loss and any defects of the talus and the subtalar joint. In addition to the flat supportive shelf at the implant–bone interface, the talar stem achieves stable fixation by engaging not only the remaining body of the talus but also the inferior talar cortex, the superior calcaneal cortex, and the supportive cancellous bone in the calcaneus. A stemmed tibial implant can provide stability by engaging the distal diaphyseal and metaphyseal bone. The stems and body sections have a porous coat to facilitate bony ingrowth (Figures 25-17 and 25-18). It is not always necessary to use a custom stem for failure of a stemmed component. Once the stemmed component has been loosened, it is possible to make an osteotomy of the front of the tibia, and remove the prosthesis. The stem cut can be made under fluoroscopic imaging. Figure 25-19 illustrates management of a failed Buechel-Pappas ankle joint replacement. In this case, laminar spreaders were used to aid in distraction of the joint, and the position of the tibial osteotomy was confirmed fluoroscopically. This was a good option for revision using the Agility prosthesis, which permitted a press fit of the tibial component. Bone graft was then impacted above the tibial component, and the slot from the stem was closed with the bone wedge removed during the osteotomy.

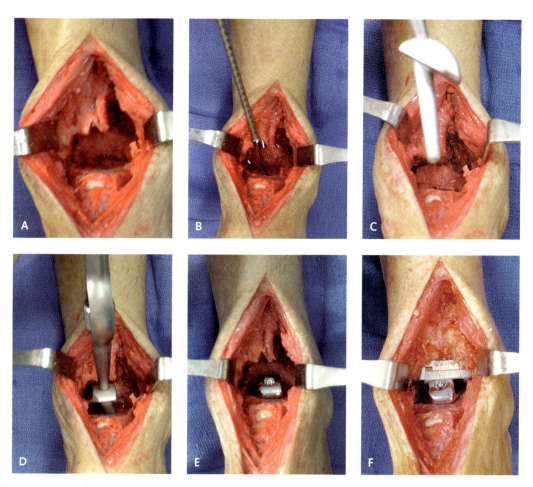

Figure 25-8 A, Massive cyst formation 7 years after an Agility ankle replacement. **B** and **C,** After removal of the implants, a drill is inserted over a guide pin to prepare the tapered cannula for the long stem of the talar component. **D,** The talar component is attached to a custom inserter tool. **E,** The talar component is then compacted with a press fit into the calcaneus. **F,** Once the tibial component has been inserted, cancellous bone graft fills in behind the prosthesis and is compacted firmly.

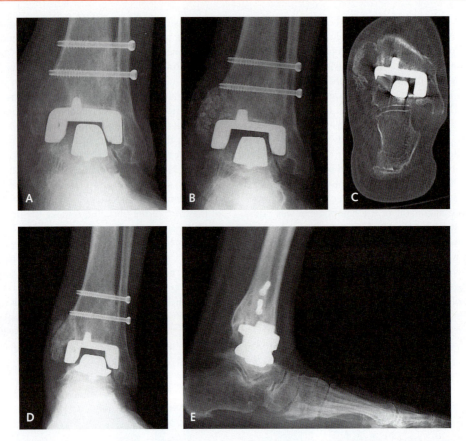

Figure 25-9 A, The patient underwent an ankle replacement 8 years earlier and presented with asymptomatic cyst formation in the medial malleolus. Initial treatment of simply bone grafting the cyst was inadequate. **B,** Radiographic appearance at 1 year. **C,** Subsequent computed tomography scan revealed recurrence of cystic degeneration. **D** and **E,** Treatment was with revision of the prosthesis and bone grafting.

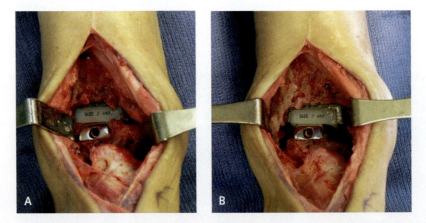

Figure 25-10 A and **B,** The patient developed pain from impingement in the gutters 5 years after the primary procedure and was treated with open arthrotomy and gutter debridement. I am not convinced that this is the correct procedure, unless true heterotopic bone formation exists and no subsidence has occurred. If subsidence of the talar component is present, removing more bone from the margins of the talus may result in additional subsidence.

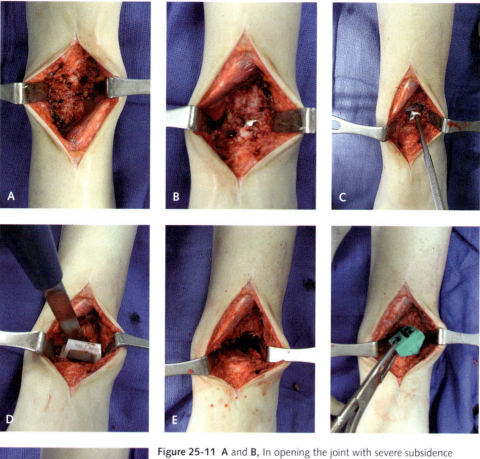

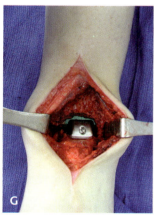

Figure 25-11 A and **B,** In opening the joint with severe subsidence and bone overgrowth, visualization of the prosthesis is difficult, and it is essential to proceed slowly. **C-E,** The talar component should first be removed **(C),** followed by the poly insert **(D)** and then the tibial component **(E).** It is difficult to insert the older versions of the polyethylene component, because they were bottom-loaded and will not slide out anteriorly until the edge rails are completely disengaged. **F** and **G,** If the tibial component is stable and does not require removal, then in order to reinsert the poly, a half-column poly liner is used.

Access to the joint should be through the previous longitudinal midline incision. If an alternative incision has been used that is not anatomically correct, care must be taken to decide on the correct course of the revision incision. If a talonavicular or subtalar arthrodesis is to be performed simultaneously, then the incisions are planned accordingly, to allow an adequate skin bridge on the lateral foot. Typically, the anterior central incision is used, and then as wide a skin bridge as possible is planned to include exposure of the subtalar joint. A short incision over the sinus tarsi is sufficient to expose the subtalar joint. Careful dissection is needed dorsally to minimize tissue trauma as this incision is prone to wound healing complications. It can be quite difficult to separate the deep neurovascular bundle owing to fibrosis and scarring, and the patient must be warned about the possibility of postoperative

dorsal foot numbness if the deep or superficial peroneal nerve cannot be preserved.

With all implant systems, it should be possible to change the size of the tibial component relative to the talus as necessary. This capability is useful if there has been increased bone loss from a loose tibial component and the talus demonstrates significant wear. If the tibial component is stable and well positioned, it should not be revised. The newer Agility LP talar component, however, has a different radius of curvature, so a mismatch poly implant will be required if an older version of the tibial component is retained to articulate with the LP talar component. The same dilemma arises with reinsertion of the poly implant, which is bottom-loading, so that it has to be inserted before the talar component. One option here is to use a half-column locking poly liner, which can be slid

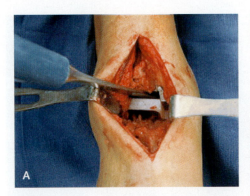
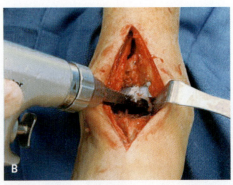

Figure 25-12 A and **B,** The older version of the Agility poly component does not disengage anteriorly and has to be slid out inferiorly. This maneuver is not easy to accomplish, and the poly insert may be cut with a saw into pieces.

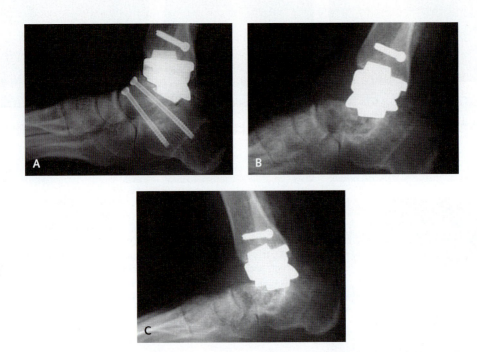

Figure 25-13 Failure in this case was due to incorrect insertion of the prosthesis and inadequate correction of the flatfoot deformity. **A,** The talar component subsided into the subtalar joint, which was then fused, but this did not stop progressive subsidence. The talar component was revised by creating a planar surface directly on the subtalar joint. **B** and **C,** Eight years later, excellent range of motion of the ankle was retained.

under the tibial component without as much joint distraction for clearance. The side columns of the poly liner are not full length, making it easier to insert. If the tibial component is unstable, loose, or malpositioned, a preferable approach is to revise the whole tibial component to the LP tibia, and the front-loading type of poly liner can be used, which is much easier to insert.

For the stemmed custom talar prosthesis, a formal subtalar arthrodesis is performed, and I use a small (2-cm) separate lateral incision over the inferior aspect of the sinus tarsi to prepare the joint surfaces. Debridement of the cartilage is performed with a curved osteotome, but the remaining talar and calcaneal subchondral bone must be preserved and is perforated with a 2-mm drill.

Once the arthroplasty components are inserted, then screws are inserted to stabilize the subtalar joint from the neck of the talus, just distal to the talar component, aiming inferiorly into the calcaneus. I use two or three 3.5-mm screws to supplement the fixation by the component stem. I do not like the idea of inserting the screw from "bottom to top." This method of placement is not precise, and repeated insertion of guide pins or drilling may compromise the talus further. It is far safer and more accurate to insert from the dorsal surface of the talus, making sure that the screw head is not impinged against the anterior aspect of the talar component.

The intraoperative sizing and tunnel preparation are done using a custom drill guide and trial component. The drill guide

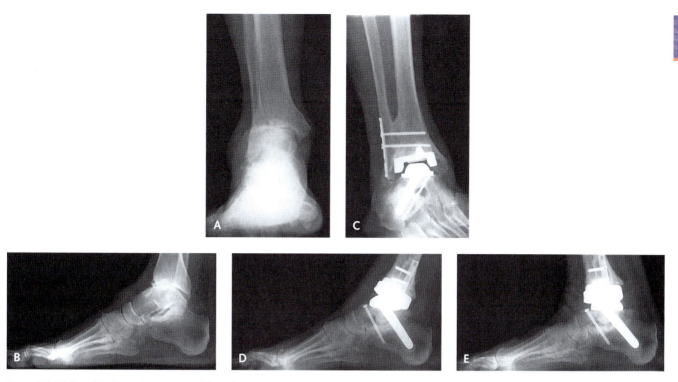

Figure 25-14 A and **B,** Avascular necrosis of the talus in a 51-year-old patient. **C-E,** For the revision procedure, a custom long-stem talar component was used in conjunction with a subtalar arthrodesis.

must be inserted into the talus and the calcaneus at the correct angle, because this is preset in the long-stem talar component. The talar component should be parallel with the plane of the floor or perpendicular to the long axis of the tibia. Because the trial talar component has a small cannulated hole to accommodate the guide pin, the pin must be inserted at the correct angle. It is easiest to align the trial talus on the surface of the base of the remaining talus, but this is not always possible, because erosion of the remaining talar body may have occurred. If the base plate of the trial talar component cannot be oriented flat with respect to the talus, the guide must still be inserted so as to position the talar component parallel with the floor; the anterior surface under the component is then filled with cancellous graft. The trial talus prosthesis is positioned on the resected talar surface exactly as the final implant is to be oriented, including the built-in 20 degrees of external rotation. It is best to confirm the correct position of the guide pin passing through the trial talar component by inserting it all the way through the skin out the bottom of the calcaneus, in order to visualize the direction and ensure that it is going to be correctly angled into the calcaneus. If the guide pin appears too lateral, then the talar component can be slightly internally rotated to ensure that the stem is completely in the calcaneus (Figure 25-20).

The talar trial is removed while the wire is left in situ. A graduated set of cannulated drills is used to sequentially enlarge the tunnel to the implant stem diameter, which is tapered. The custom trial component is then inserted to check if adequate diameter and length have been achieved. The stem of the actual component is slightly thicker because of its porous coating. The base of the talar component should be parallel with the floor. Despite careful preoperative planning incorporating appropriately "built-in" wedge augmentations, intraoperative mismatch can still exist after

debridement. Such mismatch can create a problem if a large defect is present anteriorly between the base of the talar component and the calcaneus. Rather than leaving a defect, this should be filled with bone graft (Figures 25-21 to 25-23).

After any necessary bone grafting, I have found it easiest to insert the stemmed talar component first, with the ankle in maximal plantar flexion. This is followed by placement of the tibial component if it is to be revised. The poly insert is installed last unless it is a bottom-loading poly, in which case the tibial component with the poly has to be inserted first and then the foot distracted as much as possible to permit insertion of the talar component. Additional bone graft can still be packed in between the bone–implant interface and compressed with a bone tamp.

THE SYNDESMOSIS FAILURE

Syndesmosis failure is of course relevant only with the Agility prosthesis, for which a successful syndesmosis fusion is an important consideration in stability of the tibial component and overall good outcome. Certainly, the patient for whom selection of the Agility prosthesis is easiest is one who already has a synostosis of the syndesmosis. Fusion of the syndesmosis correlates with stability of the tibial component and has the greatest influence on the outcome of the replacement. Conversely, nonunion or delayed union results in a statistically significant increase in tibial subsidence rates.

Correct technique is essential in performing the primary syndesmosis arthrodesis. For application of the fixation through the plate, a visible compression of the plate into the tibial component occurs, even though fully threaded screws are used. The significant improvement in results at my institution since the application of the plate probably has to do with distribution of the stress over the

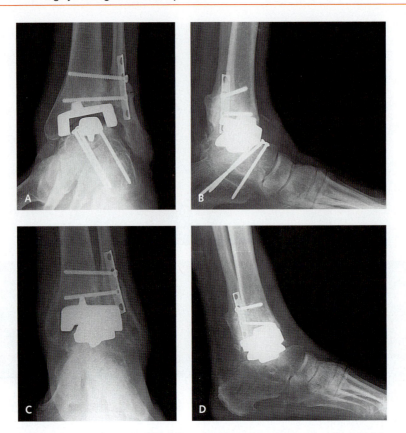

Figure 25-15 The patient underwent ankle replacement 5 years previously, when the joint became symptomatic. **A** and **B,** Obvious nonunion of the syndesmosis and lateral subsidence of the tibial component with valgus deformity. **C** and **D,** Revision was accomplished using a larger prosthesis, with cancellous bone grafting behind the prosthesis. The graft was mixed with an iliac crest aspirate, and bone morphogenic protein was applied to the anterior surface of the tibia.

distal fibula and with compressing the fibula into the lateral margin of the tibia and tibial component. Use of a laminar spreader is helpful in exposing the fibula for preparation but can easily overdistract the syndesmosis, hindering correct fit of the tibial component. The tibial component should not push the fibula away. If this sign of incorrect fit is recognized, either more bone must be cut from the fibula or a smaller-sized tibial component must be inserted. A solid fusion mass between the distal tibia and fibula should be radiographically evident by the fourth postoperative month. Patients with persistent ankle pain and swelling but inadequate radiographic evidence of union by this time require surgery. I have not found that an external bone stimulator is very helpful if an established nonunion is present. Persistence of the nonunion beyond 6 to 9 months necessitates a revision of the arthrodesis with placement of supplemental cancellous bone graft. If a nonunion develops, I recommend revision of the arthrodesis with cancellous bone graft supplemented with any variety of bone stimulants. The procedure is relatively simple, involving exposure of the syndesmosis with roughening of the cortical bone, followed by insertion of cancellous allograft or autograft. When the syndesmosis fails to fuse, a revision procedure with bone graft and more rigid fixation is advisable, using a semitubular plate on the fibula combined with stabilization of the syndesmosis with two or three fully threaded cancellous

screws gaining purchase on four cortices. Occasionally, a nonunion may result with erosive changes in the syndesmosis, avascular sclerotic changes of the lateral tibia, and valgus subsidence of the tibial component. This is the most difficult scenario to manage and must be revised promptly (Figure 25-24).

ARTHRODESIS AFTER PROSTHESIS FAILURE

Conversion to arthrodesis in the setting of significant bone loss is complicated and carries a high rate of nonunion, in addition to the associated problems of stiffness and progressive degeneration of the adjacent joints of the hindfoot and transverse tarsal joints. The inherent problem with salvage is the loss of structural bone support resulting from osteolysis or subsidence, such that an in situ arthrodesis invariably is not possible. A large structural bone block arthrodesis generally is needed and frequently has to include both the ankle and subtalar joints to ensure rigid fixation and solid fusion (Figures 25-25 to 25-27). This tibiotalocalcaneal arthrodesis (or if the bone loss is more severe, a tibiocalcaneal arthrodesis) is obviously not as functional or physiologic as a mobile ankle joint. Nevertheless, bone block arthrodesis must remain an option in cases with gross massive bone loss, severe osteopenia, compromised skin, recent infection, or unreconstructable deformity. For the

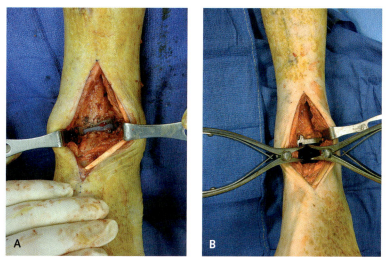

Figure 25-16 A and **B,** Laminar spreaders are useful to aid in alignment and compression of the tibial component against the bone graft.

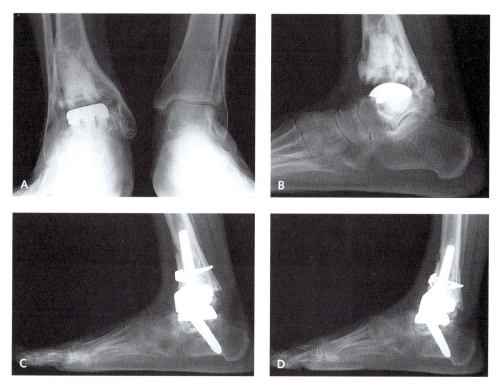

Figure 25-17 A and **B,** Ankle replacement had been performed 25 years earlier using cement, with consequent gross bone loss. **C** and **D,** Revision was accomplished using a custom prosthesis with a long-stem tibia and talus component. To allow insertion of the long-stem tibial component, an osteotomy of the anterior tibial cortex is required.

symptomatic patient, before any decision to proceed with primary or revision replacement, various factors must be taken into consideration. Although today's surgeons may have the technical ability and the wherewithal to perform a joint replacement, the question to ask first is whether the patient would be better off with an arthrodesis. In some patients with poor bone quality, for example, perhaps an arthrodesis may be a better choice. Thus, it is important to avoid introducing personal bias into the surgical decision-making

process. Surgeons have a tendency to favor their preferred procedure without adequate patient evaluation and counseling. This is a particularly important consideration with these patients, who have potentially already undergone devastating prosthesis failure, only to deal with another prolonged surgical recovery. A complex bone block tibiotalocalcaneal or tibiocalcaneal arthrodesis may not be for every surgeon to attempt, and this applies as well to use of the custom ankle prosthesis (see Figures 25-25 and 25-26).

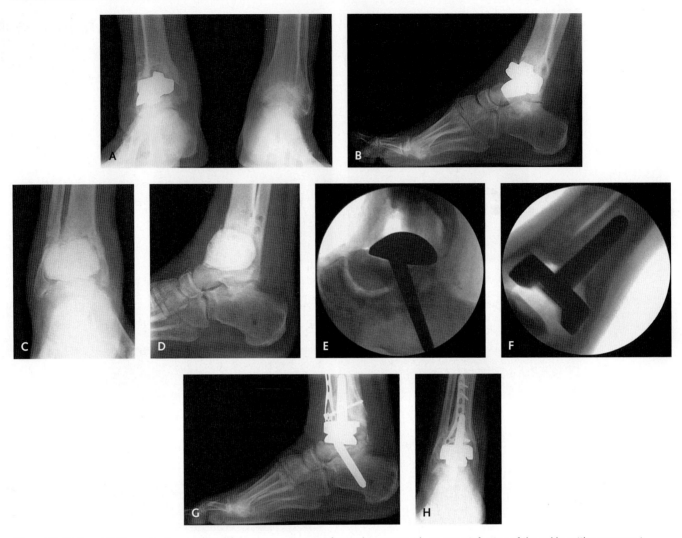

Figure 25-18 A and **B,** The patient was referred for treatment 2 years after replacement with an acute infection of the ankle, with consequent implant dislocation. **C** and **D,** The prosthesis was removed, and an antibiotic impregnated cement spacer was used and then repeated at 4 weeks. **E** and **F,** After 6 weeks of intravenous antibiotic treatment, followed by a 1-month "holiday," a long-stem custom tibia and talus replacement procedure was performed. **G** and **H,** Note the use of the tibial osteotomy followed by application of a plate over the tibia.

I use a large structural allograft to correct the deformity. An anterior incision is used, and the entire joint is exposed following removal of the prosthesis (see Figure 25-27). The defect can be quite massive and will require the insertion of an entire femoral head. I use a technique that was described to me by Bryan den Hartog, using a 34-mm acetabular reamer in the defect. The distal tibia is prepared with the reamer that fits in the ankle defect and is then turned around to ground down the talus if any is still present, to create a contoured defect. A reciprocal female reamer is then used to contour the femoral head graft. The graft is firmly held in a clamp (the Allogrip—DePuy Orthopaedics, Inc., Warsaw, Indiana), and the reamer is used to contour the head to fit the round shape of the ankle defect. The femoral head graft is then perforated with a 2-mm drill and then infused with a concentrate of an iliac crest marrow aspirate. I generally use an intramedullary rod to fuse the joint; however, this is not always necessary, and if the ankle alone is involved, a similar technique can be used, sparing the subtalar joint (see Figure 25-27).

In certain circumstances, an ankle replacement may not be indicated because of bone quality or patient age and activity level,

but the alternative of an ankle arthrodesis is not ideal because of other factors, such as the need for flexibility. Figure 25-28 demonstrates such a case. The patient, who worked as a carpenter, sustained a severe ankle injury, with subsequent development of avascular necrosis of the talus and fixed deformity. The foot was stuck in varus, and there was no motion in the ankle at all. He was unable to work, not only because of pain but also because of the limited ankle motion. Although a pan-talar arthrodesis was a consideration, this repair was considered to be too disabling for his occupation, and a total talus replacement procedure was performed. This was a staged procedure, and the varus deformity was corrected simultaneously with the collapse, distracting the ankle out to length, and then when the distractor was removed, the talar implant was inserted. The prosthesis was designed with an arthrodesis of the subtalar joint, and screw holes were predrilled in the implant to facilitate the subtalar arthrodesis.

Not all visible ankle replacement failures require revision. Despite the appearance of the radiograph in Figure 25-29, the patient was asymptomatic. She was 49 years of age when the replacement was performed, and at the time the ankle had

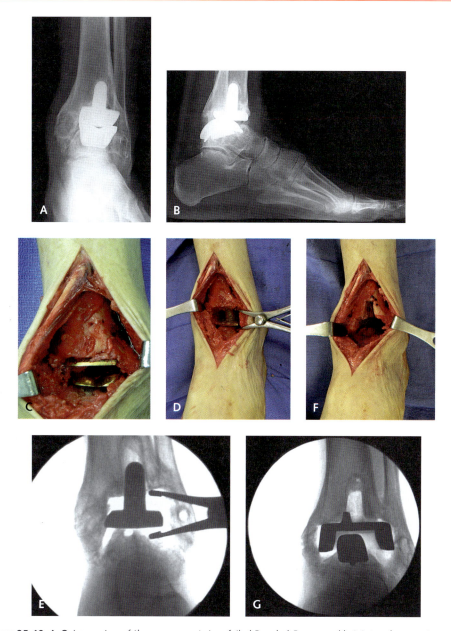

Figure 25-19 A-C, Loosening of the components in a failed Buechel-Pappas ankle joint replacement. **D** and **E,** Note the use of the laminar spreaders to aid in distraction of the joint and the fluoroscopic confirmation of the position of the tibial osteotomy. **F** and **G,** The prosthesis was removed and the Agility prosthesis inserted, which permitted a press fit of the tibial component, and the slot from the stem was closed with the bone wedge removed during the osteotomy.

approximately 35 degrees of motion. Note the progressive heterotopic bone formation around the ankle both anteriorly and posteriorly. When she presented for the most recent follow-up evaluation, 7 years after the replacement, there was no motion in the ankle, and she was minimally symptomatic. This patient probably would not improve much with revision surgery. A point worthy of emphasis is that a very stiff ankle stays stiff after surgery; some motion will be gained but not of sufficient degree to warrant a revision procedure in a patient who is not that symptomatic to begin with.

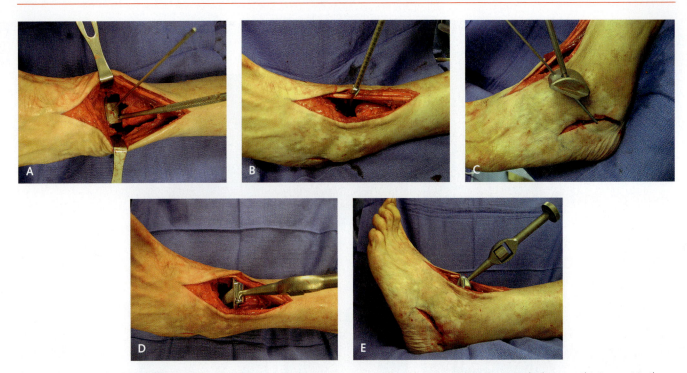

Figure 25-20 A and **B,** The drill guide is inserted into the talus trial component and the calcaneus at the correct angle, because this is preset in the long-stem talar component. **C-E,** The trial talus component is positioned on the resected talar surface exactly as the final implant is to be oriented, including the built-in 20 degrees of external rotation.

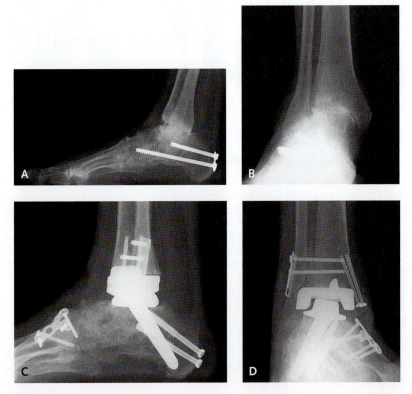

Figure 25-21 A and **B,** The patient presented at 53 years of age with ankle arthritis and avascular necrosis of the talus after a failed hindfoot procedure for hindfoot valgus deformity. **C** and **D,** Ankle replacement with a custom long-stem talar component was performed in conjunction with a medial translational osteotomy of the calcaneus. The osteotomy was performed first, and guide pins were inserted to maintain the position of the calcaneus but out of the way of the stem of the talar component. Once the talar component was in place, the guide pins were exchanged for screws.

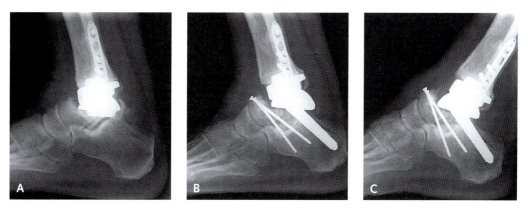

Figure 25-22 **A,** The patient was referred for treatment of severe subsidence after a failed agility prosthesis. The reconstruction was converted to a long-stem talar component replacement. **B** and **C,** Radiographic appearance on flexion and extension views 3 years after revision.

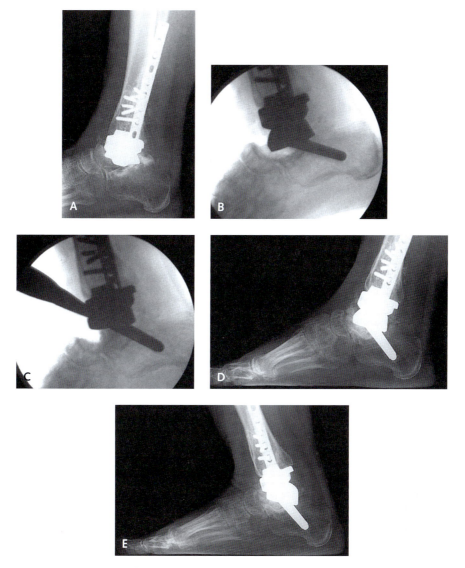

Figure 25-23 **A,** Very severe collapse and subsidence in the ankle of a 54-year-old patient. **B** and **C,** The custom replacement had to be designed to be supported completely by the calcaneus, with back-fill of the anterior aspect of the subtalar joint with cancellous bone graft. **D** and **E,** Lateral flexion and extension radiographs at 3 years after revision.

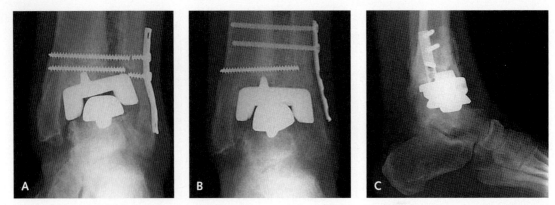

Figure 25-24 A, A nonunion of the syndesmosis featuring erosive changes in the syndesmosis, avascular sclerotic changes in the lateral tibia, and valgus subsidence of the tibial component. The most important aspect of this revision is to keep the tibial component aligned perpendicular to the axis of the tibia; the syndesmosis is back-filled with cancellous bone grafting. **B** and **C,** Radiographic appearance at 6 years after revision.

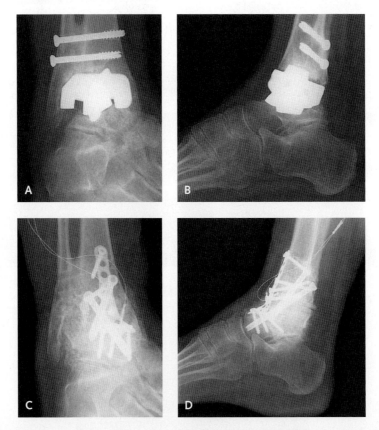

Figure 25-25 A and **B,** Although the overall alignment of this prosthesis is reasonable, the patient experienced chronic pain and had little motion in the joint. **C** and **D,** A decision was made to convert this to an arthrodesis, performed through an anterior incision, and structural bone grafting. Anterior plate fixation was used to control the sagittal plane instability inherent in this type of arthrodesis.

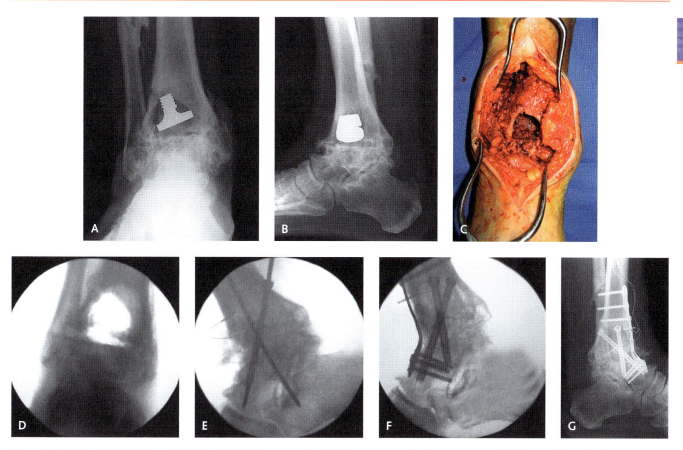

Figure 25-26 A and **B,** A Smith prosthesis implanted 25 years previously. There was not subtalar joint pain, and inclusion of the subtalar joint in the arthrodesis was not considered to be necessary. **C** and **D,** Note the significant defect in the ankle following removal of the prosthesis. **E,** After insertion of the femoral head allograft, crossed guide pins were inserted, followed by cannulated screws. **F** and **G,** These screws are not sufficient to control rotation and motion across the joint, and an anterior plate was used to control sagittal plane movement successfully.

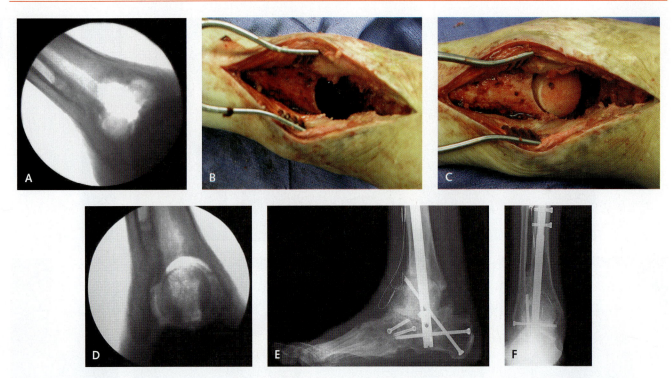

Figure 25-27 A and **B,** An anterior incision was used to expose the joint after failure. The defect in the joint is filled with a structural graft, but the size and shape of the graft are difficult to mold to the ankle. A 34-mm acetabular reamer is inserted into the defect in the ankle to grind down any remaining talus, resulting in a more precisely shaped and contoured defect. A reciprocal female reamer is then used to contour the femoral head graft. **C** and **D,** The femoral head graft is then perforated with a 2-mm drill and infused with a concentrate of an iliac crest marrow aspirate. **E** and **F,** An intramedullary rod (Biomet, Parsipanny, New Jersey) was used to fuse the joint.

25

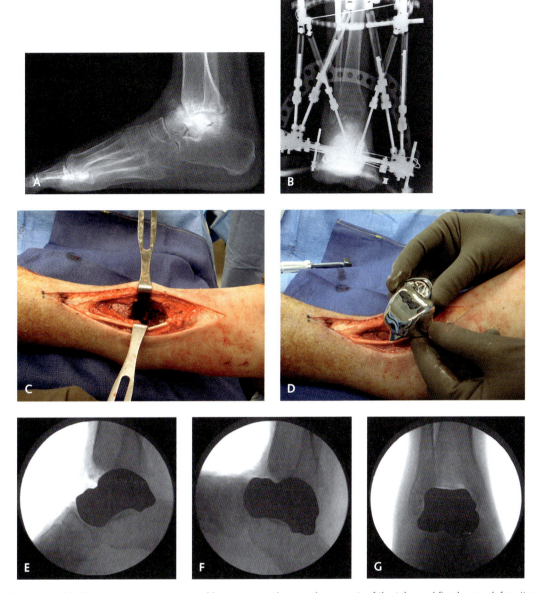

Figure 25-28 A and **B,** The patient was a 41-year-old carpenter with avascular necrosis of the talus and fixed varus deformity of the hindfoot. **C,** The varus deformity was corrected simultaneously with the collapse of the ankle, distracting the ankle out to length using a Taylor spatial frame. **D** and **E,** When the distractor was removed, the total talar implant was inserted. **F** and **G,** The intraoperative fluoroscopic images with flexion and extension of the ankle.

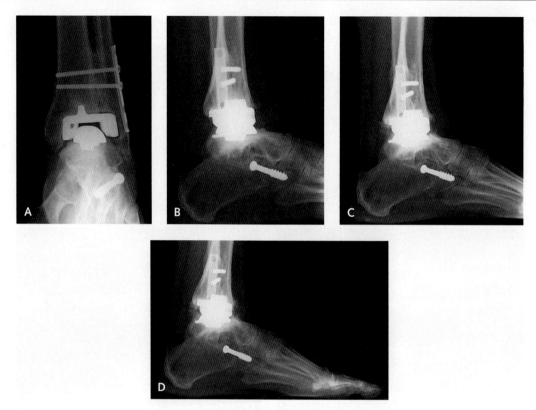

Figure 25-29 Postoperative anteroposterior and lateral radiographs after revision ankle replacement surgery: **A** and **B,** at 5 years after replacement; **C,** at 8 years; and **D,** at 11 years. Significant heterotopic bone formation around the ankle was associated with no range of motion; pain was minimal, however, so no further treatment was recommended.

CHAPTER 26

Osteotomy of the Tibia and Fibula

INDICATIONS

Indications for the supramalleolar osteotomy are numerous and include correction of deformity, joint preservation, and as a staged procedure that leads up to other operations, including total ankle replacement. Osteotomy is performed for correction of a malunion of a distal tibia fracture, with or without ankle joint arthritis, to redistribute or beneficially alter the contact pressures on the degenerated cartilage with mechanical realignment. Osteotomy can be used for preservation of limb alignment as a prelude to a total ankle replacement. One of the prerequisites for a successful total ankle replacement is a balanced mechanical axis of the foot with respect to the lower leg, and a supramalleolar osteotomy works well as a staged procedure for the appropriate patient (Figure 26-1).

The goal of osteotomy in the treatment of ankle arthritis is to shift the loads and redistribute stresses to a part of the ankle joint that is not involved in the degenerative process. The redirection of forces around the tibiotalar joint can be effected from either above or below the ankle with osteotomy of the tibia or the calcaneus, respectively. If either subtalar or supramalleolar deformity is present, the increased stresses on the tibiotalar joint may increase the likelihood of failure. The same concepts of realignment of the tibia apply to malunion after ankle arthrodesis. With the ankle joint fused in equinus, a leg length discrepancy is present because the involved leg is lengthened. This disparity leads to a genu recurvatum thrust on the knee joint, an uneven gait pattern, and increased stress concentration across the midfoot. With the ankle fused in dorsiflexion, repetitive calcaneal impact and stress concentration on the heel pad during the heel strike phase lead to chronic heel pain and gait impairment.

Varus malunion of the ankle fusion causes the patient to walk on the lateral aspect of the foot. This inverted position of the subtalar joint increases the rigidity of the transverse tarsal joints, with substantial increase in stress concentration and subsequent degenerative changes and pain. Additionally, stress is increased under the fifth metatarsal head or base, and development of painful calluses or stress fractures is not uncommon. Valgus malunion of an ankle arthrodesis generates increased stresses along the medial aspect of knee and hindfoot joints. In such a valgus position, the foot

becomes more flexible, resulting in flatfoot posture. For all of these deformities, a revision of the ankle arthrodesis malunion is required but not at the level of the ankle itself. On the basis of the mechanical axis, a supramalleolar osteotomy is recommended.

PREOPERATIVE PLANNING

The opening wedge osteotomy has the advantage of avoiding leg shortening, but delayed union or nonunion may result. Although the leg length change may not seem significant if only 1 cm of shortening is performed with the wedge resection osteotomy, such change does become significant if an opening wedge osteotomy is performed with a 1-cm graft, when the height differential is almost 2 cm once the graft has healed. With any skin-related problems (previous incisions with scar formation or previous infection) or the potential for vascular compromise, a closing wedge procedure must be performed. The closing wedge osteotomy has a major disadvantage of limb shortening but generally is easier than the opening wedge procedure, particularly if both the fibula and the tibia are included.

Use of wedge modifications allows correction of biplanar deformities. For example, a recurvatum-varus deformity can be corrected either with a posterolaterally based closing wedge osteotomy or with an anteromedially based opening wedge osteotomy. The size of the wedge is determined by drawing the desired correction angle on the preoperative radiographs, measuring the wedge size on a template, and taking magnification into account.

Measuring the center of rotation of angulation (CORA) of the deformity is important. The CORA is located at the intersection of two lines representing the mechanical axes of the proximal and distal segments of the deformity. A closing or opening wedge osteotomy at the level of the CORA leads to complete realignment of the foot and ankle. If the osteotomy is made proximal or distal to the CORA, the center of the ankle translates relative to the mechanical axis of the tibia and creates an unnecessary shift of loads and a clinically obvious zigzag deformity (Figure 26-2).

The osteotomy line should be translated and angulated so that a secondary translational deformity is not created when the osteotomy is intentionally made at a different level from that of the CORA

Figure 26-1 The patient was a 57-year-old woman with good but painful ankle motion who did not want an ankle arthrodesis performed. She already had shortening of the ipsilateral tibia. **A** and **B,** Clinical and radiographic appearance of the ankle. **C** and **D,** Because of the shortening of the limb, an opening wedge tibial osteotomy with structural allograft was performed. Note the use of a laminar spreader under fluoroscopic control to position the plafond perpendicular to the tibia.

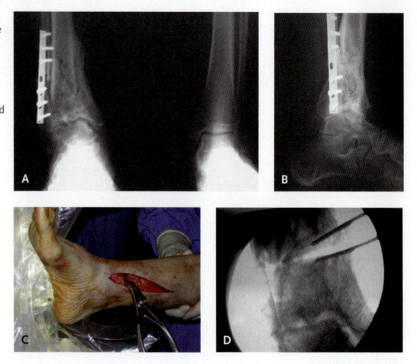

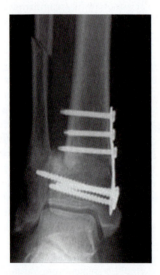

Figure 26-2 The radiograph demonstrates incorrect correction of a closing wedge lateral supramalleolar osteotomy. The ankle joint is correctly aligned with respect to the floor, but the center of the talus has been translated laterally relative to the axis of the tibia.

Deformities in the coronal plane are well compensated by subtalar joint motion, and deformities in the sagittal plane are well compensated by ankle joint motion. For example, a varus deformity of the tibia is compensated by eversion of the subtalar joint. The ability of the hindfoot to compensate for a distal tibial deformity depends on whether it is in varus or in valgus. Because the hindfoot is able to invert far more than to evert, it can compensate for a valgus deformity far better, and the foot may still be plantigrade despite tibial deformity. This may not, however, be the case with a varus deformity, because the capacity of the hindfoot to evert is more limited.

SURGICAL TECHNIQUE

Correction of Varus Deformity

For the correction of a varus deformity, I use either a medial opening wedge osteotomy or a lateral closing wedge osteotomy. For the medial opening wedge osteotomy, I use an anteromedial and a small lateral incision (for the fibular osteotomy). Which cut is made first is a matter of preference, but leaving the fibula intact provides some stability while the tibial cut is completed. When the deformity is minimal, then a greenstick cut of the tibia is made, in the hope that a fibular osteotomy may not need to be performed. This greenstick cut markedly increases the stability of the osteotomy, and the tibia can be opened with a laminar spreader to the desired amount. The advantage of this sequence is that the tibia does not move around after the cut is made, and movement may compromise stability. Another alternative is to apply a three-hole plate to the lateral aspect of the distal tibia at the level where the osteotomy exits. With this technique, the osteotomy cut does not open, and the correct tension on the osteotomy can be applied until the ankle is plantigrade. The plate is applied just before the osteotomy cut exits the lateral tibial cortex.

(Figure 26-3), as with correction of an equinus malunion of an ankle arthrodesis. In this deformity, the position of the forefoot is fixed relative to the axis of the tibia. The simplest method of correction is to remove an anteriorly based wedge from the distal tibia and then close the osteotomy while maintaining the posterior cortex intact in a greenstick-type maneuver. The problem with this type of correction is that the foot is translated anteriorly relative to the tibia, and then the mechanical limb axis is no longer aligned or efficient for ambulation.

An important consideration is the extent of compensation that can be achieved by the ankle and subtalar joints after correction.

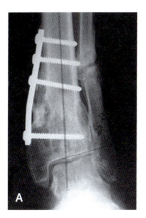
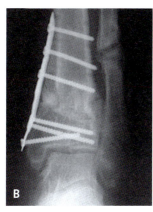

Figure 26-3 **A,** Valgus deformity associated with posttraumatic arthritis. **B,** Correction was accomplished with a medial closing wedge supramalleolar osteotomy. The center of rotation of angulation of the ankle was maintained.

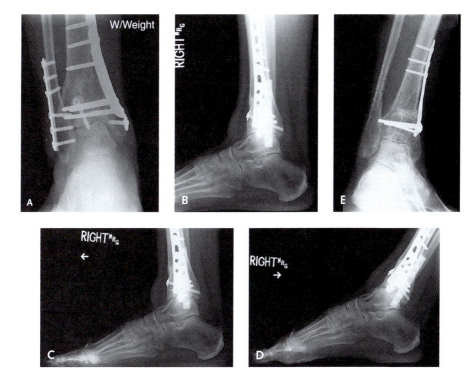

Figure 26-4 **A** and **B,** Correction of varus deformity in a patient with ankle arthritis was an important part of staged repair before ankle replacement. **C** and **D,** Note the excellent range of motion of the ankle joint preoperatively. **E,** Indeed, despite the presence of arthritis, the function of the ankle was good at 4 years after osteotomy, and no further treatment was necessary.

The opening wedge osteotomy is performed 4 cm proximal to the medial malleolar tip in metaphyseal bone (Figures 26-4 and 26-5). Once the skin incision is made, minimal periosteal stripping that is sufficient only to complete the osteotomy is performed. The cut is planned in the metaphysis. I apply the selected plate on the surface of the tibia before the osteotomy is made, ensuring that sufficient space is maintained to obtain fixation with three screws distally, mark the osteotomy, and complete it. I keep periosteal stripping to a minimum when the bone cut is made perpendicular to the tibia with a broad oscillating saw, and I preserve the

opposite cortex and periosteal sleeve to act as a fulcrum for the opening wedge and to enhance stability. If nothing more than uniplanar angulation is required, then a small plate over the lateral tibia is useful to prevent overcorrection. If translation and rotation also are necessary, then the opposite cortex must be cut to allow the distal segment to move. The fibular osteotomy is performed with the lateral incision at the same level as that for the tibial osteotomy, although this location is not critical. A wedge osteotomy of the fibula can be performed if marked angular deformity is present and when a closing lateral wedge osteotomy of the tibia

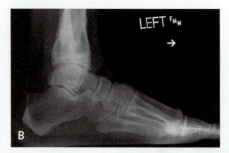
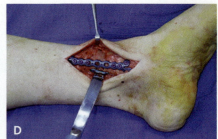
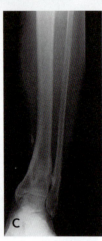
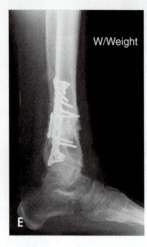
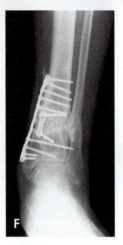

Figure 26-5 A-C, Marked varus deformity of the ankle and hindfoot associated with posttraumatic arthritis, exacerbated by a preexisting distal tibia vara. Although arthritis was present, ankle function was good, and minimal pain was present. **D-F,** An opening wedge medial osteotomy was performed with plate fixation (Orthohelix, Akron, Ohio).

is performed. I prefer to use a structural allograft from a femoral head to fill the defect. Once the osteotomy has been performed, a laminar spreader is inserted to gradually distract the osteotomy to the desired level. This is checked fluoroscopically. The structural bone graft provides immediate mechanical support, with little likelihood of collapse even after resorption, which occurs during revascularization. Some structural integrity remains during the process of bone graft incorporation, to allow the graft to withstand loads. After the deformity has been corrected, the osteotomy is provisionally secured with Kirschner wires (K-wires), and the plate is applied to the tibia at this time. The alignment is assessed with fluoroscopy.

In certain circumstances, the preservation of limb length is not necessary or desirable, so a closing wedge lateral osteotomy of the fibula and tibia is performed (Figures 26-6 to 26-8). Figure 26-6 presents an example of chronic lateral ankle instability associated with a varus distal tibia deformity. I previously used a lateral closing wedge osteotomy for correction of this type of deformity, but over the years, I have recognized that a defect of the medial distal tibia persists, so that recurrence of ankle varus is likely (see Figure 26-6, *D*). Although symptoms are markedly decreased and stability is regained, these intraarticular deformities require a different approach to osteotomy, as outlined further on. When performing a lateral closing wedge osteotomy of the tibia and fibula, I add a separate incision in a medial location to permit application of a small plate to the tibia, which prevents overcorrection. The osteotomy can be tensioned against the fixed fulcrum medially with this technique (see Figure 26-7).

I perform supramalleolar osteotomy whenever possible to preserve hindfoot alignment in cases of deformities secondary to

neuroarthropathy or avascular necrosis of the distal tibia. Correction of neuropathic deformity with distal tibia osteotomy is an excellent alternative to a more extensive hindfoot and ankle arthrodesis, particularly in the setting of neuroarthropathy. Whenever possible, arthrodesis should be avoided in patients with Charcot deformity, to prevent added stresses on the remaining hindfoot joints. A good example of such a clinical scenario is presented in Figure 26-8. In this case, the patient had profound neuropathy with peripheral vascular disease, so an opening wedge osteotomy was not a realistic choice for an optimal outcome despite the magnitude of the wedge removed.

Correction of Intraarticular Varus Ankle Deformity and Ankle Instability

As noted earlier, patients with chronic ankle instability often present with arthritis of the medial compartment of the ankle, associated with an erosion of the distal medial tibia, and a dysplastic medial malleolus (Figure 26-9). In the past, I have attempted many different types of procedures to avoid an ankle arthrodesis. These included a lateral ligament reconstruction, peroneal tendon repair or transfer of the longus to the brevis, calcaneus osteotomy, lateral closing wedge osteotomy of the tibia and fibula, and even opening wedge medial osteotomy. Although many of these procedures corrected one component of the problem, deformity frequently persisted or recurred because of the intraarticular element of the deformity. Chronic varus instability is associated with erosion of the medial distal tibia; eventually, the talus falls into the defect thus created, creating the ankle varus. In addition, the medial malleolus begins to erode, and instead of being vertically oriented, it is medially inclined. Both of these anatomic abnormalities add to

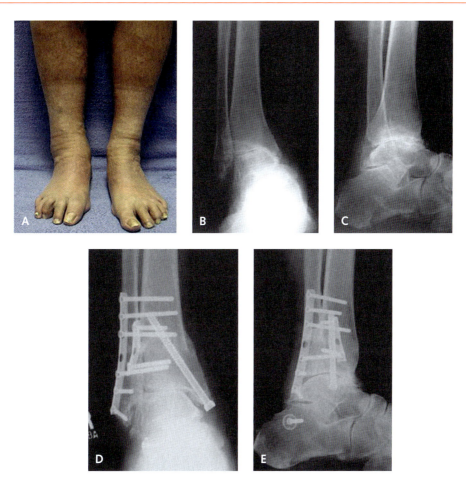

Figure 26-6 A-C, A closing lateral wedge supramalleolar osteotomy combined with ankle ligament reconstruction was performed for management of varus deformity of the hindfoot and ankle associated with ankle instability in a 60-year-old patient. **D** and **E,** Despite the slight improvement in the appearance of the alignment of the ankle joint, arthritis is still present. Attempting correction of the ankle with a supramalleolar osteotomy is unrealistic when a defect is within the distal tibial articular surface.

the likelihood of recurrent deformity. Obviously, the repair could commence with an arthrodesis of the ankle, but surprisingly, many patients maintain some range of motion of the ankle, despite the presence of arthritis, so joint preservation is desirable. I now perform an intraarticular osteotomy called the "plafond-plasty" for correction of this deformity. This procedure is performed in conjunction with additional hindfoot alignment and stabilization of the ankle as required.

For the plafond-plasty, the medial distal tibia is exposed, and a guide pin inserted to mark the plane of the osteotomy, and checked fluoroscopically. The guide pin should terminate at the start of the intraarticular defect of the tibia. Two additional guide pins are then inserted immediately above the ankle joint to function as a buttress and prevent the saw cut from entering the joint. A saw is used to perform the osteotomy along the plane of the guide pin, stopping immediately above the joint line. The osteotomy is then gradually opened using a broad osteotome, levering the distal tibia open. The joint is protected by the periarticular guide pins, which were inserted before the osteotomy. Cancellous bone graft is then used to fill the osteotomy, and fixation is achieved with a plate. When I originally began using this osteotomy, I used an external fixator to distract the joint for 6 weeks postoperatively, but I have since

discontinued this step, which I have not found to add much benefit (Figures 26-10 to 26-12).

Correction of a Valgus Deformity

The identical concepts apply to correction of a valgus ankle deformity and to ankle varus repair. An opening wedge lateral osteotomy or a closing wedge medial osteotomy is performed. If the fibula is short as a result of stress fracture or trauma, an opening wedge osteotomy is preferable to correct the valgus. Although a closing wedge medial osteotomy will correct the alignment of the ankle joint, it will not address the problems presented by the shortened fibula, and the mechanics of the ankle may continue to be abnormal. By and large, the closing wedge medial osteotomy technique is used when the skin condition is not ideal, when minimal correction is required, and when limb shortening is not an issue.

The opening wedge osteotomy commences with a single lateral incision over the fibula. After the lateral part of the tibia has been exposed and the osteotomy level has been determined, a K-wire is inserted to the tibia perpendicular to the mechanical axis. Adding a plate on the medial aspect is useful because it prevents overcorrection and allows the osteotomy, under tension, to be positioned correctly against the fixed medial tibia (Figure 26-13).

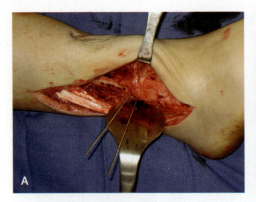
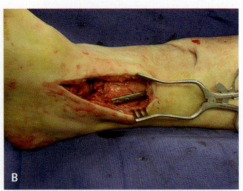
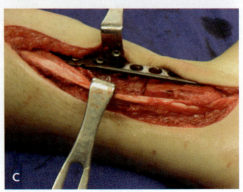

Figure 26-7 A, The exposure for a lateral closing wedge osteotomy. Retraction of the peroneal tendons is followed by application of a plate on the medial aspect of the ankle to add a tension side to the osteotomy. **B,** The incision was extended distally to debride the ankle and remove intraarticular loose fragments. **C,** Application of a plate on the lateral aspect.

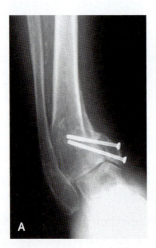
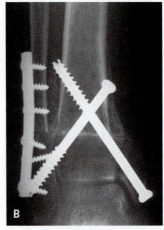

Figure 26-8 A, Despite the marked deformity present, the patient, who had neuropathy, was prepared to accept the shortening required to perform a lateral closing wedge osteotomy of the tibia and fibula to treat this severe malunion. **B,** Despite the malunion of the medial malleolus, alignment is acceptable.

If the valgus deformity is predominantly the result of shortening of the fibula, and no associated tibial deformity is present, then lengthening of the fibula may be all that is necessary, as demonstrated in Figure 26-14. In this interesting case of a fibula stress fracture associated with valgus deformity of the ankle, no tibial osteotomy was required for the correction.

The closing wedge osteotomy frequently is used to correct valgus deformity of the distal tibia or ankle. Exposure is achieved by means of the same incision as that used for a medial opening wedge osteotomy. In such cases, the fibula usually has to be cut and

is done so generally at the level of or slightly proximal to the tibial osteotomy (Figure 26-15). The key to this osteotomy is to maintain a slight cortical bridge on the lateral tibia, which will markedly facilitate correction and maintain alignment. If a secondary translational deformity is created by the osteotomy, the lateral cortical bridge must be cut to shift the tibia laterally. The guide pins for the osteotomy are inserted perpendicular to the axis of the tibia and parallel with the ankle joint, and the cut is made either inside or outside the guide pins, according to the amount of bone to be resected. Additional pins are inserted after removal of the bone

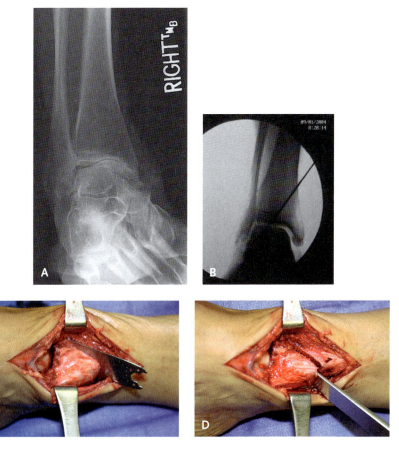

Figure 26-9 A, Medial intraarticular osteotomy with plafond-plasty to correct chronic ankle instability and varus deformity of the ankle in a 41-year-old patient. **B,** The osteotomy line is marked out with a guide pin, which stops at the apex of the intraarticular deformity. **C** and **D,** A saw is used to perform the osteotomy, which stops above the plafond **(C)** and is gradually opened with an osteotome **(D).**

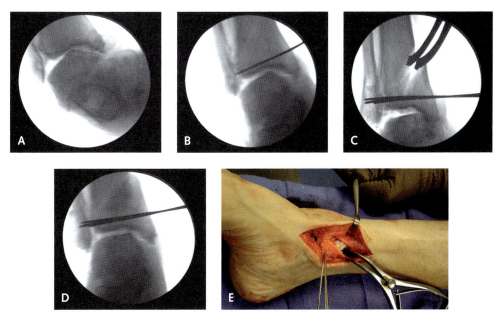

Figure 26-10 A, A typical deformity for correction with plafond-plasty. **B,** The guide pins above the plafond were inserted to prevent cracking of the osteotomy into the joint. **C-E,** A laminar spreader was used to open the osteotomy, followed by insertion of cancellous bone graft.

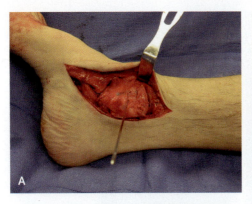
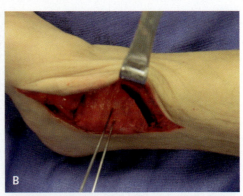
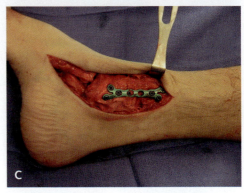

Figure 26-11 The incision was extended distally in this plafond-plasty to perform additional midfoot procedures. Note the position of the juxtaarticular K-wires **(A)**, the opened osteotomy **(B)**, and the application of the plate after cancellous bone grafting **(C)**.

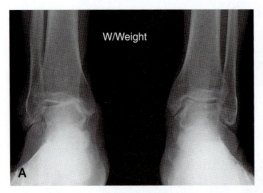
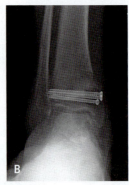
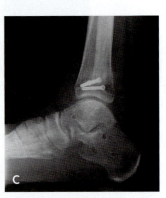

Figure 26-12 This varus deformity with ankle instability in a 44-year-old patient was treated with an intra-articular plafond-plasty. **A,** Preoperative radiograph. **B** and **C,** Postoperative radiographs.

wedge to hold the position of the osteotomy, which is checked fluoroscopically, and in particular to ensure that the alignment is correct in both the coronal and the sagittal planes. The stability of the ankle is then checked, because an additional lateral plate or crossed cannulated screws may be used at this point as required. If the tibia is shifted laterally to avoid a secondary medial translational deformity, the osteotomy of the fibula will show a gap, which should be fixed with a two- or three-hole one-third tubular plate following the tibia fixation.

Correction of ankle valgus deformity in patients with a ball-and-socket ankle joint deformity resulting from an extensive tarsal coalition is best accomplished with a closing wedge supramalleolar osteotomy. Valgus instability of the ankle is always present with the ball-and-socket ankle joint deformity. Correction of the valgus hindfoot deformity associated with the ankle instability is best accomplished with a closing wedge medial osteotomy of the distal tibia for

realignment. Additional procedures may be considered, including medial sliding translational calcaneus osteotomy to improve the mechanical axis of the subtalar joint (Figures 26-16 and 26-17).

The medial closing wedge osteotomy is used for patients with avascular necrosis, neuropathy, and valgus deformity, just as for those with a varus deformity. Joint preservation in patients with neuropathy is important (Figure 26-18).

Correction of Multiplanar Deformity

Although a biplanar opening or closing wedge osteotomy may correct multiplanar deformity, I have found that a dome osteotomy is particularly useful in patients with deformities of this type. The osteotomy can be combined with ankle replacement using an anterior approach to the joint (Figure 26-19). The incision is deepened to periosteum, which is reflected, and the dome cut is marked out with electrocautery in the metaphysis. I ensure that the oste-

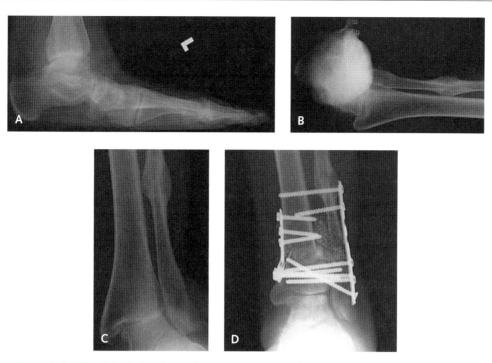

Figure 26-13 A-C, This painful foot and ankle deformity was associated with flatfoot, which was worsened by a stress fracture of the fibula. The patient already had a painful contralateral foot after a pan-talar fusion, and an arthrodesis of this ankle was not thought to be ideal. **D,** An opening wedge osteotomy of the tibia and fibula was performed by lengthening the fibula and the tibia with a structural allograft, and then an arthrodesis of the tibiofibular syndesmosis was created.

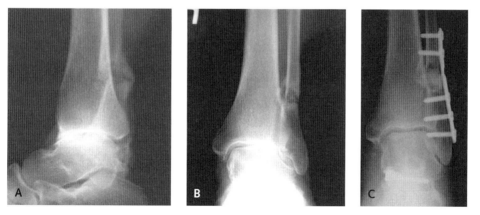

Figure 26-14 A, Stress fracture of the fibula resulting from the valgus ankle deformity. **B,** Over a short period, despite immobilization, a nonunion developed, with further deformity. **C,** The nonunion was treated with a lengthening osteotomy of the fibula with interposition bone grafting, but without an osteotomy of the tibia.

otomy is made in the metaphysis, leaving sufficient bone distally for fixation with a plate. This is particularly important when the osteotomy is combined with an ankle replacement. A 2-mm drill is now used to perforate the tibia along the cautery line. It is important to drill the tibia through the posterior cortex, because the osteotomy will break out in the incorrect location if unicortical drill holes are made. Once drilling has been accomplished, a small osteotome is used to complete the osteotomy in a dome configuration. If the fibula requires osteotomy, it can be performed at the same level laterally, or obliquely more proximally. The ankle is then manipulated, rotated, translated or angulated in any plane until the desired correction is obtained. This osteotomy is particularly useful to correct deformity when the CORA is further away from the ankle joint, as seen in Figure 26-20.

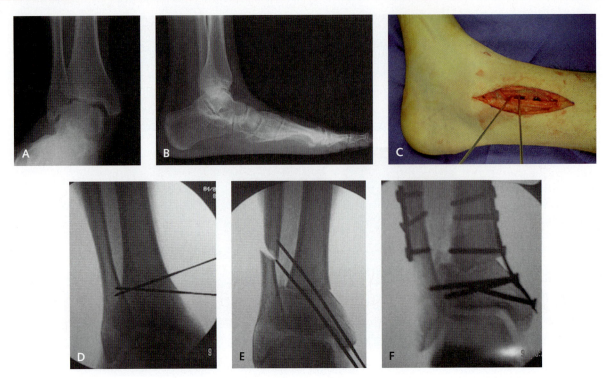

Figure 26-15 A and **B,** A medial closing wedge supramalleolar osteotomy was performed for management of premature lateral physeal closure (the patient was an adolescent), with severe subsequent valgus of the ankle associated with a flatfoot. **C** and **D,** Two guide pins were inserted, one perpendicular to the tibia and the other parallel with the articular surface of the tibia. **E** and **F,** For the tibial alignment to be maintained over the center of the talus, the tibia was slightly translated laterally, and an oblique osteotomy of the fibula had to be performed.

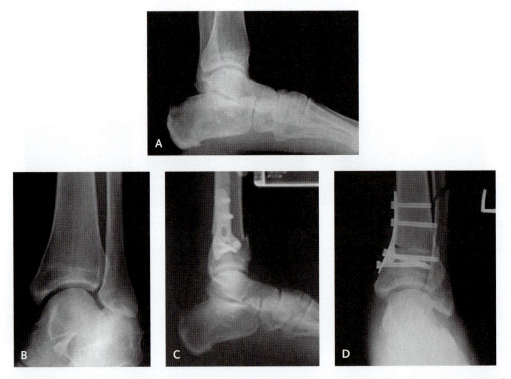

Figure 26-16 A and **B,** This ball-and-socket ankle joint deformity caused by a talonavicular coalition was associated with typical hindfoot valgus, subfibular impingement, and pain. **C** and **D,** This deformity was corrected with a medial closing wedge supramalleolar osteotomy. Note the marked improvement of the axis of the tibiotalar-calcaneal alignment **(C)** and the improvement in the height of the arch of the foot **(D).**

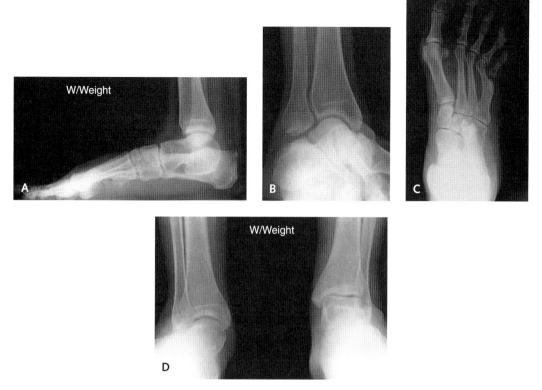

Figure 26-17 A-D, A typical ball-and-socket unstable valgus ankle deformity associated with a talonavicular coalition. Note the valgus deformity of the ankle, the flatfoot deformity, and the dysplastic fifth ray.

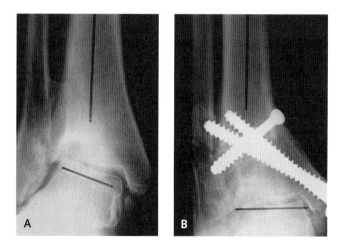

Figure 26-18 A, Valgus deformity and early ulceration over the medial malleolus associated with severe diabetic neuroarthropathy. **B,** Although an arthrodesis of either the ankle or the hindfoot was an option, a medial closing wedge supramalleolar osteotomy was performed to preserve motion. Note that the goal of surgery was accomplished, although a secondary medial translational deformity of the foot was created. This deformity was, however, asymptomatic.

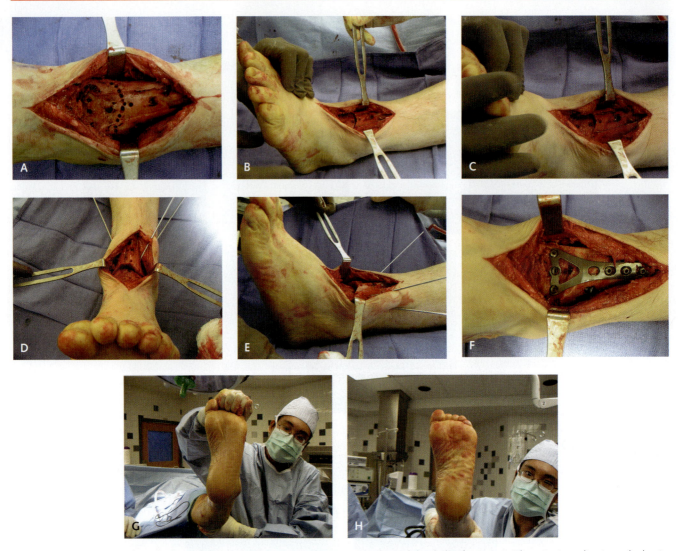

Figure 26-19 Correction of a multiplanar distal tibial deformity consequent to a malunited distal tibia fracture. **A,** The osteotomy line is marked out with a cautery, and 2-mm drill holes are made in a curved dome shape. **B** and **C,** The cut is completed using a small osteotome. **D** and **E,** The distal tibia is then rotated, angulated, and translated until correction is obtained. **F,** The repair is secured with Kirschner wires, followed by plate application. **G** and **H,** Preoperative and postoperative axial views of the heel.

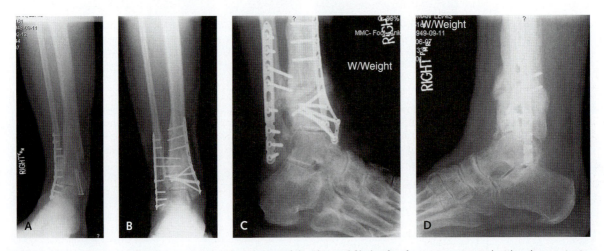

Figure 26-20 A, This multiplanar deformity associated with malunion of the tibia and fibula after fracture was treated with a dome osteotomy. **B-D,** The osteotomy was performed through a single anterior incision, with the dome reaching into the syndesmosis and the fibula, followed by revision of the fibula plate fixation, creating a tibiofibular synostosis, and plate fixation of the tibia.

TECHNIQUES, TIPS, AND PITFALLS

- Double osteotomies may be required to correct multiplanar deformity. In the case illustrated in Figure 26-21, the patient had both a nonunion and a malunion involving the tibia as well as the medial malleolus, and a double osteotomy procedure was required to correct the deformity.

- For a closing wedge medial or lateral osteotomy, it is useful to apply a small plate on the tension side of the deformity to prevent overcorrection. For a lateral closing wedge, the plate is on the medial tibia, and for a medial closing wedge, on the lateral tibia. This plate can be applied only if the osteotomy is performed at the CORA, and if no additional translation must be performed.

- I generally prefer to perform a medial closing wedge rather than a lateral opening wedge osteotomy. This cut heals well, the result is a little more predictable, and no bone grafting is required.

- An osteotomy may be required in conjunction with an arthrodesis of the ankle. In cases of very severe supramalleolar deformity, an arthrodesis alone will not correct deformity (Figure 26-22). It is important to consider the use of osteotomy in conjunction with arthrodesis of the ankle as well as ankle joint replacement depending on the needs of the patient.

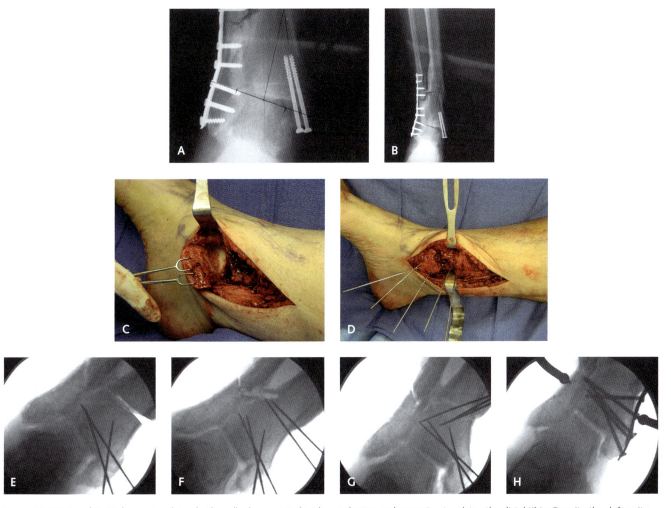

Figure 26-21 **A** and **B,** Malunion involving both malleoli associated with a malunion and nonunion involving the distal tibia. Despite the deformity, good range of motion of the ankle was retained, and preservation of ankle function was a main concern, especially because the patient was a young man. **C** and **D,** The approach used medial and lateral incisions, commencing with an osteotomy of the medial malleolus and temporary fixation with K-wires. **E** and **F,** An osteotomy was then performed through the malunion and nonunion of the tibia, with removal of avascular bone. **G** and **H,** This was followed by plate fixation of the tibia and fibula.

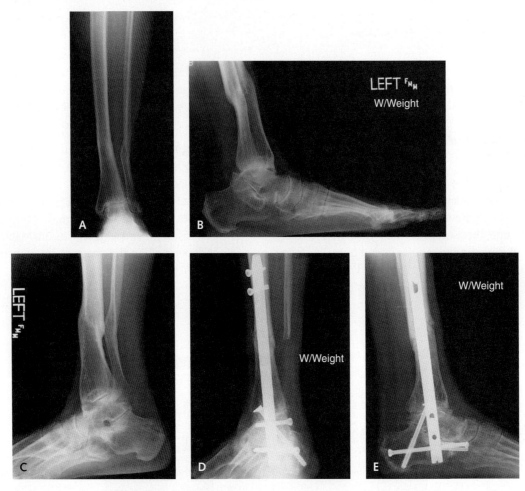

Figure 26-22 A-C, The patient presented with painful arthritis of the ankle and subtalar joint, in addition to a malunion of a previous tibia fracture. **D** and **E,** Treatment consisted of a tibiotalocalcaneal arthrodesis with simultaneous osteotomy of the tibia, using a slightly longer intramedullary rod.

CHAPTER **27**

Disorders of the Achilles Tendon

INSERTIONAL ACHILLES TENDINOPATHY

Once nonoperative methods for treatment of insertional Achilles tendon disease have failed, the next decision to be made is the type of incision used for the surgical approach. I make this decision according to the extent of the underlying disease, the presence of tendon degeneration, and the location of maximum tenderness. If osteophytes are present on the posterior central aspect of the heel, then I use a central splitting incision of the posterior Achilles tendon and calcaneus. This incision works well, and the entire broad plate of the osteophyte can be removed. Use of this Achilles splitting incision is advantageous because it allows direct visualization of the disease and ease of dissection of the torn portion of the tendon with removal of the osteophyte. This invasion is associated with a more prolonged recovery, however (Figure 27-1).

If the pain is not posterocentral, the incision should be made medially or laterally, because the irritated or torn portion of the tendon may not be visible from the central or posterior splitting incision. If no large osteophyte is present in the posterior calcaneus and thickening and degeneration of the tendon are diffuse, then a medial or lateral incision is made to debride the retrocalcaneal space, thereby decreasing the impingement of the calcaneus against the Achilles tendon (Figure 27-2).

The operation is performed with use of local anesthesia and the patient in a prone position. A 4-cm vertical incision is made directly over the tendon extending toward the junction of the plantar heel skin. The incision is deepened through the tendon, which is split longitudinally, and the incision is deepened directly onto bone, even inferiorly. The central portion of the tendon is the location of maximum degeneration, and this area can be exposed either through a vertical ellipse or by splitting the tendon and separating it with a retractor. The enlarged osteophyte is visible below the central portion of the degenerated tendon, and this is excised with an osteotome. The dorsal posterior surface of the calcaneus must be smoothed down to remove any potential source of irritation on the anterior aspect of the Achilles tendon insertion. The tendon must

be repaired with a running locking suture. If significant degeneration and tearing of the tendon that could lead to its separation off the calcaneus are noted, a suture anchor can be used to help with the reattachment of the tendon. Usually, however, placement of an anchor is not necessary, because wide bands of the tendon, inserted both medially and laterally, prevent rupture. Removal of up to one third of the central aspect of the tendon does not disrupt its attachment whatsoever, and possibly up to half of the tendon insertion can be detached (Figure 27-3).

For treatment of many severe forms of degenerative tendinopathy, the entire tendon is removed by either splitting the tendon or detaching it completely. In such cases, a decision must be made regarding whether the tendinopathy is severe enough to warrant transfer of the flexor hallucis longus (FHL) tendon, to supplement the strength and vascularity of the Achilles.

The only clinical concern that I have with this condition (whether or not it is related to the use of the central splitting incision) is the prolonged recovery time. Up to 1 year may be required for the patient to recover completely and return to full function. The advantages of the central splitting incision are the direct access to the degenerative disease and the removal of the hypertrophic osteophytes; whether the disease or the approach used is responsible for this delayed return to full, painless activity is unclear.

Careful attention to postoperative care is essential during healing of central splitting and other incisions that are used to expose the distal Achilles tendon. Healing invariably occurs uneventfully provided that the foot is held immobilized to prevent formation of a hypertrophic scar, which could be catastrophic. Formation of scar directly over the heel will lead to problems with shoe wear. The foot must therefore be immobilized postoperatively until full wound healing has occurred. Rehabilitation of the Achilles tendon is important, requiring strengthening modalities, heel elevation, and orthotic arch support. Generally, I recommend use of a removable range-of-motion walker boot for approximately 6 to 8 weeks after surgery, allowing plantar flexion but blocking dorsiflexion, to facilitate physical therapy and treatment.

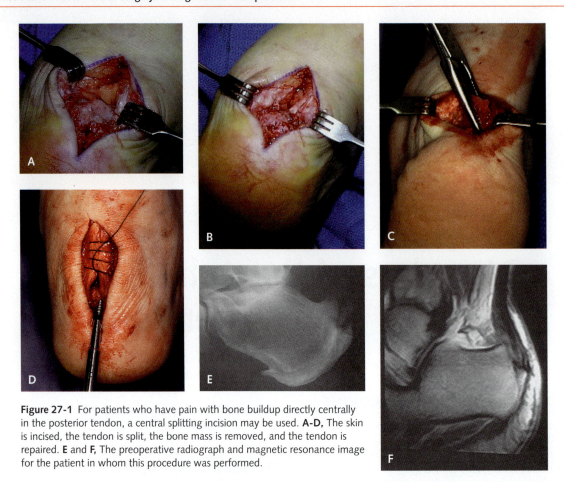

Figure 27-1 For patients who have pain with bone buildup directly centrally in the posterior tendon, a central splitting incision may be used. **A-D,** The skin is incised, the tendon is split, the bone mass is removed, and the tendon is repaired. **E** and **F,** The preoperative radiograph and magnetic resonance image for the patient in whom this procedure was performed.

Insertional tendinopathy should be distinguished from Haglund's syndrome and retrocalcaneal bursitis. In patients with these latter conditions, the bursitis occurs as a result of enlargement of the dorsal superior lateral aspect of the calcaneus. The dorsolateral tuberosity causes impingement against the lateral insertion of the Achilles tendon, and retrocalcaneal bursitis develops. If the bursitis is refractory to nonoperative treatment, the best approach is through a short dorsolateral incision just anterior to the Achilles tendon (Figure 27-4). The incision is deepened through subcutaneous tissue, the retrocalcaneal bursa is excised, and the insertion of the Achilles tendon and the enlarged posterolateral bone are exposed. Only a lateral ostectomy is performed; a more medial extension of the ostectomy is unnecessary. In the event that bilateral bone prominence is present, I prefer to use a more extensile J-incision. Strictly speaking, the latter condition is not true Haglund's syndrome, but this anatomic variant does occur (Figure 27-5).

Haglund's syndrome commonly is associated with retrocalcaneal bursitis, but the retrocalcaneal bursitis may indeed be present without a lateral bone prominence. The bursa is irritated as a result of impingement between the Achilles tendon and the posterior dorsal surface of the tuberosity, causing the inflammatory change. If surgery is required, the bursa is excised along with any bone prominence as previously described.

Alternative incisions may be used to correct insertional tendinopathy, including an extended J-incision. The advantage of this type of incision is that it gives complete access to the entire insertion of the tendon. I use this incision for more severe diffuse insertional tendinopathy when I do not think that I can access the entire tendon through either a central splitting incision or bilateral

incisions. With use of the extended J-incision, the tendon is completely detached from its insertion, the offending bone is debrided, the retrocalcaneal space is denuded, and then the tendon is reattached with a suture anchor (see Figure 27-5).

In addition to the debridement of the insertion of the tendon with bursectomy and ostectomy, the Achilles tendon needs to be repaired for management of severe insertional tendinopathy with loss of the integrity and function of the tendon (Figure 27-6). Generally, the tissue is insufficient in amount or of such poor quality that a simple debridement cannot be performed. The management of these more severe forms, as discussed later in the section on management of noninsertional tendinopathy, consists of resection of the insertion of the Achilles tendon with either a flexor hallucis longus (FHL) transfer or an Achilles tendon allograft (Figure 27-7). These more extensive procedures are distinguished from the simple superolateral exostectomy (Figure 27-8). The use of the FHL as a tendon graft for insertional tendinopathy is not as common as for more extensive noninsertional tendon disease, but certain circumstances will necessitate use of either the FHL tendon, a tendon graft, or a V-Y advancement (Figure 27-9). The choice will depend on the extent of the disease, the ability to use the remainder of the distal Achilles, and the activity or athletic needs of the patient.

MANAGEMENT OF PARATENDINITIS

Recognized as a separate disorder from the degenerative tendinopathies, paratendinitis is an inflammatory condition, typically occurring in athletes, and usually associated with hyperpronation

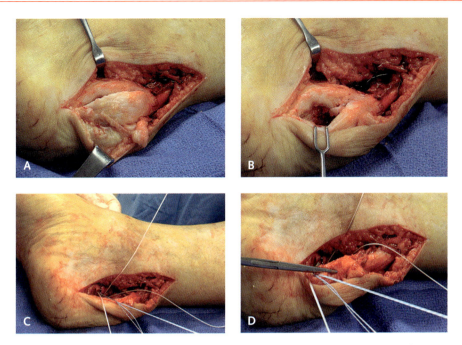

Figure 27-2 A, A more extensive lateral incision was used for the approach to this extensive degenerative tendinopathy. **B,** Note the marked degeneration in the tendon, mostly in its posterior half. **C** and **D,** No augmentation of this reattachment with a flexor hallucis longus tendon transfer was thought to be necessary, and the repair was performed with a suture anchor used to obtain the correct tension on the tendon.

of the foot in conjunction with a mild gastrocnemius muscle contracture. The usual nonsurgical methods of treatment, including contrast bathing, physical therapy, orthotic arch support, and gastrocnemius muscle stretching, usually are sufficient to alleviate symptoms. If the paratendinitis is persistent, a brisement of the paratenon is performed, beginning with injection of 3 mL of lidocaine. The No. 20 needle is inserted just underneath the paratenon, advanced into the tendon, and then backed off so that it lies indirectly under the paratenon. Injection of the anesthetic not only confirms the diagnosis and the correct location of the needle but also elevates the inflamed, scarred paratenon off the tendon. This technique works well enough that it should be tried before surgery.

The surgical procedure for paratendinitis involves a short incision on the medial aspect of the tendon over a length of 2 cm (Figure 27-10). The subcutaneous tissue is elevated, and then the paratenon is identified and incised. The paratenon is then elevated off the Achilles tendon and stripped by excising the superficial anterior sheath of the paratenon medially, dorsally, and laterally as one sleeve (Figure 27-11). The deep ventral surface of the Achilles tendon is left intact, to leave the blood supply undisturbed. The foot should be immobilized for a short period to prevent any hypertrophic scar formation, and then therapy with cross-training and modalities used in rehabilitation after boot immobilization can proceed for approximately 3 weeks.

MANAGEMENT OF NONINSERTIONAL TENDINOPATHY

The main considerations in surgical management of noninsertional tendinopathy are where and what to debride, how much to debride, and then how to do the repair. If noninsertional tendinopathy is considered to be a degenerative hypovascular condition, an

approach consisting of excision of the degenerated tendon, in the expectation that the repair process will result in improved tendon function, makes sense. Achieving this outcome, however, is easier said than done. Although noninsertional tendinopathy remains a clinical diagnosis, I like to use magnetic resonance imaging (MRI) preoperatively to locate the point of maximum degeneration.

As an alternative to an open invasive procedure for the treatment of the Achilles tendinopathy, performance of multiple percutaneous tenotomies may be effective. This procedure is indicated for patients in whom nonsurgical care has failed but in whom a more extensive reconstruction is not thought to be necessary or appropriate. If the percutaneous tenotomy approach fails, then a specifically reconstructive procedure, as described further on, is performed. Creating the percutaneous tenotomies induces a hypervascular response, which theoretically facilitates tendon healing. The other possible explanation for the success of this procedure is the slight lengthening of the Achilles tendon presumably produced by the longitudinal tenotomies. In my experience with this procedure, results have been fair and unpredictable. Some patients improve by 8 weeks, and although swelling is present, they are functionally improved. Others have persistent pain for many months, and I am not certain if it is the continued therapy, inactivity, or time that eventually results in healing.

For the *multiple tenotomy* procedure, after local anesthesia has been obtained, a No. 15 knife blade is introduced posteriorly, and multiple slits in the tendon are made. The knife blade is inserted perpendicular to the axis of the tendon, and then the foot is passively dorsiflexed while the knife blade is pushed up against the tendon proximally. A second and a third incision are made percutaneously with the foot moved distally while the knife blade is pushed in toward the distal aspect of the tendon. The tenotomy incisions can be closed with absorbable sutures, although suturing is not really necessary (Figure 27-12).

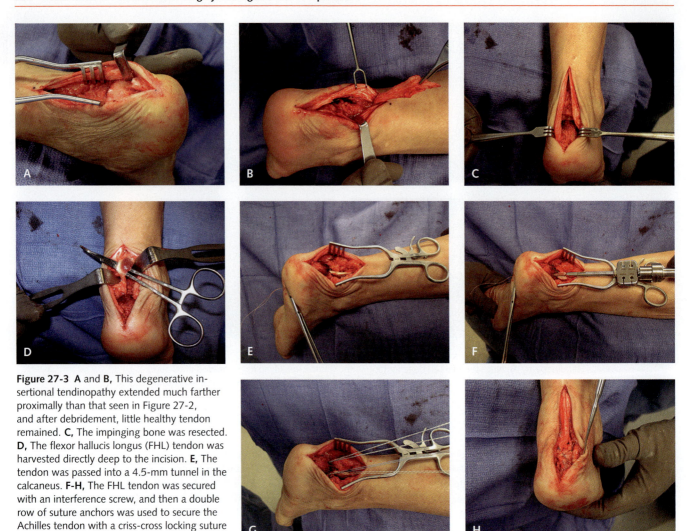

Figure 27-3 A and **B,** This degenerative insertional tendinopathy extended much farther proximally than that seen in Figure 27-2, and after debridement, little healthy tendon remained. **C,** The impinging bone was resected. **D,** The flexor hallucis longus (FHL) tendon was harvested directly deep to the incision. **E,** The tendon was passed into a 4.5-mm tunnel in the calcaneus. **F-H,** The FHL tendon was secured with an interference screw, and then a double row of suture anchors was used to secure the Achilles tendon with a criss-cross locking suture over the tendon.

After these manipulations, the Achilles tendon swells, and this swelling may be even more significant than that associated with the degenerative tendinopathy. The swelling is the result of a hypervascular reaction with fibrosis and is to be expected. Patients will continue to have symptoms for 3 to 6 months after this procedure, but most can perform activities, including exercise, comfortably by that time.

The *reconstructive* procedure for debridement of diseased tendon begins with a more extensive, medially based incision, approximately 6 cm long. I prefer to avoid a lateral incision, to prevent any inadvertent injury to the sural nerve. The incision is deepened onto the paratenon, which is inspected for any thickening or inflammation, which will necessitate debridement or excision. Removal of the paratenon is followed by inspection of the tendon. Grossly identifying the area of tendon degeneration is not easy. In patients with severe tendinopathy, with fusiform thickening of the tendon, the bulge in the tendon may be visible. The tendon is incised longitudinally, and the yellowish, mucinoid degenerative intrasubstance portion of the tendon is excised. I excise a vertical ellipse of tendon, removing approximately 50% of the cross-sectional diameter of the tendon in the area of the maximum fusiform degeneration. Knowing where to start and stop with this debridement is difficult because no clear demarcation exists between healthy and diseased tendon. With excision of the tendon,

repair is performed with a running stitch of 2-0 absorbable suture, and the knot is tied inside the tendon to prevent any friction subcutaneously (Figure 27-13).

With more advanced degeneration, particularly that involving the more distal insertion, recent interest has centered on the use of the FHL tendon to augment or replace the degenerated portion of the Achilles tendon. The rationale for this procedure is to bring the muscle belly of the FHL tendon adjacent to the avascular Achilles tendon, thereby facilitating a process of healing by proximity. The addition of the FHL tendon also unloads the Achilles tendon and supposedly increases push-off strength. Although this operation has its merits, I think that it is a case of "robbing Peter to pay Paul." Certainly, if the Achilles tendon is totally disrupted and irreparable, then the addition of autogenous tissue, including the FHL tendon, may have merit. Harvesting the FHL tendon is not without morbidity, however, and even though patients tolerate the loss of flexion of the interphalangeal joint, this is definitely noticeable with weakness of the hallux, particularly on walking barefoot.

The FHL tendon transfer is performed through a vertical incision made immediately anterior to the Achilles tendon. A curved incision along the path of the FHL tendon behind the medial malleolus is not necessary, because the tendon is easily harvested through a vertical incision. The incision is deepened through subcutaneous tissues, and then the interval between the neurovascular

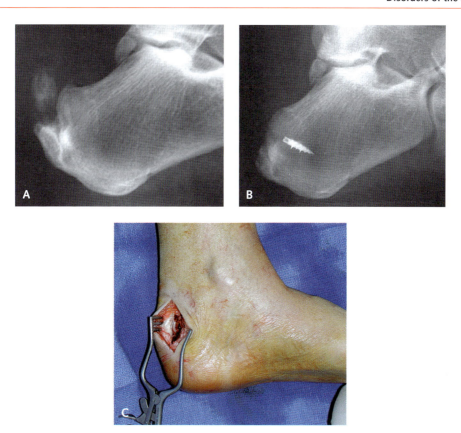

Figure 27-4 A-C, A small lateral incision can be used to debride chronic insertional tendinopathy successfully. The bone was excised through this lateral incision, and the anchor was inserted to hold the lateral border of the tendon attached. This is a satisfactory alternative; however, a more direct approach posteriorly is techincally easier.

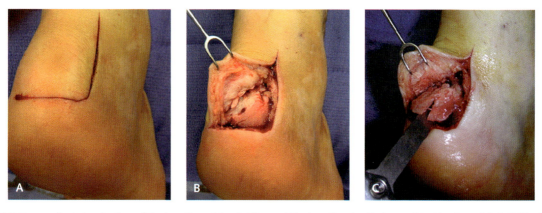

Figure 27-5 For excellent visualization of the insertion of the Achilles and the insertional pathology, a J-incision is useful. **A-C,** The tendon is elevated off the bone, tendon debridement is performed, and reattachment is made quite directly with a suture anchor.

bundle and the FHL tendon is used to identify and harvest the tendon. The incision of the flexor retinaculum and the anterior retraction of the tibial neurovascular bundle expose the deep fascia over the FHL tendon, and the retinaculum is split distally with scissors. The tendon in the arch of the foot does not need to be harvested, because a long piece of FHL tendon is unnecessary. Once the retinaculum over the FHL tendon is open, I grasp the muscle with a retractor and then cut the tendon at the level of the sustentacular tunnel under direct vision. Usually a stump of approximately 2 to 3 cm of tendon that is distal to the musculotendinous junction is present and is all that is needed for the tendon transfer. The tendon is anchored into the calcaneus using a trephine hole technique. An 8-mm trephine hole is made from the dorsal aspect of the tuberosity and extends down inferiorly. The entry point for this hole is made posteriorly at the insertion point of the Achilles tendon.

The bone plug is withdrawn, and the tendon is now advanced into the tunnel using a straight needle and suture, which are pulled out through the plantar aspect of the heel. If the tendon is too long, then the tension cannot be set correctly on the transfer unit in the bone tunnel. I pull the suture out through the heel, and then by pulling on the suture with the foot in maximum equinus, I get a sense of the resilience of the transfer unit with the foot in passive dorsiflexion. Some tension on the tendon should be evident when the foot is in approximately 20 degrees of equinus (e.g., for repair of a ruptured Achilles tendon). Usually, the musculotendinous junction is at the margin of the bone tunnel superiorly. The tendon is then secured to the bone with a suture anchor supplemented by the bone plug, which is placed back in the tunnel to give a good bone-tendon-bone interference fixation. The foot should be left in

equinus during bandaging and rehabilitation. As an alternative to the bone plug, a bioresorbable interference screw may be used to secure the tendon to the calcaneus.

Should the remaining gastrocnemius muscle be used to supplement the flexor tendon transfer? If this transfer is performed for severe degenerative tendinopathy, then a choice can be made about excising the entire degenerative portion of tendon, usually the distal 6 cm of the tendon. If a strip of the Achilles tendon is left behind, the correct tension can be maintained on the gastrocnemius muscle, in the absence of any contracture. The problem with leaving behind diseased tendon in this setting is that pain may continue as

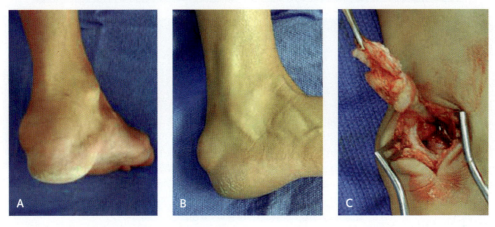

Figure 27-6 **A** and **B,** Swelling over the Achilles tendon associated with boggy tender inflammation in the retro-calcaneal space. **C,** The tendon was viable, and minimal bone impingement was noted after the bursectomy and ostectomy, which were performed through a lateral incision.

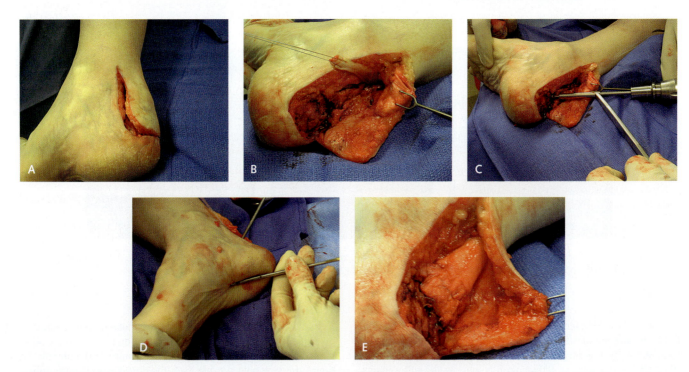

Figure 27-7 The J-incision gives excellent exposure of the distal tendon and insertion. **A** and **B,** This incision was used in a patient who presented with pain over a broad area of the insertion with enlargement of the entire tuberosity. The patient had severe insertional tendinopathy with complete loss of the function of the Achilles tendon, with gradual weakening and eventual partial rupture. **C** and **D,** Little functional Achilles tendon remained distally, and because of the severe degeneration after tendon debridement, the flexor hallucis longus (FHL) tendon was transferred into the calcaneus, through a 4.5-mm drill hole made for this purpose. **E,** Once the FHL tendon has been secured with an interference screw, the Achilles tendon is attached with a suture anchor.

a result of the degenerative process. Because revascularization of some sort is essential to healing, a portion of this tendon can be left behind with the FHL muscle belly lying up against it. Suturing the FHL muscle to the Achilles tendon stump is not easy, because this usually is at the level of the musculotendinous junction; the best result that can be obtained is with use of small 4-0 sutures to tack down the FHL muscle through its musculotendinous junction onto the Achilles tendon.

ACUTE RUPTURE OF THE ACHILLES TENDON

Over the years, cycles of operative and nonoperative management of rupture of the Achilles tendon come and go. Certainly in this age, operative management seems to be the ideal treatment to rapidly rehabilitate the patient and restore maximum function of the

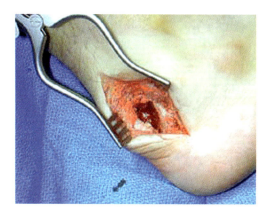

Figure 27-8 A short vertical longitudinal incision is all that is necessary for removal of a superolateral bone prominence (Haglund's deformity).

limb in the absence of weakness and the potential for re-rupture. Although nonoperative treatments are still advocated, the correct anatomic position of the tendon is impossible to obtain with these modalities, and elongation of the musculotendinous unit occurs with associated limb weakening.

To achieve the goals of treatment, which are to maximize limb function with minimal morbidity and to rapidly return the affected structure to isokinetic strength, some form of surgical treatment is necessary. The surgeon must decide which type of surgical correction is ideal, including the extensile open and percutaneous methods. Regardless of which procedure is actually used, the repair must be performed with the tendon *in an anatomic position*. This is certainly attainable with all methods, provided that the tendon ends can be inspected (i.e., a true percutaneous method of treatment is not used).

Perhaps the most significant change in my approach to management of these ruptures has been to make sure that the foot is positioned in more equinus than I anticipate will be necessary. Traditionally, both limbs were surgically prepared and included in the operative field, to permit assessment of the dynamic resting position of the contralateral limb and comparison of the normal foot with the one with the ruptured Achilles tendon, so that as the sutures were being tightened, the position of the feet was observed and the tension on the repair adjusted accordingly. Although these methods are useful, they provide only a general guide to the optimal resting position of the foot. The problem is that some stretching out of the Achilles tendon always occurs during the recovery process, regardless of the type of immobilization and rehabilitation used. Many surgeons have moved away from rigid immobilization of the limb to a functional rehabilitation program, which includes weight bearing and motion of the foot. The motion is protected in plantar flexion, and blocked dorsiflexion ensures that stretching out does not occur. It is far worse and more debilitating to have a foot that dorsiflexes excessively, because power will never be restored.

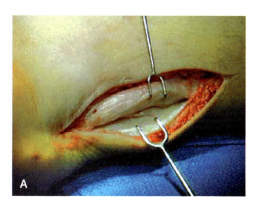

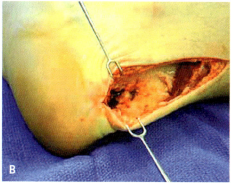

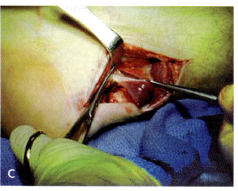

Figure 27-9 The patient had been treated with three previous operations for chronic tendinopathy. Infection followed two of the operations, and the gastrocnemius-soleus muscle did not function. **A-C,** At surgery, severe scar was identified, with no excursion of the gastrocnemius muscle. The flexor hallucis longus (FHL) tendon was harvested and transferred into the calcaneus for salvage. Note that the FHL tendon is cut just distal to the musculotendinous junction.

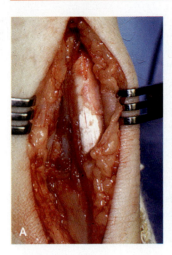
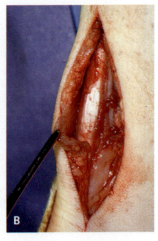

Figure 27-10 A and **B,** The typical appearance of the inflamed paratenon, which was subsequently removed.

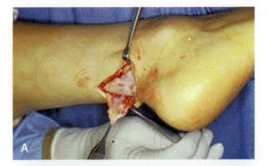
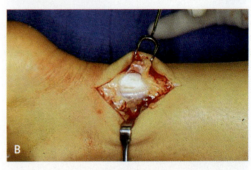

Figure 27-11 A and **B,** The paratenon is incised and clamped, and the stripping is gradually performed by retracting the paratenon over the superficial (anterior) tendon, leaving the deeper surface undisturbed.

Finally, additional concerns arise regarding the types of incisions used and the potential for wound breakdown and sural neuritis. The open extensile approach permits maximum exposure to the tendon but is associated with a greater likelihood of wound breakdown, and I now never find it necessary to use this extensile open incision (Figure 27-14). Although breakdown does not occur frequently, nonetheless this possibility is of sufficient concern that modified incisions and "mini" approaches with modified percutaneous approaches have been developed. The problems are related to not only the length of the incision but also the location, the tension on the skin from the repaired tendon, and the vascular dermatomes.

The ideal incision does not disrupt the dermatomal blood supply, which has been noted to have a watershed in the center of the limb so that an incision based centrally on the tendon has the least likelihood of disrupting this blood supply. The biggest problem with these incisions is that after repair, the subcutaneous tension is considerable because the retinaculum does not hold the tendon in its anatomic position. Thus the skin is under tension from the repaired tendon. This tension, which is readily apparent intraoperatively, can be lessened by positioning the foot in equinus. If the foot is in dorsiflexion at the completion of the repair, the skin will be under considerably more tension during skin closure. A fasciotomy of the deep compartment, which increases the transverse (cross-sectional) diameter of the posterior leg and facilitates closure without tension, has been described for use with an extensile incision. This fasciotomy is easy to perform: Once the tendon has been exposed, the deep posterior compartment becomes visible, the fascia is incised, and then the fascia is split vertically both proximally and distally with scissors. Fasciotomy is not necessary when mini open approaches and modified percutaneous approaches are used for repair.

I now rarely use an extensile incision for repair and prefer a modified approach using the Achillon system (Wright Medical Technology, Inc., Arlington, Tennessee). This modified percutaneous method of treatment is reliable and allows apposition of the frayed tendon ends in the desired position with minimal exposure of the ruptured tendon. A short transverse or a longitudinal incision is made, centered on the middle of the leg and based over the rupture. The rupture usually occurs 4 to 6 cm proximal to the insertion, and the incision is made over a length of 14 cm. The incision is deepened through the subcutaneous tissue, and the retinaculum and the paratenon are incised longitudinally (Figures 27-15 and 27-16). The hematoma is evacuated, and the ends of the tendons are identified and delivered into the incision. Severe fissuring and fraying of the tendon ends typically are seen. With a skin hook, the tendon ends are then lifted out of the bed, and the deep compartment is identified. An incision is made over the deep fascia with a knife, and then the fascia is stripped longitudinally both proximally and distally with scissors until the entire compartment is visible. I like to sweep my finger under the paratenon to free up the tendon and facilitate the insertion of the Achillon arms on both sides of the tendon.

If I use an open approach without the Achillon system, then a short (4-cm) incision is all that is necessary to visualize the ruptured tendon ends for the repair. The type of sutures used does not matter as much as the specific location for insertion of the suture and the tension of the repair once suturing is complete. I start with the proximal suture, and a running whiplock stitch of 2-0 braided nonabsorbable material is used. The sutures are locked at each corner, and three to four passes in the tendon are made until each strand of the suture is pulled distally. The entrance point for the suture is *not* where the fissuring of the rupture is noted but is located more proximally. Avulsion of tendon strands from the distal stump of the tendon is always present, and with the foot in maximum equinus, the overlapping of these strands can be seen. The same principle applies for the insertion point of the distal strand of the suture. With the patient's knee now bent and the tension applied to both ends of the sutures, until the foot is in gross equinus; the tension is then slightly released until the foot remains in approximately 20 degrees of equinus. As noted previously, I prefer to use more equinus in the repair than seems to be necessary.

Usually one strand of suture material is sufficient for the repair. The knot must be tied posteriorly deep to the Achilles tendon; otherwise, the strands will become markedly irritating if left in a

27

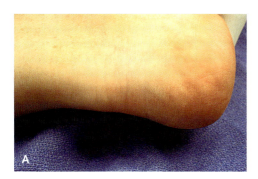

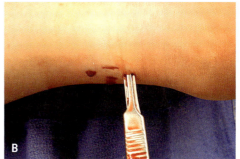

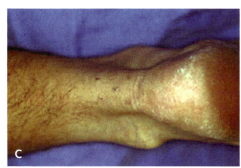

Figure 27-12 Treatment of a chronic degenerative tendinopathy with percutaneous longitudinal tenotomies, consisting of multiple punctures of the Achilles tendon. **A,** Characteristic swelling of the tendon. **B,** The punctures were made using a No. 15 blade. **C,** Appearance of the Achilles tendon 2 months later.

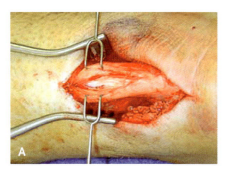

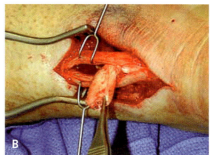

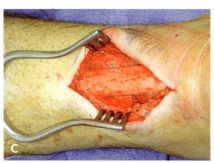

Figure 27-13 A, The degenerative tendinopathy was not extensive in this case. The diseased tendon was identified and repaired. **B,** Excision of a vertical ellipse. **C,** The repair was accomplished using a buried running suture.

subcutaneous position. The one side of the suture is tied while tension is maintained on the opposite side, and then the second side is used to set the tension on the repair. At the completion of the repair, the foot should be in 20 degrees of equinus, and with gentle pressure exerted on the foot in a plantar direction, the repair should not have a tendency to stretch out. Always check the repair by pushing fairly hard on the foot to check the quality of the repair. Now is the time to note suture failure, not during the recovery.

The mini approach with the Achillon system has been effective. This device minimizes exposure, decreases the incidence of wound complications, and facilitates end-to-end apposition of the tendon, with a modified percutaneous approach. The incision is centered over the rupture and is made over a length of 2 cm vertically, or transversely, in the center of the leg posteriorly. Locating the position of the rupture is important; otherwise, the incision will be off plane and the repair will be more difficult. Once the incision is deepened through subcutaneous tissue, the peritenon is incised transversely and then tagged for later repair. The tendon ends are identified but do not need to be pulled out into the incision. In fact, it is preferable not to deliver the frayed tendon end into the incision, and leave the strands of the tendon lying where they are (see Figure 27-16).

The fins for the Achillon system are inserted under the paratenon and on the sides of the Achilles tendon and advanced proximally. The percutaneous side pins are now introduced with an attached No. 2 braided suture in the eye of the guide pin. The sural nerve, which lies slightly more laterally and centrally, depending on where the needles are passed percutaneously, does not appear to be in any danger in this location. The sutures should be passed through the center of the musculotendinous unit. If the needle is advanced too deep, it will be in the muscle itself, which can cut through when the suture is pulled on distally. The six strands of the suture are now lifted out from the incision and clamped while the Achillon device is withdrawn; the suture strands are left directly on top of the tendon. The procedure is now reversed, again with care taken to ensure that the plane of the fins of the Achillon device is the same as the plane of the tendon. Once the sutures are withdrawn from the distal tendon segment, the one side is sutured while the other set of three suture strands is held. With the patient's knee bent, the second set of sutures is now tied, and tension is set so as to leave the foot in approximately 20 degrees of equinus. If the suture knot is anterior, it can be irritating, and the suture knot must be tied deep, behind the tendon.

Acute avulsion of the Achilles tendon must be managed differently from an acute rupture because avulsion is associated with degenerative insertional tendinopathy. The distal-most portion of the Achilles tendon usually is fibrillated, necrotic, and partially ossified. Avulsion usually is "clean" in that not much fibrillation is associated with this tearing, and it is torn out of a sleeve of its insertion. A cavity with synovium is left behind (Figures 27-17 and 27-18). I occasionally use a "hockeystick" incision (J-incision) to approach this repair. A central longitudinal incision also can be used, but exposing the entire attachment and performing the debridement of the tuberosity are easier with the J-type incision (Figure 27-19). Once the incision has been deepened down onto bone, the entire remnant of the attachment including the dorsolateral tuberosity is debrided, and then an ostectomy is performed to remove the dorsal posterior surface of the tuberosity. The ostectomy technique is similar to that used for a painful insertional tendinopathy: A raw bleeding surface is created for reattachment of the Achilles tendon. The ruptured tendon is now debrided sharply. This tendon cannot be debrided back to normal, healthy tissue because then it would be abnormally short, preventing reattachment. Instead, the margin is debrided obliquely, with as much of the superficial tendon left intact as possible.

Reattachment is performed with suture anchors, with two suture strands attached, and the tendon is approximated to the bone. Obtaining a firm attachment of the tendon to the bone with a suture anchor is difficult. One of the sutures is used with criss-cross through the tendon to try to pull the tendon down distally against the bone. The second suture is used at the loop anterior and superficial to the tendon and then tied deep to the tendon so that the criss-crossing strand pulls the tendon down against the bone.

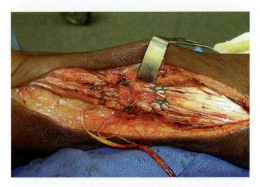

Figure 27-14 An extensile incision for repair of an acute Achilles tendon rupture is rarely used today.

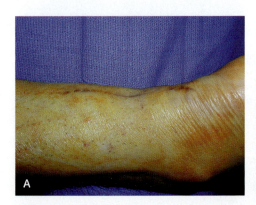

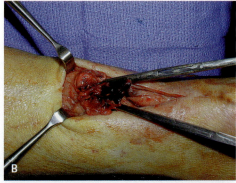

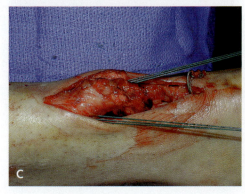

Figure 27-15 A-C, Treatment of re-rupture using the modified percutaneous Achillon system. The incision is slightly longer than that normally used, to expose the tendon thoroughly.

RECONSTRUCTION FOR CHRONIC ACHILLES TENDON RUPTURE

The approach to repair of a chronic Achilles tendon rupture is determined by the size of the gap between the tendon ends, the presence of a functioning (preferably strong) gastrocnemius-soleus muscle, and the age and activity level of the patient. An end-to-end repair is ideal because only with direct reapposition will the tendon return to maximum isokinetic strength; reattachment in this manner is the goal if at all possible, even if it necessitates positioning of the foot in slight equinus. An end-to-end repair can be performed only when the gap is approximately 1 to 2 cm in width, because some freshening up of the tendon ends needs to

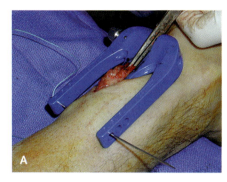
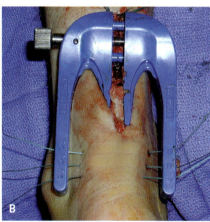
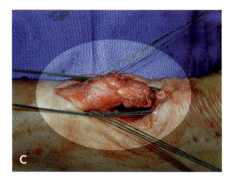

Figure 27-16 A, The fins of the Achillon device are inserted under the paratenon and on each side of the tendon, which is clamped distally. **B,** An inserter is used to push each suture pin through the body of the tendon proximally, and three sutures are used. **C,** The Achillon, including the three suture strands, is withdrawn, turned around, and inserted distally in the same manner and then is withdrawn proximally as the three sutures are pulled out. The repair is then performed with the tendon unit under appropriate tension as previously described.

be performed; subsequently, the gap may be wider by an additional 1 cm, which makes the end-to-end repair difficult. The dilemma with this method of repair arises in the delineation of normal and abnormal tissue. If a rupture is complete with atrophic ends, seeing where the tendon end lies is easy, and after debridement, the repair is performed. With many chronic degenerative ruptures, however, a degenerative scar is present in the center of the tendon, and the scar makes this type of repair implausible. In such cases, options include an end-to-end repair with tendon shortening, use of a tendon allograft, a V-Y advancement, and a transfer of the FHL, or combinations of these procedures.

As an alternative to the FHL tendon as a local autogenous graft, I have used an Achilles tendon allograft with a bone block attached to the calcaneus for management of degenerative tendinopathy or after infection. The rationale here is to obtain maximum use of the existing gastrocnemius soleus muscles in a patient who is otherwise healthy and who desires a return to athletic activity. It is never possible to return to full activity with the FHL transfer, nor is full strength regained with a V-Y advancement. If the disease process involving the Achilles tendon is extensive, the alternative of an allograft tendon remains an option. Use of the allograft, however, does not "burn any bridges," because the FHL tendon transfer can always be performed at a later date should the allograft fail.

I use either of two types of allografts, depending on the status of the calcaneus and the musculotendinous junction. If no tendon is left at all, then the full Achilles allograft is not ideal, because it is difficult to attach proximally. In such instances I use a hamstring graft. An example of this repair is shown in Figure 27-20, in which the patient presented with infection after operative treatment for tendon rupture, with extensive debridement of the entire tendon .

The Achilles allograft procedure is performed through a vertical incision made centrally down the back of the leg onto the posterior aspect of the calcaneus. If any Achilles tendon is present, this is excised except for a healthy portion left behind proximally, to which the graft is attached. The Achilles allograft bone is now fashioned into a block, which will fit into the posterior aspect of the calcaneal tuberosity. After the insertion of the Achilles tendon has been debrided, excised, and removed, a slot is cut out of the posterior calcaneus to facilitate insertion of the block of the allograft. I generally use two fully threaded cancellous 4.0-mm screws for fixation. Once this slot has been created, the key to the success of this operation is the tension on the repair (Figure 27-21).

The repair never seems to have enough equinus tension. Because this repair is performed with the patient in the prone position, I bend the patient's knee and flex the foot down into maximum equinus and pull proximally on the allograft tendon into equinus. Only while tension on the graft is maintained can the repair be performed. A running nonabsorbable 2-0 whip suture is inserted on either side of the allograft on the undersurface of the indigenous Achilles tendon. If only the distal portion of the Achilles tendon is involved and excised, an end-to-end repair, rather than a "vest over pants" repair, can be considered, but this decision will depend on the integrity and quality of the host Achilles tendon. Not surprisingly, healing takes longer than with a primary end-to-end repair.

For patients who have sustained a rupture that initially was treated nonoperatively, some elongation of the tendon often occurs during healing, with resulting weakness in peak torque, power, and strength. For these patients, although the tendon has healed, it has done so in an elongated position. In these symptomatic patients, excision of a segment of the Achilles tendon, followed by primary end-to-end repair, works well (Figure 27-22). For this central excision to be performed, the tendon is cut transversely 6 cm proximal

Figure 27-17 Acute rupture in a patient with chronic painful insertional tendinopathy. **A** and **B,** Note the bone lump at the insertion of the tendon and the degeneration at the tendon insertion. A small bone avulsion often occurs with this rupture. **C,** The posterior tuberosity is shaved to prepare the attachment for the tendon. **D,** The tendon is maintained in position with a suture anchor.

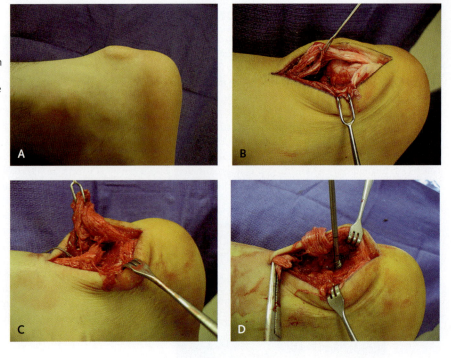

Figure 27-18 A and **B,** The patient was a 54-year-old man who had experienced 2 years of pain in the distal Achilles tendon and presented with an acute rupture of the Achilles tendon that had occurred 1 week earlier. **C** and **D,** The tendon could be advanced back to the calcaneus with the foot in equinus; however, owing to the degeneration present, after calcaneus ostectomy, transfer of the flexor hallucis longus tendon was performed in addition to the reattachment of the tendon.

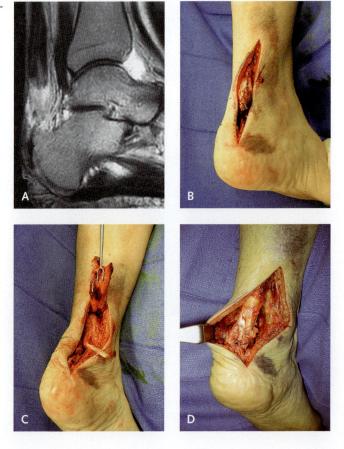

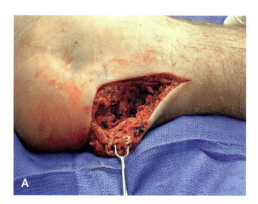

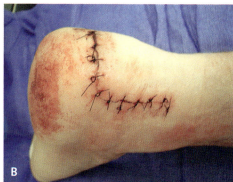

Figure 27-19 A and **B,** Note the hemorrhage in the tendon associated with this distal rupture. A J-incision was used for the approach to the tendon. The calcaneus then was debrided and the tendon reattached with an anchor.

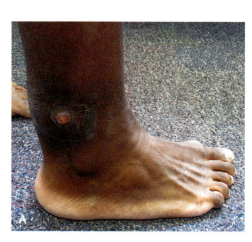

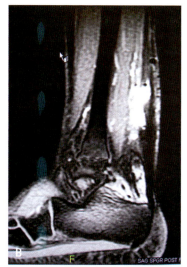

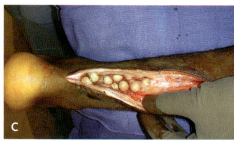

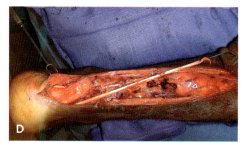

Figure 27-20 The patient was a 32-year-old athlete in whom operative treatment of a rupture of the Achilles tendon was followed by infection. **A** and **B,** At 1 year after the initial rupture, he presented with pus draining from two sinuses. **C,** The tendon was debrided, and antibiotic-impregnated cement beads were inserted for 6 weeks. **D** and **E,** On removal of the beads, a double-strand hamstring graft was used for reconstruction.

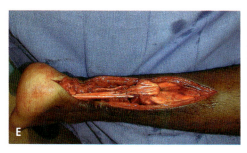

to the insertion. Two skin hooks are then placed on either end of the tendon, and the tendon is retracted proximally and distally. With the patient's knee flexed, the overlap of the two tendon ends is measured when the foot is held in 20 degrees of equinus. This overlap usually is approximately 1 to 2 cm; this segment is then cut out, followed by an end-to-end repair as described for the acute rupture.

The repair procedure is determined by the length of the gap. As a rule, if it is less than 2 cm, I repair the tendon end to end with the foot in slightly more equinus. Between 2 and 5 cm, a V-Y advancement works well, sometimes supplemented by the FHL tendon. For defects greater than 5 cm, then a tendon transfer or graft is required. For a gap in the tendon between 2 and

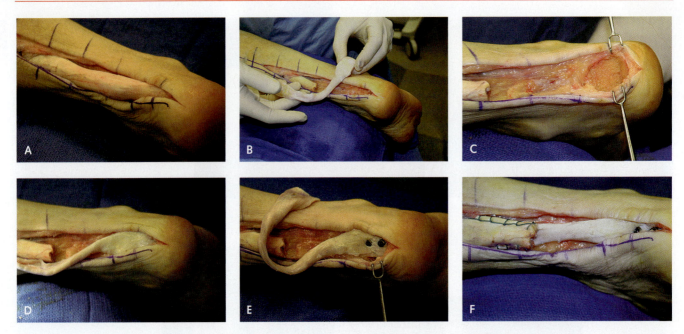

Figure 27-21 The patient was a 29-year-old athletically inclined woman who had sustained a rupture 2 years earlier. Nonoperative treatment at that time was followed by severe weakness and inability to return to function. **A,** At surgery, no viable tendon at all was present. **B,** The diseased tendon was excised. **C-E,** An Achilles bone tendon allograft was used for reconstruction. A bone defect was created in the calcaneus to receive the bone block graft, which was attached with two screws. **F,** The repair was sutured under tension.

5 cm, a V-Y tendon advancement works well. If the gap is greater than 5 cm, an adequate excursion of the tendon is difficult to obtain, and some detachment of the muscle then occurs, with a corresponding decrease in strength. A V-Y advancement is performed by measuring the gap and then doubling the length of the segment of the tendon to be advanced. The base of the V is distal, and the apex is extended proximally all the way up into the musculotendinous junction. The incision starts proximally at the musculotendinous junction at the apex of the V, and then the fascia is sharply cut but the muscle is less intact (Figures 27-23 and 27-24).

If the gap is greater than 5 cm, the V-Y advancement probably will not be sufficient on its own. Although the advancement procedure can still be used, a transfer of the FHL tendon, performed in the same manner as described previously for chronic tendinopathy, can be added. The alternative is to use an Achilles tendon allograft when no functional tendon is present, and the attachment of the graft is performed in the same manner as that described for tendinopathy (Figure 27-25).

The foot is immobilized in equinus in a removable boot for approximately 10 weeks, during which time active and passive range-of-motion exercises in the equinus position are performed, including swimming. Wound problems may occur during healing and must be promptly treated (Figure 27-26). If only an eschar is present, then I am not as concerned, although the skin should be kept as dry as possible. A wound vacuum-assisted closure (VAC) device is a very useful tool regardless of the appearance of the incision. Swimming is an excellent exercise for rehabilitation and can be done early on, approximately 3 to 4 weeks after repair once the incision is healed. The use of fins is encouraged for swimming in a pool, and a block to dorsiflexion can be constructed out of Orthoplast splint molded to the anterior ankle.

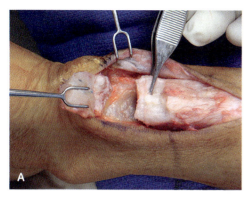

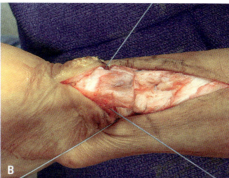

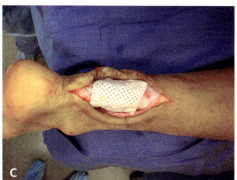

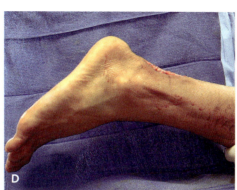

Figure 27-22 The patient was a 31-year-old man in whom an infection developed after attempted repair of an Achilles rupture 1 year earlier, resulting in marked scarring in the skin with functional lengthening of the tendon and weakness. **A** and **B,** To preserve function, the tendon was shortened with a "vest over pants" repair. **C** and **D,** The repair was covered with a biologic graft **(C)** under tension with the foot in equinus **(D)**. This was not successful, and reinfection occurred, necessitating use of a free flap and further surgery.

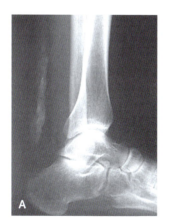

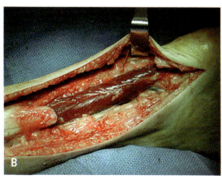

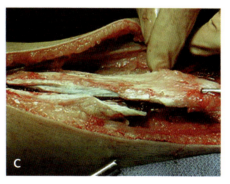

Figure 27-23 The patient was a healthy 42-year-old man who had experienced pain in the Achilles tendon for 20 years after a rupture of the tendon, which was treated nonoperatively. **A** and **B,** Such ossification of the tendon usually is not painful, but in this case, although good strength was noted at push-off, severe pain was present over the mass of calcified tendon, which was excised. **C,** The muscle was healthy, and although the flexor hallucis longus muscle could have been used here on its own, it was supplemented with a V-Y advancement to gain the necessary length for the reconstruction.

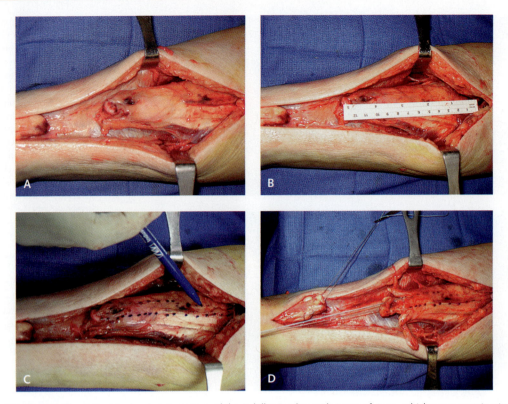

Figure 27-24 A-D, The patient had a chronic rupture of the Achilles tendon with a gap of 4 cm, which was reconstructed with a V-Y advancement of the tendon harvested from the musculotendinous junction, with repair under tension.

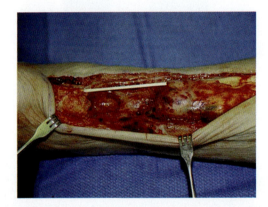

Figure 27-25 The gap in this chronic rupture measured 8.5 cm. Note the presence of the plantaris tendon. The options for treating this chronic rupture are limited. Although a tendon transfer with a flexor tendon such as the flexor hallucis longus can be used, the gap in this case is too great for repair by a V-Y advancement alone; an allograft was used to bridge the defect.

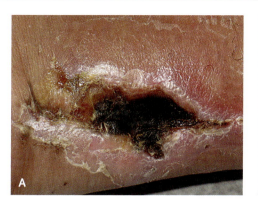
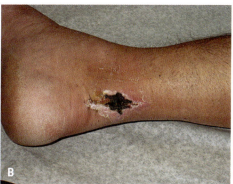
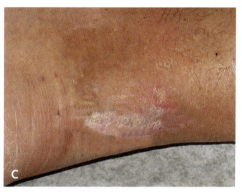

Figure 27-26 A-C, An infection occurred in the skin after repair of an acute rupture. A healthy eschar was present, so a wound vacuum-assisted closure (VAC) device was used to decrease drainage even though this was a closed wound. It took 7 weeks for the eschar to peel off uneventfully.

SUGGESTED READING

Assal M, Jung M, Stern R, et al: Limited open repair of Achilles tendon ruptures: A technique with a new instrument and findings of a prospective multicenter study, *J Bone Joint Surg Am* 84-A:161–170, 2002.

El Shewy MT, El Barbary HM, Abdel-Ghani H: Repair of chronic rupture of the Achilles tendon using 2 intratendinous flaps from the proximal gastrocnemius-soleus complex, *Am J Sports Med* 37:1570–1577, 2009.

Feibel JB, Bernacki BL: A review of salvage procedures after failed Achilles tendon repair, *Foot Ankle Clin* 8:105–114, 2003.

Heckman DS, Gluck GS, Parekh SG: Tendon disorders of the foot and ankle, part 2: Achilles tendon disorders, *Am J Sports Med* 37:1223–1234, 2009.

Jarvinen TA, Kannus P, Paavola M, et al: Achilles tendon injuries, *Curr Opin Rheumatol* 13:150–155, 2001.

Kann JN, Myerson MS: Surgical management of chronic ruptures of the Achilles tendon, *Foot Ankle Clin* 2:535–545, 1997.

Krahe MA, Berlet GC: Achilles tendon ruptures, re-rupture with revision surgery, tendinosis, and insertional disease, *Foot Ankle Clin* 14:247–275, 2009.

Maffulli N, Kader D: Tendinopathy of tendo Achilles, *J Bone Joint Surg Br* 84:1–8, 2002.

Mandelbaum BR, Myerson MS, Forster R: Achilles tendon ruptures: A new method of repair, early range of motion, and functional rehabilitation, *Am J Sports Med* 23:392–395, 1995.

Myerson MS: Achilles tendon ruptures, *Instr Course Lect* 48:219–230, 1999.

Myerson MS, McGarvey W: Disorders of the insertion of the Achilles tendon and Achilles tendinitis, *J Bone Joint Surg* 12:1814–1824, 1998.

Paavola M, Kannus P, Jarvinen TA, et al: Achilles tendinopathy, *J Bone Joint Surg Am* 84-A:2062–2076, 2002.

CHAPTER **28**

Rupture of the Anterior Tibial Tendon

The management of rupture of the anterior tibial tendon (ATT) depends almost entirely on the size of the gap present. Generally, ruptures occur in older persons as a consequence of degeneration and friction underneath the extensor retinaculum. The rupture is followed by a variable degree of retraction of the tendon. A small stump of tendon usually is left distally under the retinaculum, and the proximal stump retracts between 2 and 10 cm. The options for correction include an end-to-end repair, transfer of the extensor hallucis longus (EHL) tendon, a tendon graft interposition, and a V-Y lengthening advancement of the proximal ATT. The decision regarding which of these is performed depends on the strength of the limb, the presence of an equinus contracture, and the presence of any accessory claw toe deformities as a result of the rupture of the ATT or additional foot deformities. Even with early prompt diagnosis, degeneration of the tendon usually is present, with fraying of the tendon ends and retraction, and augmentation or supplementation of the tendon repair will be necessary. If the tendon exhibits minimal retraction, ideally it should be reattached to the medial cuneiform.

A very reasonable alternative is to insert the tendon into the navicular. For some years I performed a rerouting of the ATT (a modified Young procedure) for management of the adult flatfoot deformity. This was particularly useful if previous surgery for a flexible flatfoot deformity had failed. In this procedure, the ATT is not detached distally but is rerouted under the navicular to support the medial arch of the foot. What I observed is that there is no loss of dorsiflexion strength, and the transfer takes advantage of the slight inversion function of the ATT. Therefore, in the presence of a rupture of the ATT, and particularly if the foot is flat, I am inclined to insert the tendon into the navicular. This repair is very effective in cases in which retraction of the tendon is minimal but not enough length is available to reattach it distally into the cuneiform (Figure 28-1).

With this technique, I make a 2-cm incision over the dorsum of the midfoot in order to retrieve the stump of the anterior tibial tendon. A puncture is then made over the navicular to insert a suture anchor, which is done under fluoroscopic guidance to ensure correct positioning of the anchor. The sutures at the tip of the stump of the tendon are then passed subcutaneously out of the puncture incision used for the anchor. The sutures from the anchor are then passed subcutaneously into the longitudinal incision, with needles attached, and through the tendon. The tension on the tendon is

maximized by simultaneously pulling the sutures on the stump out distally through the puncture (see Figure 28-1).

If fixed clawing of the hallux is present as a result of accessory use of the EHL and extensor digitorum longus (EDL) tendons, then an arthrodesis of the hallux interphalangeal joint is ideal, and the EHL tendon can be used to augment the repair (Figure 28-2). A tendon graft works well in this instance, but it should be supplemented possibly with an EHL tenodesis to strengthen the repair. Positioning the foot in at least 10 degrees of dorsiflexion at the completion of the repair regardless of the technique is important.

The main problem with the final repair is the potential for wound dehiscence. Bowstringing of the repair always occurs, and because the extensor retinaculum is potentially deficient at the completion of the repair, the underlying skin is subjected to increased pressure from the repaired tendon. For this reason, I make the skin incision more lateral than the underlying repair and then raise the skin flap so that with closure, no pressure from the tendon is on the actual incision (Figure 28-3). Although bowstringing inevitably occurs, pressure from the tendon repair on the incision itself should be avoided. The other problem that occurs with all repairs is slight oversupination of the foot—an inevitable consequence of tightening the repair. This should not be of concern initially, although the foot position must be monitored during the recovery and rehabilitation phase. An Achilles tendon lengthening may be necessary to regain adequate dorsiflexion and to correct the position of the foot during the repair. The repair should be performed with minimal tension on the tendon, and the position of the foot *must* be passively correctable to at least 10 degrees of dorsiflexion without much resistance. Immediately postoperatively, use of a cast, rather than a splint, is preferable to hold the foot in dorsiflexion.

An incision is made along the central aspect of the foot at least 1 cm lateral to the position of the ATT and is deepened through subcutaneous tissues, and the nerves are retracted. The skin is retracted medially, the extensor retinaculum is incised longitudinally, and the tendon ends are visualized. Depending on when the rupture occurred, fibrillation and fraying of the tendon with degeneration at both ends are present. Frequently, the extensor retinaculum has to be incised distally to be able to identify the stump of the tendon. The proximal tendon is sutured with a No. 2 whip suture, and the tendon is then pulled distally. Maximal tension is applied to the tendon for 10 minutes to determine the mobility of the muscle and then obtain some relaxation with elongation of the tendon. The biggest challenge

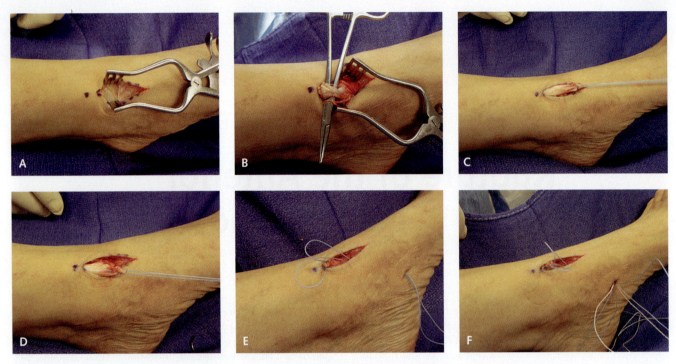

Figure 28-1 A and **B,** In this acute rupture, the anterior tibial tendon (ATT) could not reach the cuneiform. A graft was not thought to be necessary. **C-F,** The tendon stump was sutured, and a second incision made medially over the navicular for insertion of a suture anchor. The ATT suture was then pulled percutaneously out of the medial incision so that the appropriate tension on the repair could be generated, and the tendon was attached to the navicular.

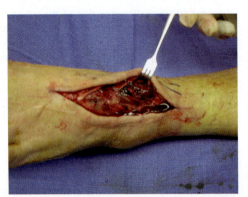

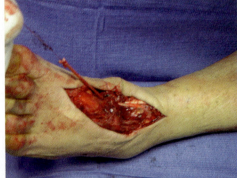

Figure 28-2 Acute-on-chronic rupture in a 73-year-old patient with a claw hallux deformity. **A,** Note the hemorrhage in the tendon. **B,** The tendon could not be repaired without a graft, and the extensor hallucis longus (EHL) was cut distally and passed deep to the retinaculum. **C,** The EHL was attached to the medial cuneiform under tension with the foot supinated and then woven through the anterior tibial tendon in a double thread to reinforce the repair.

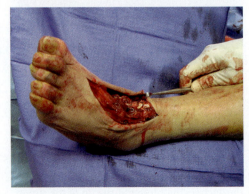

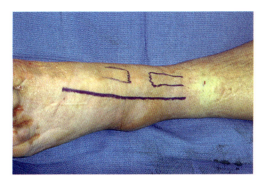

Figure 28-3 Note the planned incision, lateral to the path of the anterior tibial tendon, which will not place any pressure on the skin sutures.

with this repair is to obtain the correct tension; unless constant tension is applied at this time, elongation of the muscle develops later on, along with dorsiflexion weakness and a partial footdrop.

If an EHL tendon transfer is to be performed in conjunction with an interphalangeal joint arthrodesis, the arthrodesis is performed first. The EHL tendon is then cut on its distal portion and pulled distally to lie adjacent to the insertion point of the ruptured tendon. The length usually is sufficient for a double strand of the EHL tendon. The tendon is pulled distally and then secured over the distal stump or the medial cuneiform with a suture or suture anchor (see Figure 28-2). The distal portion of the EHL tendon is then pulled back up as a second strand and sutured down onto the proximal ATT under tension. Under usual circumstances, I do not like to harvest a normal, healthy, functioning tendon, and the only time the EHL tendon is used is when a fixed claw hallux deformity is present or if no other tendon tissue is available.

A turndown technique for repair of the ATT, as performed occasionally for the Achilles tendon, is not possible here because of the bulk of the tendon in the distal leg and ankle. Performing a V-Y advancement lengthening of the tendon is possible, however, provided that the muscle and proximal tendon are healthy. If a V-Y procedure is performed, the incision has to be made approximately 8 cm further proximally to facilitate exposure of the musculotendinous junction. The V-Y advancement is done in a standard fashion, with the amount of advancement double the length of the tendon gap after débridement of the tendon edges. The apex of the advancement is made in the extensor of the proximal tendon just at the musculotendinous junction and then is cut in a long V distally, with the base exiting at the tip of the stump of the ruptured tendon. Knowing the correct length is important, because the tip of the stump, if chronically ruptured, has to be debrided back to

reasonably healthy tendon. The suture is inserted after the distal tip of the tendon is debrided with a lock suture; then, by pulling on the sutures at the tip of the tendon, the V is advanced to the adjusted correct length. The V-Y limbs are now sutured with a running stitch of 2-0 fiber wire, and then with the foot in maximal dorsiflexion, the repair is performed distally.

If the tendon is chronically ruptured, then it is unlikely that the tendon remnant will be of any value in the repair. In such cases, a tendon graft is very useful. Usually, if I need to bridge the gap, I use a hamstring allograft. Two or three tendon strands are used and sutured in a routine manner under tension, as shown in Figure 28-4. In the case illustrated, the scarring of the tendon gives the erroneous impression of continuity of the ATT with other foot structures. For this repair, the hamstring graft was doubled up distally and then anchored with sutures into the cuneiform. Most important was the final closure of the retinaculum over the tendon repair, preventing bowstringing of the tendon into the subcutaneous tissue.

Management of an acute rupture that is diagnosed early on is far easier than treatment for one in which retraction of the tendon stump has occurred. Some organization of the tip of the tendon usually is seen after 2 weeks, which actually makes it easier to repair (much as with the Achilles tendon). In Figure 28-5, the patient was 66 years of age, and the repair was performed 2 weeks after rupture occurred. Slight hemorrhage in the tendon may be present. The suture anchor is inserted under fluoroscopic imaging. As noted, the rupture often occurs in an older patient, and degenerative changes of tendinopathy are characteristic. If the tendon is healthy, there is no need for augmentation, transfer, or grafting (Figure 28-6). If there is slight retraction only but the tendon cannot reach the cuneiform, then reattachment into the navicular is a reasonable option, particularly if there is an associated flatfoot deformity, as in Figure 28-7. In the case illustrated, note the use of a more medial incision, which was not directed over the substance of the ATT, thereby preventing compression from bowstringing of the tendon against the skin. The foot also was supinated at the completion of the procedure, and the ATT supported the medial arch much as in a modified Young procedure.

Regardless of the type of suture repair, the foot must be immobilized in dorsiflexion to at least 10 degrees and preferably 20 degrees during recovery. A cast is preferable to a postoperative splint, and this is split in the recovery room after surgery. Patients can start weight bearing in the cast at approximately 2 weeks once wound healing is apparent. A boot with a plantar flexion stop also is permissible, but any plantar flexion beyond neutral must be avoided during the recovery process for the first 8 weeks. Aggressive physical therapy with rehabilitation is important once the cast is removed, for the muscle to regain strength.

TECHNIQUES, TIPS, AND PITFALLS

- MRI is a useful imaging technique to identify the stump of the tendon. This is helpful in planning the type of necessary reconstruction, if any (Figure 28-8).

- The diagnosis of ATT rupture is easy if both feet are examined side by side, to detect the associated footdrop (Figure 28-9).

- Reattachment of the ATT to the cuneiform is ideal. If this is not possible then attachment into the

dorsomedial navicular is a good option, particularly if there is an associated flatfoot deformity, which the ATT repair will then correct.

- Tendon grafts are used for management of a large defect, when use of other adjoining tissue such as the EHL is not a good alternative solution.

Figure 28-4 A, Note the length of the post-rupture scar, which has the appearance of a stretched-out anterior tibial tendon but has no substance to serve as part of the repair. **B,** The extent of the rupture is evident. **C,** The suture anchor was inserted distally. **D** and **E,** The tendon graft was attached to the cuneiform by means of the suture anchor; a double strand was used **(E)**. The final repair was performed side to side. **F,** Note the excellent coverage of the reconstruction with the retinaculum.

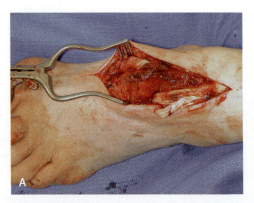
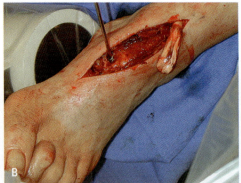
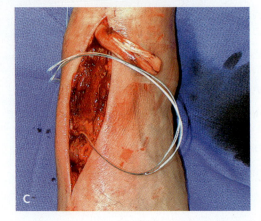

Figure 28-5 Spontaneous anterior tibial tendon rupture in a 68-year-old man, which was diagnosed 7 weeks later. **A,** Note the proximal splitting in the tendon with retraction. **B** and **C,** The medial cuneiform was identified fluoroscopically, and a suture anchor was inserted for direct repair and reattachment into the cuneiform.

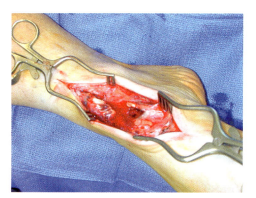
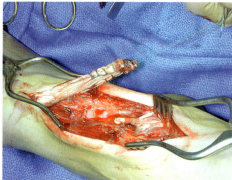
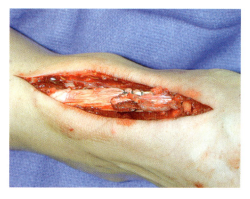

Figure 28-6   Acute traumatic rupture of the anterior tibial tendon in a 57-year-old patient, which was treated within 1 week. **A,** Although some degeneration of the tendon is evident, not much retraction of the tendon has occurred proximally. **B** and **C,** An end-to-end repair was performed without the need for augmentation.

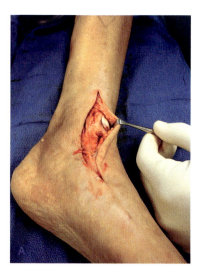
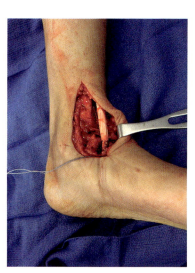
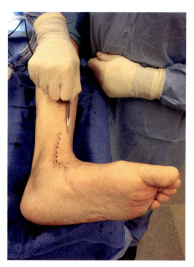

Figure 28-7   A and **B,** This rupture occurred with retraction of the tendon but not so much as to require a graft. The patient already had a flatfoot deformity, so attachment of the tendon to the navicular had the added benefit of treating the flatfoot by supporting the medial arch in a modified Young procedure. Note the medial incision, which is not directly over the anterior tibial tendon. **C,** The foot is supinated at the completion of the procedure.

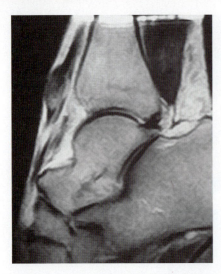

Figure 28-8 A chronic rupture of the anterior tibial tendon in a 67-year-old man. On magnetic resonance imaging, a bulge in the distal leg is visualized just proximal to the ankle, where the tendon has bunched up on the anterior aspect of the joint. Note also the talonavicular arthritis, with dorsal osteophytes on the distal talus, which probably was responsible for the attritional tear in this case.

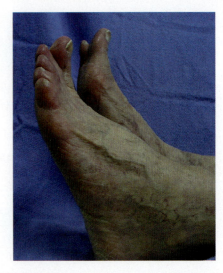

Figure 28-9 Footdrop associated with rupture of the anterior tibial tendon.

CHAPTER **29**

Peroneal Tendon Injury and Repair

Management of disorders of the peroneal tendons is not difficult, yet the results of treatment are not as predictable as expected. With peroneal tendon injury, prompt operative intervention seems to be more critical to a good outcome than with other tendon disorders—for example, injury to the posterior tibial tendon, for which a plethora of effective nonoperative treatment alternatives are available.

I have not found prolonged nonsurgical methods of treatment to be very successful with peroneal tendon disorders. Tenosynovitis may settle down (if the underlying cause is a self-limited process or one amenable to treatment by noninvasive means), yet progression to more extensive tears of the involved tendons is common. With such tears, the likelihood is that the pathologic changes will progress, leading to a far worse clinical condition with deformity and fewer options for reconstruction.

Magnetic resonance imaging (MRI) might be expected to be a useful diagnostic modality in the management of this spectrum of disorders. This has not been my experience, however, and I rely more on clinical evaluation than on MRI for decision making.

MANAGEMENT OF TENDINITIS

There are many causes of tendinitis or inflammatory-type symptoms related to tendon disease. If a patient presents after injury with pain behind the fibula or a fullness over the tendons associated with pain on resisted eversion, then either a tear or tenosynovitis is present. The cause may have been not a discrete injury but rather repetitive episodes leading to the presenting clinical problem. If the injury is not acute, then the likelihood is that either inflammation, constriction, or infiltration of the tendons is present. A common presentation may be that in which an area of pain behind the fibula is worsened by passive dorsiflexion of the ankle. Instead of a tear of the tendon, a low-lying muscle belly of the peroneus brevis is present, causing symptoms by virtue of the volume effect in the retinaculum (Figure 29-1). As the foot dorsiflexes, the tendons are sucked into the fibula groove, and if the muscle volume is increased, pain will develop from impingement.

Another, less common cause of pain other than acute inflammation is chronic fatty infiltration of the tendon (Figure 29-2). A typical clinical manifestation to be aware of is chronic pain distal to the tip of the fibula along the lateral calcaneus, where the tendons may be constricted as they pass in their separate sheaths along the peroneal tubercle. Although the tubercle may enlarge for no particular reason, enlargement definitely is more common in patients with heel varus or a cavus foot deformity. The pathomechanism

in such cases may be chronic friction and pressure of the tendons on the tubercle, causing hypertrophy. This constriction will cause thinning and narrowing of the tendons (Figure 29-3). The tendon changes will in turn be worsened by the increased stress on the tendons incurred when the heel is in varus. Insertional peroneus brevis tendinitis can occur but is surprisingly not very common. One unusual cause of insertional tendinitis has been identified as an unossified os vesalianum (Figure 29-4).

REPAIR OF ISOLATED TEARS OF THE PERONEAL LONGUS AND PERONEAL BREVIS TENDONS

For repair of isolated tears of the peroneal longus and peroneal brevis tendons, an incision is made along the length of the posterolateral ankle extending along the course of the tendons behind the fibula. The proximal and distal extent of the incision is determined once the disease is identified after the retinaculum is opened. Preserving the extensor retinaculum, particularly at the margin of the distal fibula, is important. If the superior peroneal retinaculum is not adequately preserved, dislocation of the peroneal tendon with recurrent tendinopathy and tearing will occur. The tendon generally is seen to be split longitudinally with tears within the substance of the tendon and those that are posteriorly located. Longitudinal splitting is especially likely when the tear is associated with ankle instability.

The decision has to be made whether to repair the split or to excise a portion of the tendon. Considerations in this decision include the size, length, and extent of the split. If at least 50% of the tendon can be preserved, then the split portion may be excised longitudinally. The remaining tendon can be left intact; if further splits are encountered, the tendon is "tubed" with a running absorbable suture (Figure 29-5). If ankle instability and peroneal splits are associated with heel varus, then all three components of the deformity can be addressed simultaneously using one extensile incision, through which the tendon repair, the ankle ligament reconstruction, and the peroneal repair can be performed (Figure 29-6). If the tear of the brevis tendon is extensive, reaching both proximal and distal to the fibula, a portion of the tendon may still be excised or even used as part of a nonanatomic ankle ligament reconstruction (Figure 29-7).

Tears of the peroneus longus generally occur distal to the fibula and are commonly constricted, split, or torn alongside the peroneal tubercle (Figure 29-8). Presence of focal pain along the

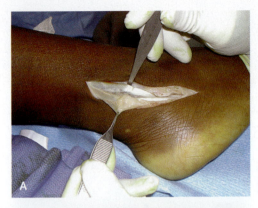

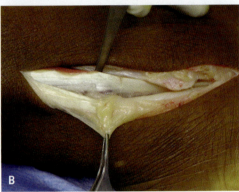

Figure 29-1 A and B, The patient experienced a persistent clicking and locking sensation proximal to the fibula. At surgery, fatty infiltration of the tendon sheath and brevis tendon was evident.

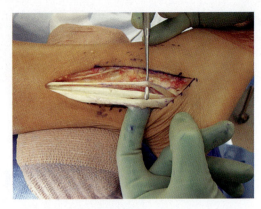

Figure 29-2 This patient presented with retrofobular pain and at surgary a peroneus quartus was idenfified under the clamp.

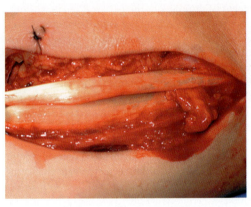

Figure 29-3 Tenosynovitis without rupture was noted in this patient following a hypesiflexion injury.

lateral margin of the calcaneus in proximity to the peroneal tubercle warrants prompt exploration, because a tear of the tendon can be prevented by releasing the retinaculum and removing the peroneal tubercle. If additional procedures are not required simultaneously, the peroneal sheath can be released endoscopically without excising the tubercle, but constriction may recur. The longus and brevis tendons distal to the fibula have a separate sheath, and both tendons should be opened with small scissors. The split in the tendon is identified under the separate retinaculum, and the peroneal tubercle is debrided if it is seen to be enlarged. I use bone wax on the raw abraded surface under the peroneal tubercle once the repair is done.

The cuboid is the more frequent location for a peroneus longus tendon tear in association with various pathologic conditions of the os peroneum as the tendon winds underneath the cuboid (Figure 29-9). Occasionally the os peroneum is visible radiographically, and its more proximal location from the undersurface of the cuboid indicates the rupture. Long-standing tears cannot be repaired in end-to-end fashion because the retracted portion of the tendon is difficult to reattach distally under the cuboid. The same limitation applies for a rupture that occurs at the junction of the os peroneum, because excision of the os peroneum frequently leaves a defect greater than 1 cm, which is difficult to repair. For a more acute injury, however, with careful excision of the os peroneum, the shell of the remaining longus tendon can be repaired by "tubing" the tendon as it passes under the cuboid (Figure 29-10). A decision has to be made, however, whether this atempt at repair is worthwhile (i.e., whether the tendon should be cut distally) and whether a tenodesis should be performed to the adjacent pero-

neus brevis tendon. This side-to-side tenodesis of the peroneus longus or peroneus brevis tendon is an acceptable procedure (see Figure 29-9); however, insertion of the peroneus longus into the cuboid is preferable. Although transfer of the longus to the brevis is commonly performed to realign a cavovarus foot deformity, I worry that scarring may cause symptoms distally in the normal brevis tendon. Generally, therefore, unless I specifically want to rebalance the hindfoot in a cavovarus deformity, a ruptured peroneus longus is inserted into the cuboid with an interference screw (Figure 29-11).

REPAIR OF BOTH THE PERONEUS LONGUS AND PERONEUS BREVIS TENDONS

More complex is the treatment of ruptures of both the peroneus longus and peroneus brevis tendons. These ruptures are difficult to repair, and the approach to combined tears will be determined by the presence of functioning tendon(s), the mobility of the remaining peroneal musculature, ankle stability, and the position of the heel. Peroneal muscle weakness often is associated with a cavovarus foot, and injury to the tendons of these muscles has a similar effect on the structural balance of the foot. A tear of the peroneus longus tendon with or without a concomitant peroneus brevis tendon tear results in net inversion of the hindfoot by the tibialis posterior muscle. In long-standing cases, this scenario

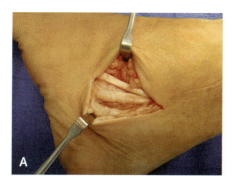
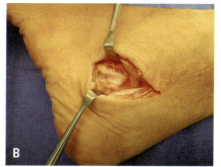
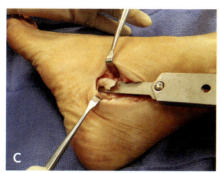

Figure 29-4 The patient experienced pain over the lateral calcaneus for 2 years. The diagnosis was correctly made on the basis of the size and prominence of the peroneal tubercle. **A,** At surgery, an enlargement of the longus tendon was noted. **B** and **C,** The enlarged tubercle was identified and removed.

results in a fixed varus hindfoot deformity, which also must be corrected.

As with an isolated rupture of either the longus or brevis tendons, any additional deformity must be addressed. Ankle ligament instability needs to be corrected, and if a varus heel is present, a biplanar or triplanar calcaneal osteotomy should be performed to decrease the force on the heel and protect the repair. It does not make any sense to perform a repair of the peroneal tendon in the setting of heel varus, which could lead to recurrent hindfoot instability and recurrent tearing of the tendon.

Although preoperative MRI is helpful, the true extent of the tendon disease generally is revealed only at the time of surgery. The condition of the tendons should be noted intraoperatively; when both are ruptured, an estimation is made of the type of rupture and the affected percentage of cross-sectional tendon area. If both tendons are grossly intact, then they are repaired in a standard manner by excision of the longitudinal tear and tubularization of the tendon using a running stitch of absorbable braided suture. If one tendon is completely torn and irreparable but the other tendon is considered functional or usable, then a tenodesis is performed proximally, with at the least the musculotendinous tissue or the healthy tendon distal to the muscle used for the tenodesis. The decision to include a tenodesis should be based on the health of the muscle, because no tenodesis should be performed if the excursion of the muscle of either tendon is absent as a result of scarring or presumed fibrosis. Alternatively, repair of one of the two tendons can be attempted, if the other is not salvageable, by either tendon grafting or a tendon transfer. A tendon graft can be used only if the peroneal muscles are healthy and demonstrate good excursion proximally. If the musculotendinous junction is scarred and has no mobility, then adding a tendon graft to a nonfunctioning muscle does not make sense. In

such cases, a transfer of the flexor digitorum longus (FDL) tendon is performed. A good example of this clinical problem is demonstrated in Figure 29-12. The patient had undergone two previous surgeries, resulting in severe scarring and tearing of both tendons. Neither tendon was reparable, so the brevis was completely excised and the longus was cut distally; then the stump of the longus tendon was attached to the brevis tendon distally to create a single tendon out of the two.

Another option for treatment of ruptures of both tendons is to perform a transfer of the FDL tendon to the peroneus brevis tendon, as in the case presented in Figure 29-13. The patient had undergone multiple previous surgeries, so after excision of the remnants of the tendons, significant scarring was present. In such cases, the FDL transfer can be performed immediately or as a staged procedure once scarring has settled. As stated quite correctly in a time-honored tenet of reconstruction, more surgery generally leads to more scarring; here, however, a silicone rod can be inserted in the retrofibular space, which will create a synovial lining, with the tendon transfer performed as a delayed operation. With this approach, at 6 weeks, when the second surgery is performed, the FDL tendon is attached to the tip of the silicone rod, which can be pulled distally without opening the entire incision. By this time a synovial lining to the tendon sheath has formed. Patients are encouraged to walk as soon as possible after the first procedure. The distal end of the silicone rod is attached to the stump of the brevis tendon, but the proximal end is left free to glide. At the second, staged procedure, the FDL tendon is attached to the tip of the silicone rod, and pulled distally to be sutured to the brevis tendon. This repair is illustrated again in Figure 29-14, in a patient with no peroneal tendons had a very unstable ankle but with no tissue that could be used for repair of the ankle ligaments. In addition to a

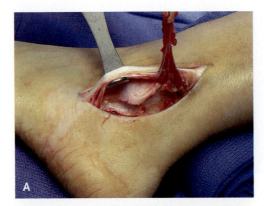

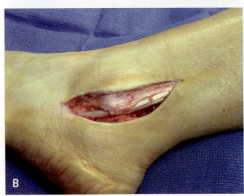

Figure 29-5 The patient presented with retrofibular pain of 6 months duration after sustaining an injury while playing basketball. The clinical findings were suggestive of a tendon tear. **A** and **B,** At surgery, an enlarged muscle was found, which was debrided, with subsequent resolution of symptoms.

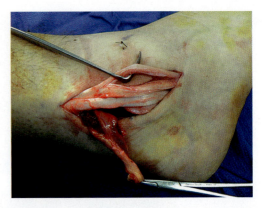

Figure 29-6 The intraopenative findings here were a split in the peroneus brevis tendon as well as an enlaiged hypertrophied musele, which was excised.

transfer of the FDL tendon, a free tendon graft was used to reconstruct the ankle ligaments.

In patients in whom both tendons are torn, but the muscle is healthy, with good excursion elicited by pulling on the musculotendinous junction, then a tendon graft can be performed. The free graft is first attached proximally to the healthy tendon or at the musculotendinous junction (Figure 29-15). When it is attached distally, the correct tension on the graft must be applied. The optimal degree of tension may be difficult to determine because no retinaculum is present, and the tendon graft may have a tendency to subluxate from behind the fibula. Once the suture attachment is performed distally, the retinaculum must be repaired to prevent dislocation. Two tendon grafts also were used for reconstruction in the case illustrated in Figure 29-16, which featured ankle instability and absence of ligamentous tissue suitable for repair; a graft reconstruction restored function of both tendons.

If a tendon transfer is indicated, I perform a FDL tendon transfer to the stump of the peroneus brevis tendon or the base of the fifth metatarsal. This transfer is preferable if there is no proximal muscle function or excursion. If, however, excursion of the proximal muscle is present, use of a tendon graft (with a hamstring allograft) seems more logical, but tendon grafting is contraindicated in the presence of muscle fibrosis. With either repair, it is important to determine the condition of the tissue bed. If active inflammation or fibrosis exists, then a nonfunctional result is likely as a consequence of scarring and limited tendon

excursion. The tendon transfer or graft procedure can be performed at the same sitting if there is minimal scarring. The silicone rod is inserted and attached to the distal stump of the brevis tendon or the base of the fifth metatarsal but is left free proximally. With this technique, passive range of motion performed postoperatively helps form a healthy synovium-lined tissue bed for the tendon graft or transfer. When the second-stage surgery is performed, a small incision is made proximally to attach the FDL tendon to the silicone rod, which can then be pulled out distally without another long incision. The FDL tendon always provides enough length.

Correcting any deformity of the hindfoot or ankle that could lead to recurrent tendon injury is important. Repair of an unstable ankle must be performed as a planned procedure that is based on preoperative symptoms of instability of the ankle confirmed with stress radiographs. If present, associated hindfoot varus is corrected with a closing wedge biplanar calcaneal osteotomy, and the same incision is used for the peroneal tendon repair as for the osteotomy. Peroneal tendon subluxation or dislocation without ankle instability is treated by a groove-deepening procedure. If peroneal tendon dislocation is present, in addition to ankle instability, then the ankle ligament reconstruction is performed with a modified Chrisman-Snook procedure, with the anterior split portion of the peroneus brevis tendon used for the reconstruction. The fibula groove is deepened, and the posterior limb of the split tendon, which passes through the fibula, is passed superficial to the remaining peroneal tendon(s) to maintain reduction of the tendon(s). Any tear or redundancy of the superior peroneal retinaculum is repaired.

REPAIR OF DISLOCATION OF THE PERONEAL TENDON(S)

Common to all repairs of a dislocated peroneal tendon is a groove-deepening procedure. An interesting dilemma arises with an acute dislocation in which the retinaculum is torn but the groove is reasonably well preserved. In this instance, and with other pathologic conditions such as snapping, subluxating, or "perching" tendons or chronic pain and tenosynovitis, I always consider deepening the groove (Figure 29-17). The simplest approach to correcting the dislocation is a deepening of the groove of the posterior fibula, by means of one method or another. My own preference is to use a large, oval-shaped burr.

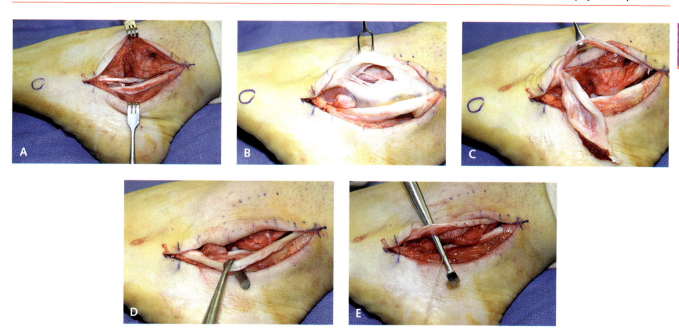

Figure 29-7 Repair of an isolated rupture of the brevis tendon. **A,** The lateral incision. **B** and **C,** Multiple splits in the tendon were present, and the bulk of the torn tendon was excised. **D** and **E,** This excision left approximately one third of the tendon, which was then repaired with a running stitch of 2-0 monofilament suture.

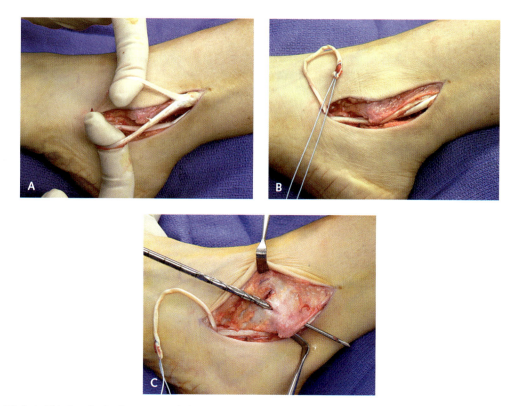

Figure 29-8 A, This longitudinal tear extended proximal and distal to the fibula. This was associated with ankle instability, (**B** and **C**), the anterior half of the tendon was used to augment ankle stability.

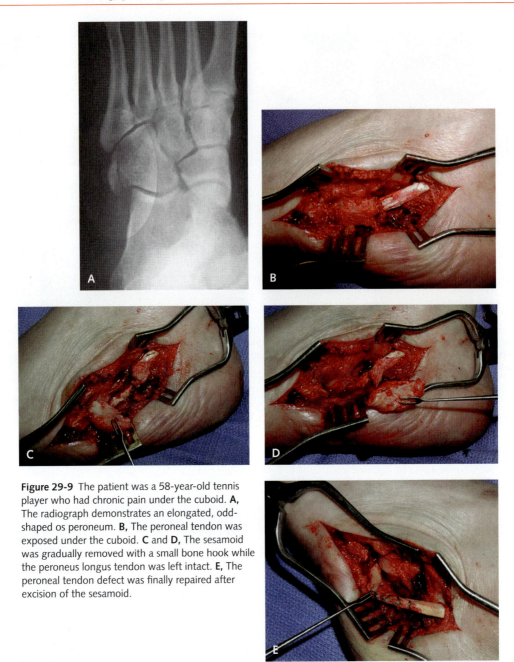

Figure 29-9 The patient was a 58-year-old tennis player who had chronic pain under the cuboid. **A,** The radiograph demonstrates an elongated, odd-shaped os peroneum. **B,** The peroneal tendon was exposed under the cuboid. **C** and **D,** The sesamoid was gradually removed with a small bone hook while the peroneus longus tendon was left intact. **E,** The peroneal tendon defect was finally repaired after excision of the sesamoid.

The incision for the dislocation must be made carefully, and the tendons must be palpated in the dislocated or subluxated position above the fibula. With location of the tendons thus confirmed, the superior peroneal retinaculum can be cut on the fibula itself; then, as the retinacular and periosteal flap is raised off the fibula, the flap serves as part of the soft tissue repair once the groove is deepened (Figure 29-18). The soft tissue and periosteal flap are raised off the fibula completely, and then the peroneal tendons and the periosteal flap are reflected posteriorly. Some surgeons recommend a tamp-type procedure wherein a periosteal flap is raised off the fibula, and then the fibula is tamped down deep in the groove. With this procedure, however, the fragment of the bone commonly remains slightly loose and does not adhere to the edge of the fibula adequately. I prefer to perform a simpler deepening of the groove using a burr. Once the groove is created, the distal tip of the fibula should not have a rough edge because of the associated potential for additional tearing of the tendon as it winds under the fibula.

With the foot in dorsiflexion, the tendons should sit behind the fibula without any tendency to subluxate whatsoever. The roughened groove is smoothed with bone wax, and all loose pieces of wax should be removed; then the retinaculum is reattached to the underside of the fibula (Figures 29-19 and 29-20). This reattachment must be fairly snug; otherwise, the tendons have a tendency to subluxate into a pouch created by the redundant retinaculum. Therefore cutting the retinaculum so it fits directly underneath the trough created by the groove-deepening procedure is frequently necessary. The retinaculum is reattached through Kirschner wire (K-wire) holes. Two pairs of K-wire holes are made so that pairs of sutures can be inserted through the fibula into the retinaculum; then the retinaculum is pulled in underneath the fibula, as depicted in Figure 29-21.

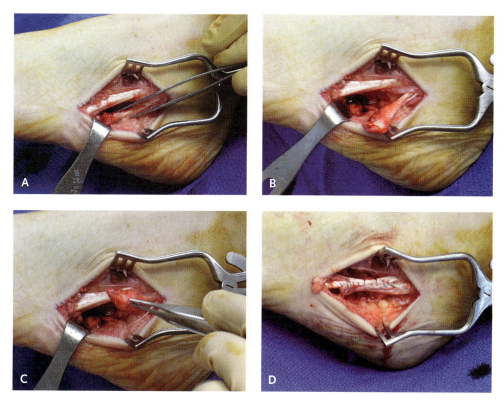

Figure 29-10 **A** and **B,** An acute rupture of the peroneus longus tendon at the level of the os peroneum. **C,** The os peroneum is held in the forceps. The tendon could not be repaired, **(D)** and a side-to side tenodesis to the peroneus brevis tendon was performed.

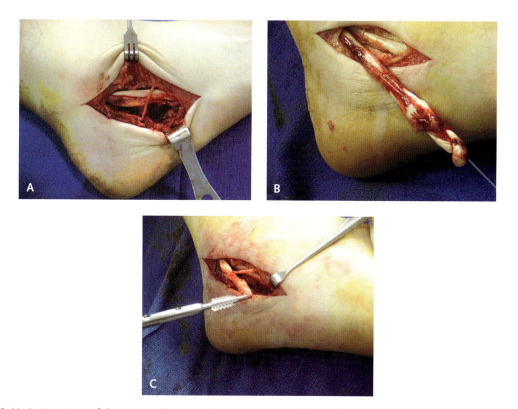

Figure 29-11 Acute rupture of the peroneus longus tendon in a professional baseball player. **A,** Note the hemorrhage in the tendon. **B,** The tendon was cut and shortened. **C,** It was then reattached to the cuboid in a tunnel with an interference screw.

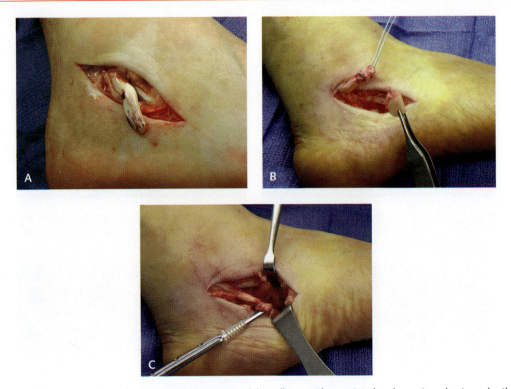

Figure 29-12 The patient sustained an acute inversion injury while walking, with associated ecchymosis and pain under the cuboid. **A,** Note the slight hemorrhage in the distal tendon. **B,** Rupture occurred at the os peroneum. **C,** The os peroneum was excised, and the peroneus longus was inserted with an interference screw into the cuboid.

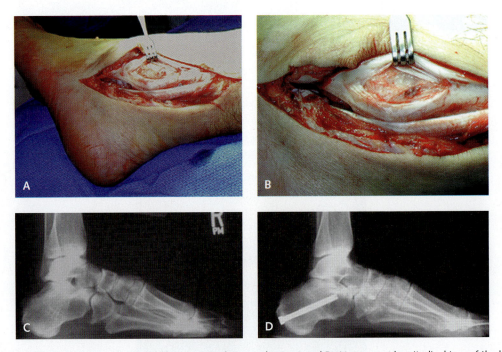

Figure 29-13 This patient presented with hindfoot varus and peroneal pain. **A** and **B,** At surgery a longitudinal tear of the brevis was noted, the split tendon was excised, and the remaining half of the tendon repaired with a running suture. A calcaneus osteotomy was then performed. **C** and **D,** The preoperative and postoperative radiographs following osteotomy are presented.

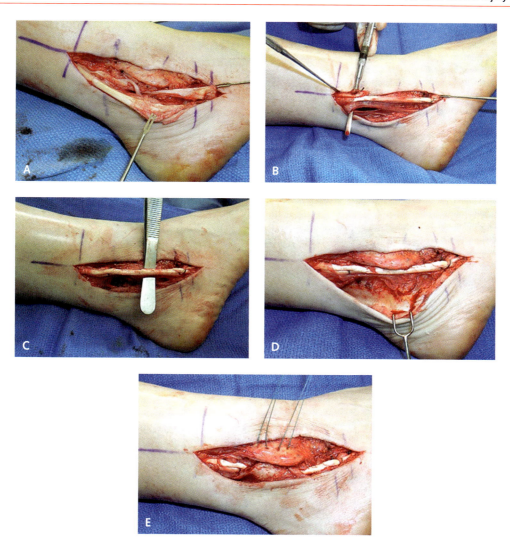

Figure 29-14 A, In this case, both brevis and longus tendons were torn; however, the muscles of both tendons were still capable of excursion. **B** and **C,** The torn longus tendon was cut distally and transferred into the stump of the torn brevis tendon distally, and a tenodesis of the longus tendon to the muscle of the brevis tendon was performed proximally. **D** and **E,** The fibula groove was deepened, and a retinaculum was created from the retrocalcaneal tissue and brought up into the fibula through K-wire holes.

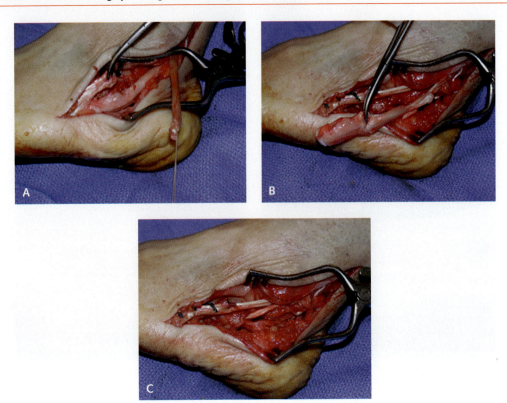

Figure 29-15   A-C, Exposure required for insertion of a hamstring graft to reconstruct complete loss of both peroneal tendons. The graft was attached proximally, using a weave into the peroneals, and then placed under appropriate tension distally.

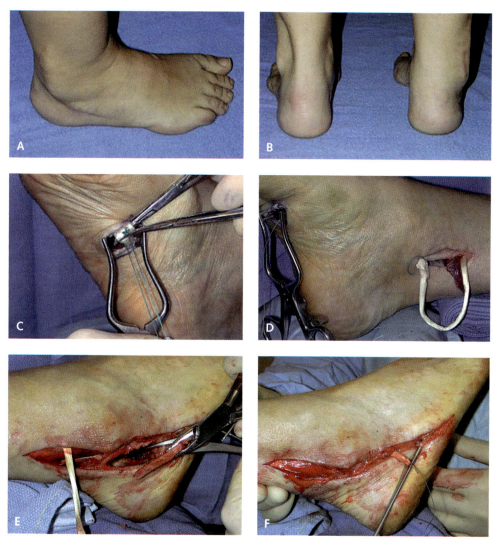

Figure 29-16 A and **B,** This patient presented after failed surgery to repair the torn peroneal tendon. Note the varus deformity of the hindfoot. **C** and **D,** The flexor digitorum longus was harvested from the arch of the foot and a side-to-side tenodesis performed to the flexor hallucis longus. The flexor digitorum longus was not pulled into the medial incision on the distal leg. **E** and **F,** The tendon was transferred from the tibia and fibula to be inserted at the base of the fifth metatarsal using a suture anchor. Note the addition of a calcaneal osteotomy to correct the varus deformity.

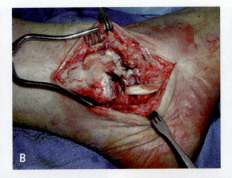
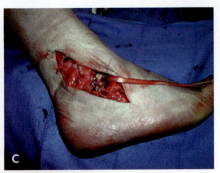
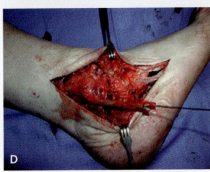
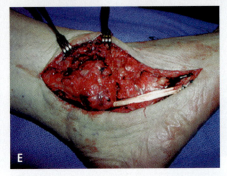

Figure 29-17 **A,** Severe ankle instability in a patient with no functioning peroneal, and marked hindfoot varus deformity. **B,** Note the appearance on dissection with the scarred stump of the peroneus longus and brevis tendons. **C,** A hamstring allograft was used to perform a reconstruction of the unstable ankle. **D** and **E,** A transfer of the flexor digitorum longus tendon was then performed and attached to the stump of the brevis tendon.

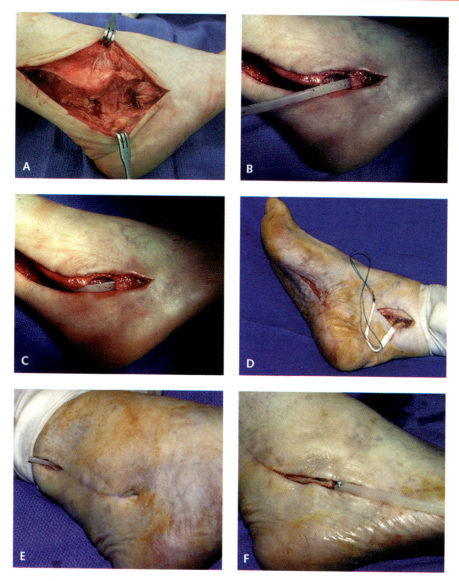

Figure 29-18 Staged flexor digitorum longus (FDL) tendon transfer. **A** and **B,** At surgery, absence of both peroneal tendons was noted, with severe scarring of the retrofibular space. **C,** A 20-cm silicone rod was attached to the stump of the peroneal brevis tendon, but it was left free proximally for use in FDL tendon transfer at 6 weeks. Until the second-stage surgery, active movement of the foot and ankle was encouraged. **D** and **E,** At the second procedure, the FDL tendon was harvested **(D)** and attached to the proximal end of the silicone rod and then pulled out distally in the synovium-filled tunnel created by the silicone foreign body, and the FDL tendon was attached distally **(E** and **F).**

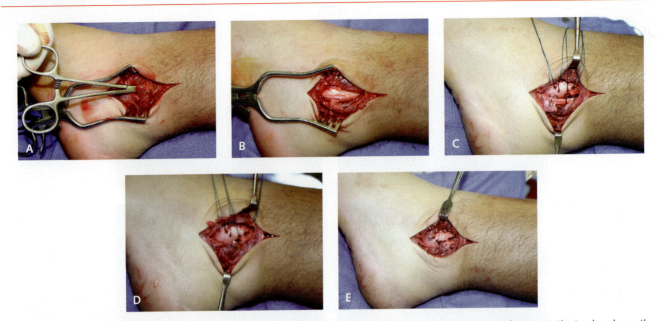

Figure 29-19 An acute dislocation in a young patient. **A,** A clamp was inserted under the retinaculum, to prevent damage to the tendons beneath. **B,** The tendons were exposed. **C-E,** The retinaculum was repaired using two pairs of sutures passed through drill holes in the fibula.

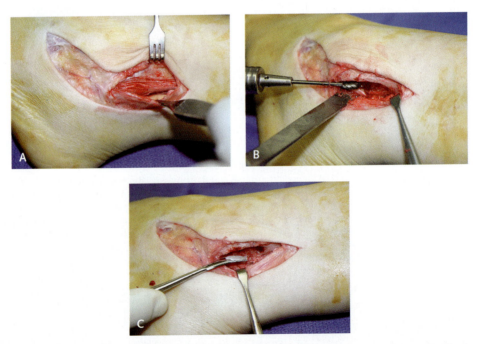

Figure 29-20 A, Chronic recurrent dislocation without tendon tearing. **B,** The fibula groove was deepened with a burr, and then a tamp was used to compress the cancellous bone. **C,** Before repairing the retinaculum, bone wax was applied to the roughened fibular surface.

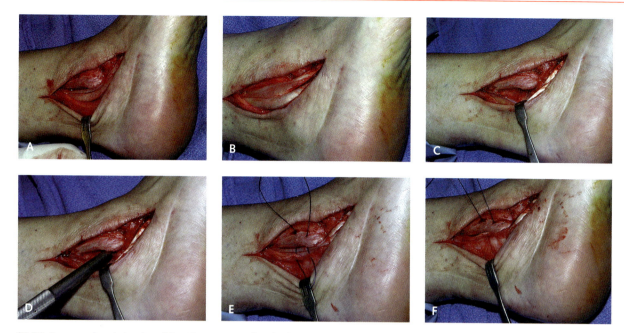

Figure 29-21 Peroneus brevis tendon dislocation associated with chronic pain. **A,** The retinaculum was opened and found to be quite redundant. **B,** By rotating the ankle, the tendon could easily be dislocated. **C** and **D,** The groove was deepened with a burr and then by tamping the posterior fibula. **E** and **F,** The tendons are now reduced but are maintained in the reduced position through securing the retinaculum with sutures under the fibula.

TECHNIQUES, TIPS, AND PITFALLS

- Determination of the extent of the tearing of the tendon ahead of surgery often is not possible. Although MRI is useful, it does not play a role in clinical decision making.

- A rupture of the peroneus brevis tendon frequently is associated with ankle instability, and manual stress testing of the ankle should be performed in conjunction with the repair.

- If the ankle is unstable and a longitudinal split or tear of the peroneus brevis tendon is present, the split can be extended distally and proximally, and then the anterior limb of the peroneus brevis tendon can be used to perform a reconstruction by means of a Chrisman-Snook procedure.

- Rupture of either peroneal tendon occurs commonly in association with an enlarged peroneal tubercle and is particularly large in patients with a varus hindfoot.

- With any repair distal to the fibula, both tendon sheaths must be opened to rule out stenosis as each tendon passes in a separate sheath. In particular, the peroneal tubercle must be debrided if prominent. This tubercle often is the source for isolated stenosis and tearing distal to the fibula.

- Distal tears of the peroneus brevis tendon are relatively uncommon. Isolated insertional peroneus brevis tendinopathy does occur in conjunction with varus hindfoot or recurrent trauma to the base of the fifth metatarsal.

- If either the peroneus brevis or the peroneus longus tendon is completely torn and not salvageable, a decision must be made about the potential use of the remaining tendon, as indicated by excursion of the muscle. If, for example, the peroneus longus tendon is completely torn and irreparable but muscle function is still adequate and excursion of the longus tendon is noted, then a tenodesis of the distal stump of the longus tendon to the brevis tendon is performed.

Continued

TECHNIQUES, TIPS, AND PITFALLS—cont'd

- Occasionally the enlarged peroneal tubercle may be the source of the tear of the peroneus brevis tendon. This pathomechanism seems to be fairly common in a cavus or varus hindfoot. As the tubercle enlarges, the retinaculum tightens, causing a constriction with consequent rupture. Removing the enlarged tubercle with a chisel followed by application of bone wax on the roughened bone surface is useful.

- Rupture of both tendons associated with a varus hindfoot deformity is preferably treated with a transfer of the FDL tendon and an osteotomy of the calcaneus (Figure 29-22).

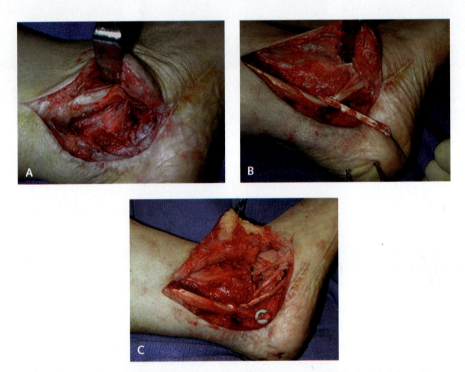

Figure 29-22 A, Dislocation of the peroneal tendons occurs commonly after untreated fractures of the calcaneus, with widening of the tuberosity. **B** and **C,** After a subtalar arthrodesis (shown here), a modified Chrisman-Snook procedure was performed, and the tendon was attached to the calcaneus with a screw and a spiked ligament washer.

SUGGESTED READING

Baumhauer JF, Nawoczenski DA, DiGiovanni BF, Flemister AS: Ankle pain and peroneal tendon pathology, *Clin Sports Med* 23:21–34, 2004.

Clarke HD, Kitaoka HB, Ehman RL: Peroneal tendon injuries, *Foot Ankle Int* 19:280–288, 1998.

Krause JO, Brodsky JW: Peroneus brevis tendon tears: Pathophysiology, surgical reconstruction, and clinical results, *Foot Ankle Int* 19:271–279, 1998.

Molloy R, Tisdel C: Failed treatment of peroneal tendon injuries, *Foot Ankle Clin* 8:115–129, 2003:ix.

Pelet S, Saglini M, Garofalo R, et al: Traumatic rupture of both peroneal longus and brevis tendons, *Foot Ankle Int* 24:721–723, 2003.

Raikin SM: Intrasheath subluxation of the peroneal tendons. Surgical technique, *J Bone Joint Surg Am* 91(Suppl 2 Pt 1):146–155, 2009.

Redfern D, Myerson MS: The management of concomitant tears of the peroneus longus and brevis tendons, *Foot Ankle Int* 25:695–707, 2004.

Squires N, Myerson MS, Gamba C: Surgical treatment of peroneal tendon tears, *Foot Ankle Clin* 12:675–695, 2007.

Walther M, Morrison R, Mayer B: Retromalleolar groove impaction for the treatment of unstable peroneal tendons, *Am J Sports Med* 37:191–194, 2009:Epub Oct 16, 2008.

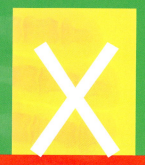

Ankle Instability and Arthrodesis

X

CHAPTER **30**

Tarsal Coalition

OVERVIEW

Regardless of the type of tarsal coalition present, once the condition becomes symptomatic, it rarely resolves with nonoperative care. Traditional management has been with immobilization of the foot to decrease symptoms, but the beneficial effects thus obtained usually are not long-lasting. Although this treatment may temporarily decrease the soreness in the foot, the reactive tenderness in the lateral calf musculature, and the generalized lower limb dysfunction and aching, symptoms recur. Rarely, therefore, do I recommend immobilization of the limb in either a child or an adult for definitive treatment purposes. If marked foot and limb tenderness is present, immobilization can be used initially until definitive surgical plans are put into effect.

EXAMINATION AND DECISION MAKING

Tarsal coalition is one condition that the clinician can diagnose standing at the door of the examination room. Typically, when the patient is seated, the foot normally drops into a position of equinovarus. With a rigid hindfoot, the foot is held in valgus; if the deviation is unilateral, it is particularly easy to diagnose. Examination of the foot while the patient is standing, walking, sitting, and lying down is recommended. When a person with a normal foot is sitting, a natural equinovarus posture is present in the foot as it relaxes. This is not the case with a tarsal coalition because the foot is held in a more rigid position of neutral dorsiflexion with slight valgus (Figure 30-1). The peroneal tendons often are visible because of ongoing contraction, but true peroneal "spasm" does not occur. The peroneal musculature may be tender and certainly tight as a result of subtalar joint irritation, but true spasm does not occur. The decision for surgery, and for a specific type of surgery, is based on the flexibility of the foot, the presence of arthritis, the type of coalition, and function of the remaining foot. The spectrum of clinical deformity associated with coalition is very broad, and when rigidity is present, marked compensatory changes may be seen in the hindfoot and forefoot (Figure 30-2).

Arthritis of the foot is rare in a child in association with either a subtalar or calcaneonavicular coalition. The beaking of the talonavicular joint appears naturally as a result of traction on the anterior capsule of the ankle on the neck of the talus and does not in any way imply the presence of arthritis. Arthritis can occur, however, as indicated by the common finding of subtalar arthritis in adults with a middle facet coalition. Early arthritis is caused by previous surgery or may be associated with extreme rigidity, even in the child. An important point in this context is that presence of motion in the hindfoot does *not* rule out a coalition. Careful examination of the foot will show that most of this motion originates from either a transverse tarsal or the ankle joints. True subtalar motion is not normal and usually is absent, particularly with a middle facet coalition.

It is not easy to examine the hindfoot for true motion when the peroneal tendons are contracting. In patients who have severe stiffness, determination of how much true motion is present in the foot and how much the peroneal muscles are limiting subtalar motion is worthwhile. If the peroneal muscles are tight, I block the peroneal nerve at the fibular neck with a short-acting local anesthetic and then reexamine the foot. After peroneal nerve blockade has been achieved, the foot frequently is much easier to examine, the rigidity of the hindfoot previously noted is no longer present, and the surgery can be planned correctly. A diagnostic blockade of the subtalar joint or the sinus tarsi is not very helpful in these patients. Sometimes the coalition is not visible on radiologic evaluation, and, rarely, even with magnetic resonance imaging (MRI) and computed tomography (CT) scanning, the coalition is difficult to visualize (Figure 30-3).

Whenever possible, I attempt resection of a coalition rather than an arthrodesis. Certainly, in the presence of arthritis of the hindfoot joints, an arthrodesis will be necessary, but in my experience, the arthrodesis is overused as a treatment modality in both adults and children. If arthrodesis is performed, a triple arthrodesis is indicated only with extensive deformity, which includes the subtalar and transverse tarsal joints as well as arthritis. A triple arthrodesis is therefore not required for correction of a middle facet coalition unless additional disease is present in the transverse tarsal joint. An interesting example of this problem, occurring in an adolescent patient with severe bilateral coalition, is presented in Figure 30-4. Not only was the hindfoot fixed in valgus, but the midfoot also was severely abducted. This was a double middle facet–calcaneonavicular coalition (see Figure 30-4). Rarely do I perform an arthrodesis for a calcaneonavicular coalition, even in adults.

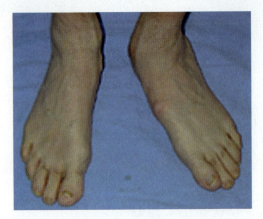

Figure 30-1 Note the severe unilateral flatfoot deformity. In children, very little other than a rigid tarsal coalition will be associated with or cause this unilateral deformity.

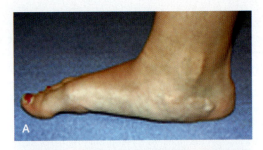

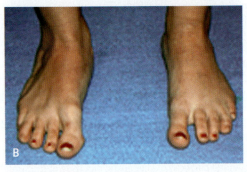

Figure 30-2 The spectrum of deformity with coalition is considerable. **A,** The right foot in this adolescent was rigid. **B,** Note, however, the marked elevation of the first metatarsal and the compensatory flexion of the hallux. Once the hindfoot deformity is corrected, the forefoot supination will worsen, and additional correction must be anticipated.

The onset of pain in adults with a calcaneonavicular coalition often follows a minor episode of trauma. This condition is the subject of frequent dispute in worker's compensation claims. Imaging studies in affected patients clearly show a tarsal coalition, which was previously asymptomatic; as a result of a minor twist or trauma, the condition becomes symptomatic. Excision of a calcaneonavicular coalition in the adult is still worth the effort. Provided that no degenerative changes are present and the foot is not too rigid, resection can restore a surprising degree of mobility, with good relief of symptoms. This procedure is not appropriate, however, for symptomatic subtalar coalition in the adult, which usually requires a subtalar arthrodesis.

It has been stated that "a middle facet coalition in a child can be excised if it involves less than 50%." I do not agree with this statement, and regardless of the extent of the coalition, I perform a resection of the entire coalition. The outcome with resection of the middle facet coalition depends more on the flexibility and deformity of the remainder of the foot. The problem with a complete coalition is not with the ability to resect it but with the adaptive changes that have taken place over time in the subtalar joint and the remainder of the foot (Figure 30-5).

The question, then, is not whether to resect the coalition but which additional procedures need to be performed to maintain motion and improve function, including calcaneal osteotomy, subtalar arthroereisis, Achilles tendon lengthening, and medial cuneiform osteotomy. The more unusual coalitions, either talonavicular or calcaneocuboid, also are encountered, and not infrequently. These present a unique set of problems, including stiffness of the hindfoot, planovalgus deformity, and a ball-and-socket ankle. The foot is always pronated, the hindfoot is fixed in valgus, and the ankle is in valgus as well.

RESECTION OF A MIDDLE FACET COALITION

As noted earlier, I attempt a resection of a middle facet coalition regardless of the extent noted on the radiograph or CT scan. This decision is based, however, on other factors as well, including the age of the patient, the shape of the foot, the extent of rigidity, and presence of associated deformity of the rest of the foot. An incision is made medially and extends from the undersurface of the medial malleolus distally and beyond the talonavicular joint. The incision is deepened through subcutaneous tissue, veins are cauterized, and the sheath of the flexor digitorum longus (FDL) tendon is opened (Figure 30-6). This tendon forms the upper boundary of the coalition, and the tendon is retracted dorsally. Inferior to this and under the sustentaculum tali, the sheath of the flexor hallucis longus (FHL) tendon is now carefully opened and identified. The tendon is retracted inferiorly; the FDL and FHL tendons mark the boundaries for dissection of the coalition. Elevation of all of the soft tissue, including a large periosteal flap from the sustentaculum, is useful to adequately visualize the bone to be resected. If necessary, the surgeon can proceed more distally to the talonavicular joint and then work back posteriorly after opening up the joint, but this precaution usually is not necessary.

The sustentaculum is now gradually removed until the scar of the original middle facet is visualized, which is seen slightly more posteriorly. A large, pineapple-shaped burr can be used above the sustentaculum; my own preference, however, is to use a combination of a rongeur, curette, and chisel. One way of identifying the location of the anterior aspect of the coalition is to make a lateral puncture in the sinus tarsi and then insert a probe, which is advanced and pushed medially. The exit point of this probe marks the anterior aspect of the coalition. If the probe does not expose the margin of the coalition, I use a cannulated sizer from the arthroereisis screw set, and as this is advanced across the tarsal canal, the coalition opens up quite easily and the margins of posterior facet become more visible. As the bone is gradually debrided, a rongeur is now inserted once fatty tissue is observed on the medial aspect of the sinus tarsi. This point represents the apex of the cone of the tarsal canal. Once this apex can be identified, then the rest of the procedure is much easier, because movement of the subtalar joint directs the dissection.

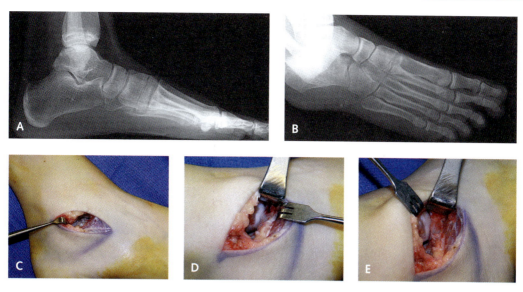

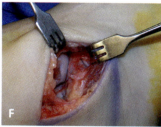

Figure 30-3 The patient was a 14-year-old girl who experienced constant pain in the sinus tarsi. **A** and **B,** Appearance of the foot on the plain radiograph and magnetic resonance imaging scan (not shown) was normal, with no evidence of a calcaneonavicular coalition. **C,** At surgery, the standard approach to the sinus tarsi was used. **D,** The head of the talus was identified. **E** and **F,** The large fibrocartilaginous band extending from the neck of the calcaneus to the navicular was then easily identified and resected.

A laminar spreader is inserted into the tarsal canal from the medial side, and then, with gradual distraction, the middle facet and ultimately the posterior facet become visible. Removal of most, if not all, of the middle facet is necessary until the entire posterior facet is visible. Perfect, unrestricted motion of the posterior facet should be present; passive rotatory motion is performed as a visual check.

Once the resection of the coalition is completed, the foot must be inspected and any deformity assessed. Some heel valgus with abduction across the transverse tarsal joint often is present, and additional procedures need to be planned carefully. If the hindfoot is left in valgus, medial stress increases, and with the lack of support of the sustentaculum, gradual collapse of the midfoot will occur, with increasing pes planus. If heel valgus and not midfoot abduction is present, I add an arthroereisis to the excision of the middle facet coalition (Figure 30-7). This procedure can be done almost under direct visualization, because the medial aspect of the subtalar implant is visible and protrudes from the resected portion of the coalition. In addition to slightly inverting the heel, this arthroereisis slightly opens up the posterior facet, which is desirable. I try to leave these implants in for at least 6 months in the child so that as the foot grows, an adaptive change, which is helped along with a good orthotic arch support, takes place in the hindfoot.

Excision of the middle facet coalition works well for adolescents. The age limit for excision is not clear, and although I have performed resection in the young adult, the results are less predictable. Certainly, arthrodesis is to be avoided in the younger child, and although an extraarticular arthrodesis may be performed (Figure 30-8), this is not my preferred procedure. If the foot is extremely rigid, then arthrodesis of the subtalar joint may have to be performed. It is worthwhile to resect the dorsal osteophyte off the neck

of the talus simultaneously, because this may cause impingement against the deep peroneal nerve and pain. In order to correct the deformity, if the subtalar arthrodesis is performed from a standard lateral approach, the entire coalition must be loosened. If the middle facet is not opened, then the hindfoot deformity cannot be corrected. From the lateral aspect of the sinus tarsi, an osteotomy is performed across the middle facet until the entire joint can be opened with a laminar spreader. The joint is debrided in standard manner, and then the hindfoot valgus is corrected by internally rotating the foot on the calcaneus. This rotation automatically improves the pitch angle of the calcaneus as well as the talocalcaneal axis. The maneuver also may cause the forefoot to supinate, in which case an opening wedge osteotomy of the medial cuneiform will need to be performed simultaneously (Figure 30-9).

EXCISION OF THE CALCANEONAVICULAR COALITION

An incision is made in the sinus tarsi and is extended from the tip of the fibula over toward the base of the fourth metatarsal. After resection of the coalition has been accomplished, either the extensor brevis muscle can be inserted as an interposition soft tissue flap, or copious bone wax can be applied to the resected surfaces. If the brevis muscle is used as an interposition flap, the condition of the skin over the lateral aspect of the foot will be fairly tenuous, and care must be taken with skin closure. This insertion has the advantage of presence of a large muscle surface, preventing bone formation. The disadvantage of this technique is that it leaves a rather substantial hollow on the lateral aspect of the foot, which may not be cosmetically desirable. Nonetheless, some covering of the bone becomes necessary.

Figure 30-4 Certain deformities defy resection. **A,** Bilateral rigid foot deformities with a double coalition (calcaneonavicular and middle facet) in a skeletally mature adolescent patient. **B,** Radiographic changes were confirmed by a computed tomography scan *(not shown)*. **C,** A triple arthrodesis was the only realistic surgical alternative. The osteophyte present on the dorsal neck of the talus, which should have been removed at this procedure, and was resected subsequently owing to impingement against the deep peroneal nerve and discomfort with shoes.

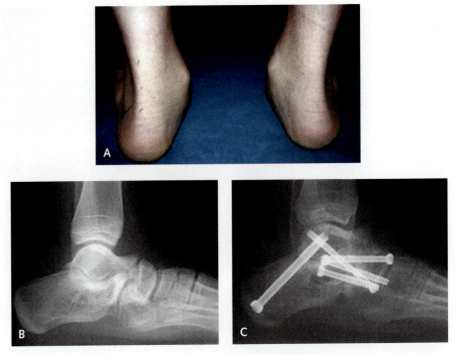

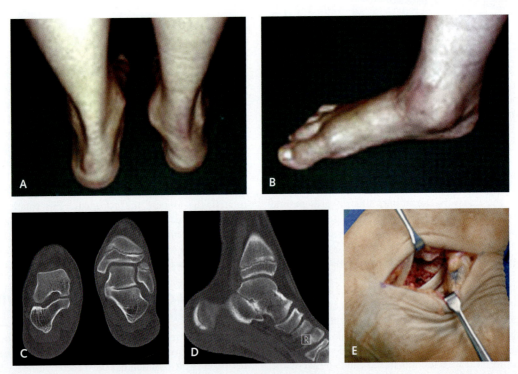

Figure 30-5 A middle facet coalition can manifest as a mass on the medial hindfoot. **A** and **B,** In this adolescent patient, the mass was so large that the presenting clinical manifestation was not a stiff foot but a tarsal tunnel syndrome secondary to compression of the tibial nerve. **C** and **D,** Appearance on computed tomography scans. **E,** At surgery, the large bony coalition was excised. Note the retraction of the flexor digitorum longus and flexor hallucis longus to expose the joint after removal of the coalition.

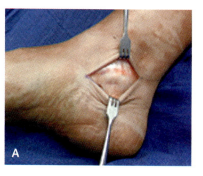
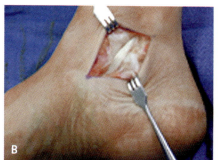
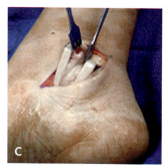
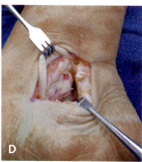
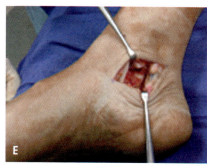

Figure 30-6 The sequence of steps in excision of a middle facet coalition. **A,** Subcutaneous dissection is performed above the flexor digitorum longus (FDL) tendon. **B,** The tendon sheath is opened. **C,** The FDL and the flexor hallucis longus (FHL) tendons are retracted on either side of the sustentaculum. **D,** With the tendons retracted, the coalition is now visible and is gradually removed. **E,** At the completion of resection of the coalition, the posterior facet is visible; the FHL remains under the sustentaculum.

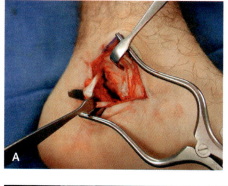
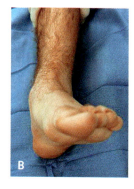
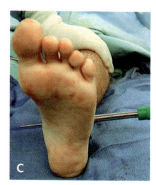
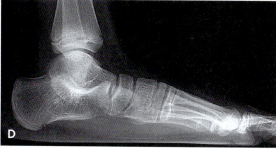
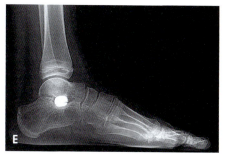

Figure 30-7 A, Resection of a middle facet coalition. **B,** The significant hindfoot valgus deformity was corrected with a subtalar arthroereisis. **C,** The correction was accomplished with insertion of the subtalar broach and sizer. **D** and **E,** The preoperative and postoperative radiographs. Good restoration of the arch of the foot has been achieved.

The extensor brevis muscle is identified and then carefully elevated off the floor of the sinus tarsi and the dorsal surface of the calcaneocuboid joint. Tagging this muscle as it is elevated from the floor of the sinus tarsi is helpful. Once the entire muscle and its proximal periosteal attachment are elevated, a small tag suture is inserted, and this suture then facilitates further dissection of the muscle off the calcaneocuboid joint (Figure 30-10).

A laminar spreader is inserted into the sinus tarsi and intermittently distracted until the anterior aspect of the subtalar joint is visible. The lateral aspect of the talonavicular joint capsule must be incised until the articular surface is visible, because this surface serves as a guide to the required extent of the dissection. The coalition is not always that easily visible. For this reason, I start at the edge of the calcaneocuboid joint, and using a half-inch straight

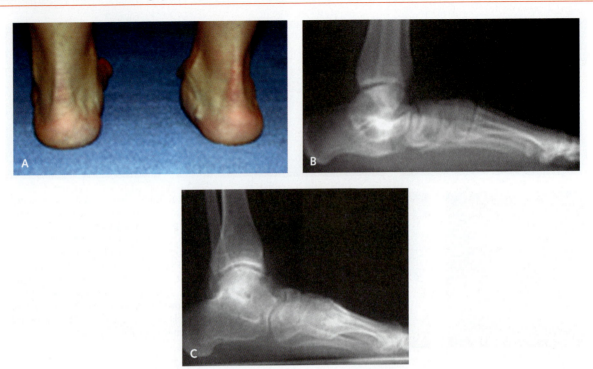

Figure 30-8 A and **B,** Severe rigidity of the hindfoot in a 15-year-old boy was due to a middle facet coalition. **C,** The rigidity was not thought to be correctable with resection of the coalition, so an extraarticular subtalar arthrodesis was performed.

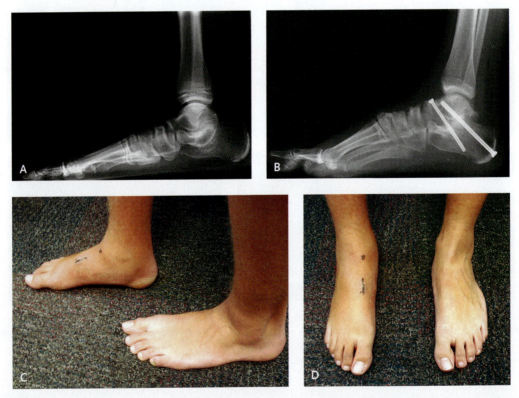

Figure 30-9 Marked rigidity and structural compensation of the midfoot and forefoot associated with a severe middle facet coalition in an adolescent patient. **A,** Note the pes planus, the metatarsus elevatus, and the hindfoot valgus, which was associated with the fixed hindfoot deformity seen on the radiograph. **B-D,** This deformity was corrected with a subtalar arthrodesis followed by an opening wedge osteotomy of the medial cuneiform, which was performed to reduce the metatarsus elevatus.

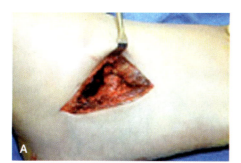
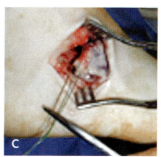
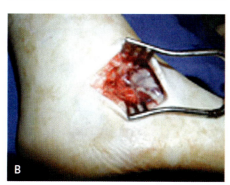

Figure 30-10 The steps in resection of a calcaneonavicular coalition. **A,** The extensor brevis muscle is elevated off the floor of the sinus tarsi. **B,** The elevated extensor brevis muscle is tagged with a suture. **C,** At the completion of the coalition excision, the extensor brevis muscle is inserted into the void, with the tagged suture inserted percutaneously through to the medial surface of the foot.

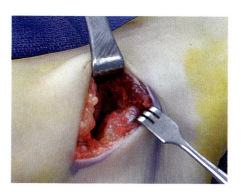

Figure 30-11 See Figure 30-10: At completion of removal of the calcaneonavicular coalition, a rectangular defect should be readily apparent, with the articular surfaces of the talus and navicular and the calcaneus and cuboid well visualized.

osteotome, I cut the bone. This piece of bone includes the portion that extends from the calcaneus up to the navicular, but usually a large protruding piece that abuts the talonavicular joint is present as well. Here, I use either a half-inch or quarter-inch osteotome to remove a rectangular rather than a triangular piece of bone.

The coalition extends far medially, and if either a triangular or trapezoidal piece of bone is taken out, the coalition will persist on the medial aspect of the joint complex. Excision of the coalition must be verified fluoroscopically. The range of motion of the peritalar joints is assessed to ensure that adequate decompression has been performed. Rarely, the foot is still stiff, and possibly a combination calcaneonavicular–middle facet coalition is present. In such instances, a second incision has to be made medially, and the approach should be as previously outlined. Before conclusion of this procedure, a laminar spreader is inserted into the sinus tarsi to open up the subtalar joint itself. The entire subtalar joint

should move freely, and the middle facet should be visible and mobile. At the completion of the procedure, I use bone wax on the resected bone surfaces. Once the coalition has been resected, a substantial tunnel should be visible in the lateral foot, created by the articular surfaces of the talus, calcaneus, cuboid, and navicular (Figure 30-11).

TREATMENT OF MORE EXTENSIVE COALITIONS

More complex or extensive forms of tarsal coalition that may be encountered in clinical practice include those with more than one pathologic fusion of discrete foot structures—for example, a middle facet coalition plus a naviculocuneiform coalition (Figure 30-12). It is not possible to anticipate the presence of more than one coalition on the basis of the rigidity of the foot. Certainly, if the foot is extremely rigid, this possibility should at least be considered, but other than the appearance on the plain radiograph and CT scan, it is only persistence of stiffness of the foot after excision of the coalition that reveals the true extent of the problem. Therefore, if on adequate resection of either a calcaneonavicular or a middle facet coalition, the foot remains stiff, then presence of an additional coalition should be considered. The treatment principles are the same as for excision of the single coalition, with even more emphasis on rehabilitation.

Other odd coalition variants include those of the talonavicular and calcaneocuboid joints and the entire posterior facet. The affected foot is always very rigid, is pronated, and exhibits a fixed heel valgus and a flattened calcaneal pitch angle. Patients with such coalitions have symptoms of aching, fatigue, and soreness along the medial arch of the foot with sinus tarsi pain. The goal here is not to create a normally shaped foot but simply to restructure the hindfoot to decrease the abnormal forces on the ankle. When possible, osteotomies are performed through the coalition, although arthrodesis of the adjacent joints may have to be performed.

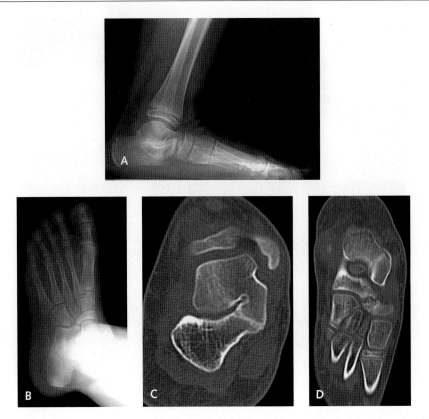

Figure 30-12 A and **B,** Radiographic appearance of a very severe rigid deformity, associated with pain in the feet and legs, in a 9-year-old girl. **C** and **D,** Both the calcaneonavicular and the middle facet coalitions were noted preoperatively on computed tomography scans, and both were removed.

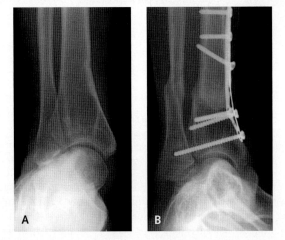

Figure 30-13 A, This severe hindfoot deformity with a fixed heel valgus and a ball-and-socket ankle was caused by a talonavicular coalition. This was corrected with a medial closing wedge supramalleolar osteotomy and an oblique fibular osteotomy. **B,** Note the marked improvement in the tibiotalar axis and the position of the hindfoot.

The talonavicular coalition as well as these other, more extensive coalitions usually are associated with a ball-and-socket ankle. This deformity is extremely unstable, and the patient presents with medial arch pain and subfibular impingement. It is preferable to avoid performing an ankle arthrodesis, because all of these patients have excellent range of ankle motion, although the foot is always medially unstable. The hindfoot is always in marked valgus. Rather than approaching the problem through the hindfoot, it is treated with a medial closing wedge supramalleolar osteotomy in conjunction with a calcaneus osteotomy or a medial cuneiform osteotomy (Figures 30-13 and 30-14). The goal of treating the talonavicular coalition is to create as much stability in the ankle as possible without arthrodesis. If the deformity is severe, then an arthrodesis, usually a tibiotalocalcaneal arthrodesis, should be considered (Figure 30-15).

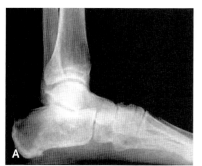

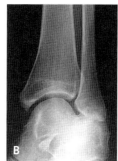

Figure 30-14 A and B, Talonavicular coalition created a ball-and-socket ankle, causing subfibular pain from the valgus ankle instability. C and D, Treatment consisted of a closing wedge supramalleolar osteotomy, with good realignment obtained.

30

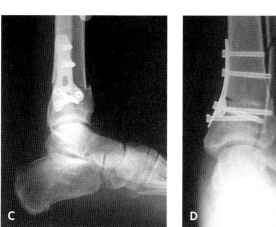

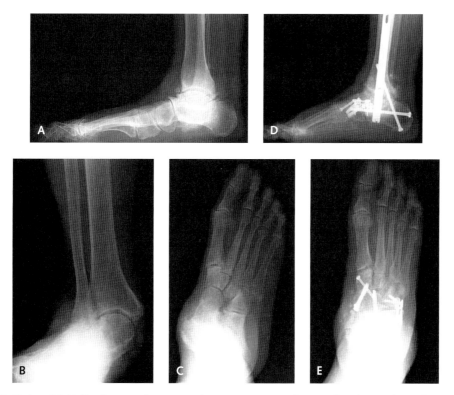

Figure 30-15 A and B, Unlike the examples presented in Figures 30-13 and 30-14, the talonavicular coalition and the ball-and-socket ankle shown here were associated with ankle pain from arthritis, in addition to the hindfoot impingement and pain, in a 67-year-old patient. Treatment was with a pantalar arthrodesis. The tibiotalocalcaneal arthrodesis was performed first using the intramedullary nail (Biomet, Parsipanny, New Jersey). C-E, Correction of the hindfoot and ankle resulted in severe midfoot supination deformity, which was then treated with an arthrodesis of the calcaneocuboid and naviculocuneiform joints.

TECHNIQUES, TIPS, AND PITFALLS

- Range of motion is the key to the success of this operation. If the foot is stiff at the completion of excision of the coalition, it will be permanently stiff after the operation, and arthrodesis would have been a preferable procedure.

- If an occult double coalition is suspected after resection of the calcaneonavicular coalition and the hindfoot remains stiff, try to open up the subtalar joint with a laminar spreader in the sinus tarsi to completely visualize the middle facet.

- Excision of the calcaneonavicular coalition must be done by resection of a rectangular piece of bone, not a trapezoidal or triangular piece of bone, because the latter leaves behind part of the coalition medially.

- Additional procedures commonly are performed in conjunction with resection of either coalition.

- Obtaining a sense of the extent of rigidity of the foot before the start of excision of the coalition is helpful. With a common peroneal nerve block performed in the office or after administration of a general anesthetic, the foot is manipulated, and the extent of the rigidity (or reactive contracture of the peroneal muscles) can be more accurately appreciated.

- Resection of the middle facet coalition *can* be performed for extensive (including 100%) coalitions. However, the hindfoot must be mobile after resection; adjunctive procedures should be performed; and postoperative rehabilitation, including use of orthotic arch supports, should be vigorous.

SUGGESTED READING

Cohen BE, Davis WH, Anderson RB: Success of calcaneonavicular coalition resection in the adult, *Foot Ankle Int* 17:569–572, 1996.

Drennan J: Tarsal coalitions, *Instr Course Lect* 45:323–329, 1996.

Vincent KA: Tarsal coalition and painful flatfoot, *J Am Acad Orthop Surg* 6:274–281, 1998.

CHAPTER **31**

Ankle Instability and Impingement Syndromes

LATERAL ANKLE LIGAMENT RECONSTRUCTION

In planning procedures for reconstruction of the lateral ankle ligament, considerations include the type of instability (whether in the ankle, the subtalar joint, or both), the presence of pain, and the exact location of symptoms. Pain associated with instability suggests either a rupture of the peroneal tendon or other intraarticular pathology, such as synovitis or an osteochondral injury. Isolated ankle instability does not cause pain. The preoperative assessment should ascertain whether symptoms are present when the patient walks on a flat surface or whether they occur only when the patient walks on uneven ground surfaces. If the patient experiences symptoms intermittently on flat-surface walking, then the need for reconstruction is increased.

When present, pain must be characterized by its location. If the pain is located behind the fibula, then I routinely use an open and not a percutaneous approach for the reconstruction. With this open approach (either an anatomic repair or a modification of the Elmslie procedure), the incision needs to be more directly over the fibula, to facilitate inspection of the peroneal tendons as well as the ankle joint if necessary. A more anterolateral location of the pain can be associated with an anterior capsular impingement syndrome or an intraarticular process, which would warrant further investigation with magnetic resonance imaging (MRI) or computed tomography (CT) studies. Sinus tarsi pain dictates evaluation for the possibility of combined ankle and subtalar instability, which is unusual, and also for an unrecognized injury to the lateral process of the talus or the anterior process of the calcaneus. With isolated sinus tarsi pain associated with ankle instability, the source of the pain may be related to subtalar joint rather than ankle instability. In this setting, evaluation and treatment for a sinus tarsi syndrome with diagnostic injection, MRI, and subtalar arthroscopy may be required.

The triad of recurrent ankle sprains, heel varus, and stress fracture of the fifth metatarsal should always be taken into consideration when treatment is planned in the sedentary or athletic patient (Figure 31-1). The case illustrated in Figure 31-1 represents a good example of failure of treatment if the underlying biomechanical and anatomic process is ignored. A calcaneus osteotomy, in addition to a stronger ankle ligament repair, which might have prevented the subsequent problems, would have provided improved correction.

An ankle ligament reconstruction can be performed without correcting the heel varus, but the outcome will depend on the flexibility of the subtalar joint and presence of additional symptoms.

If, for example, the patient has symptoms while walking on a flat ground surface and heel varus is present, then my inclination is to correct the calcaneus at the same time. If a patient has undergone previous ankle ligament reconstruction and has recurrent symptoms, I always look for unrecognized heel varus or mild tibia vara as a source for the failure. In most patients with heel varus, the deformity is bilateral. I have not, however, seen any biomechanical problem with correction of the hindfoot varus on one heel alone. Patients seem to adapt to this correction fairly well, and if contralateral symptoms develop subsequently, the correction can be done at a later date.

Usually an orthotic arch support with correct posting is sufficient to alleviate any minor symptoms of heel varus in the asymptomatic ankle. If a calcaneal osteotomy is necessary, it is performed in either one or two planes, depending on the pitch of the calcaneus. A lateral closing wedge osteotomy is always performed. Then the calcaneus can be translated slightly laterally and then shifted cephalad if the calcaneal pitch is markedly increased. For some patients with more severe heel varus associated with ankle instability, a plantar fascia release may need to be performed simultaneously.

The radiographic evaluation should routinely include weight-bearing radiographs, particularly if pain associated with the symptoms of instability is present. In addition to routine radiographs, I obtain MRI and CT scans as needed on the basis of additional disease present.

Assessment of the strength and function of the peroneal tendons in all patients who have recurrent ankle instability is important. Generally, these tendons are weak, and peroneal tendon rehabilitation is useful, even before the ankle ligament reconstruction is started. An appropriate rehabilitation regimen will facilitate functional recovery with a return to sports activities. I do not generally obtain an MRI study of the ankle even in patients who have peroneal tendon symptoms, because the incision is simply modified, as noted previously, and the peroneal tendons are inspected.

Operation Selection

Ankle ligament reconstruction in the high-performance athlete must be approached differently. The peroneal tendon should not be sacrificed as part of a reconstructive procedure, and even

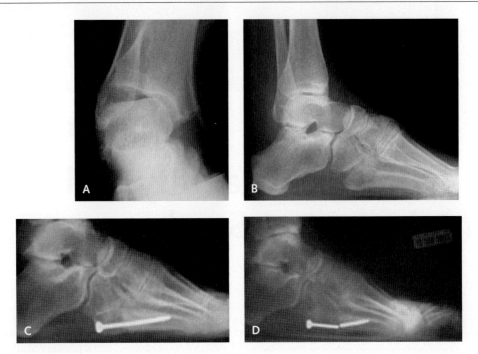

Figure 31-1 A and **B,** This patient with marked ankle instability and a cavus foot was treated incorrectly for a stress fracture of the 5th metatarsal. **C,** A screw was used to fix the metatarsal fracture, without correcting the ankle instability, and not surprisingly **(D),** the screw broke. All components of deformity should be addressed when treating a stress fracture of the 5th metatarsal.

using a strip of the peroneus brevis tendon is not warranted in the high-performance athlete. In this context, *high performance* refers also to the gymnast, the ballet dancer, and other athletes for whom pivoting on the pointed foot is important. If a patient has gross ankle instability and an anatomic repair is not thought to be sufficient, then augmentation of this anatomic repair with a hamstring graft can be performed. Under these circumstances, my preference is to perform a percutaneous hamstring allograft procedure in these athletes and not to resort to an open procedure.

Although a hamstring autograft reconstruction has been popularized recently, this reconstruction should be avoided in athletes who run and in those who participate in ball and racket sports. This reconstruction is particularly relevant in the sprinting athlete, in whom terminal flexion torque will be compromised if the hamstring is sacrificed.

When should an anatomic repair be performed as opposed to a reconstruction? I am inclined to perform a percutaneous procedure using a hamstring allograft with biointerference screws whenever possible. The percutaneous procedure is very close to being an anatomic procedure, and although of course the graft is not inserted at the kinematic points on the fibula, this repair is an acceptable alternative in certain active and athletic patients. If a graft is not available, then either of two alternatives have to be considered: a modification of either the Elmslie or Chrisman-Snook procedure, or the hamstring procedure with an autograft. Although in the past I routinely used an anatomic repair of the Broström procedure for most reconstructions, for certain patients—the heavyweight athlete, such as a boxer or body builder, and the patient with any heel varus of any degree—who are not ideal candidates for this repair, I elected to use a tendon graft procedure. Whenever a tendon reconstruction procedure is performed, maintaining the correct kinematics of the ankle, which is impossible with use of a slip of the peroneal tendon, is important.

Accordingly, a free tendon graft is preferable. Even with the allograft hamstring procedure, careful attention to selection of the entrance and exit points of the graft in the fibula is essential. As noted earlier, caution is indicated with the use of hamstring autograft in the sprinting athlete, which causes a deficit in terminal flexion torque.

In the patient with intraarticular ankle disease, the timing of the surgery is always a concern. For example, if an osteochondral defect requiring treatment is present, how should this operation be performed, in addition to ankle ligament reconstruction? (Figure 31-2). In patients with such defects, ankle arthroscopy, in conjunction with the ligament reconstruction, is recommended.

Traditional rehabilitation after ligament reconstruction, however, consists of immobilization for up to 6 weeks, presumably with considerable negative effects on recovery and rehabilitation after debridement for an osteochondral defect. Use of immobilization in this setting is essentially outmoded and should be discontinued except in rare instances. Although immobilization in a boot or brace can be used for comfort purposes, as a practical matter, if fixation techniques are used correctly, immobilization should not be needed at all. After any ankle ligament reconstruction, passive range-of-motion exercises are begun at 2 weeks, and the patient is permitted to walk out of the boot with a stirrup brace at 5 to 6 weeks, with physical therapy and rehabilitation started as early as possible.

Nonetheless, it is something to consider when combined diseases are addressed. The other issue pertaining to the intraarticular disease concerns the type of reconstructive procedure used. After ankle arthroscopy, interstitial tissue edema is always present, with fluid leakage into the soft tissues, and finding the correct anatomic plane—for example, for reconstruction using a Broström procedure—can be more difficult because of the tissue edema. I do not believe that performing an ankle arthroscopy is necessary in the absence of intraarticular disease or symptoms of ankle pain.

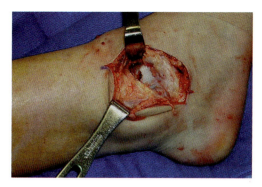

Figure 31-2 An incidental finding of an osteochondral defect of the talus noted at the time of a ligament reconstruction.

The Broström Procedure

I do not use the traditional "hockey stick", or J-type, incision for the Broström procedure, because it does not permit visualization of the peroneal tendons. I use a more longitudinal incision located over the anterior fibula, inspecting the peroneal tendon simultaneously and facilitating repair of the calcaneal fibular ligament (Figure 31-3). This incision affords ready access to the anterior ankle and can even be extended to perform an open cheilectomy.

Care must be taken to avoid the superficial peroneal nerve anteriorly in the terminal portion of the incision. The soft tissue is reflected and the extensor retinaculum identified as a separate layer before the ankle joint is opened. This extensor retinaculum can be used to strengthen the anatomic repair (Figure 31-4). The inferior root of the extensor retinaculum inserts into the neck of the calcaneus just anterior to the subtalar joint, and can be used to stabilize both the ankle and subtalar joints in cases of combined instability.

The extensor retinaculum is not strong enough on its own to correct instability, and repair based on this structure should be combined with the anatomic procedure described. The incision through the anterior talofibular ligament must be made carefully. Sometimes a bony avulsion is present off the tip of the fibula; therefore the incision through the ligament must be as close to the fibula as possible. The original description of this procedure included a "vest over pants" repair of the anterior talofibular ligament, which is almost impossible to perform correctly because of the paucity of adequate ligamentous tissue. For this reason, I make the incision through the anterior talofibular ligament as close to the fibula as possible and dissect the ligament off the tip of the fibula. The periosteal tissue is then raised with a small cuff of the remnant of the anterior talofibular ligament off the fibula, and this can then be used to lie over the anatomic repair once the anterior talofibular ligament has been pulled up into the fibula. I generally debride the edge of the fibula, using either a rongeur or a small burr, to create a bleeding trough for reattachment of the ligament.

The same principle applies with use of the calcaneal fibular ligament. Detaching it directly from the fibula is easier than cutting it in its central body and then attempting a repair of a short ligament. Attachment of the anterior talofibular ligament to the fibula can be done either with a suture anchor or with sutures passed through Kirschner wire (K-wire) holes through the fibula. I prefer the latter technique because these holes can be made in pairs and the suture can be inserted through the ligament as a Y-shaped suture, pulled up, and imbricated with the ligament into the prepared trough on the tip of the fibula. Two sets of sutures are used to reattach the anterior talofibular ligament. When the ligament is tied down, the knot should not be placed over the fibula. The knot is invariably prominent, which can be irritating and painful, particularly in patients who have thin subcutaneous tissue. The knot should therefore always be tied on the ligament side of the repair, rather than on the bone. I use a nonabsorbable suture on a stout-tapered needle, passed through the predrilled holes in the fibula.

The peroneal tendons must be retracted completely to visualize the calcaneal fibular ligament. It is useful to prepare the sutures for both the anterior talofibular and calcaneofibular ligament before tying off the anterior talofibular ligament. Afterward, the ankle needs to be moved around, and the suture repair on the anterior talofibular ligament should not be disturbed when the calcaneofibular ligament is tied off. The anterior talofibular ligament is tied off first, with the foot in neutral dorsiflexion and slight eversion. Overtightening the ligaments with this technique is possible, and the foot should not be in dorsiflexion or forced eversion during the repair. At the completion of the repair of the anterior talofibular and calcaneofibular ligaments, the extensor retinaculum can be pulled up and sutured to the prepared flap of the periosteum and remnant of the anterior talofibular ligament over the fibula. Not all patients have a well-defined extensor retinaculum, and this part of the procedure is not always feasible. These final sutures must be buried; otherwise, they can serve as a source of irritation. I use absorbable sutures here for this reason, because even with a buried suture, the knot can be irritating.

Modification of the Chrisman-Snook Procedure

The original description of the Chrisman-Snook procedure included a long strip of the peroneus brevis tendon, which was split in half and placed through a bone tunnel in the calcaneus. This aspect of the technique is not necessary because a short strip of the anterior third of the peroneus brevis tendon is sufficient. The incision is made paralleling the peroneal tendons and extending for no more than 6 cm proximal to the tip of the fibula. The length of tendon that is required should be measured before the tendon is cut proximally, but rarely exceeds approximately 8 cm. The advantage of this procedure is that it can be used in the presence of a severe tear of the peroneus brevis tendon, for which a split portion of the tendon can be incorporated and used for the ligament reconstruction. Splits in the peroneus brevis tendon are common in combination with recurrent ankle instability, and if these splits are present, this portion of the tendon is then cut proximally and used for the reconstruction (Figure 31-5).

Even though the quality of the tendon may not be ideal, it always provides sufficient strength for the reconstruction. The anterior third of the tendon is used. Distally, as the tendon is divided, care technique will ensure that it does not split down too far along the peroneus brevis tendon, and a suture can be inserted just distal to the peroneal tubercle to prevent such excessive splitting. This reconstruction does not reproduce the kinematics of the ankle joint. Nonetheless, it does provide stability and is a reliable procedure for most patients, particularly those who have subtalar joint symptoms, combined instability, hindfoot stiffness or deformity, dislocation of the peroneal tendons after a calcaneus fracture, and recurrent instability after unsuccessful previous surgery.

A 4.5-mm drill hole is made from the tip of the fibula extending posteriorly through the body of the distal fibula and exiting *anterior* to the peroneal tendons in the posterior half of the fibula. The tendon is passed through the fibular tunnel using a sucker tip and then passed over (on top) of the remaining half of the peroneus brevis and the peroneus longus tendons, to prevent subluxation of these tendons.

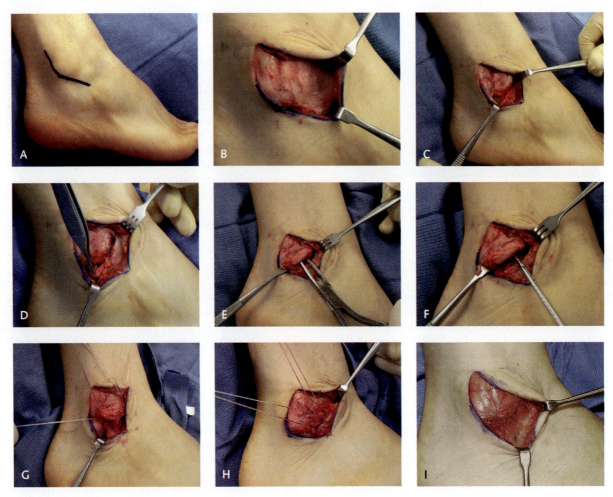

Figure 31-3 The steps of the Broström procedure. **A,** The incision is made over the fibula so as to expose the ligaments but also the ankle and the peroneal tendons if necessary. **B,** The soft tissue is retracted, ensuring that the superficial peroneal nerve is retracted medially. **C,** The margin of the extensor retinaculum is identified. **D,** The muscle is then elevated off the deeper tissue. **E,** The arthrotomy is made leaving a 2-mm cuff of tissue on the fibula, which is then débrided using a rongeur. **F and G,** Either K-wire holes or, in this case, a suture anchor is used to repair the ligaments. **H,** The calcaneofibular ligament is repaired first, and then both ligaments are pulled into the fibula. **I,** The extensor retinaculum is advanced to reinforce the repair.

A small portion of the peroneal retinaculum can be left intact when the anterior portion of the peroneus brevis tendon is harvested, to prevent subluxation of the peroneal tendon. The calcaneus is prone to fracture, so instead of passing the tendon through a complex tunnel in the calcaneus, as originally described, attaching the tendon to the bone with a screw and a spiked ligament washer or an interference screw is easier and provides a more stable repair. The tendon is inserted at the attachment of the calcaneofibular ligament just inferior to the peroneal tendons. A drill hole aimed toward the sustentaculum is made, and the screw and washer are passed through the peroneal tendon, with tension placed in the direction on the tendon to see the point at which the screw is passed through the tendon (Figure 31-6). The tendon can be split at this point with a hemostat, which simultaneously grasps the screw and pulls it through the tendon. Debriding the lateral cortex of the calcaneus is unnecessary. The tendon seems to adhere well to the periosteal tissue, and when I have had to remove the washer or screw for relief of pain, I have noted no redundancy, instability, or loosening of the attached tendon. When the screw is tightened, the foot is held in dorsiflexion and eversion, and simultaneous traction is applied to the peroneus brevis tendon. The stay

suture is pulled on while the screw is inserted. Because the washer makes contact with the tendon, minor adjustments to the tension of the tendon can be made until fixation is secure. A biointerference screw also can be used instead of the screw and spiked washer. In this case, a slightly longer piece of peroneal tendon would need to be harvested, and the same technique would need to be followed for creation of the free tendon graft as that described for the hamstring allograft procedure. Passive range of motion movement can begin almost immediately after surgery. This procedure is a strong, reliable method of fixation. Attachment of one or two sutures to the anterior aspect of the distal fibula is useful, through the old anterior talofibular ligament into the passed tendon with nonabsorbable 0-0 sutures. After 2 weeks of immobilization in a boot or a posterior splint, patients begin ambulation in a removable stirrup brace with eversion strengthening starting at this time.

Percutaneous Hamstring Reconstruction

The reconstruction is planned, and although a percutaneous approach is used, small incisions are needed for insertion of the graft. The neck of the talus should be marked with a guide pin under fluoroscopic imaging, and a small, approximately 1.5-cm incision is

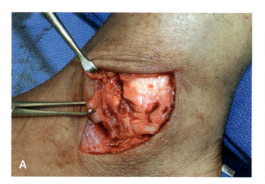
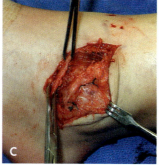
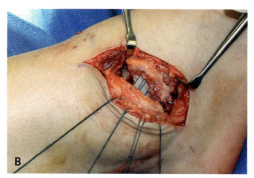

Figure 31-4 Use of the extensor retinaculum to reinforce the Bröstrum repair. **A,** After arthrotomy, the retinaculum is separated with a clamp from the deeper tissues. **B,** The sutures were inserted through small K-wire holes in the fibula. **C,** After tightening of the repair, the retinaculum is advanced as a separate layer into the fibula and secured with absorbable sutures.

made, extending from the lateral aspect of the shoulder of the talar body to the tip of the fibula. In this way, addressing the introduction and passage of the tendon graft through the same incision is possible. The incision is deepened through subcutaneous tissue with a hemostat, to avoid any injury to the superficial peroneal nerve during the dissection. The hemostat is probed down onto the bone through the extensor retinaculum.

I use the blind tunnel technique for entry into the talus. If instrumentation is unavailable for bioresorbable interference screws, then an alternative technique with a bone suture anchor can be used. A hamstring allograft is now prepared for insertion into the predrilled hole, which is directed from the lateral neck toward the body of the talus. Because of the size of the talus at the level of the anterior talofibular ligament, insertion of the tendon graft up toward the body of the talus from the anterior lateral shoulder of the talus with a blind tunnel technique is preferable, and instrumentation for insertion of the graft with biointerference screws is helpful. The drill hole is approximately 1 mm wider than the thickness of the screw, to accommodate the tendon, but with tension. I generally use a 5.5-mm drill hole, made to a depth of 17 mm. Visualizing the lateral edge of the entry hole into the talus is important both in measuring the depth of the hole and in inserting the screw, which must be flush with the edge of the talar cortex. The hamstring allograft is now cleaned, freshened, and trimmed to a thickness of 4 mm along its entire length. The length also must be measured correctly.

Measuring the length of the graft at this stage is far easier, because a whip suture is inserted into the end of the tendon for passage through the fibula into the calcaneus, and it saves a step if the correct length is cut. I lay the tendon on the skin over the course of passage on the ankle and approximate the length accordingly. A fiber wire suture knot is inserted over the tip of the tendon, and the interference screw is inserted and tightened up to the cortical margin of the talus with the inserter device. The lateral margin of the screw must be flush with the lateral cortical margin of the

shoulder of the talus. With application of considerable tension on the tendon, the graft, which is buried in the talar body, should not yield or be unstable (Figure 31-7).

From the tip of the incision at the edge of the fibula, a guide pin for a 4.5-mm cannulated drill bit is now inserted. The guide pin is inserted through the fibula from anterior to posterior, exiting just anterior to the peroneal tendon sheath, approximately 1 cm proximal to the tip of the fibula (Figure 31-8). The suture at the tendon tip is pulled through a puncture over the peroneal sheath. The tendon is passed through a subcutaneous tunnel and out a second, small, 1-cm incision, which is made inferior to the peroneal tendons and dorsal to the sural nerve. The cannulated guide pin is then inserted, and a 4.5-mm through-and-through hole is made in the calcaneus. The tendon is now pulled down, and it is passed to the medial side of the heel through a skin puncture with a suture passer. Tension is now applied to the suture, and with the ankle placed in dorsiflexion and neutral position, the correct tension is applied on the graft for the reconstruction. Once this tension has been established, the second interference screw is inserted, which must be flush with the margin of the calcaneus (Figure 31-9, *B*). The hamstring procedure may be combined with an open arthrotomy when intra articular disease is simultaneously addressed (Figure 31-10).

The foot is immobilized with a range-of-motion walker boot, which can be applied immediately after the operation. Weight bearing is permitted at approximately 10 days after surgery, followed by range-of-motion exercise and rehabilitation, which begins at 2 weeks.

DELTOID LIGAMENT INJURY AND REPAIR

Medial ankle pain with instability from injury to the deltoid ligament is an uncommon clinical entity but one that is being increasingly identified, particularly after athletic injury. Delays in diagnosis and treatment are still common. Most patients with a tear require

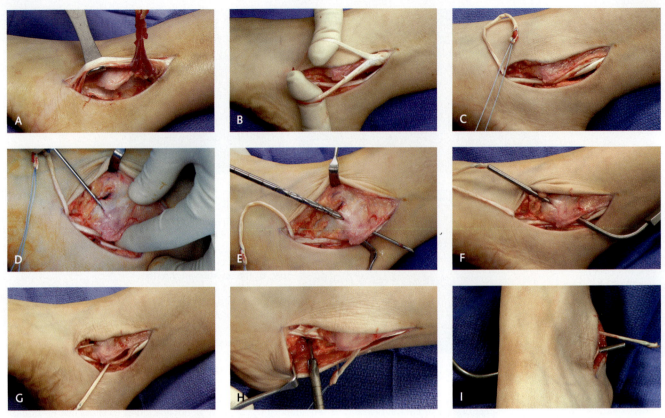

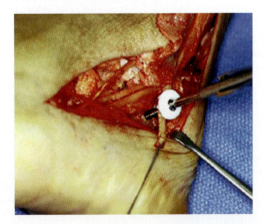

Figure 31-5 The steps in the modified Chrisman-Snook procedure performed for repair of a torn peroneal tendon. **A,** The low-lying muscle of the peroneus brevis was debrided. **B,** The tear in the peroneus brevis tendon was extended by splitting the tendon more proximally. **C,** The tip of the tendon was sutured. **D** and **E,** A guide pin was passed through the fibula, followed by a 4.5-mm cannulated drill bit. **F,** A suction device was passed back through the fibula to grasp the suture. **G,** Then the tendon was pulled through the fibula and passed dorsal to the peroneal tendons. **H,** A drill hole was then made in the calcaneus over a guide pin. **I,** The suction device was passed from medial to lateral over the guide pin to grasp the tendon. **J,** The tendon was then placed under tension medially, and an interference screw was inserted laterally.

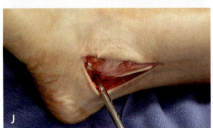

Figure 31-6 An alternative method for attaching the tendon to the calcaneus is to use a screw over a spike ligament washer.

a deltoid ligament repair that addresses the specific injury, such as ligament avulsion, bone avulsion, or a mid-substance tear. These patients, unlike those with lateral ligament injuries, require prolonged immobilization as either primary or postoperative treatment.

Of interest, although deltoid ligament ruptures associated with ankle fractures and syndesmosis injuries are routinely treated, and despite radiographic and clinical evidence of deltoid ligament injury in affected patients, uneventful healing is the expected outcome. Medial instability is uncommon after these injuries, particularly when the fibula alignment and stability have been established. Fractures with associated deltoid ligament ruptures are easily identified, and most are managed with prompt institution of prolonged immobilization, which may be why in this setting medial joint instability and chronic deltoid ligament pathology is rarely, if ever, a problem.

Degeneration and rupture of the deltoid ligament probably represent a spectrum of injury that results from a combination of both repetitive microtrauma and discrete trauma. Although eversion directly stresses the medial ankle and plays a role in deltoid ligament rupture, inversion injuries, which are far more common, also may be involved in the pathogenesis of deltoid ligament injury. The impingement of the deep posterior tibiotalar ligament between the talus and the medial malleolus during inversion trauma is the likely pathomechanism for hypertrophy and degeneration. In a series of "acute" isolated deltoid ligament injuries, inversion trauma with bony impingement of the deltoid ligament occurred in some patients without evidence of articular or lateral ligament trauma.

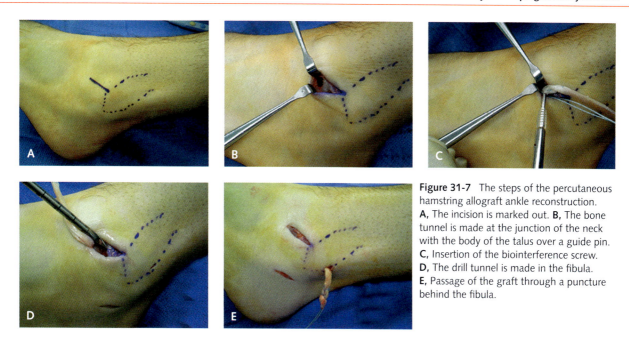

Figure 31-7 The steps of the percutaneous hamstring allograft ankle reconstruction. **A,** The incision is marked out. **B,** The bone tunnel is made at the junction of the neck with the body of the talus over a guide pin. **C,** Insertion of the biointerference screw. **D,** The drill tunnel is made in the fibula. **E,** Passage of the graft through a puncture behind the fibula.

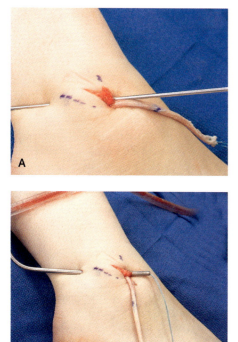

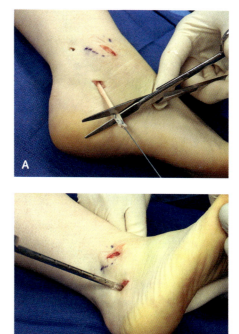

Figure 31-8 In this example of a percutaneous hamstring allograft, the graft has been anchored to the talus. **A,** The guide pin is drilled through the fibula to pass anterior to the peroneal tendons. **B,** The suction device then passed back through the tunnel over the guide pin to grasp the tendon graft.

Figure 31-9 **A,** When the tendon is passed into the foot (see Figure 31-8) it must be of correct length, otherwise it will not be secured in the calcaneus. **B,** Note the foot in dorsiflexion and eversion while the interference screw is inserted.

The isolated nature of these ligament tears may be related to underlying degeneration of the deltoid ligament, which may play a role in the limited healing potential of these injuries. Ligament degeneration may explain why the deltoid ligament readily heals in patients with ankle fractures, in whom the ligament presumably is normal, and is problematic in patients with chronic deltoid ligament injuries. The other possibility is that the acute, isolated deltoid injuries are treated as an ankle sprain, and mobilization begins too soon, resulting in a delay in healing.

Acute tension overload of the deltoid ligament from eversion injuries is the clearest mechanism of injury in these cases and probably plays some role in nearly all ruptures. The deltoid ligament also

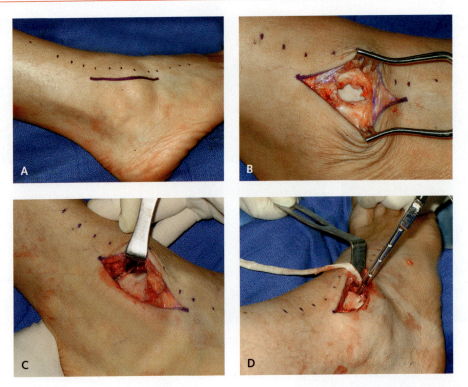

Figure 31-10 An open ankle ligament reconstruction performed to correct instability associated with anterior impingement and an anterolateral osteochondral defect of the talus. **A,** The incision is marked out. **B,** Copious synovitis is evident. **C,** The cheilectomy was performed, and the lesion was probed and treated with microfracture. **D,** This was followed by the hamstring graft reconstruction.

plays a role in stabilizing horizontal rotation around the ankle, and inversion trauma with resulting impingement of the deltoid ligament between the talus and the medial malleolus probably is also a cause of rupture. Although these inversion episodes may not result in overt failure, chronic impingement could result in partial tearing and degeneration, predisposing the tendon to rupture. In addition, chronic tension overload that occurs in the deltoid ligament associated with a posterior tibial tendon rupture again sets the stage for acute failure. This is probably the pathogenic sequence with a stage IV rupture of the posterior tibial tendon, with degeneration, rupture, and necrosis of the ligament associated with a variable degree of flatfoot and ankle instability.

Repair is carried out with the patient in a supine position with a bump under the contralateral hip to facilitate medial exposure through a longitudinal incision slightly anterior to the posterior tibial tendon sheath from proximal to the medial malleolus to the level of the talonavicular joint. The tendon sheath must be opened and the posterior tibial tendon must be checked for a tear, because associated posterior tibial tendon pathology is not uncommon. The tendon is retracted posteriorly, exposing the underlying deltoid ligament, which is now explored for the orientation, location, and extent of the tear. The posterior tibial tendon must always be carefully examined for a tear, because the mechanism of injury is similar, and the two occur concurrently (Figure 31-11).

The repair is performed in accordance with the underlying disease and the orientation of the tear, much as with the comparable Broström procedure. In cases involving avulsion of the ligament from the medial malleolus, a proximally based periosteal flap is elevated from the tip of the medial malleolus, and a trough is then made in the tip of the malleolus with a rongeur (or burr) down to

bleeding bone. The sutures are then either inserted through drill holes made with a K-wire in the malleolus or placed with a suture anchor; a 2-0 nonabsorbable braided suture is used. These sutures are placed into the trough, and the avulsed ligament is reduced with horizontal mattress stitches (Figure 31-12). The periosteal flap is brought down over the ligament in a "pants over vest" fashion and sutured. If a midsubstance tear is present, an end-to-end repair can be used, but the problem here is the degenerative nature of the tissue, which may need "freshening up" before repair. Any associated deformity should be simultaneously corrected.

Tears secondary to a chronic degenerative process, which are associated with flatfoot deformity or a stage IV flatfoot in the case of a deltoid tear, are not discussed here. In some situations, however, the foot has a preexisting planovalgus deformity, and the injury occurs to the medial ankle. Frequently this injury goes undiagnosed, and by the time the correct diagnosis is made, the medial ankle has been further compromised. In such cases I add an osteotomy of the calcaneus to support the medial repair. This additional support is particularly important when there is slight tilt of the talus; an interesting example is presented in Figure 31-13. In the case illustrated, the patient was an adult with long-standing asymptomatic rigid flatfoot deformity. A subsequent ankle sprain was followed by pain in the medial ankle only, not associated with any foot symptoms. Examination revealed slight instability of the medial ankle, with pain over the deltoid and no subtalar joint pain. The radiograph demonstrated an old middle facet coalition with associated arthritis of the subtalar joint, along with slight valgus tilt of the talus. Correction was accomplished with a medial translational osteotomy of the calcaneus and a deltoid repair as described previously (see Figure 31-13).

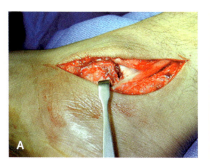
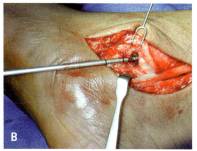
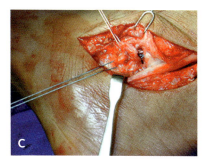

Figure 31-11 An acute rupture of the deltoid ligament occurred in a 23-year-old basketball player. After 4 months of conservative care, operative repair was performed. **A,** Note the defect in the superficial and deep deltoid ligament. **B,** The medial malleolus was débrided to bleeding bone, and the anchor was inserted. **C,** Y-shape sutures are inserted and then used to imbricate the deltoid ligament and pull it back up into the malleolus.

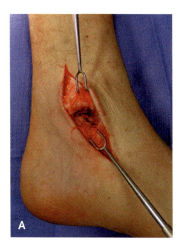
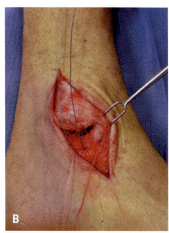

Figure 31-12 **A,** Rupture of the deep deltoid ligament, associated with avulsion of a bone fragment off the talus, in a 29-year-old tennis player. **B,** The defect was repaired with sutures attached to an anchor in the talus and then imbricated up into the medial malleolus.

ANKLE IMPINGEMENT SYNDROMES

Caution is essential in planning treatment for anterior impingement syndromes in patients with arthritis. If motion of the ankle is limited to begin with, and ankle arthritis is present, removing the impinging anterior osteophytes may increase ankle motion but simultaneously worsen pain. Whenever possible, I treat the anterior impingement syndrome arthroscopically; a large burr (a 4-mm cylindrical burr) is used to denude the anterior surface of osteophytes. Although open arthrotomy can be performed, additional disease is invariably associated with the anterior impingement, and this impingement syndrome is easier to address arthroscopically (Figure 31-14). When the osteophytes are intracapsular, however, arthroscopic treatment becomes far more difficult, and an anterolateral arthrotomy is preferable (Figure 31-15). An important consideration is that osteophytes on the tibia are predominantly lateral, and those on the talus are predominantly medial. Even if large osteophytes are present on the talus, reaching across from the anterolateral arthrotomy for resection is not always easy. Anterior impingement with osteophyte buildup also is associated with ankle instability, necessitating further evaluation. Many patients with subsequent arthritis of the ankle have recurrent instability of the ankle, which begins with instability without osteophytes. Finally in the last stages, instability becomes fixed, and the tibiotalar joint is fixed in varus, in association with marked buildup of osteophytes over its anterior aspect. Correction of the impingement syndrome

in such cases is much more difficult because the osteophyte resection is only part of a more complex realignment procedure of the hindfoot and ankle.

The anterior osteophytes are approached through an anterolateral arthrotomy, immediately lateral to the peroneus tertius tendon. The incision is deepened through subcutaneous tissue in the superficial peroneal nerve, which always lies immediately adjacent to the tendon and is identified and retracted. The extensor retinaculum is incised, and the hypertrophic capsule is incised and reflected. After a synovectomy and excision of the hypertrophied anterolateral capsule, a periosteal elevator is inserted transversely from the anterolateral distal tibia across to the more medial aspect. Under direct visualization, a large retractor is inserted into the joint over the distal tibia and a small fine chisel or osteotome is used to remove the osteophyte. The use of a curved quarter-inch or curved half-inch osteotome is helpful to perform this so that as the osteotome moves medially, it exits just anterior to the medial malleolus. Plantar flexing and inverting the ankle during this ostectomy also are helpful to prevent any inadvertent injury to the cartilage. At the completion of osteophyte removal, the stability of the ankle must be checked. As noted, many of these ankles are associated with chronic ankle instability, and some form of repair or reconstruction should be performed in conjunction with the osteophyte removal. If the osteophytes are intraarticular and not excessive or intracapsular, the osteophyte removal is then performed arthroscopically,

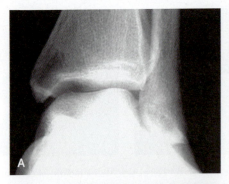

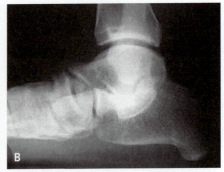

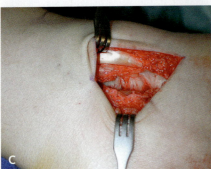

Figure 31-13 The patient, who had an asymptomatic flatfoot, sustained an ankle sprain, followed by pain on the medial ankle only, not associated with any foot symptoms. **A,** Slight valgus tilt of the talus. **B,** Middle facet coalition. **C,** Rupture of the deltoid and the posterior tibial tenosynovitis.

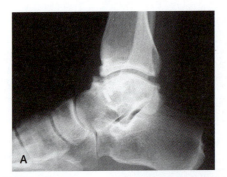

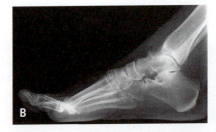

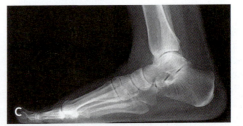

Figure 31-14 The patient was a soccer player with symptoms of anterior impingement. **A,** Note the anterior osteophytes. **B** and **C,** These are more readily seen on flexion and extension radiographs of the foot.

followed by percutaneous ankle ligament reconstruction. If a large buildup of osteophytes is noted medially, the usual location is over the talar neck, and resection must be performed through a separate arthrotomy incision medially, just medial to the anterior tibial tendon.

Large hypertrophic osteophytes associated with fixed varus and fixed tilting of the tibiotalar joint pose considerable difficulty

in management. In patients with such osteophytes, contracture occurs in the deep deltoid ligament, the posteromedial capsule, and at times even the posterior tibial tendon. These medial soft tissues undergo adaptive contracture, but even after resection of the osteophytes and lateral stabilization, the contracture is not always adequately released. A problem with anterior ankle cheilectomy is subsequent recurrence of the osteophytes, which may be limited

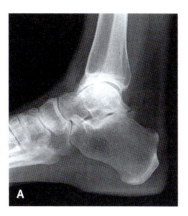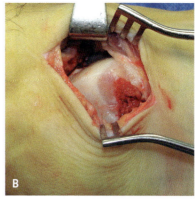

Figure 31-15 **A,** The large osteophytes on the distal tibia were not thought to be amenable to arthroscopic management. **B,** Removal was accomplished through an open anterolateral arthrotomy.

with application of bone wax over the resected portion of the ostectomy, although a beneficial effect has not as yet been proved.

The pain associated with posterior impingement syndrome is easily reproduced on examination with forced passive plantar flexion of the ankle. A decision has to be made whether the pain is arising from a hypertrophied trigonal process, from an os trigonum, or from a pathologic process involving either the peroneal or the flexor hallucis longus (FHL) tendons. In the case of posteromedial ankle pain, reproduction of the pain by forced passive dorsiflexion of the foot followed by passive dorsiflexion of the hallux usually is easy. If stenosis of the fibro-osseous tunnel is present, this combination of maneuvers pulls the FHL tendon deep into the retinacular tunnel as the flexor hallucis muscle belly is pulled distally and will reliably reproduce the pain. Pain in a directly posterior location elicited by forced passive plantar flexion is invariably the result of an os trigonum or a hypertrophic process of the talus. A passive forced plantar flexion lateral radiograph also is helpful to confirm the diagnosis (Figure 31-16), and if the specific pathologic process is still in doubt, a CT scan will delineate the size and location of the fragment (Figure 31-17).

I use a posterolateral incision to approach the decompression if the pain is directly posterior. Although a posteromedial incision can be used, this should be done only when a definite diagnosis of FHL tendon disease has been made. The morbidity associated with the posteromedial incision is considerably greater, and even with adequate retraction of the tibial nerve, irritation and scarring of the nerve may occur, with subsequent neuritis.

The posterolateral incision is made over a 3-cm length posterior to the peroneal tendons. The incision is deepened through the subcutaneous tissue, and the sural nerve is immediately identified and retracted anteriorly. The peroneal retinaculum is now incised over the muscle belly posteriorly, and the peroneal tendons are retracted anteriorly (Figure 31-18). Visualization of the posterior aspect of the ankle is impossible until the retrocalcaneal fat has been excised. Retracting the fatty tissue is simply not enough; the fat and the adjacent bursal tissue need to be excised. In addition, I find it useful to open up both the ankle and the subtalar joints before performing the ostectomy, for accurate localization of the joint margin as the ostectomy is performed. A wide periosteal elevator is used to strip the periosteum off the distal tibia, which is then left in place. A curved periosteal elevator or a Hohman retractor is inserted over the back of the tibia. Once the soft tissues are retracted, then the

excision of the os trigonum can be performed. It is then essential to identify the leading edge of the FHL tendon, which is muscular at this level because the muscle fibers blend in with the tendon distally. The exostectomy is performed from lateral to medial and is done using an osteotome. The use of a blunt osteotome here is actually helpful to prevent inadvertent injury to the FHL tendon, which lies immediately adjacent, on the medial side of the posterior tubercle. Once the process has been fractured with the osteotome, it is twisted off its pedicle using a rongeur. Subsequent to this maneuver, fibers attached to the FHL tendon typically remain medially and need to be released promptly by sharp dissection under direct visualization of the FHL tendon. In this way, both the ankle and the subtalar joints can be visualized, to identify any additional disease that may coexist in the posterior aspect of the joint.

I use an approach similar to the foregoing in high-performance athletes, dancers, and gymnasts. The only difference is that FHL tendon disease occurs with greater frequency among gymnasts and dancers than in other athletes, and I may be more inclined to use a posteromedial incision in these patients. The approach is identical, but these patients take a long time to regain full plantar flexion. During the initial phase of recovery, weight bearing is begun as soon as it is comfortable, with the foot in a walker boot in a maximally dorsiflexed position. The boot can be removed at intervals for passive range-of-motion exercises, and swimming is begun as soon as possible.

Another, less common variant of impingement pathology causing posterior ankle pain that always occurs in adolescents is a bipartite talus (Figure 31-19). The radiographic appearance of the posterior bone mass gives the impression of a very large os trigonum, but the talus is always slightly flatter on the lateral radiograph, and the fragment extends into the subtalar joint—a feature not present with an os trigonum. Flexion and extension lateral radiographs are obtained, but the diagnosis is confirmed on CT scan. In the case illustrated in Figure 31-19, the extent of the unossified posteromedial body of the talus is considerable (see Figure 31-19, *C*). Typically, approximately 20% of the surface of the posterior facet is involved, so removal will necessarily lead to some instability of the subtalar joint. I have not, however, noted subtalar joint pain in patients with a bipartite talus, who respond fairly quickly to removal of the bone mass through a posteromedial incision. The entire fragment must be isolated and probed loose with a small osteotome and then removed (see Figure 31-19).

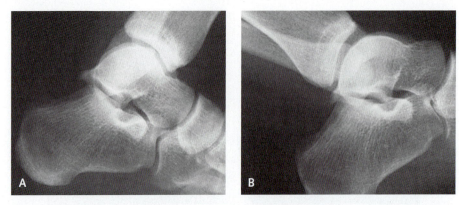

Figure 31-16 Posterior ankle pain in a gymnast was due to an os: trigonum syndrome. **A** and **B,** The diagnosis was confirmed on flexion and extension radiographs.

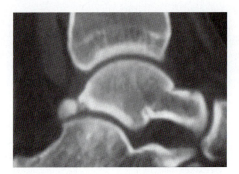

Figure 31-17 A computed tomography scan is helpful to delineate the location and size of the os trigonum.

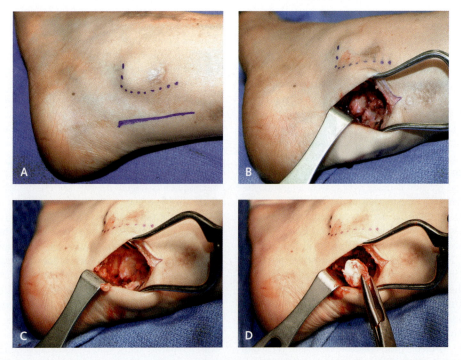

Figure 31-18 Approach to excision of an enlarged os trigonum. **A,** The incision is marked posterior to the peroneal tendons. **B,** Retrocalcaneal fat is excised to expose the bone mass. **C** and **D,** The bone mass is cut with an osteotome and twisted off its pedicle.

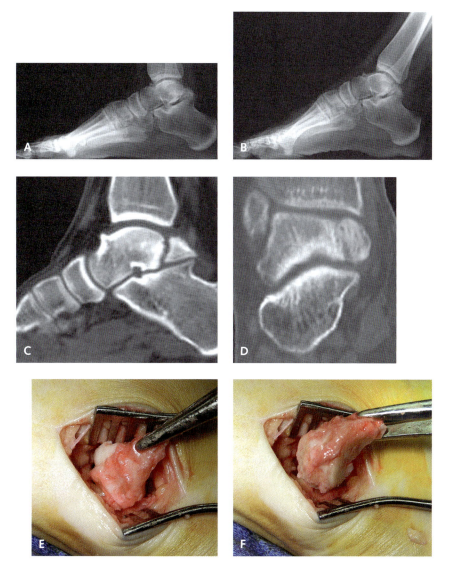

Figure 31-19 A and **B,** Flexion and extension radiographs confirmed posterior ankle impingement in a 14-year-old patient who presented with typical symptoms of this disorder. **C** and **D,** The appearance of the posterior fragment was not typical of an os trigonum, however, and the diagnosis was confirmed on computed tomography scans as a bipartite talus. **E** and **F,** The fragment was removed through a posteromedial arthrotomy.

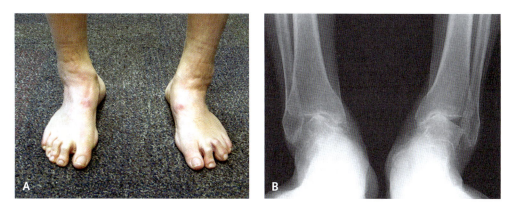

Figure 31-20 A and **B,** Varus deformity associated with bilateral severe ankle arthritis in a patient who had experienced chronic repetitive ankle sprains. This is a common outcome with repetitive untreated ankle inversion injury.

TECHNIQUES, TIPS, AND PITFALLS

- When is the Broström procedure not sufficient? What are the absolute indications for use of a nonanatomic procedure? For heavy persons and people who put a lot of demand on the ankle, the Broström procedure may not hold up, and a one-third portion of the brevis tendon can be added to the reconstruction to strengthen the repair (a Broström-Evans procedure). A nonanatomic procedure or one with a tendon graft is indicated when no tissue is available in the anterior ankle to work with, when the hindfoot is very stiff to begin with, when there is already a tear of the peroneal tendon and one half of the tendon can be used for reconstruction, and when a nonanatomic procedure will not affect the function of the ankle or subtalar joint.

- In performing a percutaneous or open tendon graft procedure, the drill hole made in the fibula must be well centered so as not to cause a fracture through the tip.

- The location of the tendon graft as it passes from the fibula down onto the calcaneus should be superficial to the peroneal tendons. This placement does not cause entrapment of the peroneal tendons, which glide under the graft, much as with a modified Chrisman-Snook procedure.

- If residual instability is present after a tendon procedure, with the ankle held in dorsiflexion and eversion, additional sutures are inserted at the anterior tip of the fibula to tighten the graft.

- Most anterior impingement syndromes can be treated arthroscopically. Very large osteophytes usually are intracapsular, and full debridement of the lesion can be difficult unless an arthrotomy is made.

- Osteophytes that are on the tibia are predominantly lateral, and those on the talus are predominantly medial.

- At the completion of debridement of the osteophytes, whether performed by arthroscopy or arthrotomy, obtaining a lateral radiograph will ensure that adequate removal has been effected.

- Osteophytes seem to recur, and application of bone wax at the completion of the ostectomy may be useful for prevention.

- Bilateral and severe ankle varus deformities are the result of chronic untreated ankle instability and do not represent primary "idiopathic osteoarthritis" (Figure 31-20).

- Ankle instability associated with ankle pain suggests an osteochondral defect of the talus. The osteochondritis dissecans lesion is most easily treated with an open arthrotomy if the ligament reconstruction is planned (Figure 31-21).

- The peroneus brevis tendon slip or tendon graft can be anchored to the calcaneus using a screw with a spiked washer or an interference screw (Figure 31-22).

- For patients with limited ankle motion and large osteophytes, removal of the impingement may be counterproductive, because the procedure will worsen the arthritis. The sudden increase in dorsiflexion merely serves to increase the range of motion, and the arthritic joint will deteriorate. Removal of osteophytes is a procedure performed for impingement, not for arthritis.

- Patients who have, in addition to the varus tilting of the talus, an indentation in the medial tibial plafond will fail to improve from an isolated ankle ligament reconstruction. The talus always falls back into this eroded tibial plafond, again pushing the talus into varus, regardless of the reconstruction performed (Figure 31-23).

- In repairing the deltoid ligament, always check for a tear of the posterior tibial tendon (Figure 31-24).

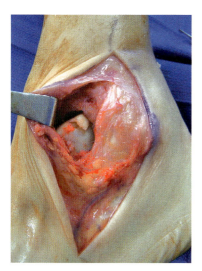

Figure 31-21 This large osteochondral lesion associated with gross ankle instability was treated with debridement, insertion of osteochondral grafts, and a Broström repair.

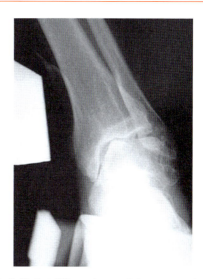

Figure 31-23 Ankle instability and varus deformity may be associated with a medial depression of the tibial plafond.

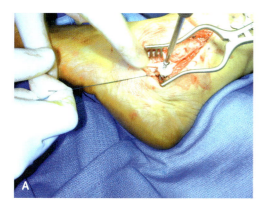

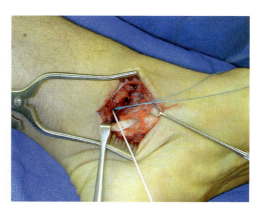

Figure 31-24 A tear of the posterior tibial tendon associated with a chronic deltoid tear.

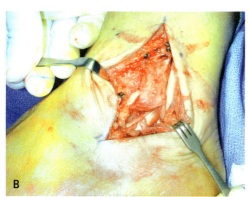

Figure 31-22 A, The attachment of the transferred split peroneus brevis tendon to the calcaneus with a screw and a spiked ligament washer. **B,** The final position of the tendon as it passes through the fibula tunnel and over the remainder of the peroneal tendons.

CHAPTER **32**

Management of Osteochondral Lesions of the Talus

SURGICAL APPROACHES TO OSTEOCHONDRAL LESIONS OF THE TALUS

With osteochondral lesions (OCD) of the talus, surgery is performed only in symptomatic cases because the lesions do not show any marked tendency for progression and typically do not lead to osteoarthritis. These lesions are a very slowly progressive condition, so there should never be any sense of urgency to treat the lesion in the absence of symptoms that warrant intervention. I generally initiate treatment with arthroscopic debridement and microfracture. The results with arthroscopic treatment of OCD lesions are good to excellent in approximately 85% of patients at initial presentation. The results with repeat arthroscopy also are fairly good, depending on the extent of the lesion. If the lesion is very large, if previous operations have failed, or if the lesion is cystic, then osteochondral autograft or allograft procedures are preferable.

Once a decision has been made to proceed with surgical treatment, several factors should be considered in selecting a particular surgical approach: the size and depth of the lesion, the exact location of the lesion (medial versus lateral, anterior versus posterior), a history of previous surgical treatment, the stage of the disease, and the viability of the articular cartilage. Whenever possible, I treat the lesion either using arthroscopy or through anterior or posterior arthrotomy. To this end, flexion-extension lateral radiographs are useful to show the location of the lesion and its accessibility by arthrotomy as opposed to osteotomy, which is associated with far greater potential morbidity.

I generally initiate treatment arthroscopically, with abrasion, drilling, and microfracture (Figure 32-1). For lesions that are large and those that have not responded to arthroscopic treatment, use of an osteochondral graft should be considered. Moderate-size defects can be filled with several small osteochondral autografts from the ipsilateral knee. Larger defects, particularly those involving the medial or lateral talar wall, may require an allograft. These marginal sidewall lesions are difficult to treat with an osteochondral autograft because the graft must be inserted perpendicular to the axis of the talar dome. With these marginal defects, a medial or lateral malleolar osteotomy must be performed.

Most anterior lesions are accessible for debridement and grafting with arthrotomy. However, if the lesion remains covered by the articular margin of the tibia, then creation of a small window in the anterior tibia is needed for further exposure. If extended visualization is required, this approach may be extended with an osteotomy of the anterior tibia, followed by replacement of the bone fragment and screw fixation.

APPROACH TO LATERAL TALAR DOME LESIONS

Most lateral talar dome lesions have a more anterior location, and if a graft is to be used, an anterolateral incision plus arthrotomy is used. The incision begins over the anterolateral aspect of the ankle, 2 cm proximal to the ankle joint, and is extended distally by 4 cm over the ankle joint (Figure 32-2). The intermediate dorsal cutaneous branches of the superficial peroneal nerve should be identified and protected. The extensor retinaculum is incised, the extensor digitorum longus tendon is identified and retracted medially, and the joint capsule is incised in line with the incision. Slight plantarflexion of the ankle will further facilitate exposure for access to debridement or grafting (Figure 32-3).

A fibular osteotomy is rarely necessary to treat a lateral talar dome lesion and is used only for very large lesions that are located centrally or posterolaterally and that cannot be accessed with arthrotomy (Figure 32-4). If a fibular osteotomy is required, then I use a 6-cm incision over the distal fibula, starting from 1 cm distal to the joint and extending proximally. The osteotomy cut is made with a microsagittal saw, oriented obliquely at an angle from lateral and proximal to distal and medial, so that the distal edge is at the level of the joint line. The advantage of the oblique osteotomy is the greater surface area for healing, as well as preservation of the interosseous ligaments. The lesion is unlikely to be visible or accessible once the osteotomy has been performed. In the rare instance in which the lateral lesion has a more central location and cannot be accessed by simply inverting the ankle, an anterolateral tibial osteotomy, in addition to the fibular osteotomy, can provide excellent visualization of the lesion.

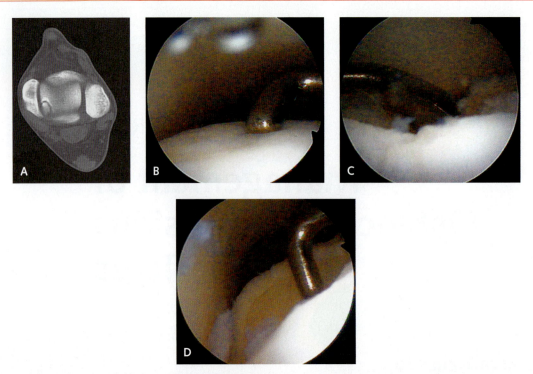

Figure 32-1 A, This is a typical posteromedial osteochondral lesion of the talus, as noted on the computed tomography scan, that is easily accessible and treatable arthroscopically. **B,** Arthroscopic view reveals softening demonstrated with use of a probe. **C,** The lesion was first debrided with curettage. **D,** This was followed by use of a shaver to create well-delineated margins.

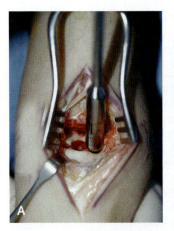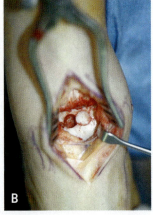

Figure 32-2 A, This large anterolateral osteochondral lesion of the talus had been twice treated with arthroscopy. **B,** An arthrotomy with osteochondral grafting was used for repair of the defect.

For any graft procedure to be performed, the lesion must be fully visible, and any graft must be inserted perpendicular to the talar surface. For this reason, an osteotomy of the lateral wall of the distal tibia often is required. The osteotomy cut must be large enough that after the graft is inserted, the piece of tibia that has been removed can be replaced and fixed with screw(s). At the completion of the intraarticular procedure, the fibular osteotomy is anatomically reduced and held with a lateral plate. The interosseous ligaments should be repaired if disrupted; likewise, if the syndesmosis was disrupted, one or more syndesmotic screws, as required, should be inserted through the plate.

For large cystic anterolateral lesions, an osteotomy of the fibula is not enough, and an osteotomy of the anterior tibia will be needed for exposure of the defect, as shown in Figure 32-5. In the case illustrated, a massive defect of the anterior talus was in a more central location and therefore inaccessible for grafting with the arthrotomy alone. The treatment plan was to use an osteoarticular allograft to fill the defect, but because the graft had to be inserted perpendicular to the axis of the talus, a tibial osteotomy was necessary. The osteotomy was made in an oblique plane (as a large fracture of the anterolateral distal tibia); 90% of the cut was made with a saw, with completion achieved by fracturing the tibia using an osteotome. The osteotomized bone was then peeled laterally, retaining the soft tissue attachments including the anterior inferior syndesmotic ligament (see Figure 32-5).

A different approach was used in another patient to fill a large, slightly more centrally located cystic defect (Figure 32-6). In this case the lesion was more longitudinally oriented, and the osteotomy of the tibia was made as a central window, followed by the graft insertion. Matching the exact size of these grafts is not easy. After removal of the necrotic center of the lesion in the talus, the talus graft is then cut to a specific size so that the margins are straight and will accept the graft. Next, I use bone wax to fill the defect and then remove the wax mold as one large piece, to get a better appreciation for the size and shape of the defect. This mold is matched as closely as possible when the osteochondral allograft is harvested (see Figure 32-6).

Central lesions are not common; when present, they are located under the tibia, making visualization very difficult without osteotomy of the tibia. In the case presented in Figure 32-7, the patient had undergone a previous medial malleolar osteotomy, which was the incorrect approach in this setting. It is important to recognize the limits of the malleolar osteotomy. After arthroscopic evaluation, anterior arthrotomy and osteotomy of the distal central tibia were performed. Once the window was removed, it was possible to insert the grafts more accurately.

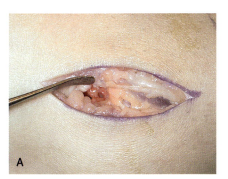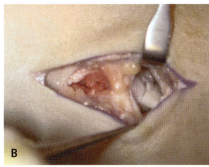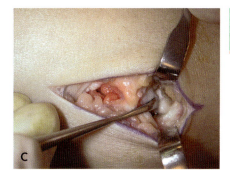

Figure 32-3 A-C, Anterolateral arthrotomy was used to treat an anterior lesion for which the patient had previously undergone unsuccessful arthroscopic debridement. (Courtesy Dr. Clifford Jeng, Institute for Foot and Ankle. Mercy Medical Center, Baltimore, Maryland.)

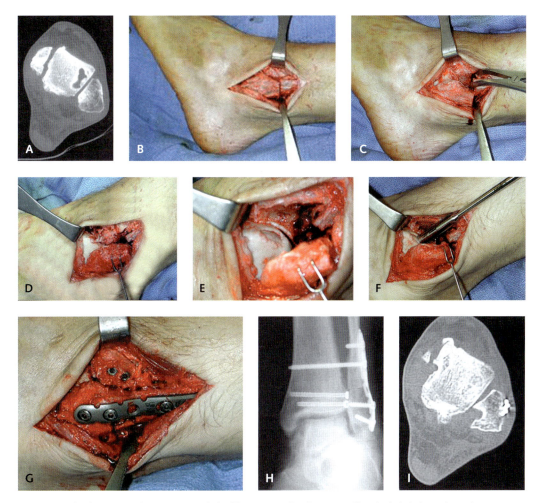

Figure 32-4 A, This large cystic lesion previously had been treated arthroscopically, which failed to relieve the patient's symptoms. **B,** An osteotomy of the fibula was used to begin definitive surgical treatment. The osteotomy shown is not in an optimal location—it is too transverse and includes disruption of the syndesmosis. **C** and **D,** The fibula was retracted laterally and the lesion exposed. **E,** An osteotomy of the distal lateral tibia was performed to obtain complete exposure of the lesion. **F,** The defect was debrided and the matched graft inserted. **G,** The osteotomy both the tibia and the fibula was then repaired, with the syndesmosis included in the fixation. **H** and **I,** Appearance of the healed lesion at 3 years after surgery.

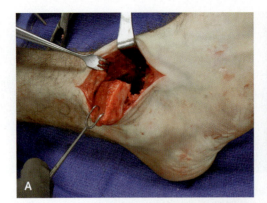
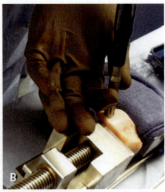
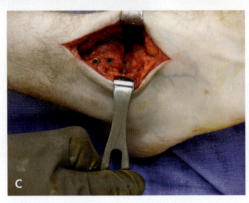

Figure 32-5 A massive anterolateral lesion in a 15-year-old patient. **A,** Treatment was begun with a standard arthrotomy. Next, the distal tibia was cut obliquely, hinging the osteotomy on the syndesmosis laterally. **B,** The grafts were harvested from a fresh osteochondral allograft. **C,** The osteotomy was repaired with screws.

APPROACH TO MEDIAL TALAR DOME LESIONS

Careful preoperative evaluation with flexion and extension lateral radiographs is essential in the management of medial talar dome lesions. For the surgical approach, if at all possible, use of a posteromedial arthrotomy is preferable to an osteotomy of the medial malleolus (Figure 32-8). Many posteromedial lesions can be completely uncovered by forcibly extending the foot passively with passive forward extension of the ankle. This same passive manipulation of the ankle can be applied intraoperatively to expose the talus.

Medial malleolar osteotomy remains a popular approach for access to medial talar dome lesions. Despite good visualization of the talus, the foot must still be forcibly everted for adequate visualization of and surgical access to the lesion, and the visualization can be improved with valgus manipulation of the foot. A saw is used to perform the first three quarters of the osteotomy cut; completion of the cut should be accomplished with an osteotome, to minimize injury to the articular cartilage. The only problem with this method is that the saw blade itself removes 1 mm of bone, so that the apposition of the osteotomy surfaces may not be perfect. Nonetheless, the osteotomy should be completed with an osteotome (Figure 32-9).

I use an oblique osteotomy that begins proximal to the tibial plafond and ends just distal to it. One problem with this technique is the potential for malunion, because as noted, apposition of the osteotomy surfaces may not be colinear with respect to the cut. This problem is compounded by the screw insertion, which should not be in the traditional plane for fixation of a fracture of the medial

malleolus, because this orientation will potentially result in a malunion (Figure 32-10). The pathomechanism presumably responsible for malunion in this setting is the creation of shear force at the osteotomy site. The addition of transverse screws perpendicular to the joint has been shown to counter this shearing force both biomechanically and clinically and helps prevent translation and malunion.

The medial malleolus is exposed through subperiosteal stripping done anteriorly and posteriorly approximately 1.5 cm above the joint line. The deltoid ligament is not disrupted. The tibialis posterior tendon must be protected at the posteromedial border of the tibia during the entire procedure. This tendon is quite vulnerable during the osteotomy. The starting point of the osteotomy is crucial to success; the cut is initiated only after insertion of a Kirschner wire (K-wire) under fluoroscopic guidance. This placement ensures that the plane of the osteotomy will be either directly on top of or lateral to the talar dome lesion. If the osteotomy is medial to the lesion, then access for grafting the defect will be insufficient, even with maximum eversion stress. The cut is made along the edge of the previously inserted K-wire either dorsal or inferior to it, depending on the position of the wire. The depth of the saw cut should be monitored fluoroscopically to ensure that a small remaining segment can be completed with an osteotome. A fine osteotome is then driven into the joint space and used as a lever, as necessary, to complete the osteotomy. The medial malleolus is reflected plantarward on the deltoid ligament, using a laminar spreader for exposure (Figure 32-11). The medial aspect of the ankle joint is exposed, and the lesion is fully visualized with forced eversion. During this stage of the repair, the malleolus needs to be kept out of the

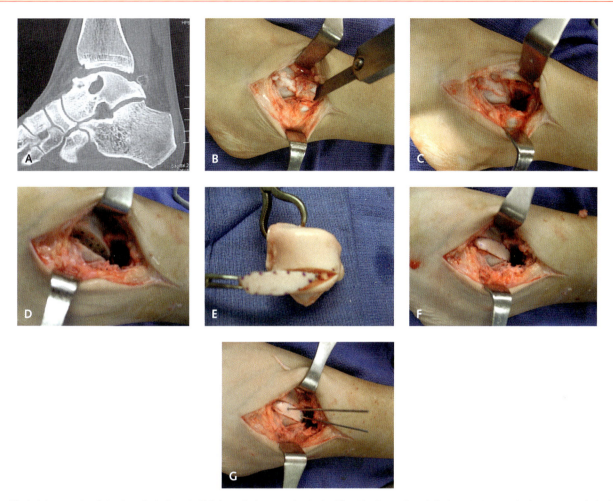

Figure 32-6 A large anterolateral cystic lesion. **A,** This large lesion was treated with arthrotomy. **B** and **C,** An osteotomy window was made in the tibia to expose the defect. **D,** The talus was cut with a chisel, and the base of the cyst was filled with cancellous graft. **E,** The graft was then harvested. **F** and **G,** After insertion of the graft, the repair was secured using absorbable pins.

way; use of a laminar spreader for this purpose may be a little too aggressive, however, so I use small skin hooks to retract and hold the bone (Figure 32-12).

Management of cystic lesions is more controversial, with numerous treatment alternatives recommended, including use of cancellous bone graft, synthetic bone graft substitutes, and osteoarticular allografts. It is always worth trying to salvage these large cystic defects as an alternative to arthrodesis. Even arthrodesis, however, is technically very difficult because of the bone loss. Accordingly, my preference is to fill the defect; then, if arthrodesis or replacement is subsequently required, the bone supportive scaffold is much improved (Figures 32-13 to 32-15).

For posteromedial lesions, I prefer to perform an arthrotomy if possible; this approach is indicated whenever the lesion is accessible using forced passive dorsiflexion of the foot. The posteromedial approach also is an excellent choice in cases of previous failed

operation or to address lesions involving the medial wall of the talus. When a small part of the medial wall of the talus is involved, treatment usually is limited to debridement of the lesion, because a graft will not hold in this location. If the entire medial wall is involved, then use of a fresh talar allograft can be considered to replace the entire medial wall. If arthrotomy without osteotomy is used, a standard posteromedial approach to the ankle joint is indicated (Figures 32-16 and 32-17). The neurovascular bundle is identified and protected with minimization of the nerve retraction. The FHL tendon is identified posterior to the neurovascular bundle and retracted posteriorly, and the tibial nerve is retracted anteriorly. The lesion is visible after capsulectomy, but the foot can be passively dorsiflexed and the posterior tibia notched with an ostectomy, with removal of a small segment of the posterior articular surface, to improve visualization of the talus and gain access for grafting.

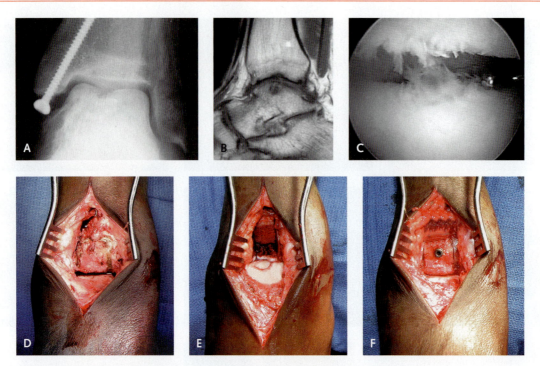

Figure 32-7 Repair after incorrect surgical approach to a large central cystic lesion. **A,** Initial approach to treatment was with a malleolar osteotomy, which did not permit adequate access to the defect because of its essentially central location. **B-D,** After arthroscopic evaluation of the joint, an anterior arthrotomy was made, and a central tibial window was cut. **E,** The lesion was grafted with biphasic synthetic plugs (Tornier, Edina, Minnesota). **F,** After replacement of the bone fragment in the window, fixation was accomplished using a single screw.

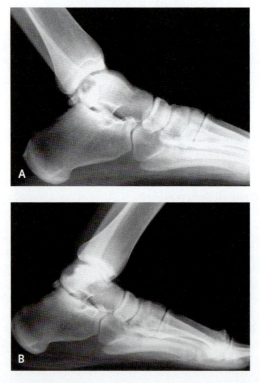

Figure 32-8 Note that the lesion is visible on the plantar flexion view **(A)** but is fully uncovered on the passive dorsiflexion lateral radiograph **(B).**

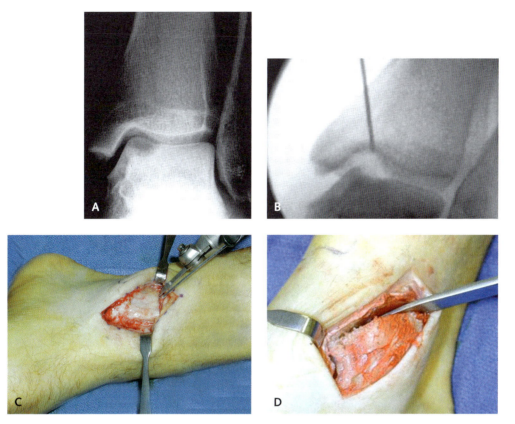

Figure 32-9 A, This medial lesion was approached with an osteotomy. **B,** The guide pin was inserted under fluoroscopic control. **C** and **D,** The osteotomy was performed mainly with a saw but was completed using an osteotome.

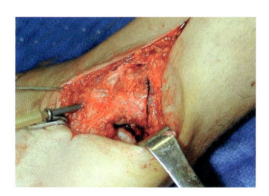

Figure 32-10 Oblique insertion of the screws after medial malleolar osteotomy, as depicted here, is not ideal, because malunion may result.

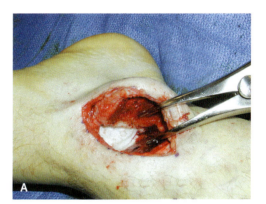

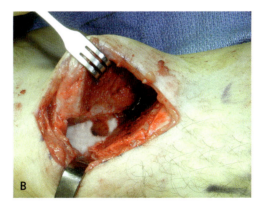

Figure 32-11 A, Use of the laminar spreader against the medial malleolus after osteotomy. **B,** The malleolus is retracted, and the graft is inserted.

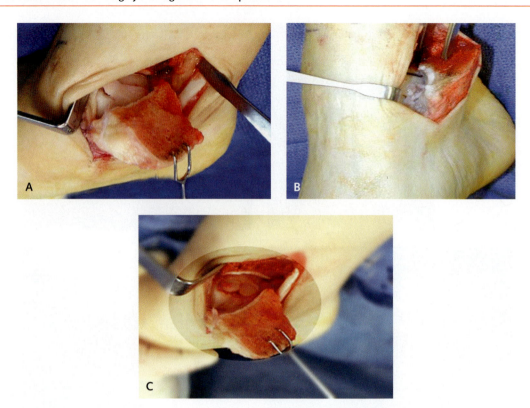

Figure 32-12 A, This very large lesion on the medial margin of the talus was approached with an osteotomy. **B,** The talus was debrided. **C,** Three bone filler plugs (OsteoCure—Tornier, Edina, Minnesota) were used to fill the defect. The advantage of use of these bone plug implants here is that unlike an osteochondral graft, they can be contoured by compression to fit the margin of the talus.

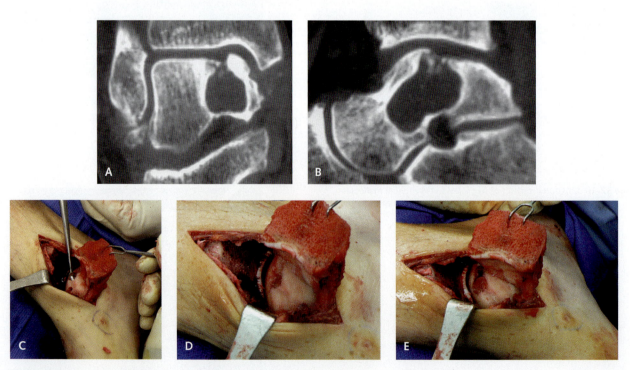

Figure 32-13 A and **B,** This massive cystic defect was approached through a medial osteotomy. **C** and **D,** The lesion was debrided with curettage, and after drilling of the sclerotic margins of the entire defect, it was first filled with cancellous bone graft mixed with a concentrate from an iliac crest aspirate. **E,** The defect was then plugged with bone filler implants (OsteoCure—Tornier, Edina, Minnesota) grafts.

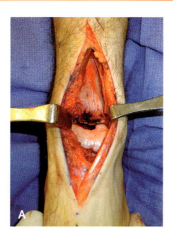
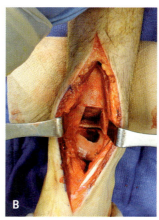
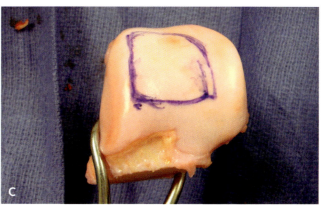

Figure 32-14 A, This central cystic defect was treated with arthrotomy and osteotomy to create a window in the tibia. **B,** This exposed the defect, which was quite large. **C,** A fresh osteochondral allograft was used to fill the defect.

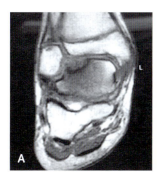
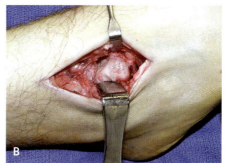
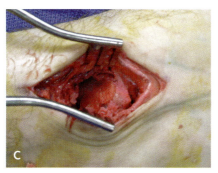

Figure 32-15 A, Large lateral lesion noted on a magnetic resonance imaging scan in a 14-year-old patient. **B** and **C,** Treatment consisted of insertion of bone filler grafts (OsteoCure—Tornier, Edina, Minnesota) through a lateral arthrotomy.

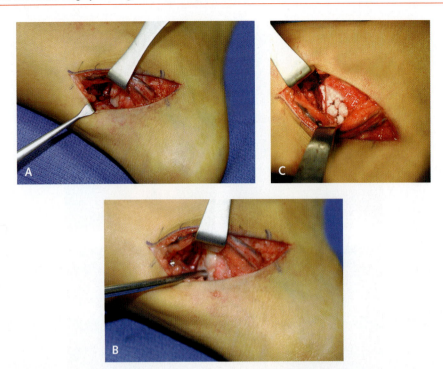

Figure 32-16 A, This posteromedial lesion was accessible with passive dorsiflexion of the ankle, and an arthrotomy was performed. **B,** The neurovascular bundle was retracted anteriorly and the flexor hallucis longus posteriorly. **C,** The lesion was debrided with curettage and then the defect was filled with multiple 6-mm osteochodral grafts harvested from the ipsilateral knee.

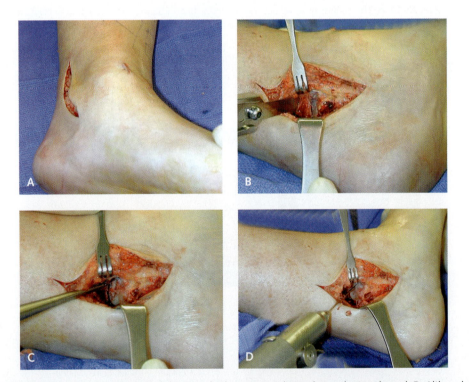

Figure 32-17 A, For the posteromedial approach, the incision is located over the tarsal canal. **B,** Although the lesion was visible, it was not entirely accessible, and a small ostectomy of the posterior tibia was performed to create a small window. **C** and **D,** Curettage **(C)** was followed by drilling and microfracture of the defect **(D).**

TECHNIQUES, TIPS, AND PITFALLS

- Almost all lesions should be treated initially with arthroscopy. In my experience, some patients with extremely large lesions do well indefinitely after arthroscopic debridement and microfracture.

- I prefer arthrotomy over osteotomy to establish access to the lesion. Whether osteotomy is performed for a medial or a lateral lesion, nonunion or malunion and further irritation of the lesion by virtue of the plane of the cut into the joint are always risks.

- A posteromedial arthrotomy works extremely well and can be used to perform debridement or osteochondral grafting.

- Marginal lesions are most difficult to treat with osteochondral autograft. Although the graft can be harvested from the margin of the femoral condyle, the shape and contour are never as well matched. If the lesion is large and on the margin of the talus, then use of a fresh osteochondral allograft may be indicated.

- Bear in mind that with use of large fresh allografts, despite correct size matching, the congruence of the graft with the articular surface of the tibia is never perfect. Each ankle joint has a unique morphology, and the match of these large grafts for marginal lesions of the talus is never perfect.

- For the medial malleolar osteotomy, insert the saw blade and check its position under fluoroscopic guidance to ensure that the saw is at the subchondral margin (Figure 32-18).

- In performing a fibula osteotomy for exposure, it is preferable to use an oblique cut, preserving the anterior syndesmotic ligament. The fibula can easily be retracted for good visualization of the lesion (Figure 32-19).

- Be careful with the orientation of the screw fixation after medial malleolar osteotomy. Screws inserted obliquely may increase shear, potentially causing a malunion (Figure 32-20, A). Correct orientation of the screws is shown in Figure 32-20, B.

- The medial malleolus osteotomy is made with the saw just to the level of the subchondral bone and then is completed using an osteotome (Figure 32-21).

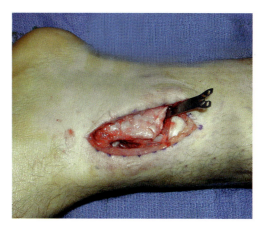

Figure 32-18 The saw blade was left in the osteotomy site, and then its position relative to the articular surface was verified.

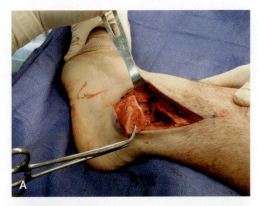

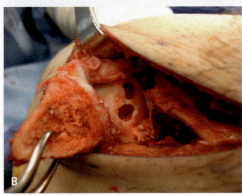

Figure 32-19 A, The oblique fibular osteotomy was used here to expose a very large lateral lesion. **B,** The defect was then debrided and prepared for grafting. (Case courtesy Dr. Rebecca Cerrato, Institute for Foot and Ankle, Mercy Medical Center, Baltimore, Maryland.)

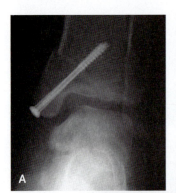

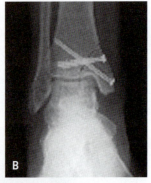

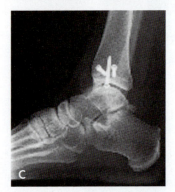

Figure 32-20 A, Incorrect use of fixation in this osteotomy, leading to a malunion and, ultimately, arthritis. **B** and **C,** The correct screw technique includes insertion of screws perpendicular to the plane of the osteotomy, thereby avoiding shear.

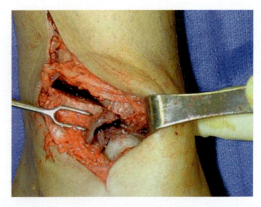

Figure 32-21 The osteotomy was performed with a saw but completed with an osteotome, to create a fractured edge more suitable for interdigitation with fixation.

SUGGESTED READING

Gautier E, Kolker D, Jakob RP: Treatment of cartilage defects of the talus by autologous osteochondral grafts, *J Bone Joint Surg Br* 84:237–244, 2002.

Hangody L, Kish G, Karpati Z, et al: Treatment of osteochondritis dissecans of the talus: Use of the mosaicplasty technique—a preliminary report, *Foot Ankle Int* 18:628–634, 1997.

Hangody L, Kish G, Modis L, et al: Mosaicplasty for the treatment of osteochondritis dissecans of the talus: Two to seven year results in 36 patients, *Foot Ankle Int* 22:552–558, 2001.

Lee CH, Chao KH, Huang GS, Wu SS: Osteochondral autografts for osteochondritis dissecans of the talus, *Foot Ankle Int* 24:815–822, 2003.

Navid DO, Myerson MS: Approach alternatives for treatment of osteochondral lesions of the talus, *Foot Ankle Clin* 7:635–649, 2002.

Schuman L, Struijs PA, van Dijk CN: Arthroscopic treatment for osteochondral defects of the talus. Results at follow-up at 2 to 11 years, *J Bone Joint Surg Br* 84:364–368, 2002.

Verhagen RA, Struijs PA, Bossuyt PM, van Dijk CN: Systematic review of treatment strategies for osteochondral defects of the talar dome, *Foot Ankle Clin* 8:233–242, 2003:viii-ix.

CHAPTER 33

Arthrodesis of the Hallux Metatarsophalangeal and Interphalangeal Joints

ARTHRODESIS OF THE HALLUX METATARSOPHALANGEAL JOINT

Approach to Arthrodesis

Arthrodesis of the hallux metatarsophalangeal (MP) joint is indicated for correction of deformity, to treat arthritis, and to address neuromuscular imbalance of the MP joint (with or without deformity). As a generalization, this is an operation that is technically easy to perform, with a predictable outcome, provided that the hallux is well positioned. Although the focus of the procedure is on the MP joint, the presence of interphalangeal (IP) joint instability, hyperextension, or arthritis may preclude a successful outcome of the arthrodesis. The key to this operation is in the correct positioning of the arthrodesis: The hallux must be slightly supinated into a neutral position, in slight dorsiflexion with respect to the correct position of the floor, and in slight valgus. Some of these parameters will need to be modified depending on patient characteristics and preferences (e.g., the running athlete, the patient who desires to wear slightly higher-heeled shoes) (Figures 33-1 and 33-2). With arthrodesis performed for correction of severe hallux valgus, a straight toe is not tolerated, and the hallux should be fused in 5 to 10 degrees of valgus (Figure 33-3).

Alignment of Arthrodesis

The dilemma always arises of how much dorsiflexion the hallux will tolerate in the fusion. Clearly, the greater the angle of dorsiflexion, the easier it will be to wear a high-heeled shoe, to perform toe-off, and to avoid any pressure on the IP joint. With a steeper MP joint angle, however, the tendency to incur rubbing on the dorsal surface of the IP joint and the nail with the underside of the shoe increases. In some patients, the tip of the hallux and the nail become painfully thickened. Furthermore, over time, if the hallux MP joint is excessively dorsiflexed, a reciprocal flexion contracture will occur at the IP joint that ultimately will become fixed and may be associated with arthritis. Conversely, too much plantar flexion of the MP joint will lead to excessive pressure under the IP joint, which is intolerably uncomfortable for the patient. Plantar flexion of the MP fusion will always lead to loosening and ultimately hyperextension of the IP joint with arthritis. The hyperextension of the hallux IP joint is a problem regardless of the status of the MP joint.

Therefore the decision regarding how much dorsiflexion to incorporate into the fusion has to be made after consideration of various factors including the presence of any preexisting hyperextension and instability of the IP joint and the patient's types and level of activity, sports interests, and shoe wear needs (Figure 33-4). Fusion of the hallux MP joint at an angle is preferable to the position of the floor rather than the metatarsal. The metatarsal declination varies considerably, and the more predictable position would be with reference to the floor. In the setting of a cavus foot or a steep plantar flexed first metatarsal, however, arthrodesis of the hallux MP joint will result in pain under the first metatarsal head and sesamoiditis. If MP joint fusion is the only possible treatment option in the setting of a fixed forefoot equinus or plantar flexed first ray, a dorsal wedge osteotomy of the first metatarsal may have to be performed before proceeding with the arthrodesis. The converse applies in a patient with severe elevatus of the first metatarsal. Here, position of the fusion relative to the metatarsal may be in neutral alignment, but the hallux remains elevated relative to the floor. Not much, if any, dorsiflexion can be incorporated in the hallux MP joint in patients with metatarsus primus elevatus.

The position of the hallux in the transverse plane can be difficult in the presence of a marked increase in the first to second intermetatarsal space (angle). After correction of hallux valgus with an arthrodesis of the MP joint, the decrease in the intermetatarsal angle will be almost proportionate to the magnitude of the deformity preoperatively. Therefore, in view of the expected decrease of this deformity, where is the hallux placed in the fusion intraoperatively? For example, if the hallux is placed in slight valgus, with the anticipation that a decrease in the intermetatarsal angle will occur postoperatively, the hallux is ultimately going to abut the second toe. For this reason, if I am dealing with severe deformity, I place a temporary lag screw between the first and second metatarsals to close down the intermetatarsal space. The deformity is thereby reduced, allowing more accurate prediction of the location for correction of the hallux with the arthrodesis. The other option is to undercorrect the hallux and leave it in a slightly more neutral position than usual, with the anticipation of the change in position of the first ray after the operation.

The alignment of the hallux in the coronal plane must be accurate. If the hallux is overpronated, pain will be present at both the medial aspect of the IP joint and the medial margin of the nail, with

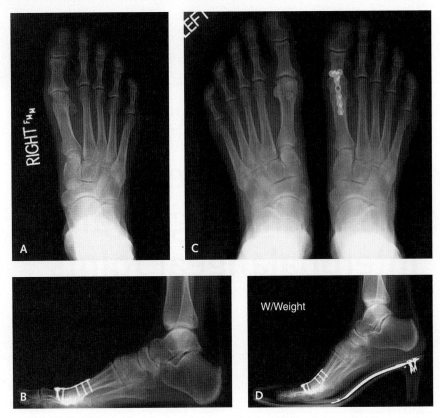

Figure 33-1 A, The patient was a recreational dancer who desired marked dorsiflexion in the hallux to enable her activities. She had undergone two previous failed surgeries and preferred the stability of arthrodesis to an arthroplasty. **B-D,** Note the position of the hallux at rest (**B** and **C**) and in a 7-cm high-heeled shoe (**D**).

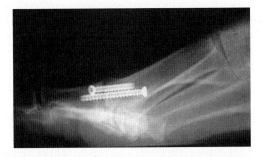

Figure 33-2 The patient was a short-distance runner who desired more dorsiflexion to permit rapid toe-off. Note the clearance of the hallux off the ground.

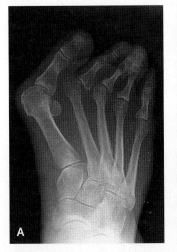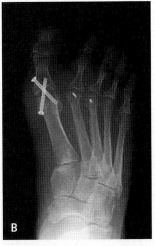

Figure 33-3 A and **B,** Correction of hallux valgus and metatarsus adductus was obtained with an arthrodesis, placing the metatarsophalangeal joint in slightly more valgus than that used for management of arthritis.

consequent ingrowth of the toenail (Figure 33-5). Pronation of the hallux MP joint fusion will lead to marked fixed deformity of the IP joint in flexion and valgus, which is very difficult to correct. If indeed this deformity develops, the MP fusion should be revised to prevent fixed changes with arthritis in the IP joint. Oversupination leads to pain on the medial or lateral nail fold, and an ingrown toenail can result as well. The best way to check alignment of the hallux is to look at the way the hallux nail lines up with the adjacent toenails.

Sesamoid Issues

Occasionally patients experience sesamoiditis after arthrodesis of the hallux MP joint. If present, this condition usually is the result of soft tissue atrophy under a plantar flexed first metatarsal, rather

than painful arthritis between the sesamoid and the first metatarsal head. If the latter occurs, it can be secondary to a hypertrophy of the sesamoid. It cannot always be anticipated, and a sesamoidectomy may need to be performed at a later date after the arthrodesis. If the patient has sesamoid pain (from pressure) preoperatively, however, the sesamoid can be resected in conjunction with the arthrodesis of

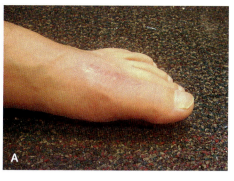

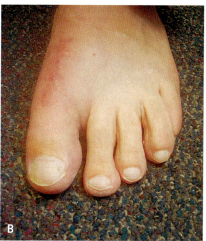

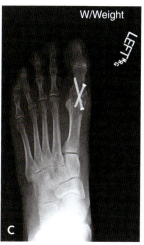

Figure 33-4 A-C, The ideal position for an arthrodesis is demonstrated with the hallux slightly elevated off the floor, correctly positioned in the coronal plane, and in very slight valgus.

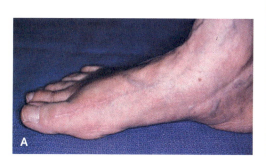

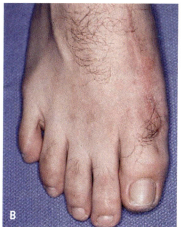

Figure 33-5 A and **B,** The hallux has been fused in too much pronation in these two patients. The nail of the hallux does not line up with the nails of the lesser toes, and development of an ingrown toenail is likely.

the hallux MP joint. It is possible to resect the sesamoid(s) through the dorsal incision. If such resection is anticipated, a medial approach to the MP arthrodesis can be used, making the sesamoidectomy easier to perform. If symptoms of pain under the metatarsal head occur after arthrodesis, removal of the sesamoid is very easy from a direct medial approach to the MP joint.

Bone Grafting

Bone graft is not used for the standard MP fusion and is necessary only when either shortening of the hallux, osteolysis, or cystic defects are present. To correct a very short hallux or one for which graft is clearly required, the decision is between fusing the hallux in situ with cancellous bone graft and using a bone block graft to

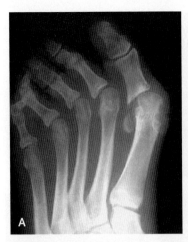 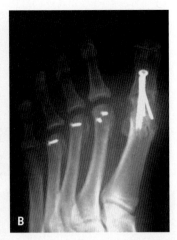

Figure 33-6 A, The patient presented with persistent pain and deformity after an unsuccessful resection arthroplasty. **B,** Despite shortening of the hallux, an in situ arthrodesis was performed.

lengthen the hallux. Clearly, if severe shortening of the hallux is present with transfer metatarsalgia, then an arthrodesis with a bone block graft would be ideal. Even with minor bone loss, although an arthrodesis is technically feasible, some further shortening of the hallux always occurs as a result of preparation of the joint surfaces; from a functional as well as a cosmetic standpoint, even minimal shortening is undesirable (Figures 33-6 and 33-7). If an in situ arthrodesis is performed when metatarsalgia is present, then either shortening osteotomies of the lesser metatarsals or metatarsal head resection should be considered. With the current custom plates designed specifically for use with a lengthening arthrodesis of the MP joint, as well as the use of orthobiologic agents, my preference usually is to lengthen the MP joint with a structural bone graft (Figure 33-8).

Approach and Joint Preparation

The technique for arthrodesis of the MP joint with standard exposure and crossed cannulated screw fixation is demonstrated in Figure 33-9. The incision is made medial to the extensor hallucis longus (EHL) tendon, over a length of 4 cm, with a small cuff of extensor retinaculum left for later closure. The extensor tendon is retracted laterally, and using subperiosteal dissection, the entire articulation is exposed. Forcibly plantar flexing the proximal phalanx is helpful; plantar flexion facilitates dissection of the periosteum off both sides of the joint. With further plantar flexion of the hallux, the undersurface of the proximal phalanx, including the attachment of the volar plate, is easily dissected. Stripping the attachment of the sesamoids is unnecessary because they retract once the volar plate is released.

The maximum length of the hallux should be preserved when the bone cuts are planned. If a saw is used to create flat cuts, apposition of the bone surfaces is not difficult, but more bone will be removed, and the hallux is shortened. Planning the ultimate position of the hallux is not as easy with flat saw cuts, and repeated shaving of either side of the joint may need to be done until the hallux is in the correct position. Alternatively, a cup and cone shape can be created to contour the joint surfaces, with use of either custom conical reamers or a 5-mm burr to denude the articular surface. I start with the hallux, burr into the phalanx, and preserve

as much of the medial cortex of the base of the proximal phalanx for later screw fixation. I try to maintain as much of the rim of the joint as possible, but it is important to burr down to healthy, bleeding cancellous bone. A reciprocal cone shape is created with the burr on the metatarsal head, and the proximal phalanx is used as a guide for the shaping of the metatarsal head. With this technique, a cock-up position of the hallux resulting from excessive dorsal bone resection should be avoided.

The hallux is reduced, and the alignment of the hallux is determined on the basis of decision making with the patient regarding shoe wear, type and level of activity, and the shape of the forefoot. The hallux is placed in 10 degrees of dorsiflexion relative to the weight-bearing surface of the floor and supinated so that the hallux nail is now parallel with the nails of the lesser toes, and slight valgus is incorporated into the position of the arthrodesis. Before reduction and fixation of the joint are performed, it is important to ensure that the head or phalanx has no bone defect. Even when good bone apposition can be achieved, if minimal bone contact is present circumferentially, a small cancellous bone graft is required; either cancellous autograft or an orthobiologic substitute can be used. Graft can be obtained from the calcaneus through a 1-cm incision on the posterior inferior heel, posterior to the sural nerve and anterior to the Achilles tendon. A small trephine can be used to harvest a 1-cm-long cylindrical tube of cancellous bone, which can be contoured and placed in the defect in the MP joint.

Fixation

For a straightforward arthrodesis with good bone support, I typically use cannulated 4.0-mm screws for fixation. Of note, use of partially threaded screws is not necessary, because broad cancellous bone surfaces are present, and the fusion requires rigidity and stability as much as compression. Nonetheless, if the bone quality is good, I currently use partially threaded screws. With the hallux in the reduced position, guide pins are introduced to cross the articular surface. The first guide pin is introduced from the plantar medial aspect of the undersurface of the metatarsal neck just proximal to the metatarsal head. This pin is aimed distally and passed out of the metatarsal head and into the lateral base of the proximal

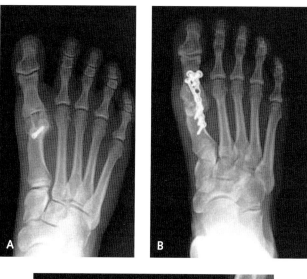

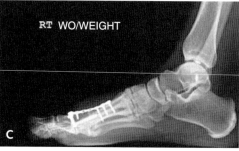

Figure 33-7 A, Avascular necrosis with shortening after bunionectomy. B and C, Treatment was with an in situ arthrodesis with plate fixation, supplemented by bone morphogenetic protein stimulation.

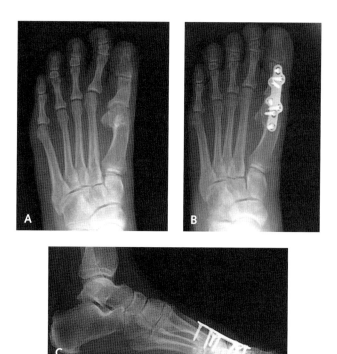

Figure 33-8 A, Avascular necrosis associated with second and third metatarsalgia and a crossover toe deformity. B and C, Treatment consisted of a bone block lengthening arthrodesis for the hallux and tendon transfers to correct the crossover toe deformity of the second toe.

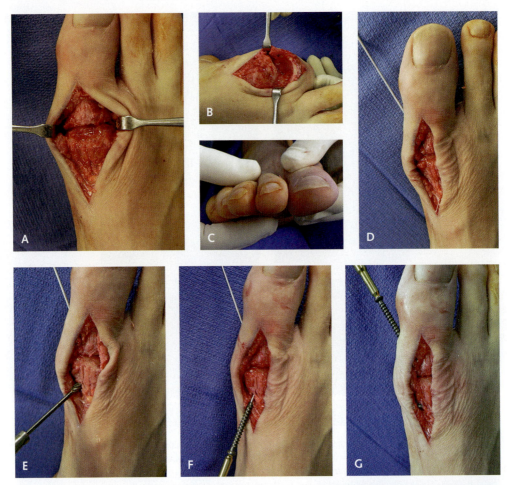

Figure 33-9 The steps for metatarsophalangeal arthrodesis.
A, A dorsal longitudinal incision is made medial to the extensor hallucis longus. **B,** The joint is plantar flexed, and a cup and cone debridement is performed using a burr. **C,** The position of the hallux is moved from neutral to a corrected position of slight supination so that the nails line up correctly. **D,** The first guide pin is introduced from the plantar-medial hallux. **E,** The countersink is prepared with a burr on the metatarsal neck. **F** and **G,** Placement of a cannulated 4.0-mm screw, followed by insertion of the second screw. **H,** The final position of the hallux is verified by pushing upward from the plantar surface; note the slight elevation of the toe.

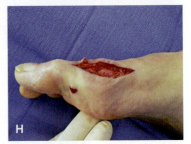

phalanx. It is useful to make a small pilot burr hole as a countersink maneuver before inserting the guide pin. The second guide pin is introduced from distal to proximal from the medial aspect of the base of the proximal phalanx across the metatarsal head and exits slightly dorsally and laterally. If the bone on the base of the phalanx or medial head is inadequate (as, for example, after bunionectomy), one of the screws is introduced from the dorsal neck of the metatarsal head distally into the phalanx.

Before insertion of the screws, the neck must be prepared with either a countersink maneuver or by creating a larger hole with a burr, to prevent fracture and to facilitate the correct angulation of the screw across the joint. The first screw is introduced from the metatarsal head going distally. During the introduction of the first screw, the hallux is compressed manually across the articular surface to provide maximum contact and compression during

the screw fixation. The second screw is introduced from distal to proximal, but before insertion the medial cortex of the base of the proximal phalanx must be prepared to prevent fracture with a cannulated drill.

Sometimes the standard screw fixation is not sufficient because of the plane of the metatarsal head or the proximal phalanx. This problem may arise, for example, after failed bunionectomy, when a medial eminence is not present and less of an anchor point is available for the head of the screw. If bone loss is a factor or if the contour of the metatarsal head does not facilitate internal fixation, other means of fixation must be used instead of screws. Alternatives include a dorsal plate, multiple threaded small K-wires, and large threaded Steinmann pins (Figure 33-10). Clearly, crossing the hallux IP joint is not desirable but is necessary with use of the larger threaded pins. Sometimes, however, the bone loss is so severe that

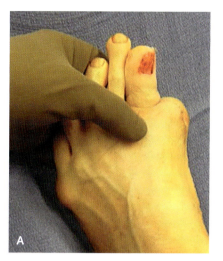
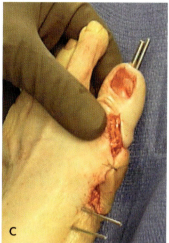
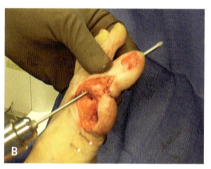

Figure 33-10 A, Severe erosive dislocation of the hallux, with no bone of substance remaining in the proximal phalanx. **B,** The arthrodesis was performed with threaded Steinmann pins inserted in antegrade and then retrograde fashion. Two transverse pins were inserted between the first and second metatarsals. There was significant diastasis between the metatarsals, and the alignment of the hallux could not be based on the relationship between the hallux and the first metatarsal. **C,** The first and second metatarsals were squeezed together, the transverse pins were introduced, and then the Steinmann pins were inserted retrograde across the metatarsophalangeal joint.

the MP joint has to be anchored with the distal phalanx for support. An anchoring method that I have found to be very stable is to use one crossed oblique 4.0-mm partially threaded screw supplemented by a custom dorsal MP fusion plate (Orthohelix, Akron, Ohio).

Correction of Deformity Associated With Bone Loss

In cases with severe bone resorption or bone loss, an in situ arthrodesis is not sufficient, and structural support with an interposition graft must be considered. With the use of custom-designed plates and added orthobiologic agents, structural grafting has now become a relatively easy procedure to perform. For selected patients, such as those with severe bone loss and erosive synovitis associated with failed implant arthroplasty, the surgery can be staged. For these patients, I remove the implant, resect the fibrinous debris, lengthen the EHL tendon, and fill the defect in the phalanx and metatarsal head with cancellous bone graft. After 6 months, once the graft has incorporated, the second-stage structural graft–fusion procedure is performed. Some patients, however, are reasonably comfortable after the first stage of the surgery, so the second stage with arthrodesis is not performed. Although the hallux remains short and weak, the pain from the inflammatory synovitis dissipates, and function is acceptable. Another alternative is to stage surgery by removing all debris, hardware, and necrotic bone, in particular when the possibility of infection is a concern. A good example is presented in Figure 33-11. In the case illustrated,

the patient underwent multiple unsuccessful surgical attempts at an MP arthrodesis, resulting in a nonunion, as well as a questionable nonunion of the tarsometatarsal joint and possible chronic infection. The hardware was removed, and after culture samples were obtained, antibiotic-impregnated cement was inserted as a spacer to maintain bone length; the second-stage surgery was performed 6 weeks later with a bone block lengthening arthrodesis.

Joint Exposure and Preparation for Distraction Bone Block Arthrodesis

The exposure for the arthrodesis is similar to that described previously, but the EHL tendon may need lengthening. There is no standard way to prepare the bone, because irregular bone defects are frequent (Figures 33-12 to 33-14). In addition to flat bone cuts, the head and phalanx can be prepared in exactly the same way as discussed previously with a burr, and then a reciprocal shape can be created with a slight contour and indentation in the bone graft.

Considerable sclerosis of the bone margins often is present, and once the sclerosis is debrided down to bleeding bone margins, the defect can be quite considerable. After the cuts at the bone ends have been fashioned, a lamina spreader is inserted into the joint space with maximum distraction, and the gap is measured using fluoroscopic imaging. While the laminar spreader is in place, it is important to check the perfusion to the soft tissues and the hallux, because ischemia may be present. I do not use a tourniquet for this

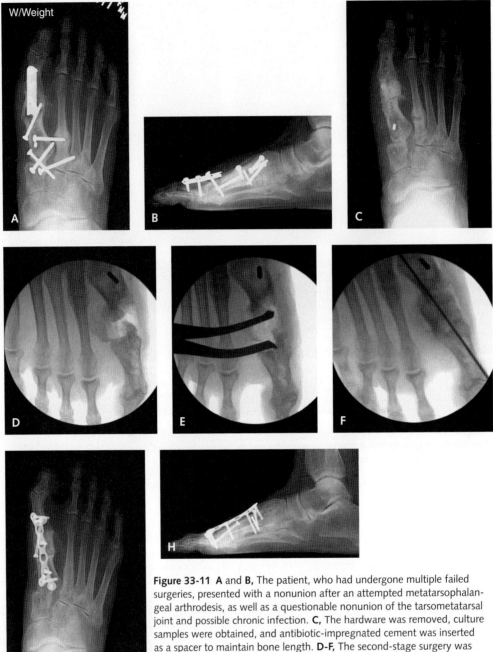

Figure 33-11 A and **B,** The patient, who had undergone multiple failed surgeries, presented with a nonunion after an attempted metatarsophalangeal arthrodesis, as well as a questionable nonunion of the tarsometatarsal joint and possible chronic infection. **C,** The hardware was removed, culture samples were obtained, and antibiotic-impregnated cement was inserted as a spacer to maintain bone length. **D-F,** The second-stage surgery was performed 6 weeks later with a bone block lengthening arthrodesis. **G** and **H,** Final postoperative appearance.

procedure, because the lengthening may have to be adjusted according to the perfusion of the hallux. Slight adjustment to the bone cuts may need to be made with a saw or burr, and the final position of the MP joint may again need to be checked fluoroscopically. I use a structural allograft, usually from a femoral head allograft, which is now shaped to fill the void in the MP joint. I try to preserve as much length of the metatarsal as possible, meaning that the phalanx and the metatarsal are not cut transversely. The shape of the graft is cut according to the shape of the metatarsal and phalanx so as to maximize bone length. It is only when the edge of the bone is very abnormal, causing instability of the graft, that I use a straight cut. A saw is used to contour the graft. Once the graft has been contoured, it is cut repeatedly until it can easily be recessed into the

prepared slot of the MP joint. Note that the allograft is cut from the femoral head at the neck, thereby incorporating slight dorsiflexion into the arthrodesis (see Figure 33-15, *C*).

A lengthening bone block arthrodesis of the hallux MP joint is not easy and is facilitated with forcible plantar flexion of the hallux and insertion of the graft under distraction. If these measures do not work, then a smooth laminar spreader can be used to recreate the gap with more tension for insertion of the graft. No tension should be on the skin, which must close easily. The graft must be intrinsically stable at this point, with minimal motion present on passive manipulation of the joint. Fixation must be stable, and a plate is invariably used. If sufficient bone is present, I try to use an oblique screw first, supplemented by the dorsal plate. At times, however, the bone of the

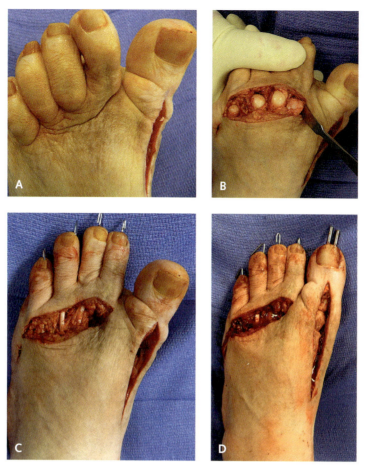

Figure 33-12 A, Gross shortening in a patient with intractable metatarsalgia and scarring after previous forefoot surgery. **B-D,** In addition to the lengthening arthrodesis, shortening osteotomies of the lesser metatarsals were performed.

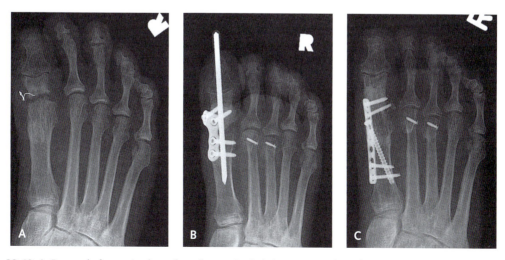

Figure 33-13 A, Removal of excessive bone from the proximal phalanx in a poorly performed resection arthroplasty resulted in a very unstable hallux. **B,** As a consequence of the bone loss, capacity for fixation was very limited, and a plate and threaded pin were used to hold the graft in place. **C,** Subsequent nonunion of the proximal segment of the graft was successfully treated with repeat plate fixation.

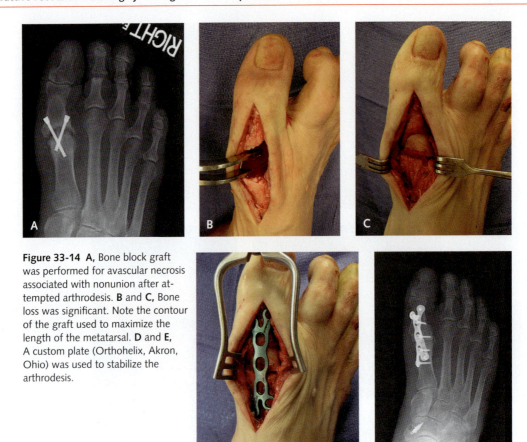

Figure 33-14 A, Bone block graft was performed for avascular necrosis associated with nonunion after attempted arthrodesis. **B** and **C,** Bone loss was significant. Note the contour of the graft used to maximize the length of the metatarsal. **D** and **E,** A custom plate (Orthohelix, Akron, Ohio) was used to stabilize the arthrodesis.

Figure 33-15 A, Lengthening arthrodesis was performed for treatment of infection with bone loss after bunionectomy. **B,** The length was established with a laminar spreader. **C,** The graft was cut from the neck of the femoral head allograft. **D,** The graft was then "press fitted" into place by forcible plantar flexion of the hallux under distraction.

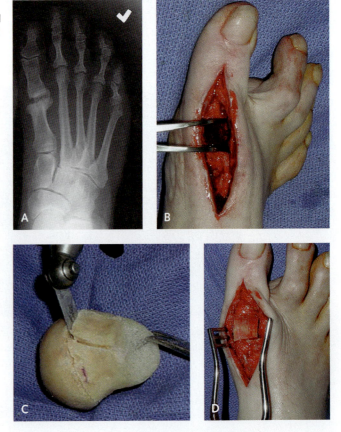

proximal phalanx is absent or insufficient for application of the plate, and large threaded pins are inserted across the IP joint. This type of fixation is difficult because the pins exit the metatarsal neck on its plantar and medial aspect, in accordance with the degree of dorsiflexion incorporated in the MP fusion. The pins must be inserted in antegrade fashion, and then, while the hallux is compressed manually, they must be redirected in retrograde manner across the MP joint.

ARTHRODESIS OF THE HALLUX INTERPHALANGEAL JOINT

33

Deformity, instability, and arthritis of the hallux IP joint can be difficult to manage, particularly if the hallux MP joint is also stiff, fused, or deformed. Although arthrodesis is the procedure of choice for correction of many of these deformities, an arthroplasty may be preferable to address instability (Figure 33-21), particularly

TECHNIQUES, TIPS, AND PITFALLS

- Arthrodesis of the hallux MP joint must be performed carefully if the IP joint is already hyperextended. Even if the hallux MP joint is correctly positioned in slight dorsiflexion, overload of the hallux IP joint may still occur. If the hallux MP joint is fused in too much dorsiflexion, the tip of the hallux is subjected to pressure on the shoe, with consequent discomfort, as a result of the preexisting hyperextension of the IP joint.

- The hyperextension of the IP joint may require correction, which can be done simultaneously or subsequently if the condition is symptomatic. In Figure 33-16, although the hyperextension was not severe, it was not tolerated by the patient because it resulted in pressure on the tip of the hallux, so correction was indicated. A malunion of an arthrodesis in excessive dorsiflexion or plantar flexion is easiest to approach from a medial incision, with use of a dome saw blade to contour and reposition the joint.

- Arthrodesis of the MP joint in the setting of a short hallux must be done carefully because the hallux will always shorten further simply from preparation of the joint surface.

- Nonunion after hallux MP arthrodesis is unusual and results from inadequate joint preparation, inappropriate fixation technique, or lack of patient compliance with mobilization postoperatively. The approach to revision can be identical to that for the primary procedure, provided that stable fixation is obtained and bone graft or bone graft substitutes are used to fill any defects or bone deficits.

- If an arthrodesis of the MP joint is performed for correction of severe hallux valgus deformity associated with arthritis, the lesser toe deformities must be corrected simultaneously. If they are not, a large, uncomfortable gap between the hallux and the second toe will occur. Release of the lesser toe MP joints does not provide sufficient correction, and relaxation of

the intrinsic tendons can only be accompanied with shortening osteotomies of the metatarsal head.

- With severe deformity of both the first metatarsal and the hallux associated with arthritis, positioning the hallux and the arthrodesis correctly is difficult. In such cases, intraoperatively realigning the first metatarsal with a compression screw inserted from the first across to the second metatarsal is helpful. This is a temporary stabilizing screw that can be removed at 3 months postoperatively. Use of a stabilizing screw is advantageous in that it realigns the metatarsal and facilitates correct positioning of the arthrodesis. Otherwise, as the position of the first metatarsal changes after surgery, the position of the hallux may change as well, potentially leading to an abutment between the hallux and the second toe.

- If bone is avascular or the success of the arthrodesis is questionable, orthobiologic agents are used to enhance the rate of fusion.

- The alignment of arthrodesis of the MP joint in the presence of hallux valgus interphalangeus is difficult, and even if positioned in slight varus, arthritis of the IP joint may ultimately occur (Figure 33-17; see also Figure 33-16). An additional osteotomy of the phalanx (a distal Akin osteotomy) should be performed to correct deformity. The alternative is to force the MP fusion into a neutral position to accommodate the valgus interphalangeus. This maneuver will work only for very mild interphalangeus deformity.

- With severe hallux valgus deformity with a widened intermetatarsal space, an osteotomy of the first metatarsal never needs to be performed because the intermetatarsal (IM) angle will decrease after the MP fusion. There is always a reduction of the valgus force of the hallux on the first metatarsal after arthrodesis. However, when the IM deformity is severe, deciding where to position the hallux in the transverse plane is

(Continued)

TECHNIQUES, TIPS, AND PITFALLS—cont'd

difficult, because some closure of the intermetatarsal space will occur after fusion, which will then lead to abutment of the hallux on the second toe. A lag screw between the first and second metatarsals is used in such instances (Figure 33-18).

● Presence of thinned-out skin under the metatarsal head may necessitate a sesamoidectomy performed in conjunction with the arthrodesis.

● The prominent medial eminence must be removed when arthrodesis is performed for correction of hallux valgus.

● Be careful with positioning of the hallux if the IP joint is unstable. Pushing up on the hallux may give a false sense of the sagittal position of the hallux, owing to the hyperextension. Measure the dorsiflexion angle off the true position of the proximal phalanx (Figure 33-19).

● Malunion of the arthrodesis in the sagittal plane is most easily corrected with a revision starting with a medial incision. An osteotomy can be performed through the arthrodesis, using a dome saw blade to rotate the hallux into the correct position (Figure 33-20).

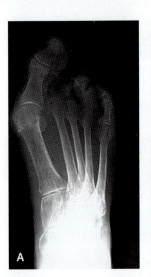 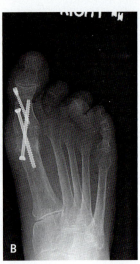

Figure 33-16 A, The deformity pictured was associated with marked hallux valgus, arthritis of the hallux MP joint, and hallux valgus interphalangeus. **B,** It was important to realign the hallux correctly, done with a distal phalangeal osteotomy in conjunction with the arthrodesis.

instability of the IP joint. Typically, the MP joint is slightly stiff or the first metatarsal is elevated, causing the instability. More severe cases are characterized by considerable arthritis at the MP joint and associated instability with hyperextension of the IP joint. I prefer not to fuse the painfully unstable IP joint, particularly in cases with any more proximal pathologic changes. Arthrodesis of the hallux IP joint is an excellent procedure for realignment, management of arthritis, or correction of a fixed claw hallux deformity or deformity in general. If the MP joint is already stiff, however, an arthrodesis of the IP joint is not ideal because the repair results in massive loading on the undersurface of the IP joint, with consequent pain.

Although arthrodesis of both the IP and MP joints is a procedure that may be necessary at times and is discussed in greater detail further on, I prefer to preserve some flexibility at the IP joint if possible. Accordingly, for patients with instability but no arthritis

of the IP joint, I advance the volar plate or tighten the flexor hallucis longus (FHL) tendon, or both (Figure 33-22). The procedure is performed through an incision medial to the IP joint, and with soft tissue retraction, the FHL tendon is exposed. A small stump of the FHL tendon is left attached to the base of the distal phalanx. The excursion of the FHL is assessed by pulling on the tendon to determine the ideal tension in the FHL tendon which will leave the joint in a neutral position. Before the tendon is cut, two stay sutures are inserted into each end (see Figure 33-22). The tendon is then cut at that level, usually with removal of a 1-cm segment. The proximal end of the cut tendon is sutured and advanced into the base of the distal phalanx. Two 2-mm drill holes are made from dorsal to plantar at the base of the distal phalanx, just distal to the joint. The drill is angled in a proximal and plantar direction. One suture is passed through the more lateral hole and then subcutaneously from lateral to medial. The second strand of suture is passed from plantar to dorsal, and the sutures are tied dorsomedially with the hallux IP joint set at the correct tension. The repair is reinforced under the IP joint with additional 2-0 sutures between the two ends of the FHL tendon (see Figure 33-22).

If instability of the hallux IP joint is present and associated with arthritis, then either of two alternative treatments—the one an arthrodesis and the other an arthroplasty—can be selected. For both of these procedures, I use a dorsal approach to the joint, exposing and protecting the extensor hallucis longus (EHL). The EHL is retracted either medially or laterally, and the IP joint is exposed. Usually, the joint is not easy to visualize well, because dorsal osteophytes are blocking exposure. These must be removed either before or after resection of the phalanx. The distal 5 mm of the proximal phalanx is now cut with a saw, with care taken not to damage the EHL tendon during excursion of the saw blade (Figure 33-23). The bone is removed and the dorsal osteophytes on the base of the proximal phalanx are trimmed. The joint is distracted and the volar plate and the FHL are grasped with a clamp and pulled into the incision. The FHL is then sutured to the undersurface of the EHL, the dorsal capsule, or the periosteum. If this method of fixation is not adequate, the suture can be inserted through K-wire holes in the proximal phalanx.

Arthrodesis of the hallux IP joint is indicated for correction of a claw hallux deformity, for correction of inflammatory or traumatic

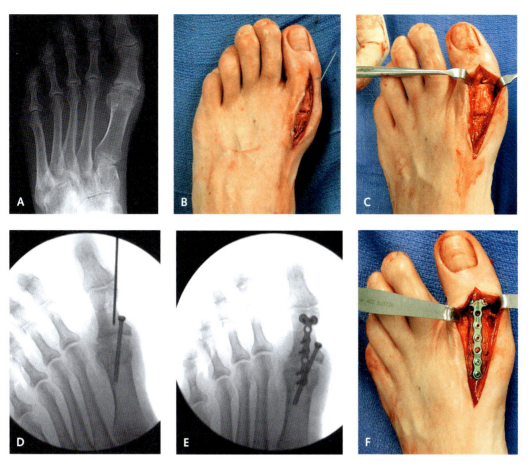

Figure 33-17 A, Severe interphalangeus deformity of the hallux in combination with arthritis of the metatarsophalangeal (MP) joint. **B-D,** The hallux cannot be fused in this position, and a distal Akin osteotomy also was performed after the MP joint was secured with a cannulated screw **(B),** the phalangeal osteotomy was performed **(C),** and temporary fixation was obtained **(D). E** and **F,** Permanent fixation was accomplished with an F3 plate (DePuy Orthopaedics, Inc., Warsaw, Indiana).

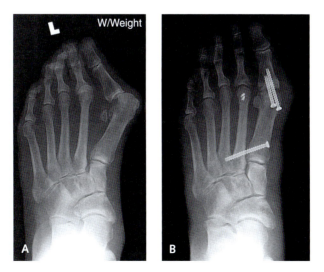

Figure 33-18 A and **B,** An arthrodesis of the MP joint was performed in conjunction with placement of a lag screw between the first and second metatarsals, to obtain better alignment of the metatarsal for positioning of the arthrodesis components.

arthritis, or for procedures that involve the harvesting of the EHL tendon for transfer. Clawing of the hallux is a common deformity and is caused by any condition that leads to atrophy, contracture, or absence of the flexor hallucis brevis. This deformity is commonly associated with overpull of the EHL and the FHL, leading to a fixed deformity at the IP joint. As noted in the chapter on claw hallux deformity, an arthrodesis of the IP joint is one option for treating this condition (Figure 33-24). In most circumstances, motion at the hallux IP joint should be maintained if possible, and if the contracture can be released, the IP joint manipulated, or balance restored to the hallux; this is preferable to arthrodesis. Lengthening of the FHL behind the ankle is a good option if the contracture is caused by tethering proximal to the ankle. The IP arthrodesis traditionally is performed when a transfer of the EHL tendon is performed, because the FHL will then cause an imbalance in the IP joint, leading to a more fixed flexion contracture. This is not always the outcome, however, and a transfer of the EHL tendon can be performed without an arthrodesis if the toe can be straightened.

In Figure 33-24, a fixed contracture in a patient with a cavus foot deformity was treated with IP arthrodesis. Another example of the use of hallux IP arthrodesis is presented in Figure 33-25; in this case, a 19-year-old patient presented with a severe fixed deformity of the hallux secondary to a tibia fracture resulting in a compartment syndrome of the leg. This deformity was not possible to treat without arthrodesis.

The IP joint may have to be included in an arthrodesis performed in conjunction with an arthrodesis of the hallux MP joint for severe forefoot deformity. This is necessary, for example, in patients with rheumatoid arthritis and certain congenital deformities. In the case illustrated in Figure 33-26, the patient presented for correction of congenital aplasia and hallux varus; an arthrodesis of the distal phalanx to the hallux was performed on one side, and a simultaneous arthrodesis of the IP and MP joints on the opposite foot. The clinical result was quite satisfactory despite the flexed position of the hallux. The problem for this patient was the extension deformity of the tip of the hallux with associated chronic nail problems,

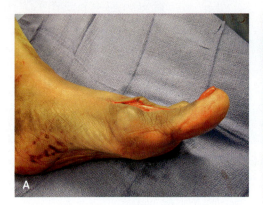
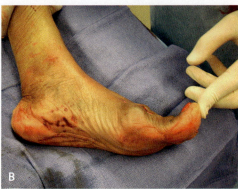

Figure 33-19 A and **B,** Position of the hallux initially was incorrect owing to the hyperextension of the hallux interphalangeal joint, and the proximal phalanx was not sufficiently dorsiflexed.

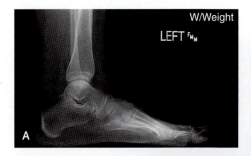
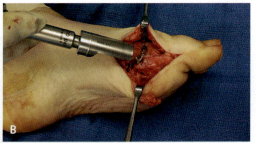
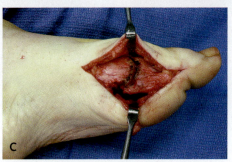

Figure 33-20 Revision of a malunion. **A,** Although the degree of dorsiflexion resulting from the arthrodesis was not significant, it was not tolerated by the patient. **B** and **C,** Correction was accomplished using a dome saw cut through a medial incision.

and the hallux had to be fused in more flexion than would normally be acceptable. Because the entire hallux was short, however, this degree of flexion was not clinically bothersome to the patient (see Figure 33-26).

Arthrodesis of the IP joint also is necessary to address gross instability of the joint that cannot be corrected with an arthroplasty or shortening of the FHL tendon as outlined earlier. A difficult such case is presented in Figure 33-27, in which the patient was referred for treatment after resection of the distal phalanx for pain, and the FHL tendon was cut at the time of surgery. There was no option other than an arthrodesis, but to restore function to the hallux, a lengthening of the hallux with interposition grafting was performed, through a dorsal incision. The distal phalangeal joint surface was prepared, and the proximal phalanx was cut straight

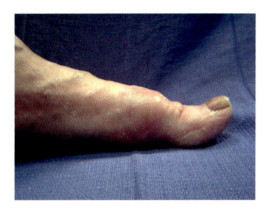

Figure 33-21 Hyperextension of the hallux interphalangeal (IP) joint associated with hallux rigidus is present with pain at the tip of the hallux, in the metatarsophalangeal joint, and on the plantar aspect of the hallux IP joint.

for insertion of the graft. An iliac crest graft, shaped to the phalanx, was used for structural purposes. Holes were then made in the graft and the distal phalanx using smooth K-wires, and the graft was held in place with one K-wire while the adjacent wire was exchanged for a threaded wire. The second wire was then used as a guide pin over which a cannulated screw was inserted (see Figure 33-27). The joint was then manually compressed, and the screw was inserted first, followed by the threaded K-wire to control rotation.

Hallux valgus interphalangeus is a common condition, and the apex of the deformity generally is centered in the distal part of the proximal phalanx. The traditional procedure of a closing wedge osteotomy of the proximal phalanx generally is recommended; however, from an anatomic standpoint, the osteotomy should be performed distally, closer to the apex of the deformity. Nonetheless, an arthrodesis should rarely be performed to correct hallux valgus interphalangeus, because some type of osteotomy is always preferable. When the deformity is fixed or associated with arthritis, then an arthrodesis may have to be the procedure of choice. In Figures 30-28 and 30-29, both patients had posttraumatic hallux valgus interphalangeus, associated with pain in the IP joint in addition to painful abutment against the second toe. Perhaps an osteotomy could have been performed, using a dome cut in the distal phalanx, thereby preserving the length of the toe, but because of the IP joint pain, I selected an arthrodesis for both patients. Another example of gross posttraumatic deformity of the hallux with interphalangeus is presented in Figure 33-30. Problems included marked enlargement of the hallux, thickening of the IP joint, and fixed valgus and flexion at the IP joint. To obtain adequate realignment, some shortening of the toe was necessary; this was accomplished with resection of a portion of the proximal phalanx.

Numerous procedures are available to correct the failed hallux MP arthrodesis associated with malunion and hallux pain. The most common cause of failure in this setting is performing the

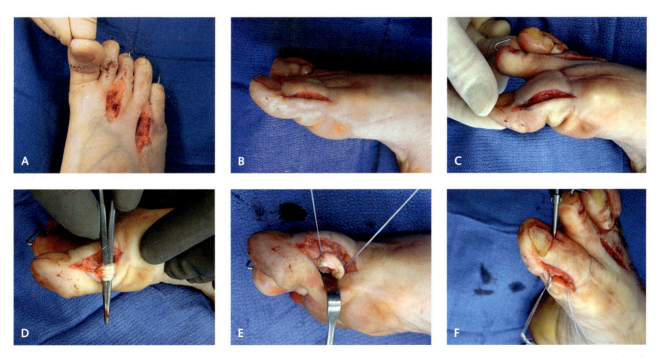

Figure 33-22 A, Hyperextension of the hallux with interphalangeal (IP) joint instability. **B-D,** An incision was made medial to the IP joint, and with soft tissue retraction, the flexor hallucis longus (FHL) was exposed. **E,** A small stump of the FHL is left attached to the base of the distal phalanx, and two stay sutures are inserted into each end of the tendon. **F,** The tendon is then cut at that level, usually with removal of a 1-cm segment of tendon. The tendon end is sutured and advanced into the base of the distal phalanx.

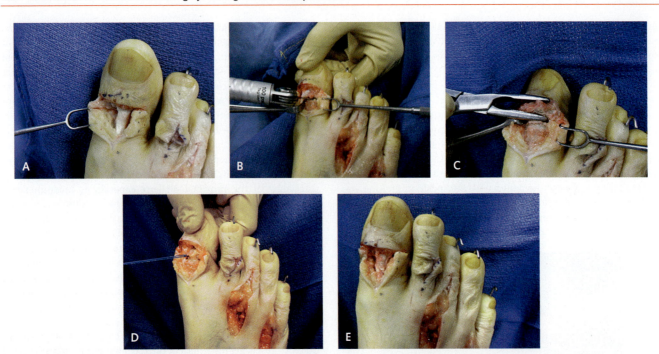

Figure 33-23 Instability of the hallux interphalangeal joint associated with arthritis in a patient with stiffness but no arthritis of the metatarsophalangeal joint. **A,** A dorsal approach to the joint affords exposure and protection of the extensor hallucis longus (EHL). **B,** The distal 5 mm of the proximal phalanx is now cut with a saw, with care taken not to damage the EHL with the excursion of the saw blade. **C,** The bone is removed and the dorsal osteophytes on the base of the proximal phalanx are trimmed. **D,** The joint is distracted, and the volar plate and the flexor hallucis longus (FHL) are grasped with a clamp and pulled into the incision. **E,** The FHL was then sutured to the undersurface of the EHL and the dorsal capsule.

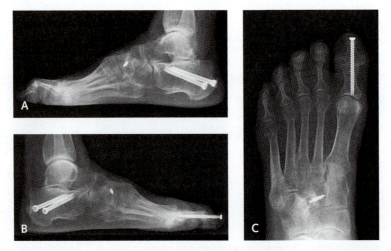

Figure 33-24 A-C, Appearance of a cavus foot with a contracted claw hallux corrected with interphalangeal arthrodesis.

arthrodesis with the joint in too-neutral a position (i.e., not in sufficient extension). This improper positioning causes overload on the hallux with instability and consequent arthritis. One option is to revise the MP arthrodesis to lift up the position of the hallux. The problem with this result is the increasing pain at the tip of the hallux, which is worsened by wearing a closed shoe without a heel. If arthritis of the IP joint is present in addition to instability, then an arthrodesis of the IP joint can be considered, but only with a simultaneous revision of the MP arthrodesis, adding extension to the joint. For this procedure, I start with the IP arthrodesis, fixing this in a neutral position, and then revise the MP arthrodesis using a dome

osteotomy to correct the alignment. It is more precise to correct the IP joint first. Fixation options are numerous, including insertion of retrograde screws across both joints, application of small plates, and use of screws supplemented with a plate applied over the MP joint (Figures 33-31 and 33-32). In Figure 33-31, the distal screws in the plate were removed in order to insert the screw across the IP joint. Because the fixation of the IP joint is more demanding, and the location of the wires or screws cannot vary very much, I begin with this joint and then proceed with whatever fixation at the MP joint is required, using instrumentation that will fit around the screw used for the IP joint arthrodesis (see Figure 33-32).

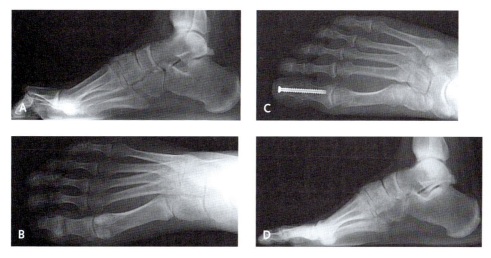

Figure 33-25 A and **B,** Severe contracture of the hallux secondary to a compartment syndrome of the leg associated with a tibia fracture in a 19-year-old patient. **C,** The treatment was with interphalangeal arthrodesis. **D,** Note the appearance of the hallux after removal of the screw and the intramedullary rod in the tibia.

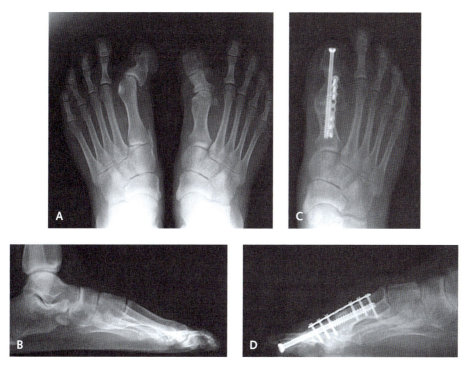

Figure 33-26 A and **B,** Congenital aplasia and hallux varus in an adolescent girl. **C** and **D,** An arthrodesis of the distal phalanx to the hallux was performed on one side, and a simultaneous arthrodesis of the interphalangeal and metatarsophalangeal joints on the opposite foot. The clinical result was quite satisfactory despite the flexed position of the hallux.

It is unfortunately a very difficult problem to correct the same deformity in the patient with rheumatoid arthritis. Erosive arthritis of the IP joint is common, and fixation options are limited. Nonunion of the arthrodesis only adds to the problem of hyperextension and instability of the toe, with further bone loss and erosion (Figures 33-33 and 33-34).

An example of a failed IP arthrodesis is presented in Figure 33-35. The patient had undergone numerous incorrect procedures

to the forefoot. The misalignment of the hallux in this patient was the result of overcorrection from an osteotomy of the hallux. The head of the fifth metatarsal had been resected in an attempt to relieve metatarsalgia. The deformity was in the hindfoot, however, and removing the fifth metatarsal is never a solution for this problem. An IP joint arthrodesis was attempted to correct the interphalangeal hallux varus deformity. This attempt also failed, and the screw migrated proximally, entering the MP joint

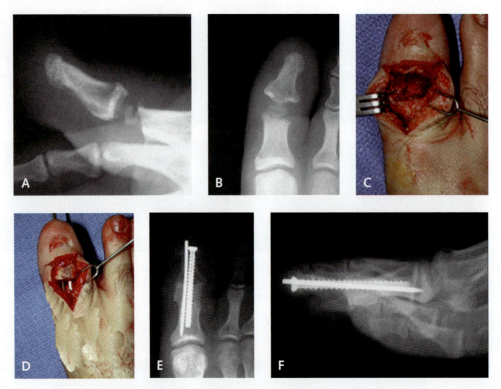

Figure 33-27 Arthrodesis of the hallux interphalangeal (IP) joint was performed after incorrect excision of the terminal portion of the proximal phalanx for plantar interphalangeal pain. **A** and **B,** Severe instability and hyperextension of the hallux were present in addition to the pain. **C,** Appearance of the IP joint with distraction. **D,** Correction was accomplished with a bone block arthrodesis with interposition of a corticocancellous graft harvested from the ipsilateral calcaneus and cut into an appropriate shape. The guide pins were advanced out through the tip of the hallux and then back into the proximal phalanx. **E** and **F,** The final radiographic appearance.

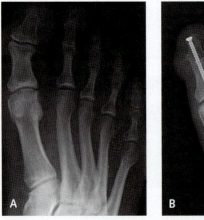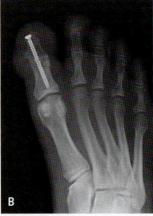

Figure 33-28 A and **B,** Traumatic hallux valgus interphalangeus was corrected with an interphalangeal arthrodesis.

and causing arthritis. At this stage, the IP joint was very stiff and not too painful, but the MP joint was more symptomatic, and a combination resection and interposition arthroplasty was performed (see Figure 33-35).

The standard approach for the IP arthrodesis is with an incision is made dorsomedial to the EHL tendon and extending distally to end just proximal to the nail fold (Figure 33-36). A second transverse incision is then made to create either an L or a T shape.

Maintaining some of the attachment of the EHL tendon is useful if it is not to be lengthened or used for a transfer. For some of the attachment to be maintained, the medial side of the joint is cut open, and then after subperiosteal dissection, a small skin hook is used to retract the dorsal tissues and the EHL tendon. Cutting the proximal phalanx to preserve the EHL tendon attachment is easy, but cutting the distal phalanx is not as easy, because of the attachment of the EHL to the base of the proximal phalanx.

Once both the collateral ligaments are cut, the hallux is plantarflexed, the EHL tendon is retracted laterally, and the distal portion of the proximal phalanx is cut with a saw. The orientation of the cut must take into consideration the plane of the deformity. If severe rigid flexion contracture is present, then slight dorsiflexion can be incorporated into the angle of the cut. Correcting the deformity with the cut on the proximal phalanx is always the easiest because less freedom is available with the bone cut distally. Once the articular surface of the proximal phalanx is resected, the hallux is now lined up and the cut is made accordingly. At this time, it is helpful to manipulate the hallux, insert a soft tissue retractor laterally to pull aside the EHL tendon, and then completely plantar flex the hallux until the undersurface of the joint is visible. The base of the articular surface of the distal phalanx curves under the proximal phalanx, and care is required in resection of this portion. Usually, the flexor hallucis longus attachment is not disturbed. Once the bone has been cut, however, the attachment of the flexor hallucis longus tendon must be in clear view to ensure that this has not been transected.

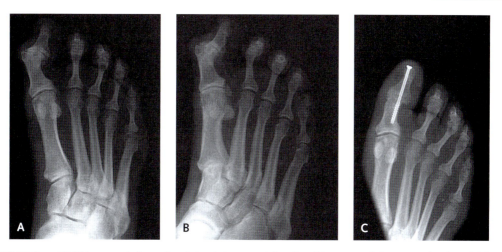

Figure 33-29 **A** and **B,** This severe hallux valgus interphalangeus deformity with erosion of the IP joint developed following trauma. **C,** This was easily corrected with arthrodesis, including slight shortening of the hallux to accomplish correction.

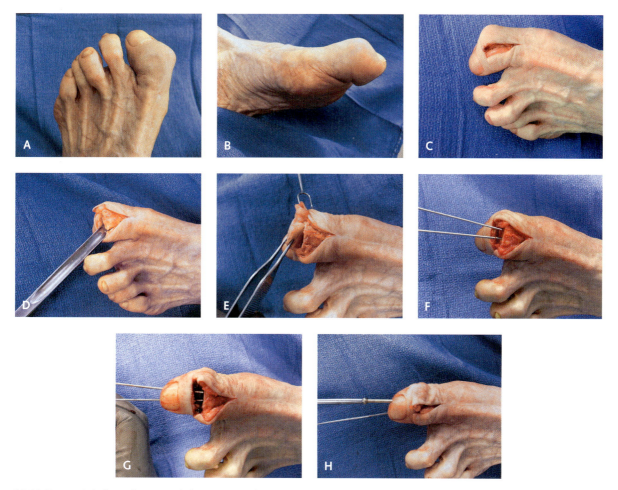

Figure 33-30 Traumatic hallux valgus interphalangeus. **A** and **B,** Note the marked enlargement of the hallux, the thickened interphalangeal joint, and the fixed valgus and flexion at the joint. **C,** A curved periosteal elevator was used to expose the condyles of the proximal phalanx. **D** and **E,** Guide pins were inserted after the bone cuts were made. **F-H,** Some shortening of the toe had to be accomplished, with resection of a portion of the proximal phalanx, and fixation with cannulated screws.

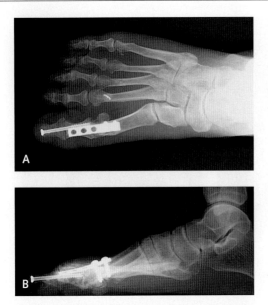

Figure 33-31 A and **B,** Interphalangeal (IP) arthrodesis was performed after a metatarsophalangeal arthrodesis for instability and arthritis. The distal screws in the plate were removed, and fixation of the IP arthrodesis performed with a cannulated screw.

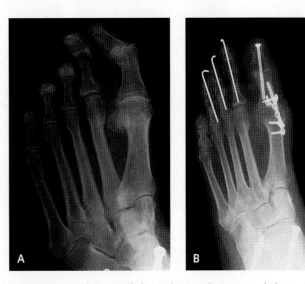

Figure 33-32 A and **B,** Interphalangeal (IP) and metatarsophalangeal arthrodesis procedures were performed simultaneously in a patient with hallux rigidus and deformity with arthritis of the IP joint.

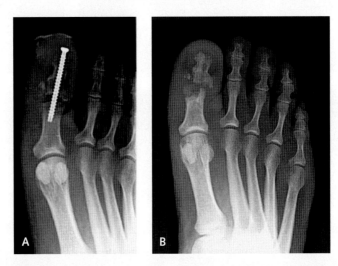

Figure 33-33 Nonunion after arthrodesis in a patient with rheumatoid arthritis.

The bone is now lined up and the cut is adjusted until complete correction of the position of the distal phalanx with reference to the hallux is present. It is important to ensure that no slight medial or lateral translation of the distal phalanx is present, because either will cause a painful subcutaneous spur. If correction is performed for hallux valgus interphalangeus, then more bone will need to be removed medially, and the distal phalanx will need to be slightly translated medially to aid correction. I use a cannulated, fully threaded 4-mm cancellous screw for fixation (Figure 33-37). The guide pin is first inserted into the center of the proximal phalanx; then a second hole is made in antegrade fashion out the distal phalanx so that it exits distally just under the nail. The guide pin is then inserted in retrograde fashion into the predrilled guide pin hole in the proximal phalanx. With this technique, the hallux can be perfectly centered over the proximal phalanx. The hallux is then manually compressed as the screw is being inserted. A partially threaded screw can be used, although I have not found this to be necessary, and a fully threaded screw is sufficient, provided that manual compression of the articulation is noted. If the joint slightly separates, then the screw is removed, manual compression is again applied, and the screw is reinserted.

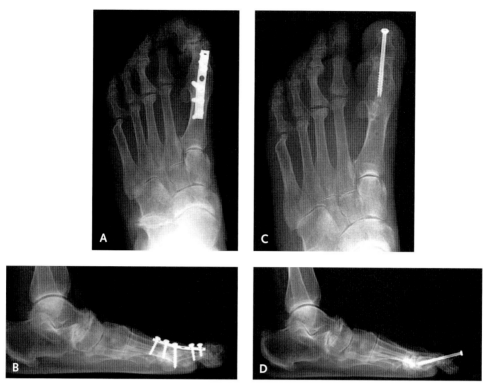

Figure 33-34 A-D, Failure of arthrodesis of the metatarsophalangeal (MP) joint in a patient with rheumatoid arthritis. Hyperextension of the interphalangeal (IP) joint was present, with painful arthritis. The plate was removed, and the IP arthrodesis performed. It would have been preferable to change the position of the MP arthrodesis simultaneously, with an osteotomy performed to place the hallux in less extension.

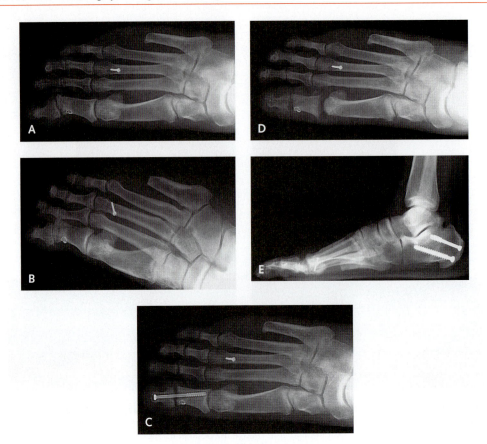

Figure 33-35 The patient had undergone numerous incorrect forefoot procedures. **A** and **B,** Note the alignment of the hallux, the result of overcorrection from an osteotomy of the hallux. The head of the fifth metatarsal had been resected in an unsuccessful attempt to relieve metatarsalgia. **C,** An interphalangeal (IP) joint arthrodesis was attempted to correct the IP hallux varus deformity. **D,** This attempt also failed, and the screw migrated proximally, entering the metatarsophalangeal (MP) joint and causing arthritis. **E,** At this stage, the IP joint was very stiff and not too painful, but the MP joint was more of a problem, so a combination resection and interposition arthroplasty was performed.

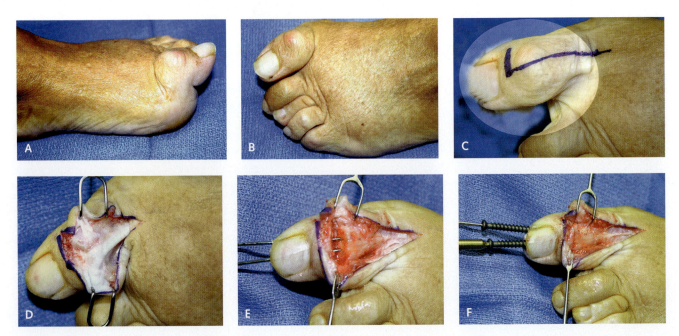

Figure 33-36 The steps in arthrodesis of the hallux interphalangeal joint. **A-C,** Claw hallux deformity requiring repair. **D,** The EHL is retracted. **E,** A saw is cut made on the phalanx. **F,** Guide pins are inserted to predrill holes in the proximal and distal phalanges. Two fully threaded cannulated screws were used to control rotational instability.

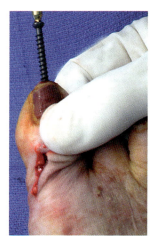

Figure 33-37 Note the manual compression of the hallux while the screw is inserted. This is an important step in gaining alignment and maintaining rotational control.

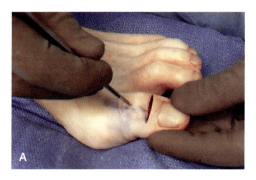
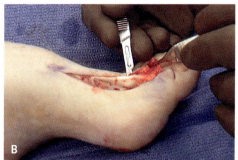

Figure 33-38 A and **B,** When an extensor hallucis longus (EHL) tendon transfer is performed, the distal cut is made below the matrix, and the EHL tendon is detached to define the transfer.

TECHNIQUES, TIPS, AND PITFALLS

- The incision for the IP arthrodesis can be made in any direction distally. The EHL tendon is always detached to some extent. Use of a straight longitudinal incision can be tried, but frequently, to facilitate exposure, this incision is extended distally into the shape of either a T or an L.

- A key principle in making this incision is to avoid the base of the nail in the germinal matrix (Figure 33-38).

- Minimal bone should be removed from the proximal phalanx. Cutting the proximal phalanx is easier than cutting the distal phalanx, which curves under the proximal phalanx, and more bone is removed from the plantar than from the dorsal distal phalanx.

- Nonunion of this arthrodesis is unusual unless there has been a previous arthrodesis of the hallux MP joint. The added stress, with a longer lever arm on the hallux, increases the force on the joint, potentially leading to failure.

- Fixation options are numerous, and the use fully threaded versus partially threaded screws does not appear to be of any importance. For patients with poor bone quality, multiple threaded K-wires can be introduced along the edges of the toe, in addition to a screw.

- Management of the painful hallux IP joint after MP joint arthrodesis is difficult. An arthrodesis including both joints is quite functional, although the toe must be perfectly aligned.

SUGGESTED READING

Brodsky JW, Passmore RN, Pollo FE, Shabat S: Functional outcome of arthrodesis of the first metatarsophalangeal joint using parallel screw fixation, *Foot Ankle Int* 26:140–146, 2005.

Brodsky JW, Ptaszek AJ, Morris SG: Salvage first MTP arthrodesis utilizing ICBG: Clinical evaluation and outcome, *Foot Ankle Int* 21:290–296, 2000.

Myerson MS, Schon LC, McGuigan FX, Oznur A: Result of arthrodesis of the hallux metatarsophalangeal joint using bone graft for restoration of length, *Foot Ankle Int* 21:297–306, 2000.

Sammarco VJ: Surgical correction of moderate and severe hallux valgus: Proximal metatarsal osteotomy with distal soft-tissue correction and arthrodesis of the metatarsophalangeal joint, *Instr Course Lect* 57:415–428, 2008.

Singh B, Draeger R, Del Gaizo DJ, Parekh SG: Changes in length of the first ray with two different first MTP fusion techniques: A cadaveric study, *Foot Ankle Int* 29:722–725, 2008.

Womack JW, Ishikawa SN: First metatarsophalangeal arthrodesis, *Foot Ankle Clin* 14:43–50, 2009.

CHAPTER **34**

Arthrodesis of the Tarsometatarsal Joint

OVERVIEW

Arthrodesis of the tarsometatarsal (TMT) joint is performed for treatment of arthritis of variable extent with or without deformity, in the setting of idiopathic osteoarthritis or posttraumatic or inflammatory arthritis, and for correction of neuropathic deformity. The arthrodesis should be limited to symptomatic joints, which are not always easy to identify. A combination of the location of the patient's symptoms, the appearance on plain radiographs and findings on clinical examination will determine the joints to be fused. The radiographic appearance of the lateral column is not always helpful with the decision-making process because the lateral column often is asymptomatic despite the radiographic presence of arthritic changes (Figure 34-1). All involved segments of the midfoot should be included in the arthrodesis, which often will extend to the naviculocuneiform and intercuneiform joints (Figure 34-2). Such extensive involvement is particularly common after trauma, when arthritis and deformity may include the intercuneiform and naviculocuneiform joints—hence use of the term *tarsometatarsal joint complex* to designate the relevant anatomy.

Common to all of these procedures is the need to correct and restore the alignment with the arthrodesis, because the functional results with arthrodesis are far better if the forefoot as well as any hindfoot deformity is corrected. The deformity that commonly accompanies arthritis of the TMT joint is abduction of the forefoot relative to the hindfoot associated with sagittal and coronal plane instability of the first metatarsal. With increasing abduction, the midfoot and forefoot pronate, creating torque on the medial aspect of the midfoot and on the hallux, with resultant hallux valgus. With increasing deformity, additional procedures must therefore be performed to obtain adequate alignment of the foot.

In some instances, as with a flatfoot deformity associated with hindfoot valgus, the hindfoot deformity is primary and the arthritis of the TMT joint is secondary; nevertheless, the hindfoot deformity must be adequately corrected in addition to the obvious painful focus, which as perceived by the patient may be only the TMT joint (Figure 34-3). In other situations, the midfoot deformity clearly is primary and the deformity of the hindfoot occurs secondarily, as in the case shown in Figure 34-4. In this example, severe dislocation involved the entire TMT joint complex including the lateral column. Although I rarely include the lateral column in the arthrodesis, here the entire midfoot required arthrodesis as a consequence of crushing of the cuboid and lateral foot pain. In order to correct this rather severe deformity, each joint was first debrided and the lateral contracture was released by lengthening the peroneus brevis tendon. Such severe deformities also may necessitate temporary lengthening of the lateral column with an external fixator, followed by reduction of the medial and middle columns (Figure 34-5). In the case illustrated in Figure 13-4, after complete "loosening" of each joint was achieved with debridement, the peroneus brevis was lengthened and the external fixator applied. The fixation was then initiated from medial to lateral, commencing with placement of temporary pins and followed by application of a combination of plates, including F3 plates (DePuy Orthopaedics, Inc., Warsaw, Indiana) for the second and third TMT joints and Maxlock plates (Orthohelix, Akron, Ohio) for the first, fourth, and fifth TMT joints.

DEFORMITY CORRECTION PRINCIPLES

Incision and Exposure

If the planned arthrodesis includes two adjacent joints, I try to use only one incision, if possible. For the middle column arthrodesis (of the second and third TMT joints), I use a single dorsal incision placed slightly more lateral than the second metatarsal, because the third metatarsal-cuneiform joint extends farther over toward the midline of the foot than is readily apparent. If the third metatarsal cuneiform joint is to be included in the arthrodesis, then the dorsal incision must be centered correctly over the midfoot, and not the second metatarsal. If the first and second TMT joints are to be fused, either one or two incisions can be used. With minimal deformity, I try to use one dorsal incision in the first TMT–second TMT interspace. If, however, both deformity and instability of the medial column are present, then I use a separate medial incision for access to permit plantar flexion of the medial column (Figure 34-6). I also use this incision when an extended navicular cuneiform metatarsal arthrodesis is performed that requires application of a plate from the medial aspect of the foot.

Once the dorsal incision has been deepened through subcutaneous tissue, the branches of the superficial peroneal nerve must be identified and then retracted. A neuroma on the dorsal surface of the foot is intolerably uncomfortable, and formation of these lesions can be avoided. The tendon of the extensor hallucis brevis is used as a guide to the location of the deep neurovascular bundle. Once

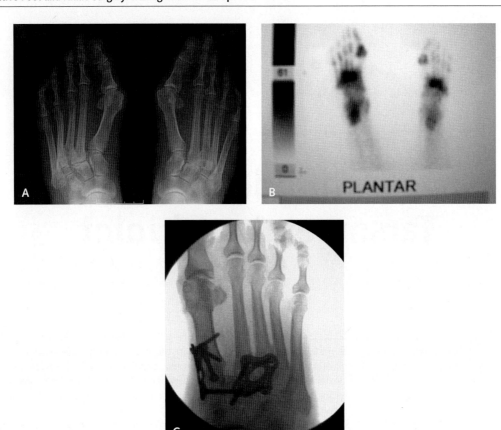

Figure 34-1 A, The patient had symptomatic arthritis of the medial and middle columns of the right foot. **B,** Radionuclide bone scan showed uptake in the lateral column. **C,** This segment of the foot was asymptomatic, however, so it was not included in the subsequent arthrodesis.

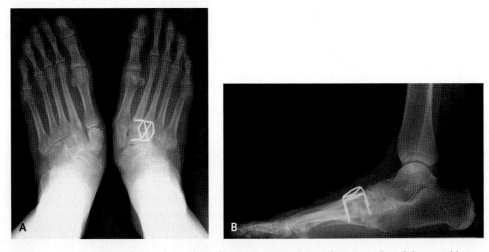

Figure 34-2 A and **B,** Failure of arthrodesis. The deformity was not adequately corrected, and the unstable segment of the naviculocuneiform joint should have been included in the fusion.

the tendon is identified, the bundle is seen to lie directly underneath it, and both are retracted medially. The easiest way to retract is to undermine the bundle from the subperiosteal tissue over the second metatarsal and then elevate the flap, which includes the neurovascular bundle, using a large periosteal elevator.

The joint is prepared by removing the remaining articular cartilage with a flexible chisel. Perhaps the most important aspect of

the joint preparation is aggressive perforation of the joint surface using a 1.5- or 2-mm drill bit, made at 1- to 2-mm intervals across the entire joint surface. I do not like to use a Kirschner wire (K-wire) for this purpose, because it seems to cause more bone burning. The only time I use a saw is for very severe deformity, as, for example, in a chronically abducted neuropathic midfoot, when I may want to correct a plantar medial rocker-bottom deformity. I prefer to keep

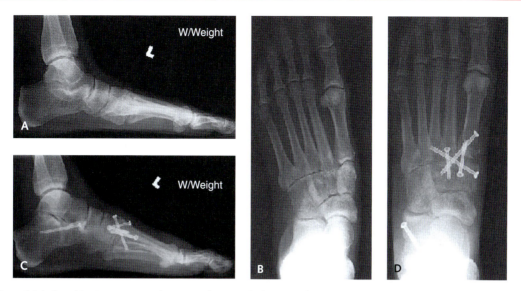

Figure 34-3 **A** and **B**, Tarsometatarsal (TMT) arthritis, probably secondary to the hindfoot valgus and abduction deformity. **C** and **D**, Correction was accomplished with a TMT arthrodesis, in addition to a lengthening of the lateral column by means of a calcaneus osteotomy.

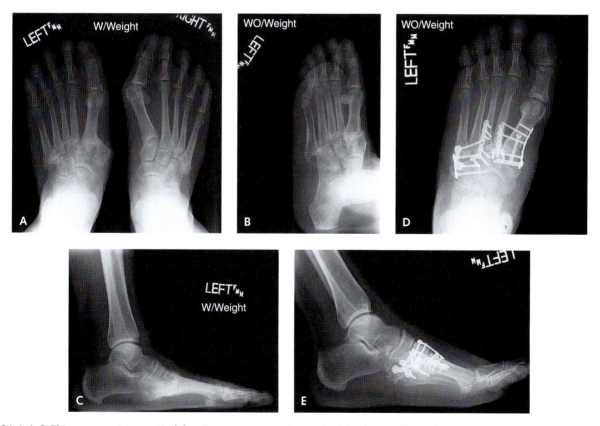

Figure 34-4 **A-C,** This severe post-traumatic deformity was symptomatic in each of the three midfoot columns. Note the severe abduction of the entire tarsometatarsal joint complex. **D** and **E,** Correction was accomplished with an arthrodesis of all three columns, with complete realignment obtained, and plate fixation.

the anatomy of the joints completely intact and remove as little bone as possible; therefore use of a saw is not ideal. The problem occurs with preparation of a hard sclerotic joint, which can be associated with posttraumatic or idiopathic osteoarthritis. The second metatarsal in particular can be quite avascular, and once this bone is debrided, the metatarsal shortens, resulting in a large gap in the

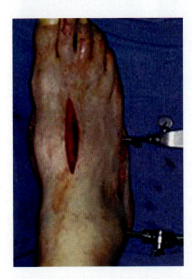

Figure 34-5 For correction of very severe abduction of the midfoot, temporary lengthening of the lateral column can be achieved by means of an external fixator with pins in the calcaneus and fifth metatarsal. This fixation device can be removed once the reduction is complete and internal fixation is secure.

joint. For this reason, aggressive perforation of the joint surface only is used to create a bone slurry, rather than debridement of the joint below the subchondral bone surface. The third metatarsal usually adheres well to the second metatarsal and will follow the second metatarsal into a corrected position. If the medial and middle columns are fused, then I try to debride the spaces between the first and second metatarsal bases and between the medial and middle cuneiforms and then place a bone graft in this location to further stabilize the arthrodesis. The metatarsals tend to dorsiflex with fixation, because debridement of the joint frequently is performed dorsally only. These are very deep joints, and the entire base of the metatarsal cuneiform joint must be completely debrided to prevent a dorsal malunion of the arthrodesis. Insertion of a smooth lamina spreader into the joint dorsally to visualize the plantar apical surface of the joint, before the arthrodesis is completed, is helpful. Frequently, small bits of bone remain on the plantar surface, which must be thoroughly cleared of such debris (Figure 34-7).

Fixation and Joint Stabilization

Arthrodesis must be performed with realignment. In situ arthrodesis is never ideal when deformity is present, and if the foot is left abducted and pronated, recurrence of symptoms is likely. After joint preparation, correction is therefore done first in the medial column, in which the first metatarsal is adducted and locked in position. For the first metatarsal to be positioned correctly, the hallux is grasped and the base of the first metatarsal is pushed inward into the medial cuneiform while the distal portion of the first metatarsal is pushed into adduction. At the same time, the hallux is dorsiflexed; this dorsiflexion forces the first metatarsal joint into plantar flexion. A guide pin or K-wire is used to lock the

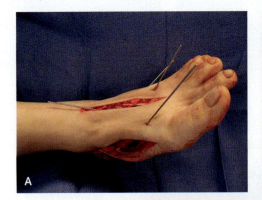
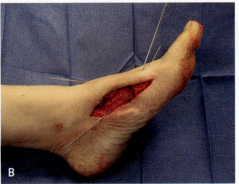
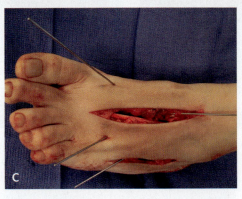

Figure 34-6 The incisions are determined by the extent of the arthrodesis. **A-C,** In this case, because all three columns were included in the arthrodesis, three incisions were used, with as large a skin bridge between each as possible.

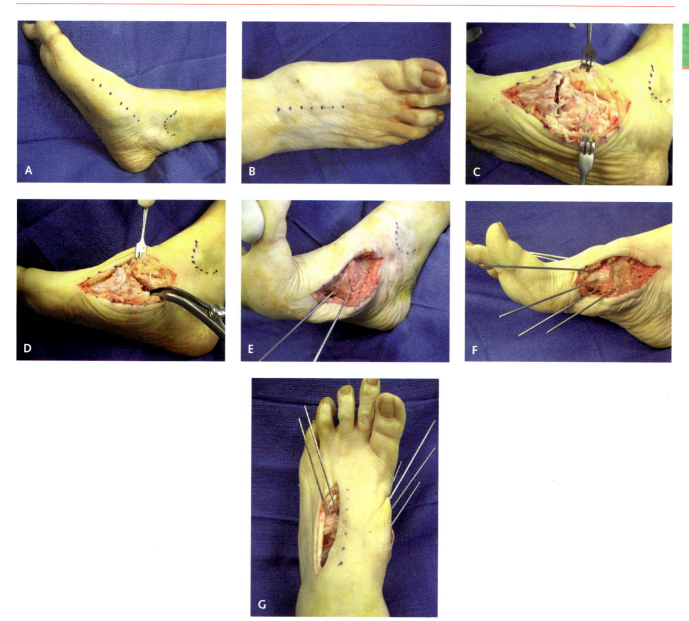

Figure 34-7 A and **B,** Surgical approach to extended tarsometatarsal (TMT) arthrodesis, with the dorsal and medial incisions marked out. **C** and **D,** The first TMT joint is opened. **E-G,** After removal of the plantar osteophytes and reduction of the midfoot malalignment, the hallux is dorsiflexed to produce plantar flexion of the first metatarsal, and guide pins are introduced to maintain reduction.

first metatarsal in the corrected position, which can then be used as a template on which to build the rest of the foot. Once the first metatarsal is correctly positioned, the second metatarsal can be reduced into its base and the mortise with a bone reduction clamp, which is applied to the medial cuneiform and the base of the second metatarsal (Figure 34-8). A guide pin is introduced through the medial cuneiform up and through the base of the second metatarsal to hold the joint in a reduced position. Alternatively, if no deformity is present, the screw fixation for the second metatarsal cuneiform joint can be performed axially. The decision of whether to use screws, staples, or a plate is determined by the anatomy, the presence of bone loss, and the joints to be fused.

Although I prefer to use screws whenever possible, sometimes they simply do not provide adequate stabilization because of either

the plane of the metatarsal or the paucity of available bone. The medial column is easier to stabilize by inserting a screw from the medial cuneiform aimed distally into the first metatarsal. Although this insertion can be made from the second metatarsal directed proximally, the screw may split the base of the metatarsal. Therefore, after drilling is completed, a careful countersink maneuver must be used to prevent splitting of the base of the metatarsal with insertion of the screw. Frequently a ridge is present on the base of the second metatarsal as a result of osteophytic hypertrophy, which can be used to advantage in positioning the screw. If, however, the entire dorsal osteophyte is left untouched, a dorsal ridge will remain, with subsequent patient discomfort. A balance has to be found between leaving behind a small ridge to facilitate screw insertion and adequate resection of the osteophyte. The configuration of fixation depends on the local anatomy.

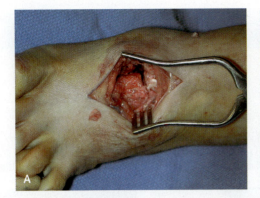
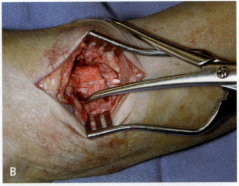

Figure 34-8 A, Midfoot deformity with chronic subluxation of the second tarsometatarsal joint. **B,** Reduction was obtained by means of an obliquely applied bone reduction clamp, followed by fixation.

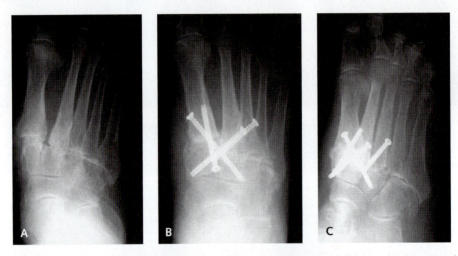

Figure 34-9 A, This post traumatic deformity involved the entire midfoot, with all three columns seemingly affected. Despite the severity of the deformity, only the medial and middle columns were clinically symptomatic. **B** and **C,** Arthrodesis was performed with realignment and screw fixation.

If the instability of the medial column is severe and the fusion is extended across to the navicular cuneiform joint, the use of a dorsally or medially applied plate should be considered. At times, I apply the plate on the tension side of the bone directly under the first metatarsal cuneiform joint, particularly in patients for whom instability and the potential for nonunion are increased (e.g., in those with neuropathy). This plantar plate has been shown to be more stable than other screw configurations for TMT joint fixation. Compression of the joint surface is desirable with fixation. Currently available fixation options such as custom anatomically designed midfoot plates can provide stability as well as providing locking and compression capability (Maxlock—Orthohelix, Akron, Ohio) (Figures 34-9 to 34-11).

I do not routinely use bone grafting to correct arthrodesis of the TMT joint unless a substantial defect is present. Insertion of small volumes of cancellous graft in the intermetatarsal and intercuneiform spaces is useful, however, if the arthrodesis incorporates more than a single metatarsal cuneiform joint. In such cases, stabilizing the medial to the middle column, to include the intercuneiform space, and using bone graft are advantageous. Sometimes, after debridement of the joint surfaces, apposition of the joint, in particular the second metatarsal cuneiform joint, is poor. This problem can be addressed by inserting a small amount of cancellous graft into the joint space with a tamp.

Management of Bone Loss and Nonunion

Whether bone loss is secondary to trauma or to erosive changes associated with osteoarthritis or inflammatory arthritis, management of such loss in the midfoot is difficult. Generally, use of structural bone grafts is required to reestablish correct anatomic relationships. These structural grafts usually are required to restore the length of the medial column, as illustrated in Figure 34-12.

One of the problems associated with idiopathic osteoarthritis of the TMT joints is the bone loss that accompanies the erosive changes of chronic arthritis, particularly of the medial column. There often is some elevation in addition to the valgus or abduction deformity of the first metatarsal. After joint preparation and debridement, further bone loss occurs, and in order to obtain a plantigrade forefoot, the first metatarsal joint has to be placed in considerable plantar flexion to align the forefoot. This positioning results in a short first metatarsal and very long second and third metatarsals, which may be quite symptomatic. One alternative to in situ arthrodesis is to lengthen the medial column with a structural bone graft, as demonstrated in Figure 34-13.

Management of Arthritis of the Lateral Column

In the case illustrated in Figure 34-14, severe adductus deformity of the entire midfoot was the result of erosive changes of the first TMT joint with consequent bone loss and recurrent stress

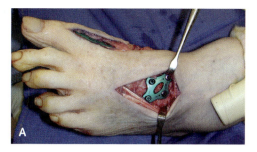

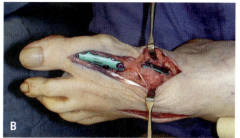

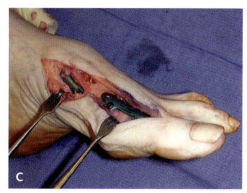

Figure 34-10 A-C, As an alternative to screw fixation, a custom midfoot plate with locking as well as compression capability (Maxlock plate—Orthohelix, Akron, Ohio) was used to secure the arthrodesis.

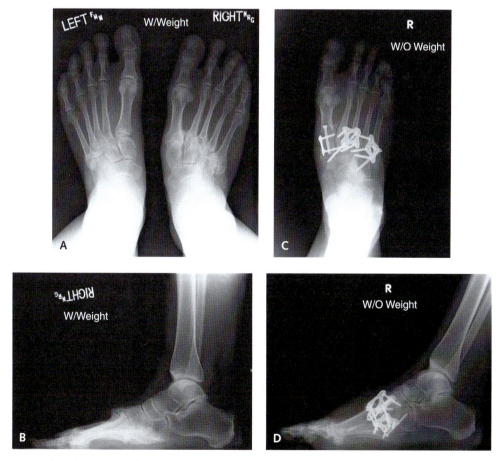

Figure 34-11 A and **B,** The entire midfoot was symptomatic in a patient with a posttraumatic deformity. Note the severe abduction deformity across the tarsometatarsal joints as well as the unstable medial column with dorsiflexion of the first metatarsal. **C** and **D,** Correction was accomplished with realignment of all three columns by means of plate fixation (Orthohelix, Akron, Ohio).

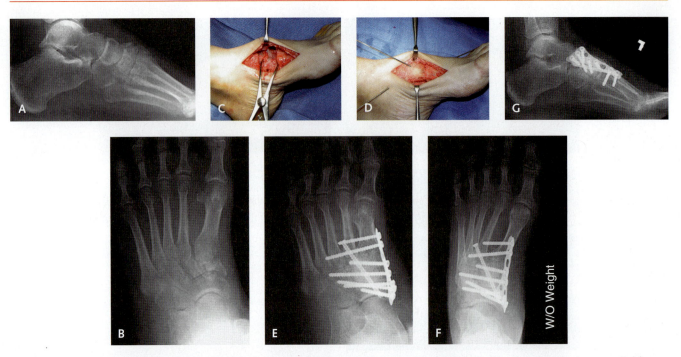

Figure 34-12 **A** and **B,** Fracture-dislocation of the tarsometatarsal complex with crushing of the medial cuneiform in a patient who presented for treatment 4 months after injury. **C** and **D,** At surgery, the cuneiform was in multiple fragments, necessitating replacement with a structural allograft in order to maintain length of the medial column. **E-G,** A plate (DePuy Orthopaedics, Inc., Warsaw, Indiana) was used for stabilization, and screws were inserted into the middle column for stability.

fractures of the lesser metatarsals (see Figure 34-14, *A-C*). The correction of this deformity began with a double osteotomy of the fifth metatarsal, removing a small lateral wedge, followed by insertion of an intramedullary guide pin (see Figure 34-14, *D* and *E*). The fifth metatarsal in corrected position was used as a template to build on for correction of the remaining deformities. An osteotomy of the third and fourth metatarsals was performed through the site of the nonunion of the original stress fractures, and the lesser metatarsal deformities were corrected by abduction against the template of the now intact fifth metatarsal (see Figure 34-14, *F*). The fifth metatarsal repair was then secured with one 5.5-mm cannulated screw crossing both osteotomies. The second and third metatarsals were stabilized with cancellous bone graft placed across both the nonunion of the stress fracture and the joint arthrodesis (see Figure 34-14, *G*). Finally, a large bicortical structural allograft was inserted into the first metatarsocuneiform joint, followed by stabilization with a plate. The final appearance of the foot 2 years after arthrodesis is shown in Figure 34-14, *H-J*.

Reconstruction after bone loss generally requires structural grafting to maintain alignment and restore the correct weight-bearing surface of the forefoot. These principles are well illustrated in Figures 34-15 and 34-16, both of which, although presenting cases of differing etiology, highlight the use of a structural graft, in the setting of trauma reconstruction (see Figure 34-15) and for reconstruction of midfoot and hindfoot deformity (see Figure 34-16).

I generally prefer not to fuse the lateral column unless the surgical problem is part of a neuropathic, degenerative, or post-traumatic process with lateral column collapse associated with a lateral rocker-bottom deformity. If arthritis of the lateral column is present and painful, arthroplasty of this joint, as opposed to arthrodesis, can be considered. The foot is extremely stiff after

an arthrodesis of all three columns, and these arthroplasty procedures work well. Either a resection arthroplasty of the joint with interposition of soft tissues or insertion of ceramic spheres with the joint under slight distraction is performed to decrease the inflammatory arthritic process. I have in the past performed either an interposition arthroplasty or insertion of ceramic spheres into the base of the fourth and fifth metatarsocuboid joints, but in my experience, the latter procedure has not reliably relieved symptoms over time (Figure 34-17). For the past several years, I have performed a cheilectomy of the symptomatic lateral joint(s) as an alternative to arthrodesis or interposition arthroplasty (Figure 34-18), with fair success. The downside to performing this cheilectomy is minimal because the option of an interposition arthroplasty or arthrodesis remains.

The approach for cheilectomy (Figure 34-19) is similar to that for soft tissue interposition arthroplasty. The procedure begins with a single incision between the fourth and fifth metatarsals. This location should be identified under fluoroscopic imaging because the tendency is to make the incision too far lateral to the fifth metatarsal. After the incision is deepened through the subcutaneous tissue, the interval between the sural nerve and the dorsal lateral cutaneous branch of the superficial peroneal nerve is used. The nerves are then retracted, and an incision is made transversely directly down onto the cuboid, with a cut through the soft tissue envelope, including the peroneus tertius tendon.

For the arthroplasty, the tendon, the capsule, and periosteum are raised as one large flap based distally. The flap is raised off the base of the fourth and fifth metatarsals, to be used later for the interposition. The joint is then opened, distracted, and debrided. The bone can be removed off either the cuboid or the base of the metatarsals; I prefer to resect the bone off the cuboid, keeping the soft tissue flap on the metatarsals intact. The attachment of

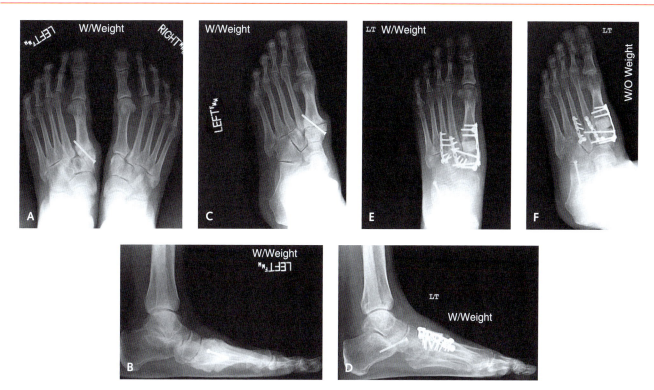

Figure 34-13 Management for a nonunion consequent to a previous attempted arthrodesis of the first tarsometatarsal (TMT) joint. **A-C,** Note the marked shortening of the first metatarsal as well as abduction and elevation of the medial column. **D-F,** The hindfoot deformity was corrected with a simultaneous lateral column lengthening osteotomy, in conjunction with arthrodesis of the medial and middle columns. Use of a structural tricortical bone graft in the first TMT joint restored the length of the medial column.

the peroneus brevis muscle is not disturbed, because this is farther proximal and more lateral than the location of the incision and dissection. Approximately 5 mm of bone is removed from the articular surface to achieve full mobility, but not instability, of the metatarsal cuboid joint. The flap of soft tissue is now inserted into the created joint space and then held secure with K-wires inserted transversely across the joint or with sutures. Weight bearing can begin at 10 days after surgery with the foot in a walker boot, with institution of passive range-of-motion exercises as soon as possible.

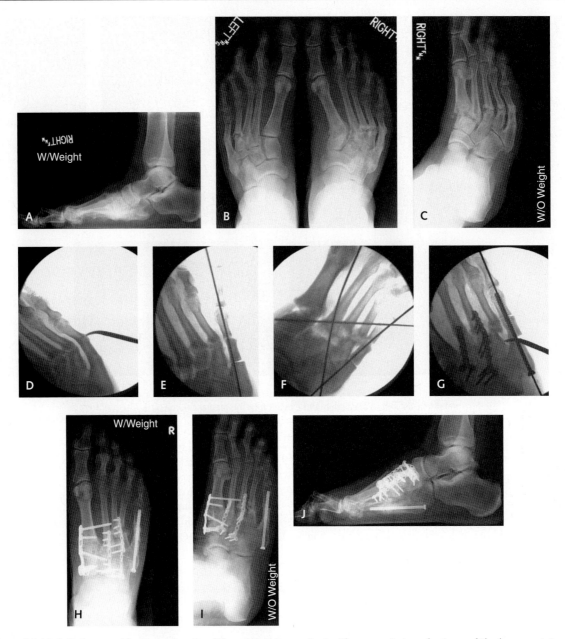

Figure 34-14 A-C, Severe adduction deformity of the midfoot in a patient with recurrent stress fractures of the lesser metatarsals. **D-G,** Correction was instituted with osteotomies of the lesser metatarsals **H-J,** Additional procedures included arthrodesis of the second and third tarsometatarsal (TMT) joints and a bone block lengthening arthrodesis of the first TMT joint.

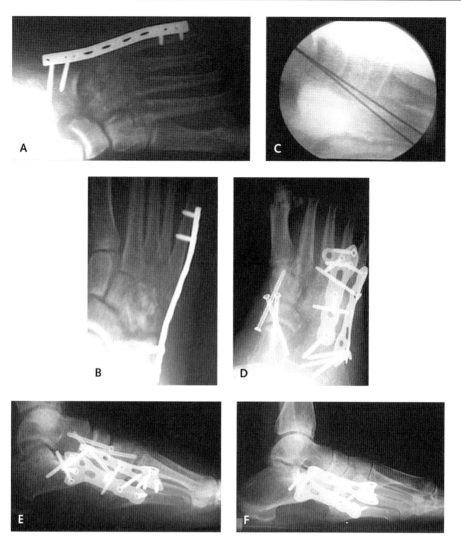

Figure 34-15 A and **B,** Failure of open reduction with internal fixation of a midfoot dislocation with persistent subluxation of the talonavicular joint and crushing of the cuboid. **C,** For reconstruction to be performed, temporary stabilization of the medial column was required. Note the intraoperative reduction of the talonavicular joint and the large void laterally where the comminuted bone was removed **D-F,** A 4-cm structural allograft was inserted laterally to replace the cuboid, and two plates (DePuy Orthopaedics, Inc., Warsaw, Indiana) were used to secure the arthrodesis. When the medial screws were removed 5 months later, fusion had been achieved.

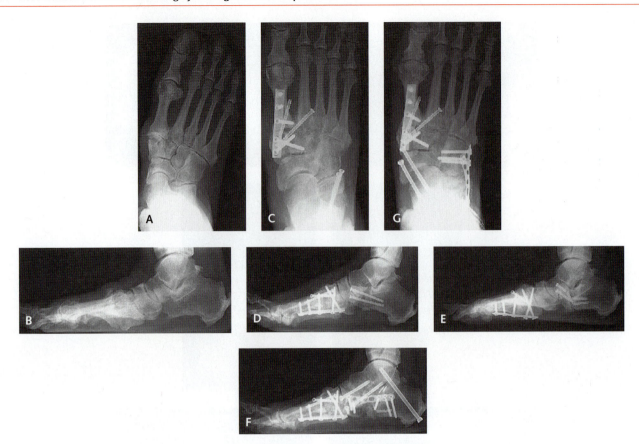

Figure 34-16 A and **B,** Hindfoot collapse with abduction of the transverse tarsal joint in a patient with symptomatic tarsometatarsal (TMT) arthritis. **C** and **D,** In addition to TMT arthrodesis, a lateral column lengthening was performed, with good realignment and healing of the fused TMT joint. **E,** Subsequently, an arthrodesis of the TMT joint was present; however, a nonunion of the lateral column resulted in worsening deformity. **F** and **G,** Correction was accomplished with structural grafting of the entire lateral column and conversion to a triple arthrodesis to improve the likelihood of a solid fusion, which was successfully achieved.

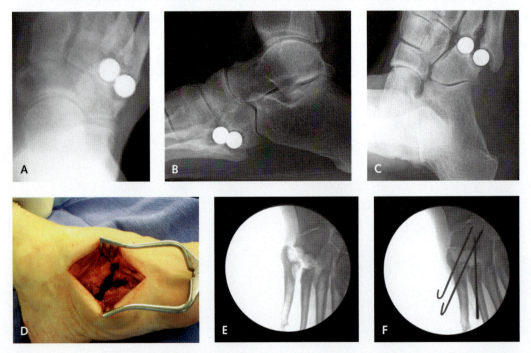

Figure 34-17 A-C, After unsuccessful ceramic sphere interposition arthroplasty, radiographs show subsequent marked erosive changes in both the fourth and fifth tarsometatarsal joints. **D** and **E,** At reconstructive surgery, erosion in the joints was evident. **F,** Repair was accomplished with interposition arthroplasty with temporary K-wire fixation.

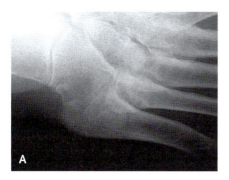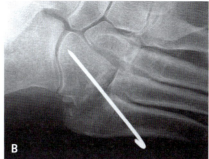

Figure 34-18 **A** and **B,** Isolated post traumatic arthritis of the fifth metatarsocuboid joint was treated with interposition arthroplasty with a temporary K-wire.

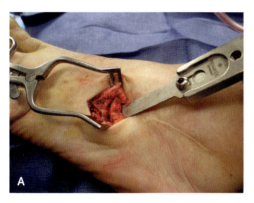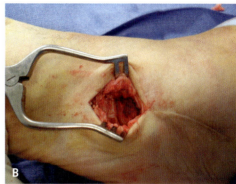

Figure 34-19 **A** and **B,** A cheilectomy of the fourth and fifth metatarsocuboid joints was performed for treatment of isolated arthritis of these joints.

TECHNIQUES, TIPS, AND PITFALLS

- Realignment in performing a midfoot arthrodesis is essential. An in situ arthrodesis in the setting of deformity leads to continued problems, including medial midfoot pain and pronation of the forefoot with hallux valgus.

- The reduction maneuver must begin with the first metatarsal, with correction of its alignment with the talus navicular and medial cuneiform. This maneuver is similar to that performed for a Lapidus-type bunionectomy.

- Be careful of the potential for deformity of the hallux after correction. With erosive osteoarthritis, the medial column shortens and becomes unstable. In order to correct the deformity, the first metatarsal should be slightly plantar flexed to establish a plantigrade forefoot. The extensor hallucis longus tendon, which often is already tight, bowstrings further, and a cock-up deformity of the hallux occurs. This deformity can be prevented to some extent by lengthening of the extensor hallucis longus tendon.

- For patients with idiopathic osteoarthritis and a plantar medial callus, a medial incision is essential to permit removal of the bone underlying the callosity (Figure 34-20).

- The superficial peroneal nerve and its branches must be retracted. If a neuroma develops, it is always painful and necessitates subsequent treatment.

- If no instability is present, then the intercuneiform and intermetatarsal spaces do not require arthrodesis.

- Bone grafting is necessary only when large defects are present, and bone graft substitutes are quite effective to fill in small defects between the metatarsals and cuneiforms.

- A simple technique to maintain reduction of the subluxated joint is to pass a guide pin through the dorsum of the foot after application of a bone reduction clamp and to hold the guide pin with a hemostat clamp to prevent loss of reduction during drilling of the bone (Figure 34-21).

- Development of a cock-up hallux deformity may follow surgical correction, as for idiopathic osteoarthritis, as shown in Figure 34-22.

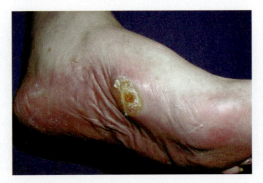

Figure 34-20 Callosity on the plantar surface of the first tarsometa-tarsal joint mandates a medial approach so that these osteophytes can more easily be removed.

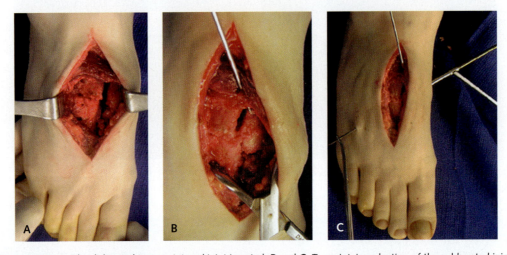

Figure 34-21 A, The dislocated tarsometatarsal joint is noted. **B** and **C,** To maintain reduction of the subluxated joint, a guide pin is passed through the dorsum of the foot after application of a bone reduction clamp and held with a hemostat clamp, to prevent loss of reduction while the bone is drilled.

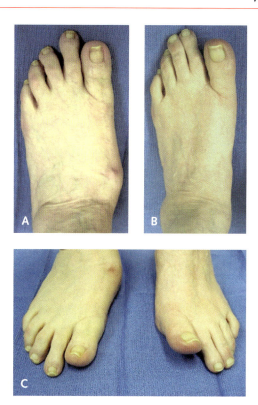

Figure 34-22 A, Clinical appearance of the affected foot before surgical treatment of idiopathic osteoarthritis. **B** and **C,** Note the postoperative changes in length and position of the hallux. Despite very good transverse plane correction, the hallux, which was short preoperatively, is now even shorter, as well as slightly cocked up. This malpositioning can cause relentless pain under the first metatarsal.

SUGGESTED READING

Aronow MS: Treatment of the missed Lisfranc injury, *Foot Ankle Clin* 11:127–142, 2006.

Chiodo CP, Myerson MS: Developments and advances in the diagnosis and treatment of injuries to the tarsometatarsal joint, *Orthop Clin North Am* 32:11–20, 2001.

Jung HJ, Myerson MS, Schon LS: The spectrum of operative treatments and clinical outcomes for atraumatic osteoarthritis of the tarsometatarsal arthritis, *Foot Ankle Int* 28:482–489, 2007.

Komenda GA, Myerson MS, Biddinger KR: Results of arthrodesis of the tarsometatarsal joints after traumatic injury, *J Bone Joint Surg Am* 78:1665–1676, 1996.

Mann RA, Prieskorn D, Sobel M: Mid-tarsal and tarsometatarsal arthrodesis for primary degenerative osteoarthrosis or osteoarthrosis after trauma, *J Bone Joint Surg Am* 78:1376–1385, 1996.

Myerson MS: Tarsometatarsal arthrodesis: Technique and results of treatment after injury, *Foot Ankle Clin* 1:73–83, 1996.

Sangeorzan BJ, Veith RG, Hansen ST Jr: Salvage of Lisfranc's tarsometatarsal joint by arthrodesis, *Foot Ankle* 10:193–200, 1990.

CHAPTER **35**

Subtalar Arthrodesis

OVERVIEW: APPROACH AND INCISIONS

The indications for subtalar arthrodesis are broad and include arthritis and deformities. Specific problems amenable to management by this method are calcaneus fracture, isolated traumatic subtalar arthritis, middle facet tarsal coalition, and calcaneovalgus deformity, among others.

The surgical approach that I use for the subtalar arthrodesis depends to some extent on the underlying pathology. Many of these procedures are performed for posttraumatic arthritis secondary to a calcaneus fracture. I generally use a standard incision across the sinus tarsi. In some cases, the patient has undergone multiple surgeries, and the incision is prone to dehiscence unless care is taken with the approach (Figure 35-1). If previous surgery has been performed, I prefer not to reopen the original incision for the open reduction with internal fixation (ORIF) procedure. Although use of the original incision is an option, considerable scarring will be encountered over the lateral calcaneus and peroneal tendons, and it is not as easy to reach the sinus tarsi and the more medial aspect of the subtalar joint through this route (Figure 35-2). The more limited incision over the sinus tarsi heals well, with no risk for compromise of the intervening skin bridge between the sinus tarsi incision and the original more extensile lateral incision (Figure 35-3).

Subtalar arthrodesis procedures are of two basic types: (1) fusion performed in situ, without changing the orientation of the hindfoot and (2) a bone block arthrodesis with structural grafting to restore the height of the hindfoot. In addition to these two basic procedures, osteotomies of the calcaneus may be added to correct additional deformity. Beyond correction of the calcaneus and subtalar joint problems, other essential considerations include the condition of the peroneal tendons, which frequently are torn or dislocated, as well as the flexor hallucis longus and the soft tissues on the medial ankle, including the tibial nerve and its branches.

Complete exposure of the peroneal tendons and adequate subfibular decompression in patients with subtalar arthrodesis after calcaneus fracture are essential. Impingement in the subfibular recess is common, and the bone must always be removed regardless of the type of arthrodesis performed (Figure 35-4). The easiest way to determine that an adequate decompression has been performed is to make sure that the lateral wall of the calcaneus is slightly medial to the undersurface of the overhanging talus. After completion of the procedure, I palpate the subfibular recess percutaneously to detect any persistent bone underneath the tip of the fibula.

The incision is made from the tip of the fibula extending distally down over the sinus tarsi toward the calcaneocuboid joint. On the inferior surface of the incision the peroneal tendon sheath is identified, and more distally in the incision the terminal branch of the sural nerve should be looked for. The nerve usually lies inferior to the peroneal tendons, but if the dissection extends more distally, the nerve can be at risk for injury.

What incision should be used after a failed ORIF of a calcaneus fracture? Reuse of these extensile incisions for a subsequent elective arthrodesis procedure typically is problematic, and visualization of the entire joint can be limited because of scarring. I do not recommend using the original incision. Provided that 6 months has elapsed since the initial ORIF procedure, a standard sinus tarsi approach is far easier. With fractures treated initially with ORIF for which the hardware is still in place, two outcomes are possible: (1) either failure of the ORIF with widening and collapse of the subtalar joint or (2) normal hindfoot anatomy with arthritis. In the first case, the hindfoot widens with collapse of the subtalar joint, and the hardware needs to be removed before the lateral wall ostectomy and arthrodesis are performed. In the second case, despite the arthritis, the overall architecture of the hindfoot has been maintained, and the hardware can be left in place. Fixation of the subtalar fusion can be a little more difficult here, but the larger screws for the arthrodesis can be inserted around the plate and original screws, as is done for a primary arthrodesis of the subtalar joint combined with ORIF for an acute fracture.

When the hardware removal is planned as a simultaneous procedure, the plate and screws should be removed percutaneously assisted by fluoroscopic imaging. Each screw can be marked with a needle, and then a 2-mm puncture incision is made directly on top of the screw through the skin and then deepened through subcutaneous tissue with a hemostat, to avoid injury to the sural nerve. The plate can then be grasped with needle-nose pliers and then twisted out the front of the incision.

The retinaculum of the undersurface of the peroneal tendon sheath is stripped and elevated off the lateral wall of the calcaneus. Depending on the nature of the underlying disease, the peroneal tendons may be left in position or completely retracted if the lateral calcaneus has widened. After a calcaneus fracture, bone builds up laterally and squeezes the peroneal tendons into the fibula. To address this problem, the lateral wall of the calcaneus is completely exposed proximally toward and then posterior to the fibula, until the impingement against the lateral wall of the calcaneus is

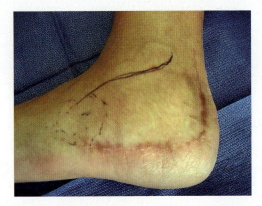

Figure 35-1 A short sinus tarsi incision is used here to perform the subtalar arthrodesis. The old incision, which was used for open reduction with internal fixation of the calcaneus, is ignored.

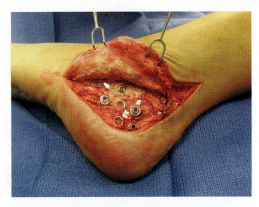

Figure 35-2 The original flap was elevated for conversion of the previous fracture repair to an arthrodesis of the subtalar joint. Note that the subtalar joint is not readily visible.

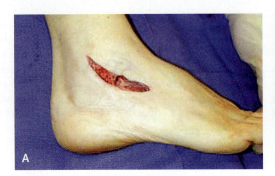

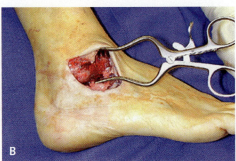

Figure 35-3 A and **B,** An alternative approach is to use a small incision in the sinus tarsi to expose the joint after a previously treated fracture.

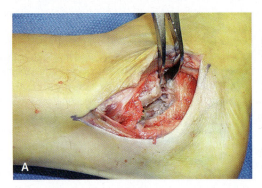

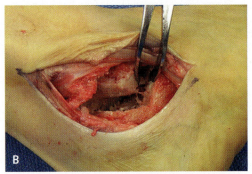

Figure 35-4 A and **B,** A laminar spreader is used to expose the posterior facet of the subtalar joint.

visible. A retractor is inserted into the soft tissue to pull the peroneal tendon sheath inferiorly and expose the entire lateral wall of the calcaneus.

For the lateral wall ostectomy, I use a 2-cm curved osteotome to remove a generous amount of bone to achieve complete exposure of the lateral aspect of the posterior facet of the subtalar joint and also remove the lateral impingement under the tip of the fibula. Slight irregularities often are present in the lateral wall of the calcaneus after this ostectomy, and the surface should be palpated through the skin to identify residual bone, which may be the source of pain. After completion of the ostectomy, the lateral margin of the posterior facet of the calcaneus should be slightly medial to the undersurface of the lateral margin of the talus. I preserve the resected bone and cut it up with a bone cutter into 5-mm fragments for later use as graft material (Figure 35-5).

The contents of the sinus tarsi are elevated off the floor of the sinus tarsi until the anterior aspect of the posterior facet of the subtalar joint is well visualized. A rongeur can be inserted directly into the posterior facet of the subtalar joint and then twisted around to loosen up the joint. The rongeur can then be pushed more medially to first open up and then debride the interosseous scar, opening up the middle facet. Once the debridement has been performed with the rongeur, a toothed laminar spreader is inserted into the sinus tarsi. With the spreader placed on stretch, the remnant of the interosseous ligament is visualized and is debrided to gain access to the posterior aspect of the subtalar joint and the middle facet. I use a flexible chisel to denude the articular surface of the posterior facet, but minimal bone is removed. The posterior facet is debrided down to bleeding healthy subchondral bone. All of the chondral fragments are removed with the rongeur. Final debridement using

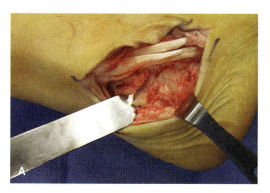
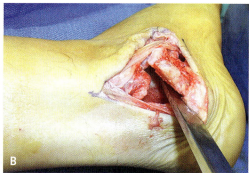

Figure 35-5 For management of dislocation of the peroneal tendons after a fracture of the calcaneus with subfibular impingement, the arthrodesis included a lateral wall ostectomy. **A,** The incision was extended more proximally to expose the dislocated tendons, and the joint was opened to reveal the impingement. **B,** The ostectomy was performed with an osteotome inserted posteriorly.

a flexible chisel is performed again on the more medial aspect of the subtalar joint, with entry into the middle facet and complete denudation of the articular surface and the undersurface of the talus, as well as the dorsal surface of the middle facet. It is important to debride the medial aspect of the joint, including the middle facet; otherwise, a gap will be present, which may not close, or the heel will tilt into valgus as the posterior and lateral aspect of the joint is compressed. Once I have removed all of the cartilage and chondral fragments, the joint is aggressively punctured or "fish-scaled" using an 8-mm curved osteotome and then perforated with a 2-mm drill bit.

The bone graft harvested earlier from the lateral wall of the calcaneus is used to augment the arthrodesis (Figure 35-6). The graft is now inserted into the sinus tarsi and the recesses in the subtalar joint and packed into place with a bone tamp. It is essential to ensure that no graft spills into the soft tissues, particularly under the peroneal recess laterally and then more posteriorly into the retrocalcaneal space. Over the past few years I have been routinely adding a spun-down concentrate from an iliac crest aspirate to the cancellous bone graft. In patients who are considered to be at higher risk for nonunion, I include use of bone morphogenic protein or an implantable bone stimulator in addition to the arthrodesis.

If I anticipate that copious amounts of bone graft will be needed, the surgical plan includes obtaining either autograft or allograft supplemented with mesenchymal cell aspirate from the iliac crest. If I anticipate that a defect will be present or that elevation of the height of the hindfoot is necessary, then I use a vertical incision. If, however, I have used the standard sinus tarsi incision, then before I complete the procedure, I make sure that the skin can be closed without tension. Removing some of the bulk of the bone graft may be necessary to achieve a tension-free closure. A defect is inevitable if avascular necrosis of the posterior facet is present: As debridement is performed, more bone loss will result. This defect can be filled with either a bulk structural graft or cancellous chips. Before the graft is inserted, a laminar spreader is placed into the sinus tarsi to check the required height, and the tension on the skin is evaluated.

FIXATION

I find it useful to secure the arthrodesis under fluoroscopic imaging using cannulated 7.0-mm screws. In the past, I inserted the first screw from the heel directed dorsally into the talus, trying to avoid

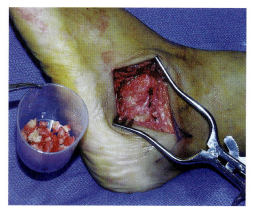

Figure 35-6 Bone graft cancellous chips were harvested from the cuts for the lateral wall ostectomy.

inserting the screw into the heel pad. The heel pad often is damaged with the impact of the hindfoot fracture, and further compromise is unwarranted with insertion of a screw too inferiorly on the heel. More recently, I have found that it is far easier to perform this maneuver using a cannulated screw (Orthohelix, Akron, Ohio), starting from the anterior aspect of the ankle in the center of the talus, immediately anterior to the ankle joint (Figure 35-7). The guide pin is inserted with the foot in plantar flexion so that the pin goes directly through the posterior facet of the subtalar joint, and is directed out the posterior heel, thereby avoiding the heel pad. This is easier than trying to aim for the center of the body of the talus from the inferior heel.

Are two screws necessary? The second screw adds to rotational stability and also may increase compression. In various biomechanical studies the addition of a second screw has been shown to be relevant, and I continue to use a second screw inserted from the neck of the talus inferiorly into the body of the calcaneus. Although a second screw can be inserted from the heel up into the neck of the talus, guiding its correct passage along this route is a little more difficult. This screw must not cause any impingement against the neck of the talus with the foot in maximum dorsiflexion. The position of the screws and the alignment of the hindfoot with respect to the forefoot are checked fluoroscopically before skin closure. It is of utmost importance to obtain an

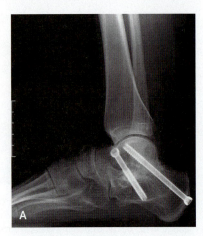
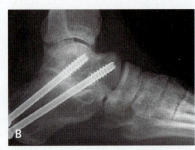

Figure 35-7 A and **B,** Two alternative methods of screw fixation to secure the arthrodesis.

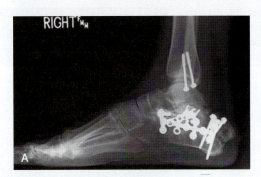
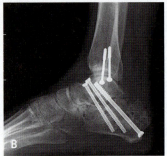

Figure 35-8 A, A nonunion of the posterior tuberosity with subtalar arthritis. **B,** This was corrected with removal of the hardware and a subtalar arthrodesis combined with repair of the calcaneus nonunion.

anteroposterior view of the ankle, to ensure that the screw(s) are actually in the talar body.

MANAGEMENT OF SUBTALAR FUSION NONUNION

Subtalar fusion nonunion is a frustratingly difficult problem that occurs in approximately 10% of the cases, depending on the underlying premorbid problems. Patients at high risk for this condition include those who smoke, those in whom calcaneus fractures have resulted in hard avascular bone in the region of the subtalar joint, and those in whom any areas of segmental avascular necrosis are present in the subtalar joint (Figure 35-8). If a nonunion in one of these high-risk categories is the surgical problem, bone graft augmentation with supplementation with bone graft substitutes or an implantable bone stimulator is recommended. The workup for a patient who has pain after a subtalar arthrodesis should include plain radiographs and a computed tomography (CT) scan. I have not found plain radiographs to be very helpful in determining the

cause of discomfort, unless an obvious deformity or nonunion is present (Figure 35-9). Sometimes the arthrodesis is solid, but the pain is due to subfibular impingement by an osteophyte on the inferior aspect of the fibula projecting off the arthrodesis either into the peroneal tendons or under the fibula. In such cases, the osteophyte is easily visible on a CT scan.

An inherent problem with treatment of a nonunion is that preparation of the joint requires further debridement, which frequently creates a larger hole or defect necessitating further bone graft supplementation (Figure 35-10). Grafting can be done with either autograft or allograft; usually cancellous bone allograft chips are used and can be mixed with a concentrate of an iliac crest aspirate (Figure 35-11). A nonunion that recurs is very frustrating and may be best treated with a triple arthrodesis to increase the likelihood of obtaining a solid union (Figure 35-12). After this procedure, patients should be kept non–weight bearing for a prolonged period of time, up to 3 months, until bone healing is evident radiographically. More important, these patients should demonstrate minimal swelling and no warmth in the hindfoot on palpation before initiating weight bearing.

TECHNIQUES, TIPS, AND PITFALLS

- Sural neuritis must be avoided. The nerve usually is immediately inferior to the peroneal tendons and must be avoided during the dissection. The dorsal lateral cutaneous branch of the superficial peroneal nerve is vulnerable in the more distal portion of the incision.

- Subfibular impingement must be treated after calcaneus fracture. The calcaneal ostectomy with removal of the lateral wall of the calcaneus is an integral part of the subtalar arthrodesis in these cases. At the completion of the procedure and when bone graft has been packed into the sinus tarsi, make sure that no graft has slipped back between the peroneal tendon and the fibula (Figure 35-13).

- A laminar spreader is very useful to open up the subtalar joint (Figure 35-14).

- In cases with long-standing subfibular impingement, the peroneal tendons may be torn or even dislocated out of the sheath (Figure 35-15). Always open the sheath under the fibula and inspect the tendons for a tear. If dislocation is present, it will be obvious, and the incision is then extended further back posteriorly behind the fibula to deepen the groove.

- If there is a tear of the peroneal tendons as well as dislocation associated with chronic impingement, a modified Chrisman-Snook ankle reconstruction can be performed. This procedure can include repair of the torn portion of the tendon, stabilization of the dislocation, and correction of ankle instability if present.

- In patients at higher risk for nonunion, I use bone graft or bone graft substitutes as well as bone morphogenic protein.

- Malunion is unusual with an in situ arthrodesis, but if it occurs, it is due to overrotation with internal rotation of the subtalar joint during internal fixation. Such overcorrection leads to adduction and slight supination of the forefoot and hindfoot varus. On careful inspection, when the hindfoot is held in the correct position, the heel should be seen to be in a few degrees of valgus and the forefoot should be plantigrade relative to the hindfoot. Caution is advised in making this determination if the patient is lying in a lateral decubitus position, which may make it difficult to visualize the relationship of the hindfoot, forefoot, and the knee. Slight valgus positioning of the hindfoot is preferable and does not cause too much of a problem unless the arthrodesis is performed for correction of flatfoot. In these cases, the subtalar joint is intentionally internally rotated, but again, care is taken to ensure that malunion with fixed forefoot has not been created.

- Subtalar arthrodesis performed for correction of a middle facet coalition can be challenging if the posterior facet is completely obliterated. Although the coalition involves the middle facet, it may be difficult to visualize the posterior facet, which has to be opened gradually. The entire joint including the middle facet coalition must be opened with a laminar spreader to correct the severe valgus that can accompany this deformity (Figure 35-16). If the posterior facet is not visible, then a small osteotome should be positioned fluoroscopically before attempting to open the joint. The calcaneus should be internally rotated slightly under the talus before fixation to correct the hindfoot valgus.

- It is not always easy to visualize the subtalar joint. Despite the correct approach to the sinus tarsi, there are cases, for example, a middle face coalition, in which it may seem that the joint is already fused. Working into the sinus tarsi and placing a small retractor over the peroneal tendons and behind the tuberosity will make the posterior facet more visible and accessible for debridement (Figure 35-17).

- A subtalar arthrodesis can be used as part of a hindfoot reconstruction for correction of a flatfoot deformity. By internally rotating the subtalar joint slightly with the arthrodesis, the arch height can be restored (Figure 35-18).

DISTRACTION BONE BLOCK ARTHRODESIS

The indications for a subtalar distraction bone block arthrodesis are fairly specific and are limited to procedures in which an arthrodesis of the subtalar joint needs to be performed but significant vertical collapse of the hindfoot is present (Figure 35-19). The traditional indication for this procedure has been reconstruction after a calcaneus fracture when shortening of the heel height with painful anterior ankle impingement and weakened push-off strength is present. An interesting point is that not all patients with collapse of the hindfoot and a horizontal talus (a negative talar declination angle) have anterior ankle pain. Indeed, although all of these

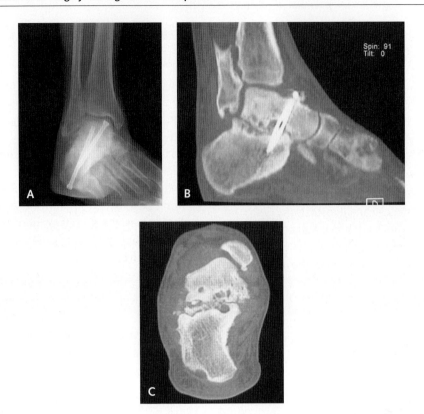

Figure 35-9 A, Nonunion after arthrodesis is not always evident on the plain radiograph. **B** and **C,** Nonunion is readily seen on these computed tomography scans of the ankle in a patient who presented with pain after a previous attempt at arthrodesis.

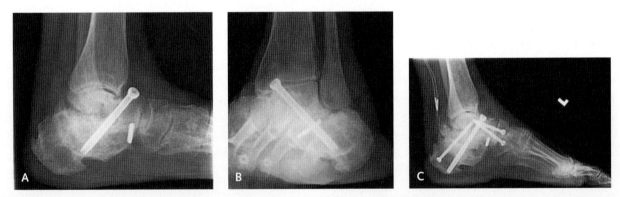

Figure 35-10 A and **B,** Persistent severe hindfoot deformity in a patient who had already undergone two previous attempts at arthrodesis. Note the marked valgus of the heel and the nonunion with subtalar collapse. **C,** A bone block arthrodesis, which included placement of an implantable bone stimulator, was performed through a vertical posterior incision. This procedure was not sufficient, however, to correct the remaining foot deformity, and a talonavicular arthrodesis was performed at the same time.

patients might be expected to have markedly limited ankle range of motion, this is also not necessarily the case. If the range of motion of the ankle is normal, and anterior ankle pain is not present, then an in situ subtalar arthrodesis can be performed. The mechanics of the hindfoot are never restored, however, and push-off strength remains weak (Figure 35-20).

In planning the bone block arthrodesis, it must be anticipated that the Achilles tendon will require lengthening. The increase in vertical height places more tension on the tendon, which will markedly limit ankle dorsiflexion if not lengthened. This lengthening can

be performed with an open technique using the same vertical incision. I try to obtain at least 10 degrees of dorsiflexion without much force on the foot after the arthrodesis (Figure 35-21).

The incision is made vertically in the posterior aspect of the ankle and extends from the inferior heel up and slightly posterior to the course of the sural nerve (Figure 35-22). The sural nerve is identified, the peroneal tendon sheath is identified more anteriorly, and the sheath and the nerve are retracted more anteriorly. The nerve can then be maintained in this position throughout the rest of the procedure. The nerve should be inspected, and if any

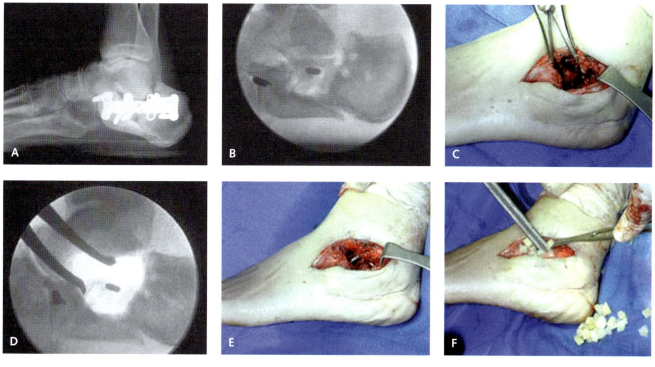

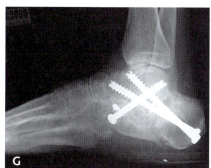

Figure 35-11 A, The patient had a severe malunion and nonunion of the body of the calcaneus after attempted open reduction with internal fixation. Despite the marked change in the talar declination, no anterior ankle pain was present, and a bone block graft was not performed. **B,** The hardware was removed percutaneously. **C,** The nonunion was approached through a short sinus tarsi incision. **D** and **E,** Realignment was achieved with use of a laminar spreader for joint distraction. **F** and **G,** Cancellous allograft chips were used to fill the defect. If the height of the hindfoot is increased with use of a sinus tarsi incision, it is essential to ensure that a tension-free skin closure can be obtained.

severe scarring is present or the patient had symptoms of neuritis preoperatively, the nerve can be transected and buried in the fibula through a drill hole made more proximally. Generally, however, I try to protect the nerve whenever possible by retraction. An important step at the end of the procedure is to ensure that the nerve is intact. If it has been damaged inadvertently, it should be transected and buried if possible.

For visualization of the posterior subtalar joint, the subcutaneous tissues are dissected deeper onto the posterior aspect of the calcaneus. Then the back of the joint can be identified with the posterior surface of the calcaneus used as a guide, proceeding anteriorly until the posterior part of the joint is identified. This portion of the procedure may be easier under fluoroscopic imaging. The posterior aspect of the retrocalcaneal space will have to be dissected out for visualization of the calcaneus. Next, proceeding laterally with subperiosteal dissection, strip the peroneal tendon sheath is stripped and the lateral wall elevated off the calcaneus. In almost all circumstances, subfibular impingement is present, and the lateral calcaneus ostectomy must be performed. This procedure may seem difficult but can be done through visualization of the hypertrophic bone laterally, with bone impingement evident under the fibula once the peroneal tendons are elevated. The ostectomy is performed

with a curved 1.5-cm osteotome. The ostectomy is started on the posterior margin of the tuberosity of the calcaneus inferior to the posterior facet. The entire bone mass must be removed, and there should be a clearance between the tip of the fibula and the calcaneus laterally. To ensure that the ostectomy is complete, palpation through the skin is performed by pressing under the fibula to feel if any bone remains prominent.

Working posteriorly in the retrocalcaneal space, I insert a curved osteotome along the posterior margin of the tuberosity of the calcaneus into the original subtalar joint. This insertion is not always easy and may have to be done fluoroscopically. If the joint is not visible, a 1-cm curved osteotome is inserted under the talar articular surface and passed down inferiorly and distally. The osteotome is now gradually worked into the original joint space in order to distract the joint. The plane of this osteotomy may go awry, so that the calcaneus is entered in the wrong direction. If this misplacement is noted under fluoroscopic imaging, the osteotome is reinserted in the correct direction. Once the joint is opened, it is possible to begin the distraction with a laminar spreader, which can then be inserted deeper into the joint. I use a combination of flexible chisels and osteotomes to decorticate the entire joint. Care is taken not to injure the flexor hallucis longus tendon on the

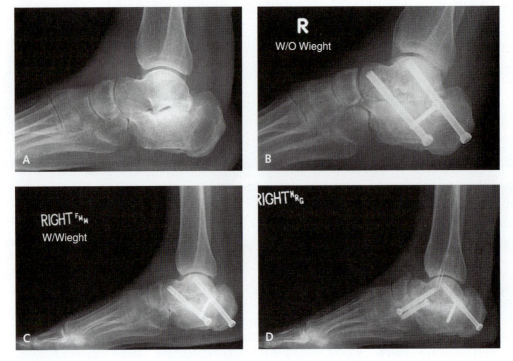

Figure 35-12 A and **B,** A nonunion developed after arthrodesis in a patient with diabetes. **C,** The nonunion persisted after another attempt at arthrodesis. **D,** Bone healing finally occurred after a repeat subtalar and calcaneocuboid arthrodesis was performed.

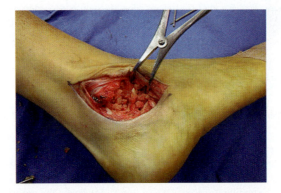

Figure 35-13 Cancellous bone graft is always used to fill the sinus tarsi.

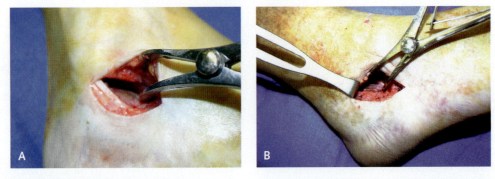

Figure 35-14 A and **B,** Exposure of the subtalar joint may not be easy until a retractor is inserted behind the peroneal tendons to obtain good visualization.

35

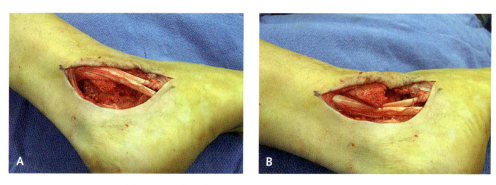

Figure 35-15 A, Dislocation of the peroneal tendons. **B,** Reduction was achieved by deepening the fibular groove after arthrodesis.

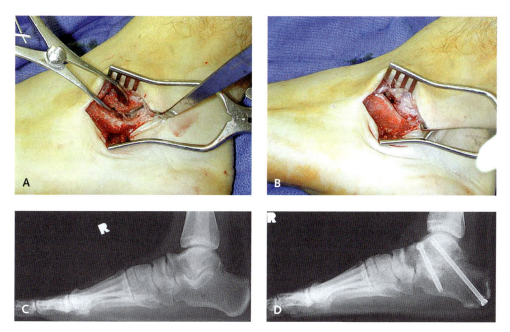

Figure 35-16 A-D, Treatment of a middle facet tarsal coalition with a subtalar arthrodesis.

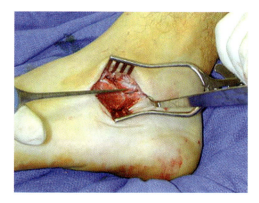

Figure 35-17 The joint was not visible in this hindfoot until the peroneal tendons were retracted and an osteome was inserted into the sinus tarsi.

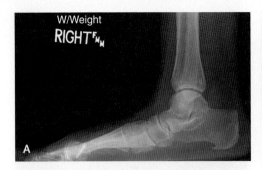
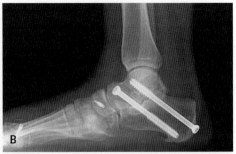

Figure 35-18 A and **B,** This adult flatfoot deformity was corrected with a modified Young suspension–anterior tibial tendon transfer combined with a subtalar arthrodesis.

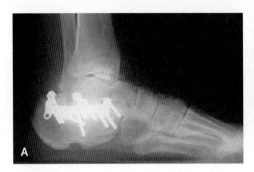
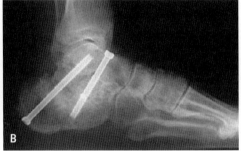

Figure 35-19 A, Note the horizontal talus after failure of an open reduction with internal fixation procedure. **B,** A bone block arthrodesis was performed to restore the height of the hindfoot.

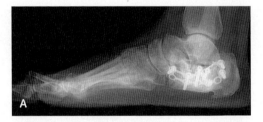
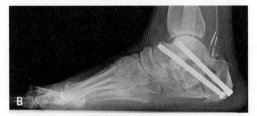

Figure 35-20 A and **B,** Despite a negative talar declination angle, no anterior ankle pain was present, so an in situ subtalar arthrodesis was performed.

posterior medial aspect of the joint. It is useful to reach with a ronguer as far forward as possible into the anterior subtalar joint, to enhance debridement.

I use structural allografting for the distraction procedure. A femoral head allograft is cut with a saw to contour its shape for insertion into the subtalar joint (Figure 35-23). The optimal shape is a trapezoid, slightly higher medially than laterally and higher posteriorly than anteriorly. The graft size can be measured fluoroscopically and will depend on the space opened by the laminar spreader. The shape of the graft will assist its insertion into the subtalar joint, where it will prevent varus deformity, which can occur

with this distraction type of arthrodesis. The graft generally is quite stable, but if it appears to wobble around, then a small notch or recess can be made with the osteotome in the posterior tuberosity of the calcaneus to promote stable insertion of the bone graft. At this time, the position of the heel should be checked, because varus tilt of the calcaneus with the laminar spreader in place is common. The heel must be in slight valgus once the graft is inserted. Before inserting the block graft, I once more debride the anterior aspect of the sinus tarsi with a curved curette and then place pieces of cancellous bone autograft more anteriorly into the sinus tarsi. Once I decide on the size of the block graft, I switch from the laminar

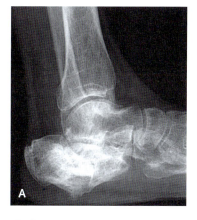
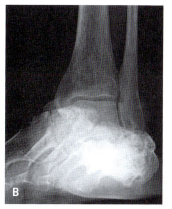
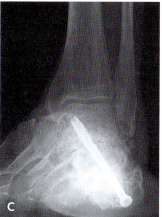
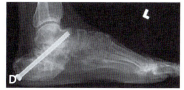

Figure 35-21 **A** and **B,** In addition to anterior ankle pain, severe lateral foot pain was present, the result of subfibular impingement. **C** and **D,** Correction was accomplished with a bone block arthrodesis.

spreader to one that has no teeth, to permit its easy extraction once the graft is inserted. The laminar spreader is now placed on maximum stretch to facilitate insertion of the graft, which is tamped into place securely. The graft only fills the space of the posterior facet and usually is not long enough to reach the sinus tarsi. Additional cancellous graft can be inserted into the sinus to augment the fusion. The laminar spreader is now gradually withdrawn, and the position of the heel noted. If a varus position of the heel persists, the lateral calcaneus can be shaved down directly under the graft with a saw.

Fixation is easier to perform with cannulated screws. I do not think that it makes much difference whether partially or fully threaded screws are used, but the height of the graft should not be lost as a result of excessive compression of the subtalar joint. The same principle of position of the screws applies here as for the in situ fusion previously described.

POSTOPERATIVE COURSE AND TREATMENT

The sutures are removed only after the wound is completely healed. The wound must be monitored carefully for problems related to stretching of the incision. The foot is immobilized in maximum dorsiflexion. If the skin's viability is in question, the foot can be positioned in slight plantar flexion to take the tension off the back of the ankle. This positioning compromises later rehabilitation, however, and once tissue healing is present, then

passive range-of-motion exercises can be started, but with dorsiflexion and plantar flexion only. Rehabilitation exercises are possible only with the foot in a boot, which must be worn at night to prevent plantar flexion deformity and equinus contracture. Weight bearing should not begin until 8 weeks after surgery. Whether the arthrodesis is done in situ or as a bone block procedure, determining whether arthrodesis is present radiographically is sometimes difficult. Frequently, monitoring of the soft tissue for swelling, pain, and in particular warmth is more helpful than the radiographic appearance, and a combination of clinical and radiographic observations is used to determine bone healing and weight-bearing status. The operated limb is immobilized in either a cast or a boot until full healing is evident both clinically and radiographically. Physical therapy with strengthening and rehabilitation is useful, particularly to maximize dorsiflexion and plantar flexion strength. Swelling usually is present for 6 to 12 months after the operation.

CORRECTION OF COMPLEX HINDFOOT DEFORMITY AFTER CALCANEUS FRACTURE

Issues unique to salvage surgery after failure of treatment for calcaneus fracture include the timing of surgery, the optimal surgical approach, the choice between ostectomy and arthrodesis, the type of arthrodesis to be performed, and the use of osteotomy in conjunction with arthrodesis to correct severe hindfoot deformity.

Figure 35-22 A, Vertical incision for a subtalar bone block arthrodesis. **B,** A laminar spreader is inserted into the incision, and the joint is distracted. Note the hemostat pointing to the flexor hallucis longus tendon on the medial aspect of the ankle. **C** and **D,** The graft is inserted and is tamped into place securely before fixation.

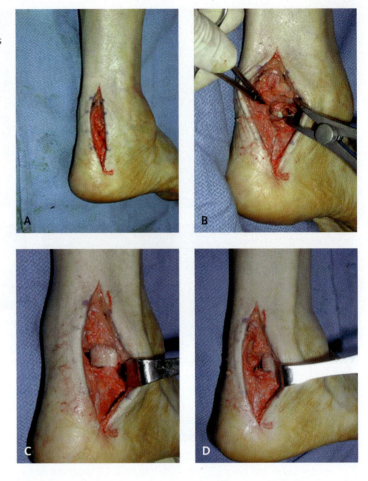

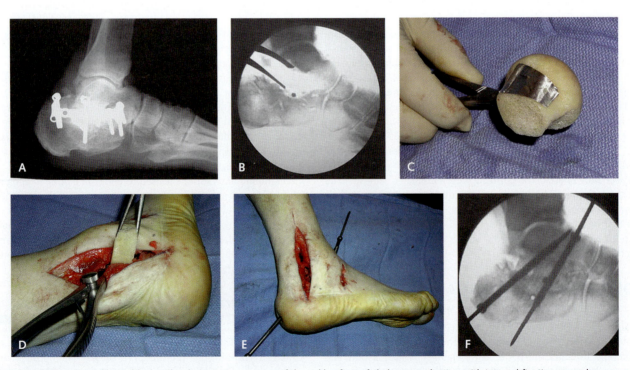

Figure 35-23 The steps of bone block arthrodesis. **A,** Appearance of the ankle after a failed open reduction with internal fixation procedure. **B** and **C,** The graft size is determined fluoroscopically with the laminar spreader in place **(B)** and then is measured on a femoral head allograft **(C).** **D,** Insertion of the graft. **E** and **F,** Cannulated screws are used for fixation.

TECHNIQUES, TIPS, AND PITFALLS

- If distraction bone block arthrodesis includes any correction of deformity, be careful with the final foot position. For example, if the procedure initially involves correction of mild subtalar valgus after debridement of the posterior facet of the subtalar joint, the heel tends to fall into more valgus. For this to be corrected, the more medial aspect of the joint, including the middle facet, must be debrided.

- If the heel tends to fall into valgus during correction, then slight internal rotation of the subtalar joint can be performed to create mild heel varus. The forefoot must not be overcorrected into supination.

- The incision for a bone block must be vertical. If any incision is placed in the longitudinal plane of the foot and an increase in the height of the hindfoot is created, a wound slough or dehiscence with likely infection will be created. With the vertical incision, the height of the hindfoot can be lengthened easily without risk for skin problems.

- The incision must be posterior to the peroneal tendons and sural nerve. The nerve is retracted anteriorly, and resection of the nerve is unnecessary unless a neuroma related to previous trauma or surgery is present. Retraction of the nerve anteriorly with the peroneal tendons is not difficult.

- The back of the subtalar joint cannot be seen initially. Locate the joint fluoroscopically with a guide pin and mark its entrance; then gradually open up the joint with a quarter-inch osteotome until entrance inside the joint is certain. At times, this procedure is difficult, and the osteotome has to be inserted fluoroscopically, corresponding to the original joint surface. Seeing the undersurface of the talus radiographically is easier than seeing the calcaneus, because the posterior facet of the calcaneus usually is severely impacted into the body of the tuberosity.

- Once the joint has been entered, gradually prying it apart, first with the osteotome and then with the laminar spreader, is helpful. This prying cannot be done initially because bone is under the fibula, and a lateral wall ostectomy needs to be performed first.

- The biggest problem with distraction of the subtalar joint is that the laminar spreader automatically tilts the heel into varus. This is an important problem that can be prevented. The graft must be shaped into a trapezoid that is higher medially than laterally, and as the graft is inserted, the heel must be manipulated into valgus before fixation.

- Once the bone block has been inserted, although the talar declination angle has been improved, the tension on the back of the ankle increases as the Achilles tendon tightens, and dorsiflexion of the ankle decreases. An Achilles tendon lengthening will often need to be performed. The foot must be positioned in 10 degrees of dorsiflexion with the bone block graft in place.

Salvage procedures for repair of complex hindfoot deformity can be divided into a number of categories. These depend on the following: (1) the presence of widening of the hindfoot; (2) the presence of varus or valgus deformity of the calcaneus; (3) the talar declination angle; (4) the presence of hardware; (5) any secondary deformities, including abduction of the transverse tarsal joint, which may be associated with crushing of the calcaneal cuboid joint; and (6) the presence of peroneal tendon dislocation.

For all of these complex deformities, a CT scan should be obtained (Figure 35-24). Although the nature of the deformity may be anticipated, the scan is helpful in planning the correction, particularly if an osteotomy of the calcaneus needs to be performed in conjunction with the realignment subtalar arthrodesis. CT scans are especially helpful when the tuberosity of the calcaneus has slid up against the fibula and the heel remains in varus. In such cases, a bone block procedure can be performed, through the original plane of the old fracture. Use of this procedure is more common in patients who have not been treated operatively because of a severe malunion of the calcaneal tuberosity.

If hardware is present, the operation may have to be staged (Figure 35-25). If the hardware can be removed percutaneously, then a bone block procedure can still be performed. A transverse incision in the plane of the hindfoot cannot be made when lengthening of the height of the hindfoot is performed, and for this reason, if a plate is present, it may need to be removed through the posterior incision in conjunction with percutaneous stab incisions directly over the screws. This is my preferred approach, rather than staging the operation. The combination of an osteotomy of the calcaneus and a subtalar arthrodesis can be performed either through a vertical incision posteriorly, as for a subtalar bone block arthrodesis, or through a more standard incision along the course of the peroneal tendons.

The latter incision is much easier to use because it permits complete visualization of the plane of the osteotomy from the site of the calcaneus. If a bone block procedure is performed in addition to the osteotomy, as illustrated in Figures 35-26 to 35-28, the osteotomy can still be performed with a large osteotome inserted in the plane of the fracture. Regardless of the type of incision used, the osteotome must be inserted fluoroscopically. After removal of the overhanging bone, which is lying underneath the fibula, a guide pin is inserted in the plane of the deformity. This usually is from dorsolateral to plantar and medial at approximately an angle of 30 degrees. The guide pin is inserted and then the position is checked with an axial view of the hindfoot on fluoroscopic imaging.

Minor adjustments are made to the position of the guide pin to place it exactly in the plane of the original fracture, and then the

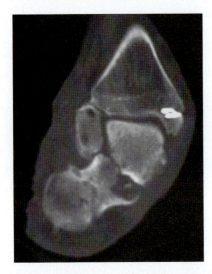

Figure 35-24 The computed tomography scan demonstrates the severity of this deformity requiring talar arthrodesis.

osteotomy is performed. I use a large broad osteotome to initiate the osteotomy, and the guide pin is then removed. The progress of the osteotomy should be checked fluoroscopically, also with an axial image of the calcaneus. Cracking open the osteotomy cut on the inferior medial aspect of the calcaneus at the completion of the osteotomy is easier than perforating through with the osteotome; such perforation risks injury to the medial soft tissues. Once the osteotomy is complete, the tuberosity now needs to be levered down inferiorly back into its corrected position. Usually the tuberosity has to be distracted distally and then pulled into valgus. The tuberosity is freed up with an osteotome, and then I insert a laminar spreader into the osteotomy site to open it up completely. The osteotome is levered laterally into the osteotomy site, and the tuberosity is forced down inferiorly. With this method, the tuberosity tends to be pushed into more varus, so use of guide pins usually is necessary to control the position of the calcaneus as it is being pulled into valgus while it attains a more normal height. Multiple guide pins are inserted into the tuberosity to maintain this position.

At times, the use of adjunctive bone graft is not necessary because of the plane of the osteotomy, which is in a sense sliding the calcaneus distally and into valgus simultaneously. This procedure is always performed, however, in conjunction with the subtalar arthrodesis, which can be done either as an in situ fusion or as a bone block procedure, depending on the extent of the subtalar collapse. If a bone graft procedure is being performed, the trick is to insert the graft and not lose the reduction of the calcaneal osteotomy. For this reason, I use multiple guide pins in the tuberosity extending up into various parts of the calcaneus and the more anterior portion of the talar neck and head, and then I insert a laminar spreader into the subtalar joint while the guide pins are

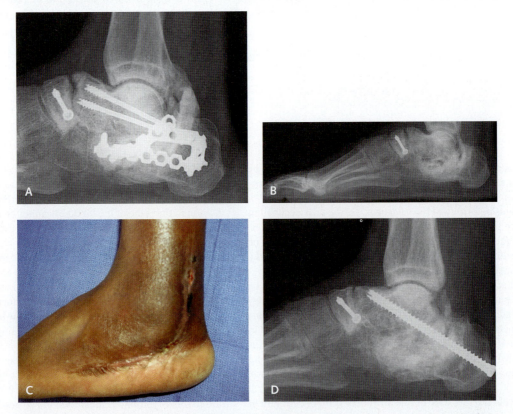

Figure 35-25 A, Repair of this severe deformity had to be staged. **B** and **C,** Hardware removal was the first step. **D,** Definitive repair was accomplished later with a bone block arthrodesis.

maintaining the reduction. The graft is inserted in much the same way as that described for the subtalar distraction bone block arthrodesis, and then some of the guide pins can be realigned to cross through the osteotomy site and the subtalar joint simultaneously.

Sometimes the deformity is severe, and in addition to a standard bone block of the subtalar joint, lengthening of the lateral column needs to be performed simultaneously with a second bone block to correct crushing of the calcaneocuboid joint. In the case illustrated in Figure 35-29, a double bone block was performed. The biggest problem with such procedures is in planning the incision. This is the one instance in which an extensile incision can be used, but the elasticity and the tension of the skin must be tested during the operation to avoid excessive tension with skin closure.

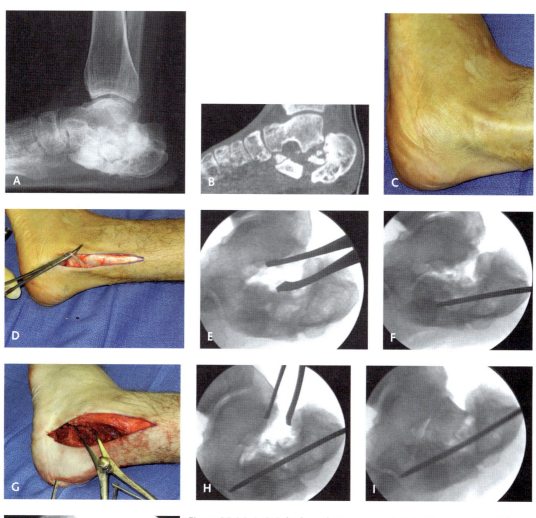

Figure 35-26 A-C, Subtalar arthritis was associated with a nonunion of the calcaneus and dislocation of the peroneal tendons. **D,** A vertical incision was used. **E,** A laminar spreader was inserted. **F,** An osteotomy was performed through the nonunion. **G** and **H,** The laminar spreader was again inserted. **I** and **J,** Insertion of a bone block graft and cannulated fully threaded screws for fixation.

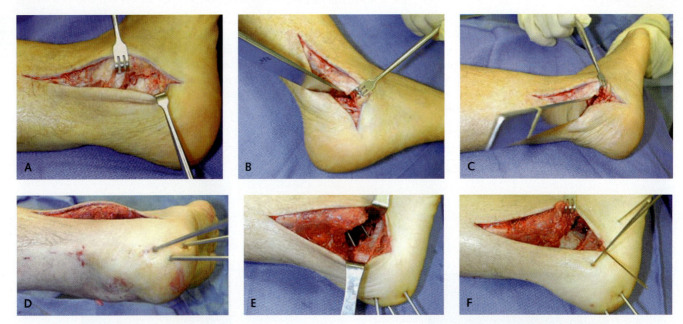

Figure 35-27 Severe hindfoot malunion after a non-surgically treated calcaneus fracture. **A,** For correction of the hindfoot collapse, a bone block arthrodesis was planned, but first a calcaneus osteotomy was performed through the original fracture plane to correct the valgus collapse of the heel. **B** and **C,** An osteotome was inserted under fluoroscopic control into the calcaneus in the plane of the original fracture line. **D** and **E,** The calcaneal tuberosity was levered inferiorly and medially with the osteotome and a laminar spreader and then held in place with multiple guide pins and Kirschner wires. **F,** Once the position and reduction were verified, a structural bone graft was inserted into the subtalar joint.

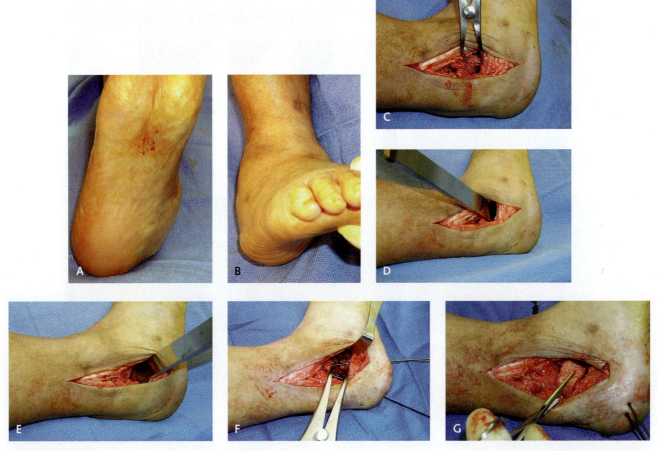

Figure 35-28 A and **B,** A very severe malunion with hindfoot valgus. **C,** Through a vertical incision, a laminar spreader was placed between the tip of the fibula and the laterally dislocated calcaneus. **D,** An osteotome was inserted along the plane of the deformity. **E,** The calcaneus was levered down into a corrected position. **F,** The laminar spreader was reinserted. **G,** A bone block graft was inserted.

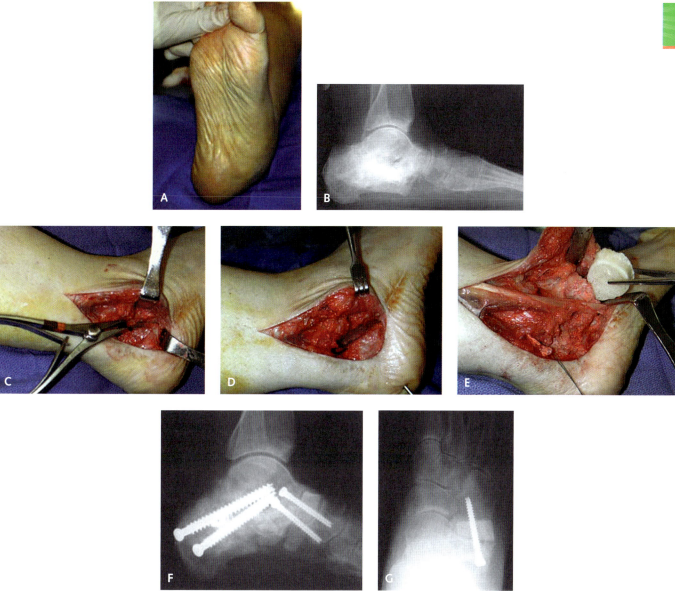

Figure 35-29 **A** and **B,** A double osteotomy–arthrodesis was performed for correction of severe hindfoot valgus associated with abduction of the transverse tarsal joint. **C,** A curved incision was used to approach the calcaneus, the dislocated peroneal tendons, and the hindfoot valgus. **D,** A calcaneus osteotomy in the plane of the original fracture was performed, and the subtalar joint was distracted. **E,** The suture under the fibula was attached to half of the peroneus brevis tendon, which was used in a modified Chrisman-Snook procedure to correct the dislocated peroneal tendons, and a second bone block graft was inserted into the calcaneocuboid joint. **F** and **G,** Final radiographic appearance.

TECHNIQUES, TIPS, AND PITFALLS

- Sometimes the calcaneal tuberosity is markedly displaced proximally and lies at the level of the talus. Correction of this type of deformity requires an open lengthening of the Achilles tendon, and the tuberosity has to be levered down inferiorly before the bone block graft can be inserted.

- A bone block graft does not always need to be performed in the setting of a decreased talar declination angle. If no anterior ankle pain is present and the pain is limited to the subtalar joint, then an in situ arthrodesis can be considered. This is a good option particularly in cases in which a nonunion is present, in addition to the vertical collapse. In such cases, correction of the nonunion takes precedence over restoring height of the hindfoot.

- I prefer to use a short sinus tarsi incision rather than the original incision for ORIF of the fracture. Elevation of the flap, which is thickened and scarred, is difficult. Exposure of the joint using the original incision also is difficult.

- Removal of hardware is not necessary before arthrodesis. If a lateral wall ostectomy must be performed, then the hardware can be removed percutaneously. This approach is particularly useful with a bone block distraction, in which the incision for hardware removal cannot be made along the length of the calcaneus.

- Obtaining a solid repair in this group of patients is not predictable. Bone sclerosis, presence of segments of avascular bone, and other factors, including threatened skin integrity, mitigate against a successful fusion. These patients should stop smoking before undergoing arthrodesis.

- Arthrodesis should be performed as soon as possible if the ankle is symptomatic. Many patients with these complex deformities associated with posttraumatic arthritis are construction workers, and the longer the interval between injury and return to work, the less likely it is that they will ever resume an active lifestyle. In my experience, these patients do not demonstrate substantial improvement beyond 9 months after calcaneus fracture.

- If a symptomatic tarsal tunnel syndrome is present, then the subtalar fusion should be performed first and the tarsal tunnel release staged to facilitate rehabilitation after the nerve operation.

SUGGESTED READING

Aminian A, Howe CR, Sangeorzan BJ, et al: Ipsilateral talar and calcaneal fractures: A retrospective review of complications and sequelae, *Injury* 40:139–145, 2009:Epub Feb 5, 2009.

Buch BD, Myerson MS, Miller SD: Primary subtalar arthrodesis for the treatment of comminuted calcaneal fractures, *Foot Ankle Int* 17:61–70, 1996.

Coughlin MJ, Smith BW, Traughber P: The evaluation of the healing rate of subtalar arthrodeses, part 2: The effect of low-intensity ultrasound stimulation. *Foot Ankle Int* 29:970-977, 2-8.

Easley ME, Trnka HJ, Schon LC, Myerson MS: Isolated subtalar arthrodesis, *J Bone Joint Surg Am* 82:613–624, 2000.

Myerson MS: Primary subtalar arthrodesis for the treatment of comminuted fractures of the calcaneus, *Orthop Clin North Am* 26:215–227, 1995.

Myerson M, Quill GE Jr: Late complications of fractures of the calcaneus, *J Bone Joint Surg* 75A:331–341, 1993.

Radnay CS, Clare MP, Sanders RW: Subtalar fusion after displaced intra-articular calcaneal fractures: Does initial operative treatment matter? *J Bone Joint Surg Am* 91:541–546, 2009.

Stamatis E, Myerson MS: Percutaneous removal of hardware following open reduction and internal fixation of calcaneus fractures, *Orthopedics* 25:1025–1028, 2002.

Trnka HJ, Easley ME, Lam PW, et al: Subtalar distraction bone block arthrodesis, *J Bone Joint Surg Br* 83:849–854, 2001.

Trnka HJ, Myerson MS, Easley ME: Preliminary results of isolated subtalar arthrodesis: Factors leading to failure, *Foot Ankle Int* 20, 1999:678-678.

CHAPTER **36**

Triple Arthrodesis

OVERVIEW AND APPROACH

In a *triple arthrodesis*, the subtalar, talonavicular (TN), and calcaneocuboid (CC) joints are included in the surgical fusion. A trend emerging over the past few years has been to try to preserve as much movement as possible in the remaining joint(s) of the hindfoot yet to create a functional plantigrade foot. Although a more limited hindfoot procedure such as a TN-subtalar arthrodesis or a subtalar-CC arthrodesis can be performed, such procedures may not reliably correct deformity. Nonetheless, as discussed further on, these more limited approaches have a lot of merit if performed in the right patient and with careful technique.

The triple arthrodesis is an extremely reliable procedure for correction of hindfoot deformity and treatment of associated arthritis. Although the approach to the procedure may have evolved or even changed technically, over the decades this has remained a standard method for correction of severe deformity regardless of the etiology. A triple arthrodesis is performed if a simpler hindfoot arthrodesis will not be sufficient; indications include a severe flexible flatfoot deformity, a rigid flatfoot deformity, posttraumatic arthritis, severe tarsal coalition associated with arthritis or uncorrectable deformity of the subtalar and transverse tarsal joint, congenital and neuromuscular deformity, and inflammatory arthritis. I try not to overuse the triple arthrodesis in the setting of the flexible flatfoot because osteotomy combined with tendon transfer usually is sufficient for correction of flexible deformity and generally can be expected to maintain joint motion. On the other hand, because a triple arthrodesis is so reliable a procedure, the indications for a flatfoot reconstruction should not be extended in order to specifically avoid an arthrodesis, because motion is not always preserved anyway. When arthritis of the tarsometatarsal or naviculocuneiform joints is present and a triple arthrodesis needs to be performed, there is obviously a considerable amount of stress on the intervening open joint, which may ultimately require arthrodesis. Nonetheless, what I refer to as an "extended hindfoot arthrodesis" must at times be performed.

Posttraumatic arthritis generally follows a talus or calcaneus fracture, but for most patients with arthritis and deformity secondary to a calcaneus fracture, a subtalar rather than a triple arthrodesis is the procedure of choice. A triple arthrodesis usually is the preferred procedure after a talar neck fracture with malunion, particularly when a varus malunion associated with arthritis is present (Figure 36-1). In the presence of a middle facet tarsal coalition, a subtalar arthrodesis is sufficient, and a triple arthrodesis is preferred only in the setting of arthritis or deformity, which typically is associated with a naviculocuneiform coalition, and when the coalition is not resectable. In patients with inflammatory arthritis, caution is indicated in selecting an isolated TN fusion, even when this is the only involved hindfoot joint. An isolated TN arthrodesis is associated with a higher incidence of nonunion, and once this occurs, correction is far more difficult because of bone loss and erosion, even with a triple arthrodesis.

SURGICAL APPROACHES

Over the years, I have been performing more hindfoot arthrodesis procedures through a single medial incision. Initially, I identified correction of a severe fixed valgus deformity as the specific indication for use of this approach, to limit the risk of lateral wound complications occurring as the hindfoot position is corrected to neutral (when using a lateral incision). This rationale still holds; nevertheless, I have been very pleased with the ability to correct deformity and associated arthritis from a single medial incision. Although the medial approach to triple arthrodesis is discussed in more detail further on, the concept of use of a single incision to perform a hindfoot correction is important. As might be expected, the inclusion of the CC joint in the fusion in performing a triple arthrodesis from the medial approach is difficult. In my own experience, both anatomic observations and outcomes in clinical series have demonstrated that the CC joint can be exposed and included in the arthrodesis with this approach. Nonetheless, as supported by results with my frequent use of the medial approach to correct deformity, it is apparent that the CC joint does not always need to be included in the arthrodesis (Figure 36-2). In performing the more limited arthrodesis (subtalar and talonavicular), however, it is important to recognize the potential for inferior subluxation of the cuboid relative to the calcaneus. This subluxation will produce a fixed rotation of the transverse tarsal joint, causing pain under the cuboid and the base of the fifth metatarsal. A good example of this potential problem is presented in Figure 36-3: After a limited arthrodesis performed using a medial approach, intraoperative fluoroscopy revealed that the CC joint was inferiorly subluxated, demonstrated by pushing up from below the cuboid to correct the subluxation, and could be corrected only by including the CC joint in the arthrodesis. There are probably fewer indications for a limited lateral arthrodesis, such as a subtalar and calcaneocuboid arthrodesis, but when the correction can be obtained, it is well worth trying to leave the talonavicular joint untouched.

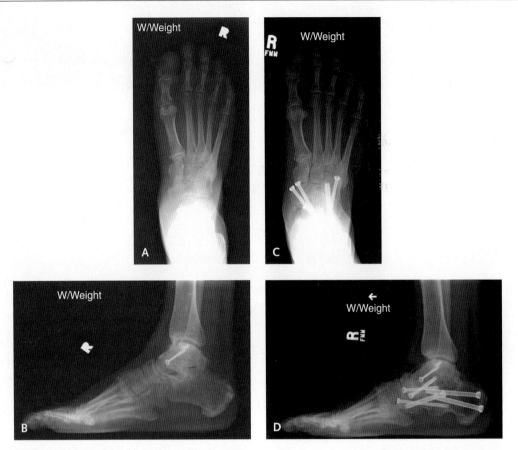

Figure 36-1 A and **B,** Malunion of a fracture of the neck of the talus treated with open reduction and internal fixation. The hindfoot was fixed in varus as a result of shortening of the medial column of the hindfoot. **C** and **D,** Correction was accomplished with a triple arthrodesis achieved by resecting a small wedge from the lateral aspect of the calcane-ocuboid joint.

The Lateral Incision

The incision is made from the tip of the fibular extending distally down over the sinus tarsi toward the CC joint (Figure 36-4). On the inferior surface of the incision, the peroneal tendon sheath is identified, and the terminal branch of the sural nerve must be looked for more distally in the incision. Both the peroneal tendons and the sural nerve are retracted inferiorly, and the incision can be deepened down on the periosteum directly over the calcaneus. The incision is extended distally toward the CC joint and then further toward the base of the fourth metatarsal. In the terminal aspect of the incision, care must be taken to ensure that no branches of either the sural or lateral cutaneous branch of the superficial peroneal nerve are present. The retinaculum of the undersurface of the peroneal tendon sheath is stripped and elevated off the lateral wall of the calcaneus. I prefer to save the contents of the sinus tarsi, because in the event of a wound dehiscence, sufficient tissue is always present for covering the peroneal tendons. The soft tissues are elevated sharply off the floor of the sinus tarsi until the anterior aspect of the posterior facet of the subtalar joint is visualized.

The incision is deepened directly onto the periosteum along the CC joint, and a large periosteal elevator is used to strip the lateral aspect of the calcaneus and then the cuboid. The peroneal retinaculum is retracted inferiorly, and a knife blade is inserted directly into the CC joint and then manipulated dorsally to cut the cervical ligament. The knife blade is swept vertically through the CC joint and then is rotated dorsally across the bifurcate ligament and directly into the posterior facet with one maneuver. The cuboid

bone should now be freely mobile, and the articular surface of the entire joint is denuded with a 2-cm flexible chisel, as well as with a rongeur and curette. Removal of more than 2 mm of bone and cartilage on either side of the joint is unnecessary. An important point here is that regardless of the type of deformity, a lateral bone wedge is *not* removed, and the position of the hindfoot is corrected with translation and rotation, not with resection of bone wedges. A laminar spreader is inserted into the CC articulation to check that all of the cartilage has been removed. Care must be taken to ensure that a minimal amount of bone is resected, to minimize any shortening of the lateral column.

A laminar spreader is inserted into the sinus tarsi, and when it is placed on stretch, the interosseous ligament is easily visualized and cut to gain access to the posterior aspect of the subtalar joint and the middle facet. A 1-cm flexible chisel is used to denude the articular surface of the posterior facet. As with the CC joint, minimal bone is removed. The posterior facet must be debrided down to bleeding, healthy subchondral bone (Figure 36-5). Care is taken with the debridement of the posteromedial corner of the joint, where the flexor hallucis longus tendon is at risk for injury from the chisel. Finally, the more medial aspect of the subtalar joint and the middle facet must be completely denuded, including the undersurface of the talus and the dorsal surface of the middle facet. Before the medial incision is made, the space between the navicular and the cuboid is debrided with a rongeur. This debridement adds another segment and bone surface to the fusion mass and converts the triple arthrodesis to a "quadruple arthrodesis" (Figure 36-6).

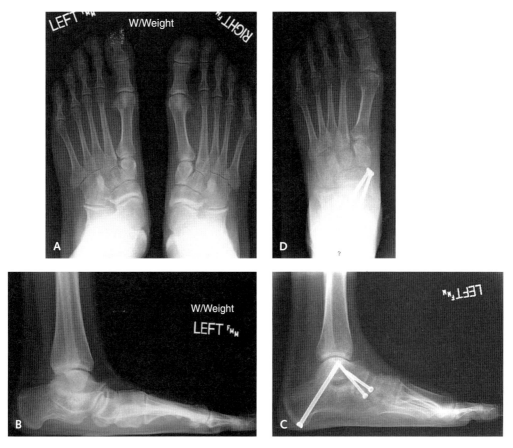

Figure 36-2 A and **B,** Weight-bearing radiographic appearance of a rigid flatfoot deformity. **C** and **D,** Treatment consisted of a double arthrodesis (talonavicular and subtalar) performed using a medial approach to the hindfoot.

The TN joint is clearly the most difficult of the three joints to visualize and to debride adequately. With either a varus or valgus deformity, the TN joint is only partly visible, but it must be distracted to permit visualization in its entirety. It may be tempting to approach the TN joint from the lateral incision, but only one third of the joint is visible from this incision, perhaps more if the hindfoot is fixed in varus. Of note, however, the TN joint is the one joint that will end up in nonunion if the joint debridement is not performed carefully. The medial incision is made medial to the anterior tibial tendon, extending from the ankle toward the medial cuneiform bone. The extensor retinaculum is incised, and the anterior tibial tendon is retracted laterally, exposing the deep subcutaneous tissue. Partially cutting into the extensor retinaculum and the medial edge of the anterior tibial tendon more distally may be necessary at times, because the tendon blends into the fibers of the retinaculum.

After the dissection, a retractor is inserted to pull aside the anterior tibial tendon and the medial soft tissues. The periosteum along the navicular bone is stripped, and then the TN joint is fully exposed with a curved periosteal elevator. Inserting an elevator directly into the joint to fully expose the head of the talus, followed by further stripping of the soft tissue dorsally and laterally, is useful. When a severe valgus deformity is corrected, pushing the midfoot into varus and then loosening the tension of the medial TN joint are helpful. I then cut around the medial joint from the outside in, through the remnant of the posterior tibial tendon and spring ligament into the TN joint. This step makes opening and distraction of

the joint far easier. A smooth laminar spreader (Figure 36-7, *A*) or rongeur is inserted into the joint and then exchanged for a toothed laminar spreader to facilitate distraction of the joint. Another option to maximize visualization of the joint is to apply distraction using pins inserted through a laminar spreader through which distraction can be applied (see Figure 36-7, *B*). The entire joint is denuded of cartilage using a 1-cm flexible chisel. An important consideration with the navicular is that because this bone can be hard, it can fragment if not debrided gently. The same contour must be maintained with debridement of the talar head while a small flexible chisel is used. Presence of osteopenia increases the risk of injury with use of the laminar spreader, which may crush into the talus. At the completion of the joint debridement, surfaces should appose well, with maintenance of the overall joint contour. If bone is resected from either joint surface, the medial column of the foot will be shortened, followed by a varus malunion.

Once the joints have been adequately visualized and their surfaces debrided, the final preparation is accomplished with a 2-mm drill bit to thoroughly perforate each bone surface. This aspect of the procedure is particularly important when the bone is sclerotic, which often is the case with the navicular.

Reduction of Deformity and Fixation

The reduction maneuver of the hindfoot relative to the forefoot is critical. For most deformities, the hinge point is the TN joint; therefore this is the joint that I reduce and fix first. The foot is rotated around the axis of the TN joint, and as the forefoot is adducted,

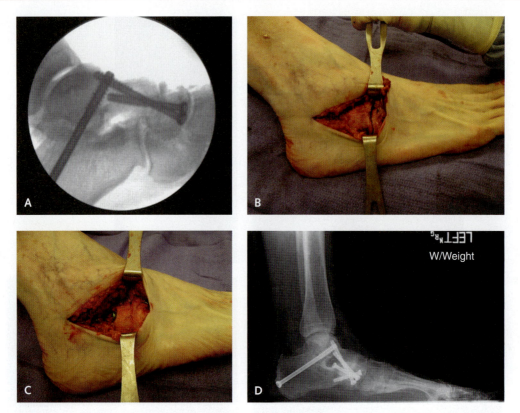

Figure 36-3 A, Fluoroscopic image, obtained at revision surgery, demonstrating the alignment of the hindfoot after an attempted double arthrodesis (talonavicular and subtalar). Note the inferior subluxation of the calcaneocuboid joint. **B,** Subluxation was confirmed on opening the lateral aspect of the foot. **C** and **D,** Correction was accomplished by including the calcaneocuboid joint in the arthrodesis.

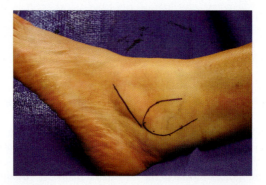

Figure 36-4 Lateral incision for hindfoot arthrodesis. The incision is marked out from the tip of the fibula across the sinus tarsi.

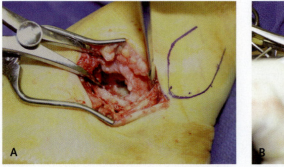
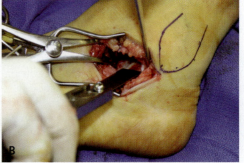

Figure 36-5 A, The subtalar joint is visible with insertion of a laminar spreader, which pushes the joint anteriorly. **B,** Debridement is performed using a flexible chisel. Note the protection of the peroneal tendons by means of a curved retractor placed behind the subtalar joint.

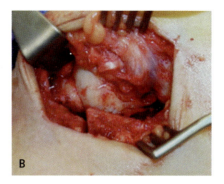

Figure 36-6 A and **B,** The local anatomy of the junction between the talus, navicular, cuboid, and calcaneus. The junction of these four bones is the fourth joint in a so-called quadruple arthrodesis.

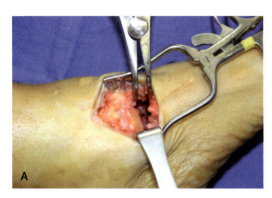
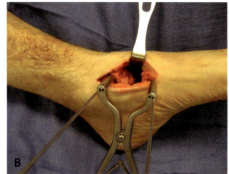

Figure 36-7 A, The talonavicular joint can be exposed by inserting a laminar spreader into the joint. **B,** Alternatively, pins can be inserted through a laminar spreader to distract the joint.

the first metatarsal is plantar flexed to correct the forefoot relative to the hindfoot (Figure 36-8). This maneuver is unsuccessful only when the subtalar joint is rigid and the calcaneus is laterally translated, in which case I fix the subtalar joint first. In the latter instance, then the TN joint may not line up perfectly, although clinically the forefoot alignment may appear to be corrected. For some very severe deformities that feature gross posterior subluxation of the subtalar joint, it is helpful to address this problem first by inserting a laminar spreader between the anterior process of the calcaneus and the lateral process of the talus. This maneuver forces the calcaneus forward, reducing the subtalar subluxation.

In the past I routinely used cannulated screws for fixation of the arthrodesis of each of the joints, and for the most part I still prefer screws for fixation. I currently use one 7.0-mm cannulated screw for the subtalar joint and one or two 5.5-mm screws for the CC and TN joints. I have noted, however, that it is difficult to obtain good placement of screws across the TN joint. One screw is easy to insert from the plantar medial aspect of the navicular, but the available space is not always sufficient for a second screw, and even use of two screws inserted from the medial aspect of the joint does not provide adequate fixation of the dorsal joint surface (Figure 36-9). The fixation of the TN joint may then be quite inadequate, because the joint is compressed predominantly medially, which may be associated with a delayed union or even nonunion of the joint fusion (Figure 36-10). If I am not satisfied with the fixation in the TN joint after placement of one or more screws, I supplement this with a dorsal two-hole locking compression plate (Figure 36-11).

I generally begin with the TN joint fixation. One or two guide pins are inserted into the TN joint, the first from the inferior medial tuberosity, and the second from a slightly more dorsal location, immediately adjacent to the anterior tibial tendon. The head of the second, more dorsal screw will be close to the naviculocuneiform joint. The heads of all screws must be well buried flush with the margin of the bone and not protrude into the naviculocuneiform joint. As noted, this configuration of screw fixation will provide fixation and compression of the medial aspect of the talonavicular joint only. An alternative method of fixation is to use crossed screws, one from the medial navicular and the other introduced percutaneously from the dorsolateral aspect of the navicular just dorsal and medial to the cuboid (Figure 36-12).

A few alternatives are available for insertion of the subtalar joint screw. The traditional method is to introduce a guide pin from the undersurface of the calcaneus, but off the weight-bearing surface of the heel. The problem with this method is that pin placement is not always accurate and the screw frequently is not exactly in the body of the talus. Another method is to insert the guide pin from the top of the talus just anterior to the ankle joint and then direct the guide pin all the way out the back of the heel. This maneuver permits determination of the exact starting position of the guide pin in the center of the talus. The pin is pulled out of the heel until the length in the body of the talus is correct, and then the screw is introduced from the heel up into the talus.

The CC joint is fixed last, using a posterior-to-anterior approach. The lateral aspect of the CC joint is flat, and screw

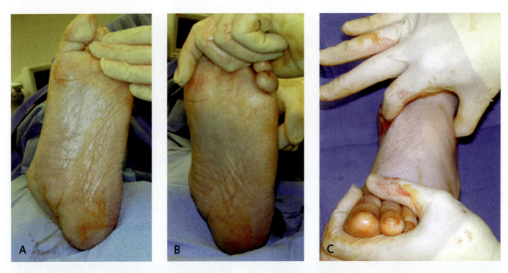

Figure 36-8 Manipulation of the hindfoot before fixation of a talar arthrodesis. **A,** Valgus of the hindfoot. **B,** With manipulation of the hindfoot around the axis of the talonavicular (TN) joint, the heel assumes a neutral position. **C,** The forefoot is adducted and pronated around the TN joint while the joint is palpated (using the index finger) for reduction.

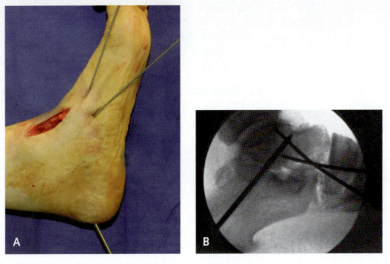

Figure 36-9 **A** and **B,** Two guide pins for cannulated screws were inserted across the talonavicular (TN) joint, and one was inserted across the subtalar joint. Despite presence of the two pins, a large segment of the TN joint is without any fixation or stabilization.

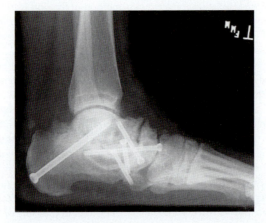

Figure 36-10 A nonunion resulted despite what appears to be satisfactory screw fixation of the hindfoot. The talonavicular joint is the one most likely to be involved in nonunion.

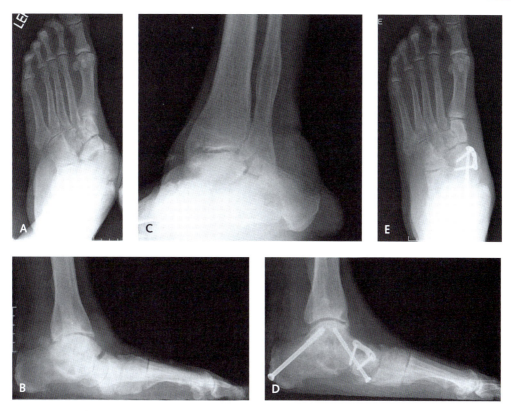

Figure 36-11 A-C, This rigid flatfoot deformity was treated with a modified triple arthrodesis (double arthrodesis). **D** and **E,** The fixation initially obtained with one screw across the TN joint was not adequate and was therefore supplemented with application of a two-hole locking compression plate (Orthohelix, Akron, Ohio) dorsally.

insertion will not be easy unless the surface of the calcaneus is prepared by making a notch with a chisel 1 cm proximal to the articular surface (Figure 36-13). This step is important in obtaining a solid fusion, and the lateral aspect of the foot must be elevated across the CC joint. Although the TN and subtalar joints are already fixed, some lateral mobility will still be present, and if the cuboid bone drops down, weight bearing will be painful as a result of a malunion. It is therefore imperative to elevate the inferior aspect of the cuboid, to create a plantigrade lateral weight-bearing surface. The guide pin for a 5.5-mm screw is inserted across the notched surface into the CC joint, followed by a 35-mm partially threaded screw. If the joint

surface is very flat and a screw cannot be easily inserted, then use of a small locking compression plate is ideal (Orthohelix, Akron, Ohio) (Figure 36-14).

Once fixation has been completed, the stability of the ankle should be checked, particularly with those procedures that are performed for a severe valgus deformity. As a result of the chronic valgus impingement between the calcaneus and the fibula, there is frequently erosion of the calcaneofibular ligament leading to ankle instability. In the case illustrated in Figure 36-15, gross instability was noted after screw fixation, and repair was accomplished with a modified Chrisman-Snook procedure.

TECHNIQUES, TIPS, AND PITFALLS

- Two incisions are ideal for complete visualization of all three joints.

- A single medial incision approach to the triple arthrodesis is useful to correct fixed hindfoot valgus deformity or when a modified triple arthrodesis with fusion of the talonavicular and subtalar joints is performed.

- The "fourth joint" of a triple arthrodesis is the recess between the navicular and the cuboid. This is the so-called quadruple arthrodesis.

- Minimal bone should be resected, and wedges of bone should not be removed, because the resulting defect will lead to shortening of the foot and possibly malunion. Correction of deformity is obtained by translation and rotation, not by resection of wedges of bone.

- Rigid internal fixation is preferable, and I have found that cannulated screws are very useful to maintain and hold reduction and are far more stable than staples.

TECHNIQUES, TIPS, AND PITFALLS—cont'd

As an alternative to screws, small locking plates are very useful to maintain the alignment of the TN and CC joints.

● As an alternative to screw fixation, consider the use of a plate for either or both of the TN and the CC joints. This also can supplement screw fixation when the joint appears to be unstable (Figure 36-16).

● I have not found it necessary to use bone graft because of the creation of good bleeding cancellous bone surfaces, which are always well apposed. Bone graft may be used in cases of severe deformity with a nonunion consequent to a previously attempted triple arthrodesis when a void exists after the debridement and realignment.

● The reduction maneuver before insertion of the cannulated guide pins is important, and the hinge of the TN joint is the key to correct alignment. If a severe fixed valgus deformity of the subtalar joint is present,

then I fix this joint first, followed by the TN joint, which then has to be more forcibly adducted and plantar flexed.

● Severe abduction of the forefoot with marked subluxation of the TN joint may require a structural bone graft with lengthening of the CC joint for correction (Figure 36-17)

● Isolated TN arthrodesis may be sufficient to correct deformity or arthritis of that joint, but complete correction of a hindfoot deformity is rarely accomplished with a single-joint arthrodesis. A modified triple arthrodesis with fusion of two joints (TN and subtalar, or subtalar and CC) can be considered.

● After the screw fixation, check the ankle dorsiflexion with the knee flexed and extended and perform a gastrocnemius muscle recession or lengthening of the Achilles tendon, as required (Figure 36-18).

The Medial Approach

For correction of severe fixed valgus deformity, particularly in the setting of rheumatoid arthritis, I use a single medial incision to perform the triple arthrodesis. Any incision on the lateral aspect of the foot in the setting of severe rigid hindfoot valgus is at risk for wound dehiscence. The approach to triple arthrodesis with a medial incision is performed through an extensile incision that begins at the naviculocuneiform joint and then extends proximally behind the medial malleolus. The incision must be dorsal to the neurovascular bundle at all times. A more precise idea of the location of this incision can be obtained by visualizing use of a portion of it for excision of a middle facet tarsal coalition and then extending it proximally and distally. The plane of the dissection runs just below the remnant of the posterior tibial tendon.

Pulling the flexor hallucis longus tendon inferiorly protects the neurovascular bundle during the dissection. Starting at the TN joint is the easiest way to identify the joints. Because of the severe abduction that is present across the TN joint, the head of the talus is always easily visible. The dissection is then deepened down onto the head of the talus, and then the middle facet can be identified by maneuvering an osteotome under the head of the talus. Once the middle facet is visualized between the talar head and the anterior aspect of the calcaneus, it should be opened with a curved osteotome. With the curved osteotome in place, the opening of the anterior aspect of the subtalar joint is then facilitated with insertion of a laminar spreader. The posterior facet is now denuded of the articular cartilage using a flexible chisel, followed by exposure of the TN joint. Stripping of the entire dorsomedial aspect of the joint is necessary (Figures 36-19 to 36-21).

By this time, the laminar spreader can be inserted into the TN joint followed by debridement as needed. Removal of a wedge from

the head of the talus is sometimes necessary to permit adduction of the foot around the transverse tarsal joint. An osteotome is used to cut all the way across into the CC joint, which can be verified fluoroscopically. A guide pin can be inserted across from the head of the talus into the CC joint to verify the position of the joint before cutting it with the osteotome. Realigning the subtalar joint is fairly easy also with the removal of slightly more bone on the medial aspect with the joint debridement, although resection of a bone wedge is rarely necessary because correction is performed by rotation and translation. If the hindfoot cannot be corrected, and remains fixed in valgus, it is helpful to release the peroneal tendons percutaneously which can be done proximally along the edge of the fibular. I correct the deformity by first bringing the heel into neutral and then securing it in this position with a cannulated guide pin. The midfoot is then passively pronated, adducted, and finally plantar flexed across the transverse tarsal joint, and the TN joint is then fixed. Extending the fixation across the navicular into the cuneiform and including the naviculocuneiform joint in the arthrodesis is sometimes necessary, because not much navicular bone is available to facilitate fixation itself (Figure 36-22).

TRIPLE ARTHRODESIS AND MEDIAL ANKLE INSTABILITY

The use of triple arthrodesis in a patient with an unstable medial ankle should be approached with caution. Such instability usually is present in the setting of a flatfoot deformity associated with a rupture of the deltoid ligament. A number of alternatives for correction of this deformity are available, including a triple arthrodesis with reconstruction of the deltoid ligament, a triple arthrodesis followed by an ankle replacement, and a pan-talar arthrodesis. With each of these procedures, medialization of the calcaneus is important

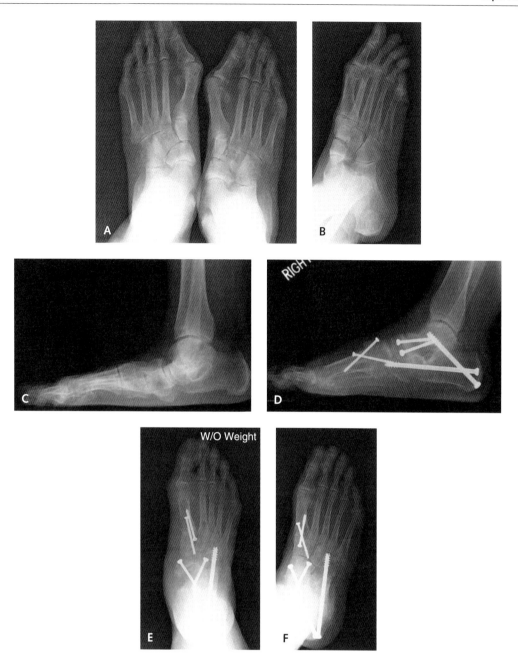

Figure 36-12 A-C, Rigid flatfoot deformity before treatment with a triple arthrodesis. **D-F,** Note the fixation of the talonavicular joint using crossed screws. The lateral oblique screw in the talonavicular joint is inserted percutaneously. (Photos courtesy Dr. John Campbell, Baltimore, Maryland.)

to balance the weight-bearing forces under the ankle more effectively. With a medial shift of the calcaneus, there occurs an increase in the contact on the medial ankle that takes stress off the deltoid ligament reconstruction. Clinical evidence suggests that a simple repair of the deltoid ligament will not be adequate, and some sort of reconstruction must be performed as discussed in the section on the adult flatfoot deformity. More important, a triple arthrodesis cannot be performed without some sort of reconstruction of the deltoid ligament. The technique that is described in the chapter on flatfoot deformity includes a hamstring allograft reconstruction of the deltoid ligament.

Laterally, the incision needs to be modified for the triple arthrodesis when a calcaneal osteotomy is performed simultaneously. I prefer to use two separate incisions (Figure 36-23). The first

is for the calcaneal osteotomy, and the second is a slightly shorter incision in the sinus tarsi but is slightly more dorsal than would normally be made. The calcaneal osteotomy is performed first, and the calcaneus is shifted medially by 10 mm. The guide pin for fixation of the calcaneal osteotomy is then inserted through the tuberosity and into the body of the calcaneus. The same guide pin, however, will be inserted across the subtalar joint once the subtalar joint has been debrided so that one screw will incorporate both the calcaneal osteotomy and a fixation for the subtalar arthrodesis.

Because of the medialization of the calcaneus from the osteotomy, the screw needs to be inserted slightly more laterally on the undersurface of the posterior heel, so that the screw enters the body of the talus correctly. I have not encountered skin healing problems with placement of these two incisions laterally. If for any reason

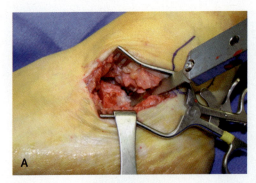
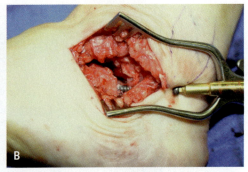

Figure 36-13 A, To permit insertion of a screw across the calcaneocuboid joint without fracture, a notch was cut in the lateral calcaneus 1 cm proximal to the joint. **B,** The screw was then inserted percutaneously into the notch.

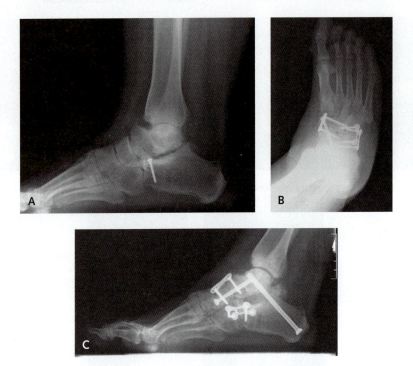

Figure 36-14 A, A triple arthrodesis was performed for management of posttraumatic arthritis of the hindfoot associated with avascular necrosis of the talus. **B** and **C,** Owing to the anatomy of the foot, it was far easier to use plates supplementing the screw fixation on the talonavicular and calcaneocuboid joints.

the use of these two incisions may be inadvisable, then certainly a single, more extensile incision can be used that is directed posteriorly underneath the peroneal tendons. My only concern with this approach is the stretch on the skin occurring as the calcaneus is shifted medially. When I use two incisions, the posterior incision for the calcaneal osteotomy is slightly more posterior and vertical so that little stress is placed on this incision with medialization of the calcaneus (Figure 36-24). After a triple arthrodesis, it is important to manually stress the ankle and get a feel for any instability. This can occur in either varus or valgus or in both planes. The multiplanar instability results when stretching or tearing of the deltoid has occurred, and as the hindfoot moves into a more fixed valgus position, the calcaneus abuts the fibula, causing an erosion of the calcaneofibular ligament. The manifestation of instability on clinical examination is important to appreciate; instead of a firm end point, a "clunking" sensation can be felt as the ankle moves into

varus or valgus. It is ideal to make the diagnosis of medial or lateral instability preoperatively, to anticipate the need for ligament reconstruction. This foreknowledge is helpful with respect to planning for the incisions and the approach to the triple arthrodesis (Figure 36-25).

REVISION TRIPLE ARTHRODESIS

The foot must be inspected immediately before the start of the revision triple arthrodesis and must be carefully examined while standing to determine the exact location of the apex of the deformity. The position of the calcaneus (neutral, varus, or valgus) and the presence of pressure anywhere along the lateral plantar surface of the foot must be assessed. The location of the apex (or apices) of the deformity also must be determined. Once this evaluation has been completed, the revision can be planned. As a generalization, for

36

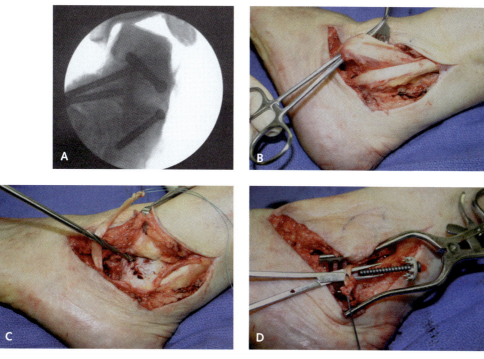

Figure 36-15 **A,** After screw fixation, gross instability on inversion stress was noted. **B,** The incision for the triple arthrodesis was extended proximally, and the peroneus brevis tendon was identified. **C,** The tendon was split, and a 4.5-mm drill hole was made in the fibula. **D,** The tendon was pulled through posteriorly, and a screw was pulled through the tendon over a spiked ligament washer. **E,** The screw was then fixed into the calcaneus with the tendon under appropriate tension.

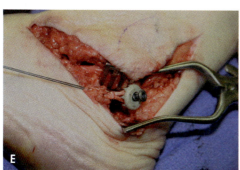

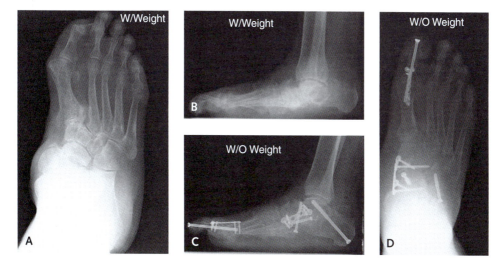

Figure 36-16 **A** and **B,** A flatfoot deformity in an elderly man with a complete dislocation of the talonavicular joint. At surgery to reduce the dislocation, a fracture of the sustentaculum tali was noted in association with the peritalar dislocation. **C** and **D,** The fixation combined the use of cannulated screws and a medially applied plate to maintain the reduction of the talonavicular joint.

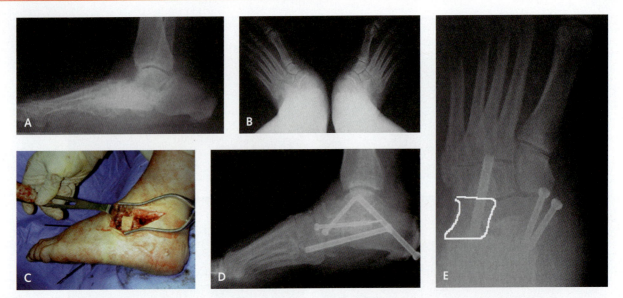

Figure 36-17 **A** and **B,** A structural bone block may be used for correction of severe deformity, as shown here. **C,** An allograft from the femoral head was cut to shape and then inserted into the calcaneocuboid joint to lengthen the lateral column. **D** and **E,** Postoperative appearance, with the bone block graft *outlined* on the anteroposterior view **(E).**

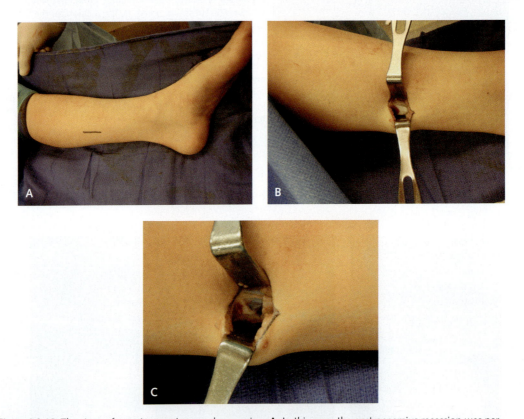

Figure 36-18 The steps of a gastrocnemius muscle recession. **A,** In this case, the gastrocnemius recession was performed after the triple arthrodesis. **B,** An incision was made laterally, and the sural nerve was identified and retracted. **C,** The fascia was cut transversely with a knife to expose the muscle belly beneath.

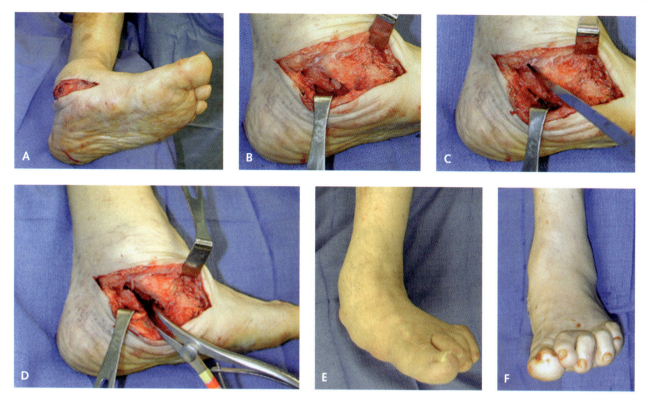

Figure 36-19 A severe rigid planovalgus deformity and arthritis of the hindfoot in a patient with rheumatoid arthritis. **A** and **B,** An extensile medial incision was used for the triple arthrodesis. **C,** The subtalar joint is opened with the osteotome. **D,** A laminar spreader is inserted to visualize the entire subtalar joint. **E** and **F,** The preoperative and immediate postoperative clinical appearance.

correction of a varus deformity, the incisions are made laterally, and for revision of a valgus deformity, the primary incision is medial.

The use of any of the original incisions is not necessary and often not advantageous, because placement of the incision is critical to gain maximum access for correction. These incisions must be extensile and often will cross the original incision. An important consideration is to locate the incision on the side of the apex of the deformity, so that with resection of a wedge of bone from that side, the chance of problems with skin healing is reduced. The incision is deepened, creating large thick skin flaps, with elevation of the entire dorsal, lateral, and plantar tissues off the hindfoot.

Malunion is the result of inappropriate intraoperative positioning of the foot with fixation. By contrast, malunion does not result from inappropriate casting in the postoperative period. Varus or valgus malunion seems to occur with increased frequency when the TN joint is not lined up correctly. Malunion is also likely if wedges of bone are resected from either the medial or the lateral transverse tarsal joint.

Correction of malunion actually is far easier than correction of a nonunion after a triple arthrodesis. After a nonunion, avascular bone loss is common, and with the consequent loosening of the fixation, the ability to secure the arthrodesis the second time around is greatly reduced. These problems do not occur, however, with a varus or valgus malunion when arthrodesis is present. In any case, with all malunions, the inevitable slight shortening of the foot occurs after treatment.

The size of the wedge of bone that is resected depends entirely on the location of the apex of the deformity. For example, if the apex of the deformity is at the base of the fifth metatarsal and the calcaneus is in slight valgus, then no wedge needs to be resected. With this deformity, an osteotomy can be made directly across the

transverse tarsal joint, and the entire midfoot can be rotated around the osteotomy without resection of the wedge. If, however, the apex of the deformity is at the level of the cuboid bone or the CC joint, then a wedge of bone usually needs to be resected. In this respect, therefore, a varus malunion and an equinovarus malunion differ. With an equinovarus deformity, the wedge that is resected will be slightly more dorsal than lateral. For correction of varus malunion, a second deformity may exist in the calcaneus itself in addition to the primary deformity, which is in the transverse tarsal joint. If a double deformity is present and the calcaneus is indeed in varus, then a calcaneal osteotomy must be performed, in addition to a transverse tarsal osteotomy.

For correction of a valgus malunion, two options are available: shortening the medial column or lengthening the lateral column. I generally base this decision on the size and shape of both feet and the overall needs of the patient, because shortening the foot may not be acceptable to some patients. It is far easier to remove a uniplanar or biplanar wedge from the medial foot than to elongate the lateral foot with bone graft and risk wound healing problems. The slight shortening that occurs with the medial shortening generally is well tolerated by the patient once the foot is plantigrade (Figures 36-26 and 36-27). The patient in Figure 36-27 presented with severe valgus deformity after an attempted triple arthrodesis. She had undergone multiple previous surgeries, and the skin over the lateral foot was particularly vulnerable. A medial approach to the revision arthrodesis was used, accomplished by resecting a wedge from the subtalar as well as the transverse tarsal joint. Resection of the wedge from the subtalar joint medially requires adequate soft tissue retraction and exposure (Figure 36-28). Although not a valgus malunion, an extremely rigid flatfoot deformity in an adolescent patient required far more than a triple arthrodesis (Figure 36-29).

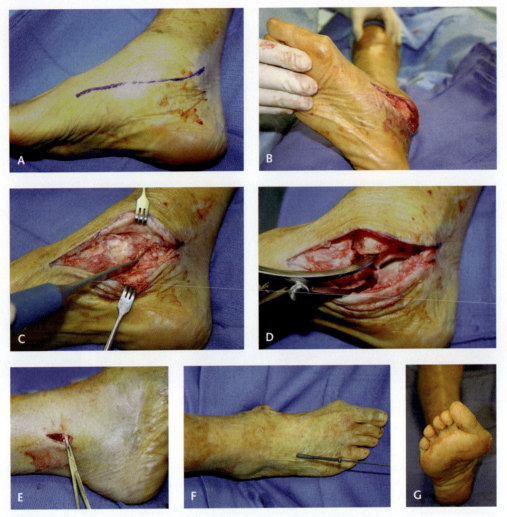

Figure 36-20 The steps of the medial approach to the triple arthrodesis. **A** and **B,** The surgical problem was a very fixed deformity of the hindfoot and a dislocation of the talonavicular joint. **C,** The head of the talus was exposed using an osteotome. **D,** A laminar spreader was inserted into the anterior subtalar joint. **E,** To permit reduction of the dislocation, a percutaneous lengthening of the peroneal tendons was performed. **F,** The calcaneocuboid joint was fixed percutaneously. **G,** Appearance of the foot at the completion of the repair.

For correction of a varus malunion, a biplanar osteotomy is performed at the apex of the deformity. A lateral incision is used and can be extended all the way posteriorly to include the calcaneus, if a calcaneal osteotomy is necessary. Because the plane of correction is from varus to valgus, an incision on the lateral aspect of the foot is not at jeopardy, and the single skin incision can be made extending from the base of the fourth metatarsal all the way to the back of the calcaneus. Before the incision is started, a decision has to be made regarding the necessity for a calcaneal osteotomy. Therefore the foot must be carefully inspected preoperatively to determine whether the calcaneus is in varus; the more significant deformity at the transverse tarsal joint also must be assessed.

If the deformity is not severe, then a more standard approach with two incisions can be used, as illustrated in Figure 36-30, in which the patient presented with avascular necrosis of the navicular and a varus deformity, the result of Müller-Weiss disease. For exposure, the incision is deepened through the subcutaneous tissue, and an extensile thick flap is created across the entire transverse tarsal joint. The peroneal tendons and sural nerve are reflected inferiorly, and a large malleable retractor is inserted underneath the calcaneus at the level of the CC joint, extending all the way underneath

the arch of the foot. The soft tissues need to be stripped off both the dorsal and the plantar surfaces of the transverse tarsal joint. The soft tissues are then protected with the malleable retractor on both of these surfaces to provide full visualization of and access to the lateral aspect of the foot for the wedge osteotomy. A guide pin is now inserted across the transverse tarsal joint under fluoroscopy. Locating the position of the osteotomy with this guide pin is important. Although the lateral foot and the apex of the deformity are easy to see, the medial extent of the wedge is not very predictable. I use two guide pins if I am performing a wedge resection or one pin if I have elected to use a rotational osteotomy across the transverse tarsal joint. The guide pins should meet at the appropriate point on the medial aspect of the foot. A triangular wedge, rather than a trapezoidal wedge, which would shorten the foot even further is resected. The osteotomy is then initiated on either the inside or outside of the guide pin, depending on its location. An important consideration is that the thickness of the saw blade itself will remove an extra 2 mm of bone with each cut. Although it may be tempting to use an osteotome for removal of the wedge, the osteotome does not afford the necessary precision for this maneuver—it cannot be controlled medially and can accidentally perforate the soft tissues. Once the

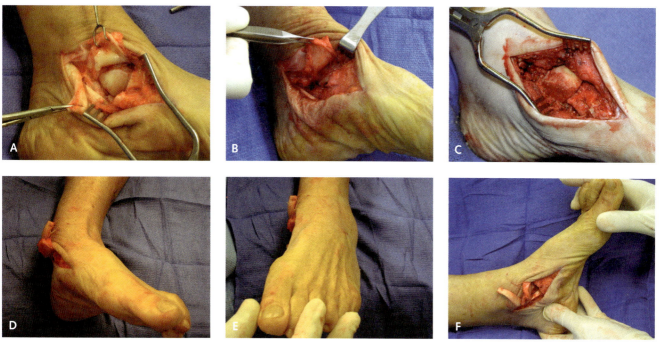

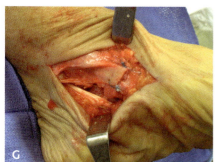

Figure 36-21 A and **B,** The medial approach was used in this patient and a complete rupture of the deltoid ligament. **C,** The subtalar joint was exposed with the laminar spreader in place. **D-F,** The deformity was corrected after the joints were debrided. **G,** The deltoid flap was finally repaired with reinforcing sutures.

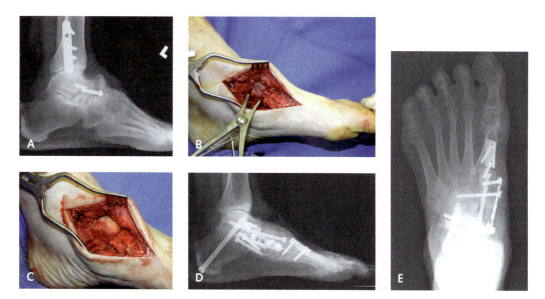

Figure 36-22 A, Necrosis involving the entire navicular after two previous attempts at a talonavicular arthrodesis. **B,** At revision surgery, a large defect was evident. **C,** This defect was filled with a structural allograft. **D** and **E,** Plate and screw fixation from the talus to the cuneiform was used to secure the repair.

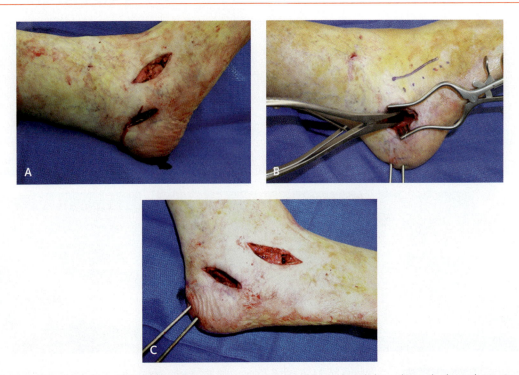

Figure 36-23 A, Location of the incisions for a combined triple arthrodesis and medial translational calcaneal osteotomy. **B,** The laminar spreader is used to check the location of the guide pins and to ensure adequate medial translation. **C,** The guide pins are finally introduced across the osteotomy and the subtalar arthrodesis.

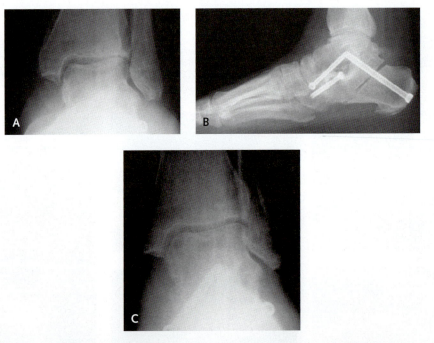

Figure 36-24 A, Valgus tilting of the tibiotalar joint is evident on the preoperative anteroposterior radiograph of the ankle. This was associated with a severe flatfoot deformity and rupture of the deltoid ligament. **B,** The triple arthrodesis was combined with a medial translational osteotomy of the calcaneus and a deltoid ligament reconstruction. **C,** The postoperative anteroposterior ankle view shows good correction of the tibiotalar alignment.

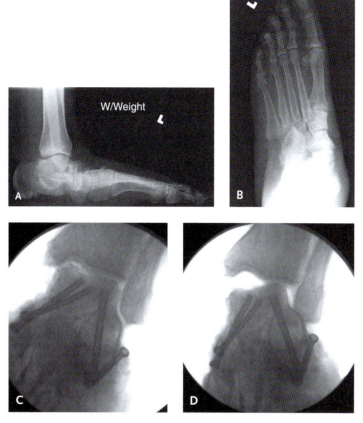

Figure 36-25 A and **B,** Triple arthrodesis was performed for a very severe but flexible hindfoot deformity. **C** and **D,** After completion of this procedure, stressing the ankle revealed marked instability, which was treated with a hamstring allograft ligament reconstruction.

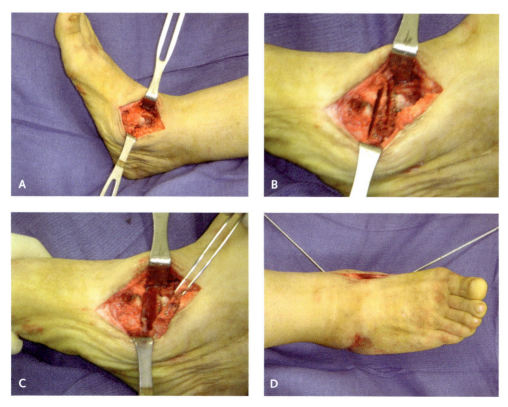

Figure 36-26 A-D, Management of a valgus malunion with a revision of the transverse tarsal arthrodesis. Note the use of a biplanar wedge resection from the medial aspect of the foot with temporary stabilization with guide pins.

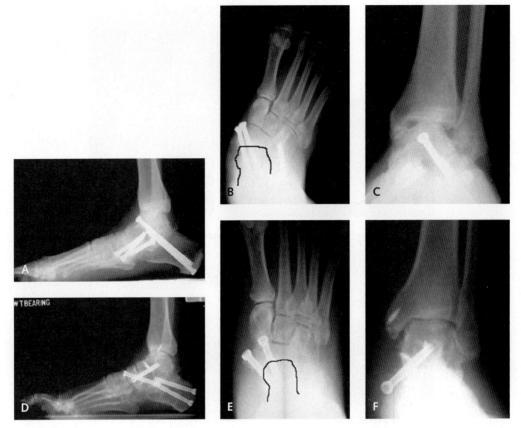

Figure 36-27 A and **B,** After a triple arthrodesis, severe abduction of this foot persisted. Note the effect of this fixed valgus on the ankle joint, which was markedly deformed. An ankle arthrodesis in this case would require a revision of the position of the midfoot as well. **C,** Once the ankle is reduced from a fixed valgus position to neutral, the forefoot supinates and has to be plantar flexed. **D-F,** Correction was accomplished with a transverse tarsal medial wedge rotational osteotomy with a medial incision and with reconstruction of the deltoid ligament with a hamstring allograft attached to the talus, medial malleolus, and calcaneus with bone suture anchors.

osteotomy is completed, the forefoot is rotated, as well as translated, to gain the correction. Of note, as the transverse tarsal joint is rotated from varus to valgus, plantar flexion of the first metatarsal will occur. The degree of this plantar flexion can be severe; in such cases, a dorsal wedge osteotomy of the first metatarsal or medial cuneiform also must be performed. Of note, however, the focus of the correction must be on the lateral aspect of the foot for correction of the hindfoot deformity; any secondary deformities are corrected subsequently.

Once the hindfoot deformity has been corrected, guide pins are then inserted to maintain the position of the foot, which should be inspected fluoroscopically before screws are inserted. Generally,

the plane of the osteotomy is such that screws will be inserted from distal to proximal across the osteotomy. For example, as the foot is rotated into pronation and translated slightly laterally, an elevated dorsolateral segment is created; this segment can be used for insertion of the guide pins and screws. Frequently, however, the pins and screws need to be inserted across additional joints, so the screws will ultimately need to be removed. The other option for fixation is to use staples. Because of the offset that usually is created as a result of this osteotomy, however, unless an offset staple is used, this method of fixation is not ideal.

Once the incision has been deepened down further through subcutaneous tissue, the entire dorsal and lateral periosteal surface

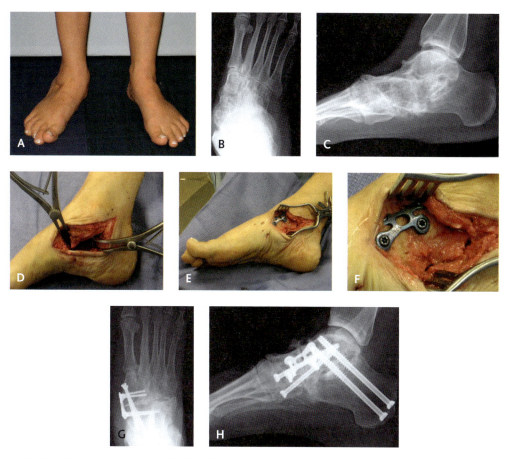

Figure 36-28 A-C, Fixed valgus deformity. **D** and **E,** Repair can be performed using a medial approach to the hindfoot. **F-H,** A biplanar wedge was resected from both the transverse and the subtalar joints, and fixation was accomplished using a combination of a locking plate and cannulated screws.

is elevated off the calcaneus and cuboid. The peroneal tendons are reflected and retracted inferiorly, and then with subperiosteal dissection the entire dorsal surface of the original CC joint and then the TN joint are exposed. The talus and navicular should be easily visible from the lateral aspect of the foot. Large soft tissue retractors are inserted on the underside of the CC joint and dorsally over the original TN joint to protect the soft tissue structures.

One or more guide pins are inserted transversely across the original transverse tarsal fusion mass to determine the location of the bone cut. Before the osteotomy is initiated, a longitudinal mark along the length of the calcaneus and cuboid bone is made with an electrocautery. After the osteotomy, when the shift of the hindfoot

position is started, the exact amount of translation and rotation can be visualized. A saw blade, rather than an osteotome, is used to cut across the original transverse tarsal joint (Figure 36-31). The first cut is made parallel with the position of the guide pin, approximately three quarters of the way across the foot. The guide pin is now removed, and the second bone cut performed. The size of the wedge cut is of course variable, but the height usually is approximately 8 to 10 mm at the apex dorsolaterally. The foot should rotate nicely out of the deformed position, and in addition to the rotation, some dorsal translation of the lateral aspect of the foot can be effected for complete unloading of pressure on the cuboid and fifth metatarsal.

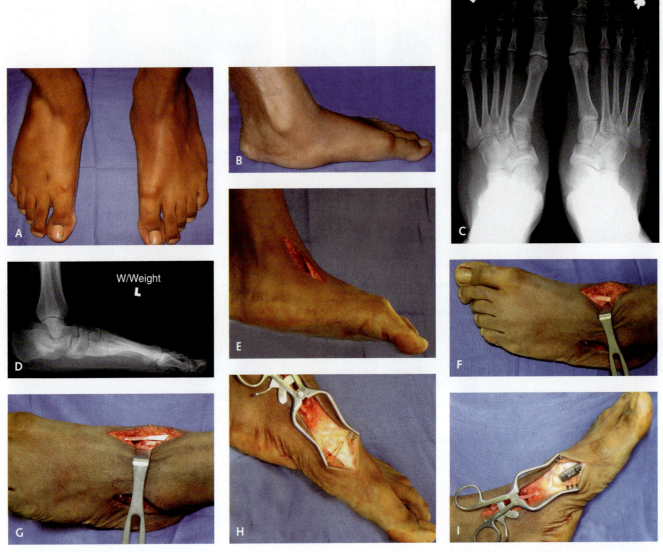

Figure 36-29 A-D, Triple arthrodesis was performed for correction of severe rigid flatfoot associated with a middle facet coalition in a 19-year-old patient. Note the marked elevation of the first metatarsal **(B)** and the fixed flexion of the hallux **(D). E-G,** After the standard medial and lateral incisions were made, the anterior tibial tendon was exposed and lengthened with a Z-step cut in the tendon. **H** and **I,** Once the fixation of all three joints was complete, the elevation of the first metatarsal was corrected with a plantar flexion osteotomy, with removal of a small wedge of bone from the base of the first metatarsal, followed by fixation with a two-hole, one-third tubular plate.

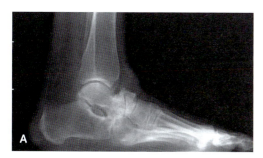
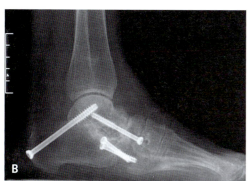
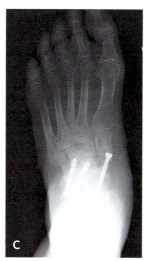

Figure 36-30 A-C, Correction of a fixed varus deformity in a patient with avascular necrosis of the navicular, the result of Müller-Weiss disease, was accomplished using a standard approach and fixation.

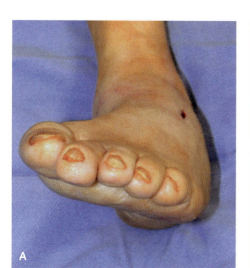
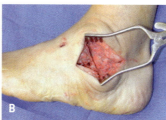
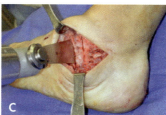
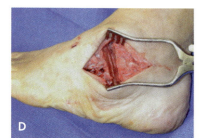
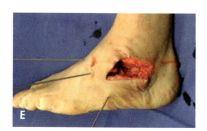
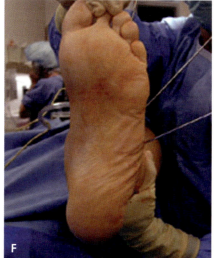

Figure 36-31 A, Severe adductovarus deformity, associated with plantar lateral foot pain, subsequent to a triple arthrodesis. The heel was not in varus, and therefore a calcaneal osteotomy was unnecessary. B-D, The apex of the deformity was dorsolateral directly over the calcaneocuboid joint, so the wedge was removed with the apex directly lateral. E and F, After reduction of the hindfoot deformity, the guide pins were inserted.

TECHNIQUES, TIPS, AND PITFALLS

- With fixation, I generally begin with the TN joint, which is the key to the reduction of any hindfoot deformity. The foot, particularly the planovalgus foot, pivots around the TN joint. Once this is locked in position, the rest of the joints fall into place. This is, however, a generalization. I do not think it is wrong to begin with the subtalar joint. Indeed, sometimes the primary fixation of the TN joint does not adequately reduce the heel valgus. In this instance, I will start with the subtalar joint fixation first. If this is done, however, the midfoot needs to be forcibly pronated around the head of the talus. If this maneuver is used for correction of severe hindfoot valgus, although the position of the foot may be correct, the anteroposterior radiograph will show slight overcorrection of the TN joint, with the navicular protruding slightly medially relative to the head of the talus. This positioning is not abnormal and results from primary correction of the subtalar joint followed by forcible pronation, adduction, and plantar flexion of the midfoot around the head of the talus.

- Under normal circumstances, because I start correction with fixation of the TN joint, I can feel with my thumb and index finger around the joint as the foot is swiveled from valgus into the neutral position. This is an important maneuver involving a "feel" for accurate positioning, and this technique must be mastered to prevent undercorrection and overcorrection in the arthrodesis.

- When naviculocuneiform arthritis or first tarsal-metatarsal arthritis is present and a triple arthrodesis is performed, the decision has to be made whether to include these joints in the arthrodesis. If they are included in the fusion, the foot will be extremely stiff, with inevitable overloading of the remaining "open" medial joint. In addition to arthritis, instability of one of these joints presumably will necessitate arthrodesis because no subluxation of the joint appears on the lateral radiographic view with a gap on the plantar surface. In such instances, I try to perform an opening wedge osteotomy of the medial cuneiform to realign either the naviculocuneiform or the cuneiform metatarsal joint *without* performing an arthrodesis. Joint instability is invariably corrected, and although (mild) arthritis may be present, it seems preferable to loss of motion with an arthrodesis. I prefer to wait and see what happens with this joint and perform an arthrodesis at a later date, if necessary.

- Although bone graft is not necessary for filling in the void in the sinus tarsi, on occasion I may use a structural bone graft for correction of severe deformity. Sometimes, because of abduction across the transverse tarsal joint with crushing of either the cuboid or the calcaneus, a structural graft inserted in the CC joint for purposes of lengthening is useful.

- A triple arthrodesis is rarely necessary after calcaneal fracture because a subtalar arthrodesis usually is sufficient. When severe collapse of the hindfoot with abduction across the transverse tarsal joint has occurred, then a triple arthrodesis is preferable. Under these circumstances, however, correcting the position of the calcaneus is necessary, and usually an osteotomy of the calcaneus in addition to the arthrodesis is required. If an osteotomy is performed, be careful with placement of the incision, because any increase in of the height or length of the foot must be in the plane of the incision itself.

- Planning the triple arthrodesis in the presence of pantalar arthritis can be tricky. The triple arthrodesis usually is done as a staged procedure to be followed by either a total ankle replacement or possibly an arthrodesis, depending on the outcome of the triple. Perfect position at the hindfoot is essential if the procedure is being planned as a staged triple arthrodesis before a total ankle replacement.

- Motion is lost after a triple arthrodesis—not only in inversion and eversion but also in dorsiflexion and plantar flexion. This outcome is inevitable whether or not the triple arthrodesis is performed for correction of a flatfoot or a cavus foot deformity. As a matter of course, significant stresses are placed on the ankle joint after a triple arthrodesis whether or not it is performed correctly. Generally, a valgus stress is placed on the ankle in the setting of a preexisting flatfoot deformity, when laxity or elongation of the deltoid ligament may have been present preoperatively.

- With severe valgus deformity, the Achilles tendon moves laterally with the calcaneus, and the gastrocnemius-soleus muscle shortens. Once the heel has been returned to a neutral position, this contracture will be unmasked. Whenever possible, I try *not* to lengthen the Achilles tendon because of inevitable weakening of the muscle. If the deformity can be corrected, I am inclined to do so without lengthening.

TECHNIQUES, TIPS, AND PITFALLS—cont'd

- Some deformities cannot be corrected with a triple arthrodesis without additional osteotomy or arthrodesis. Figure 36-29 demonstrates such a deformity, with marked rigidity in an adolescent foot associated with fixed elevation of the first metatarsal. Compensatory contracture of the hallux in plantar flexion with contracture of the short flexor of the hallux was present. In addition to the triple arthrodesis, a lengthening of the anterior tibial tendon and plantar flexion osteotomy of the first metatarsal was performed.

- Bone loss in the hindfoot that requires structural bone grafting is easier corrected with a triple arthrodesis than with an isolated hindfoot arthrodesis. This principle is well illustrated in Figure 36-22 in a patient with marked bone loss after two attempts at arthrodesis of the talonavicular joint.

- Remember to keep it simple. Although I have shown many alternative methods of fixation of the triple arthrodesis, screws provide excellent stability and afford sufficient control of deformity (Figure 36-32).

- Be careful with correction of the flatfoot deformity in an obese patient. Because of the size of the patient's thighs, walking is accompanied by a valgus thrust on the leg as well as the foot, and the foot must be placed in a greater degree of valgus than normal, to prevent lateral foot loading and pain. If the foot is placed in neutral, the degree of valgus will not be sufficient to permit the foot to clear the walking surface, with consequent discomfort for the patient (Figure 36-33).

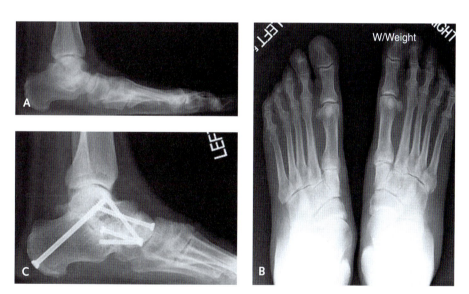

Figure 36-32 A-C, Standard cannulated screw fixation for a triple arthrodesis is simple and predictable.

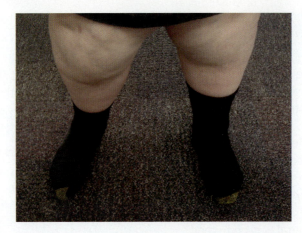

Figure 36-33 The correction of hindfoot deformity in an obese patient is difficult. The hindfoot must be positioned in slightly more valgus to accommodate the bulk of the thighs, which necessitates a wider base for walking.

SUGGESTED READING

de Heus JA, Marti RK, Besselaar PP, Albers GH: The influence of subtalar and triple arthrodesis on the tibiotalar joint. A long-term follow-up study, *J Bone Joint Surg Br* 79:644–647, 1997.

Fortin PT, Walling AK: Triple arthrodesis, *Clin Orthop Relat Res* Aug, 1999, pp 91–99.

Haddad SL, Myerson MS, Pell RF: 4th, Schon LC: Clinical and radiographic outcome of revision surgery for failed triple arthrodesis, *Foot Ankle Int* 18:489–499, 1997.

Jeng CL, Vora AM, Myerson MS: The medial approach to triple arthrodesis. Indications and technique for management of rigid valgus deformities in high-risk patients, *Foot Ankle Clin* 10:515–521, 2005:vi-vii.

Pell RF 4th, Myerson MS, Schon LC: Clinical outcome after primary triple arthrodesis, *J Bone Joint Surg Am* 82:47–57, 2000.

Raikin SM: Failure of triple arthrodesis, *Foot Ankle Clin* 7:121–133, 2002.

Saltzman CL, Fehrle MJ, Cooper RR, et al: Triple arthrodesis: Twenty-five and forty-four-year average follow-up of the same patients, *J Bone Joint Surg Am* 81:1391–1402, 1999.

Sullivan RJ, Aronow MS: Different faces of the triple arthrodesis, *Foot Ankle Clin* 7:95–106, 2002.

CHAPTER **37**

Ankle Arthrodesis

The optimal technique for ankle arthrodesis yields a predictable outcome, gives a high rate of fusion, and can be used in most patients. The repair should be secured with internal fixation, to achieve both clinical and biomechanical stability. The approach that I have found to meet these criteria is the mini-arthrotomy method with use of three crossed screws for fixation.

I originally described the mini-arthrotomy approach for use in ankles without much deformity and without bone defects or the presence of avascular segments of the talus and distal tibia. Subsequent experience, however, has shown that arthrodesis can be performed with the mini-arthrotomy technique even in the presence of significant deformity. This approach requires little periosteal stripping and is associated with rapid bone healing and an increased likelihood of a solid fusion as a result of maintaining the periarticular blood supply. I have not found that flat cuts on the ankle joint offer any advantage; indeed, such cuts require more extensive exposure and periosteal stripping. Performing a fibular osteotomy along with the arthrodesis adds an unnecessary sequence to the procedure, requiring more periosteal stripping as well as creating a larger area for the fusion with increased potential for failure with nonunion. Even less advisable in this clinical setting is the removal of both malleoli, which significantly decreases vascularity as well as the surface area for arthrodesis.

The desired position for ankle arthrodesis is with the foot in neutral with respect to the leg. There is rarely any reason to fuse the foot in equinus relative to the leg; this positioning will markedly increase the potential for complications, including subsequent arthritis of the peritalar joints as well as foot and knee pain. Much importance has been ascribed in the literature to the position of the foot and the need to translate the foot posteriorly under the tibia, which is not possible with either arthroscopic or mini-arthrotomy arthrodesis. The range of motion of the foot after arthrodesis depends on the preexisting deformity and, in particular, the motion of the remaining joints. The true sagittal motion of the tibiotalar joint accounts for approximately 70% of the sagittal plane motion. The sagittal motion after arthrodesis is in plantar flexion through the transverse tarsal joints (Figure 37-1). This motion may have a deleterious effect on both the talonavicular and the subtalar joints, as confirmed by an increase in arthritis in these joints in some patients.

INCISION AND JOINT EXPOSURE

Two incisions are used for the surgical approach to the ankle. The first is a medial incision made between the notch of the malleolus and the anterior tibial tendon, over a 2.5-cm length. On the lateral aspect of the ankle, the interspace between the peroneus tertius tendon and the fibula is identified, lateral to the lateral cutaneous branch of the superficial peroneal nerve, which is retracted medially with the peroneus tertius tendon. On the medial aspect of the ankle the incision is deepened through subcutaneous tissue through the capsule, which is incised down to the periosteum, and a retractor is inserted. Stripping the anterior distal periosteum off the tibia is helpful; then the articular debris, osteophytes, and loose bodies should be removed. Both gutters should be debrided extensively, with a focus on the lateral gutter between the talus and the fibula. I pay a lot of attention to obtaining an arthrodesis between the medial and lateral aspects of the talus and the medial malleolus and the fibula. Either a rongeur or a smooth nontoothed laminar spreader is inserted in the medial incision, followed by insertion of a toothed laminar spreader laterally (Figure 37-2).

The goal of joint debridement is to remove the joint surface down to bleeding bone. With use of the laminar spreader alternating between the medial and the lateral aspects of the joint, the articular surface of the talus and tibia is completely denuded. I use copious irrigation to ensure that good articular apposition is obtained and that good bleeding cancellous bone is present. One of the most significant changes in my preparation of the joint over recent years has been the creation of broad bleeding bone surfaces with use of a 5-mm osteotome, as well as thoroughly perforating the joint surfaces with a 2-mm drill bit. Before fixation, I check the alignment of the ankle fluoroscopically to ensure good bone-to-bone apposition. Large bone gaps are to be avoided; ideally, the prepared bone surfaces should give the appearance that the joint is already fused.

SCREW FIXATION

Crossing the plane of the screws is important. No screw construct should be created in which all of the screws are perpendicular to the axis of the joint. Parallel screw fixation should be avoided, because this technique is ineffective in controlling torsion and rotational

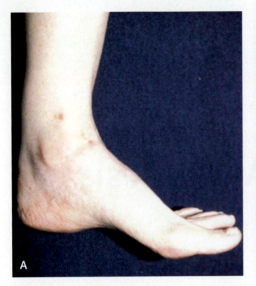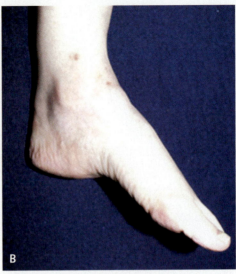

Figure 37-1 Range of motion of the ankle in dorsiflexion **(A)** and plantar flexion **(B)** after the mini-arthrotomy fusion. The motion is in the transverse tarsal joint.

forces. The fixation is performed with three screws placed over cannulated guide pins. The first guide pin is inserted from the medial malleolus to extend obliquely down toward the anterior aspect of the sinus tarsi. Why insertion in the medial malleolus first? I find that this is a more predictable placement that affords good compression of the joint. This screw is introduced from the medial aspect of the medial malleolus and extends down inferolaterally into the lateral body of the talus, directly above the lateral process of the talus. The screw must not enter the subtalar joint, and I rarely use a screw longer than 40 mm here. The foot can then be held in position while the second guide pin is introduced from the posterior leg adjacent to the Achilles tendon between the tendon and the sural nerve. The posterior axial screw is introduced next, from the posterior aspect of the tibia into the anteromedial neck of the talus; a 7.0-mm partially threaded screw, usually approximately 65 mm in length, is used.

The insertion point for the third screw is variable and depends on the anterolateral bone shape. If a ridge is observed on the distal lateral tibia, then the third screw is inserted from the anterolateral tibia immediately adjacent to the fibula into the distal medial talus. If no shoulder is present on the distal tibia, then one or two smaller screws can be inserted from the fibula into the talus, but these screws are not my preference (Figure 37-3).

In complex cases and when the bone quality is poor, the arthrodesis can be extended up into the syndesmosis, with insertion of a few extra screws from the fibula into the tibia (Figures 37-4 and 37-5). Sometimes the second posterior-to-anterior screw does not go in smoothly and hits the first medial screw. In such instances, a more lateral starting point is preferable, with the guide pin inserted through the posterolateral tibia. The three screws ideally should go through the tibia into the talus, rather than through the fibula. If, however, placement through the fibula is necessary, it should be drilled through to allow the screw to compress the fibula against the tibia. I like to use compression here if at all possible. Clearly, the first medially inserted screw gives the most compression, with less afforded with each subsequent screw, despite the use of partially threaded screws. If the bone quality is very poor, I forego compression; after making sure that the joint surfaces are very well debrided, I then use fully threaded screws (Figure 37-6).

It is imperative to check for motion in the ankle after *each* screw insertion. This series of manipulations provides a "feel" for the quality of fixation and the contribution of each screw to the arthrodesis construct. Aiming for the first metatarsal with the first posterior screw is important. The position of the guide pin should be checked fluoroscopically on the lateral view but, more important, on an anteroposterior view of the foot, to make sure that the guide pin is in the center of the talus. The pin often is inserted too far laterally, so that it may appear to be in the correct position on a lateral image but may be completely out the neck of the talus. With use of the mini-arthrotomy approach, it is possible to leave existing hardware in place unless it blocks the location of the arthrodesis screw.

CORRECTION OF DEFORMITY

If bone defects are present, they will be noticeable with the foot held in a neutral position, and a bone graft should be used. Provided that the defect is not substantial, it can be filled with cancellous chips, for which I routinely use allograft bone. I pay particular attention to placing bone graft in the medial and lateral gutters and intentionally try to obtain arthrodesis in this location.

If a large defect is present on one side of the joint after debridement, the normal side of the joint can serve as a template to lock the talus in place. This problem commonly arises, for example, when the distal lateral tibia is avascular or necrotic. I then use the medial malleolus as the point of fixation, lock the ankle in neutral, and fill the anterolateral defect with bone graft (Figures 37-7 and 37-8). Once the foot is dorsiflexed, the graft is then compressed. In patients at high risk for arthrodesis, as a consequence of conditions such as neuropathy or avascular necrosis, I add stimulation with bone morphogenic protein or an implantable bone stimulator, as needed. For bone grafting, I almost routinely include a spun-down aspirate of the iliac crest, which is then mixed with cancellous bone graft chips. This addition is particularly important in correction of avascular necrosis (Figure 37-9).

The position of the ankle is fused relative to the forefoot, not the lateral position of the talus. Equinus deformity should be corrected with the bone contour within the ankle. For correction

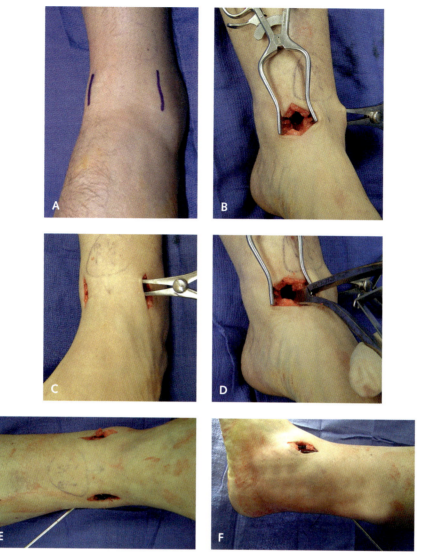

Figure 37-2 The mini-arthrotomy approach to ankle arthrodesis: **A,** the incisions; **B,** exposure of the joint with a retractor; and **C,** alternation of the retractor with a laminar spreader between the medial and the lateral incisions. **D,** The medial and lateral gutters are debrided with a rongeur. **E,** The first guide pin is placed through the medial malleolus. **F,** The second guide pin is inserted adjacent to the Achilles tendon and directed into the head of the talus toward the sinus tarsi, avoiding the posterior facet.

of severe equinus deformity, I often use an anterior approach to the ankle, with similar crossed screw fixation but with application of an anterior plate to the distal tibia. This anterior ankle plate will hold the ankle on the compression side of the joint, particularly by forcing the foot into dorsiflexion with the tightness of the posterior ankle soft tissues to create a tension band effect (Figure 37-10)

With correction of a cavus foot, extreme care is required in positioning the foot relative to the leg. As a rule, the foot should never be left in equinus. The position of the ankle is determined according to the position of the forefoot, and although this may correlate with the declination angle of the talus, such correlation does not necessarily hold with forefoot equinus or a cavus foot deformity. Overdorsiflexion of the ankle to place the forefoot in neutral position is specifically contraindicated in patients with a cavus foot. The result will be to place the hindfoot in a calcaneus

position, causing a painful heel strike. For these patients, after correct positioning of the ankle has been accomplished, a dorsiflexion osteotomy of the calcaneus can be added (Figure 37-11).

To fill a large defect in the ankle, a structural femoral head allograft is preferable to a cancellous graft. A decision often has to be made regarding subtalar joint preservation, which is always ideal, particularly if this joint is not symptomatic. In such cases, I may even use the entire femoral head, contoured with either a saw or an acetabular reamer to fit into the joint space. The same technique is used after arthrodesis for failed total ankle replacement (Figures 37-12 to 37-14).

Occasionally, when a bone defect is present, apposition of the surfaces of the ankle arthrodesis is good, and a structural graft is not necessary. Fusion of the ankle joint only, with preservation of the subtalar and transverse tarsal joints, whenever possible, is

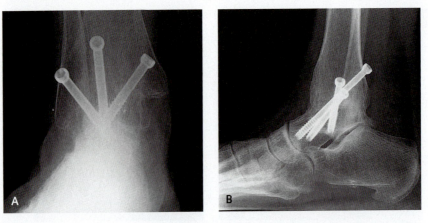

Figure 37-3 The standard screw location as seen on anteroposterior **(A)** and lateral **(B)** plain radiographs. Note that there is no screw in the fibula, and the lateral screw is inserted from the anterolateral tibia.

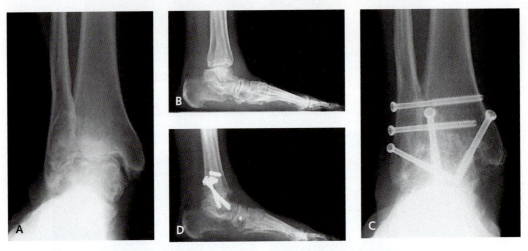

Figure 37-4 A and **B,** Arthrodesis was performed for treatment of ankle arthritis associated with a flatfoot deformity. **C** and **D,** The bone quality was particularly poor, and the syndesmosis was included in the arthrodesis.

preferable. The graft is cut, shaped, and inserted into the ankle, followed by placement of the posterior and medial screws. Because these screws usually do not provide adequate compression, an anterior plate generally is used for fixation. Need for this added fixation must be anticipated, because an anterior central incision is used when use of a plate is planned. The plate is applied to the tibia first; then the foot is forcibly dorsiflexed and the graft compressed. While the foot is held in this position, small screws are inserted through the plate into the talus (see Figure 37-13).

CORRECTION OF NONUNION AND SEVERE DEFORMITY

A definitive diagnosis of nonunion requires appropriate imaging studies. In some cases, the nonunion will be obvious, manifesting as an area of lucency on the plain radiograph accompanied by clinical findings of warmth and swelling. In other cases, the lack of bone healing will be easier to confirm on flexion-extension lateral radiographs (Figure 37-15); in still others, a computed tomography (CT) scan will be necessary for visualization.

The approach to management of nonunion must be individualized. The decision to start all over again with complete exposure of the joint, further periosteal stripping, and bone debridement will depend on the etiology. If the problem was poor fixation, then redoing the arthrodesis with good debridement and appropriate fixation is preferable. The difficulty with management of nonunion when good fixation has been used, however, is that further exposure means additional bone removal, with less mass for fixation and potentially worsening instability. If appropriate, bone stimulation modalities can be tried, particularly if the nonunion is of metabolic etiology. In such cases, I may simply make a few small incisions and aggressively perforate the joint with a 2-mm drill bit, change the screws using washers if necessary, and add some form of bone stimulation (Figure 37-16).

Attaining union is not sufficient. The foot must be correctly aligned under the leg in both the sagittal and the coronal plane (Figures 37-17 to 37-19). Treatment of nonunion associated with bone loss and deformity requires use of a more extensile lateral incision, although the medial incision may be the same as that used for the mini-arthrotomy approach. In planning correction of equinus malunion of the ankle, an important consideration is that if a wedge is removed from the anterior distal tibia and the foot is brought up into dorsiflexion, the foot will fall forward relative to the tibia, and push-off will be compromised (Figure 37-20). Before fixation and after

Text continued on p. 500

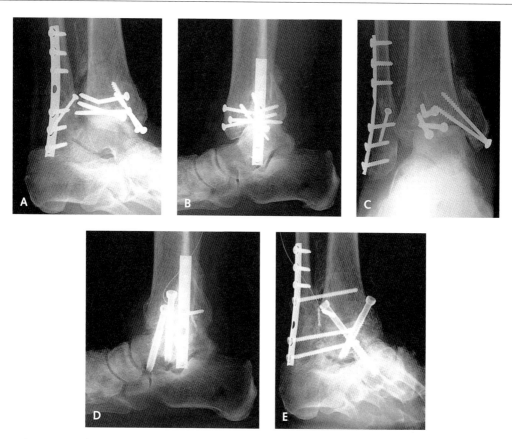

Figure 37-5 A-C, Failure of fixation of an ankle fracture associated with diastasis of the syndesmosis. **D** and **E,** The syndesmosis was included in the arthrodesis with tibia and talus pro fibula screws.

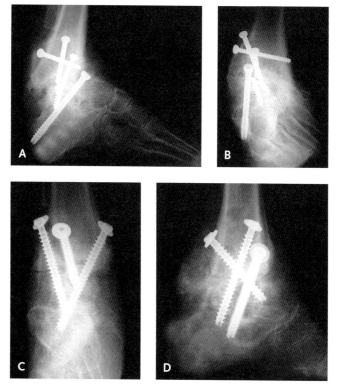

Figure 37-6 A and **B,** Severe deformity secondary to an unsuccessful ankle arthrodesis. **C** and **D,** Fully threaded screws were used to increase the bone purchase for the arthrodesis.

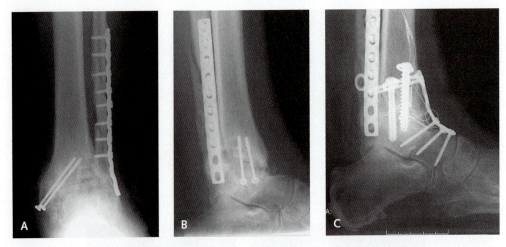

Figure 37-7 A-C, For correction of this severe deformity associated with avascular necrosis of the distal tibia, an anterior approach was used. Copious bone graft was used anteriorly, and the fixation was accomplished with fully threaded screws combined with an anterior plate.

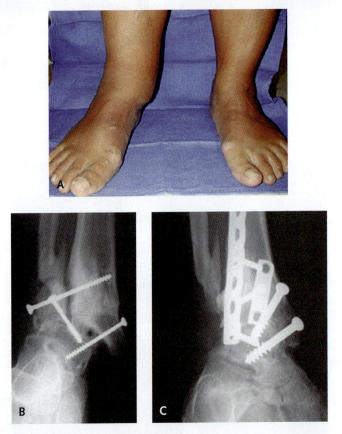

Figure 37-8 A, Clinical appearance in malunion and nonunion after attempted correction of ankle deformity. **B** and **C,** Treatment was accomplished using a laminar spreader to realign the joint. Cancellous screws and two plates were used to maintain alignment.

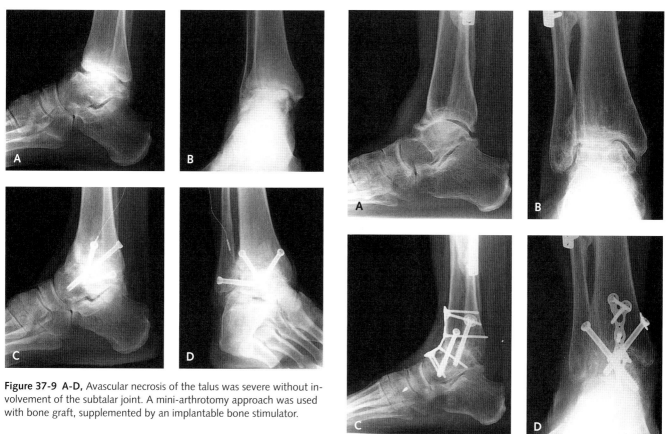

Figure 37-9 A-D, Avascular necrosis of the talus was severe without involvement of the subtalar joint. A mini-arthrotomy approach was used with bone graft, supplemented by an implantable bone stimulator.

Figure 37-10 A and **B,** Use of an anterior plate to treat marked avascular necrosis of the talus with anterior ankle instability. **C** and **D,** An anterior approach was selected, and cannulated screws combined with an anterior plate (Orthohelix, Akron, Ohio) were used for fixation.

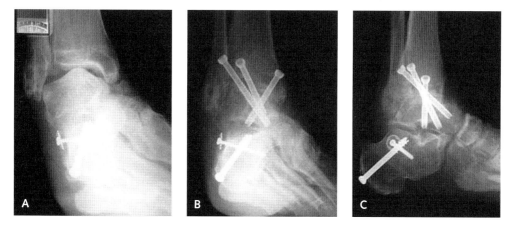

Figure 37-11 A-C, The mini-arthrotomy approach can be used for correction of deformity, as in this cavus deformity associated with marked ankle instability. Note the use of an additional osteotomy of the calcaneus to correct the heel varus and the pitch angle of the calcaneus.

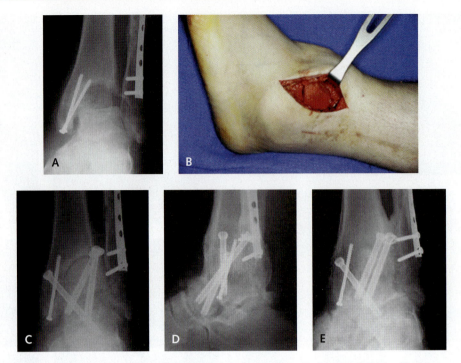

Figure 37-12 A, Ankle fusion for extensive posttraumatic bone loss. **B,** An extended lateral incision was used for insertion of a tricortical allograft from a femoral head, which was infiltrated with a spun-down iliac crest aspirate. **C,** Early radiographic appearance. **D** and **E,** Final healing occurred at 16 weeks.

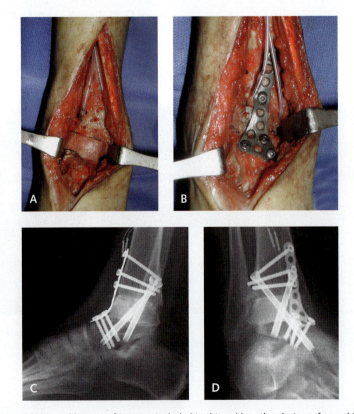

Figure 37-13 A, Structural bone grafting was included in this ankle arthrodesis performed to treat severe avascular necrosis in a patient treated with steroids for leukemia. **B-D,** The cannulated screws are inserted first, followed by the two screws through the plate into the tibia. Then the foot is forcibly dorsiflexed, compressing the ankle, and the two screws are inserted into the talus.

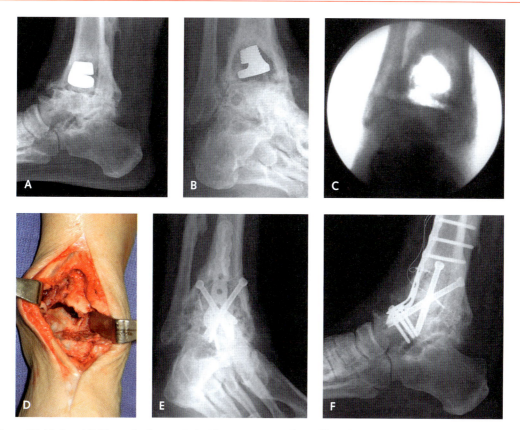

Figure 37-14 **A** and **B,** The patient presented with pain 20 years after ankle replacement. The subtalar joint was functional. **C** and **D,** Note the significant bone defect after removal of the prosthesis, which was filled with a structural allograft infiltrated with iliac crest aspirate. **E** and **F,** A combination of screw and anterior plate fixation was used to secure the repair.

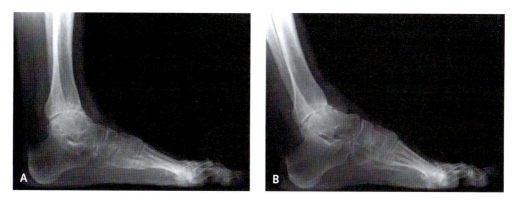

Figure 37-15 **A** and **B,** Diagnosis of a nonunion of this ankle arthrodesis was made with passive flexion and extension lateral radiographs. Note the significant movement in the joint.

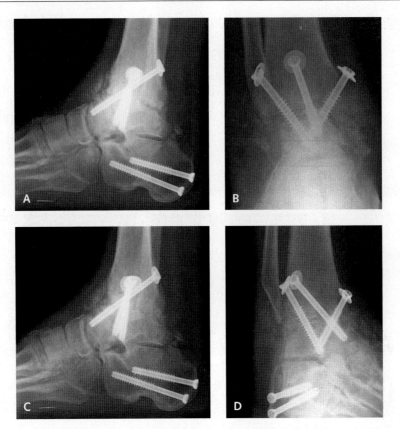

Figure 37-16 A and **B,** Nonunion of an in a patient treated with steroidal medication for a lung disorder. **C** and **D,** The revision surgery was performed through two small incisions. Multiple perforations of the joint were made using a 2-mm drill bit; cancellous graft and bone morphogenic protein were then inserted into the anterior ankle, with resultant successful arthrodesis.

removal of this wedge, the foot must be translated posteriorly under the tibia and left in a neutral position. This principle applies with revision of an equinus malunion as well as with the primary arthrodesis procedure. In correction of equinus malunion of an ankle fusion, the surgeon may be tempted to remove an anteriorly based wedge from the distal tibia, dorsiflex the foot, and complete the arthrodesis. The foot may now be in neutral position, but a secondary translational deformity will result, with consequent difficulty with gait.

An important issue here is whether an ankle or a tibiotalar calcaneal arthrodesis should be performed. The basis for this decision is not just the presence of a nonunion or malunion; additional factors to consider include associated bone loss, bone sclerosis, and possibly subtalar arthritis. If the motion in the subtalar joint is good, I try to avoid a tibiotalar calcaneal arthrodesis. With appropriate fixation, revising the ankle, even in the presence of bone loss, is always possible. The surgical plan should include preparations for the addition of bone graft and bone graft supplements, the insertion of an implantable bone stimulator, and the use of various types of instrumentation for rigid fixation. Frequently, compression across the joint is no longer possible because of screw failure leading to large voids in the tibiotalar joint space, and larger, fully threaded screws will need to be used.

Whenever possible, I preserve the fibula. If a fibulectomy previously has been performed, then a lateral approach to the nonunion or malunion may be used. If the fibula is present, however, then revision is focused anteriorly. Incorporating the fibula into the arthrodesis process is useful, particularly in the presence of bone

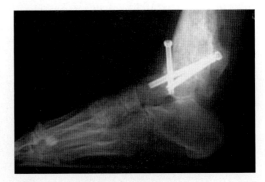

Figure 37-17 This ankle was markedly symptomatic after arthrodesis despite radiographic fusion. Note the marked anterior translation of the ankle, in addition to the equinus position.

loss in the region of the lateral tibial plafond. In this case, adding graft to the entire syndesmosis and in the fibular gutter and then adding a fibular plate with lag syndesmosis screws will increase the stability of the construct and thus of the arthrodesis. If patients undergo an arthrodesis for bone loss present anteriorly, the foot tends to dorsiflex during the fixation maneuver, and the heel is positioned in calcaneus. This heel position is difficult for ambulation, resulting in an inefficient gait. Surgical planning for an ankle fusion should always allow for additional procedures that will be required, including osteotomy, forefoot correction, and even tendon transfer (Figure 37-21).

37

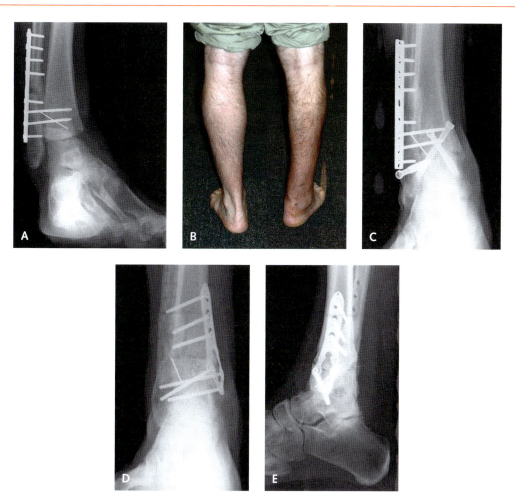

Figure 37-18 A and **B,** The patient presented with a severe varus deformity associated with absence of the medial malleolus. **C,** Despite treatment with arthrodesis, the patient remained symptomatic as a result of the varus position of the hindfoot. **D** and **E,** Correction was accomplished with an opening wedge osteotomy of the distal tibia followed by structural grafting and plate fixation.

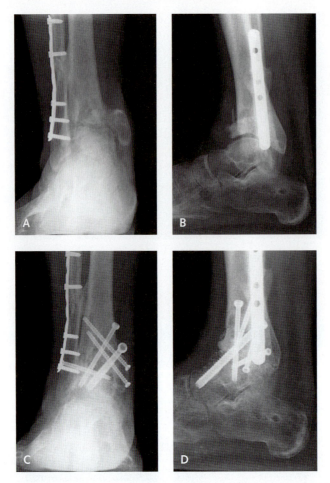

Figure 37-19 A and **B,** Note the medial and anterior translation of the talus as well as the nonunion of the medial malleolus in a patient with arthritis and deformity following ankle fracture. **C** and **D,** The nonunion was corrected and the alignment was improved after arthrodesis. Note mild persistent anterior translation of the foot under the tibia.

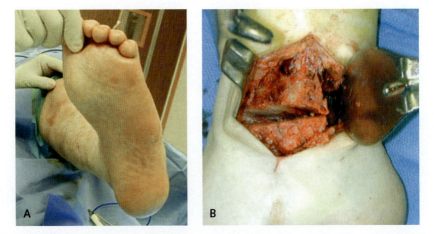

Figure 37-20 A, This severe equinovarus malunion was approached laterally with a osteotomy through the tibia. A fibulectomy had already been performed previously. **B,** A biplanar wedge was removed from the tibia, correcting the varus and the equinus and translating the foot posteriorly.

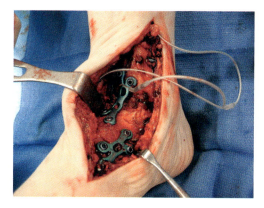

Figure 37-21 Nonunion of an ankle arthrodesis and associated arthritis of the talonavicular joint, treated simultaneously through an extended medial incision. Correction was accomplished with use of a combination of cannulated screws and a plate, and the talonavicular joint was stabilized in a similar fashion by means of a locking compression plate (Orthohelix, Akron, Ohio).

TECHNIQUES, TIPS, AND PITFALLS

- Removal of preexisting hardware before this arthrodesis procedure is unnecessary. Hardware removal will add to the required dissection and periosteal stripping, and screws can be inserted around this fixation. This procedure is much easier when cannulated screws are used, because the guide pins will facilitate the correct passage of the screws.

- Three-point fixation of an ankle arthrodesis is ideal, and the screws should be placed at oblique angles to one another. Use of parallel screws does not control the rotation or torque on the ankle, and fixation by this method has been well demonstrated to be biomechanically inferior.

- As with other arthrodesis procedures, patients should avoid postoperative use of COX-2 nonsteroidal anti-inflammatory medication. These agents have been demonstrated to inhibit bone formation, which can lead to delayed union or nonunion.

- The mini-arthrotomy approach can be applied to revision procedures for correction of nonunion of an ankle arthrodesis or even for cases in which avascular necrosis of the talus is present. In such cases, healing of the arthrodesis will therefore depend on the anterior vascularized portion of the tibia and the neck of the talus.

- I find it useful to completely denude and debride the malleolar gutters and fill this with bone graft. This procedure applies particularly to the fibula and the lateral aspect of the talus in cases of diastasis in which the fibula separates from the tibia as a result of old syndesmosis injuries.

- If ankle deformity is present preoperatively, the mini-arthrotomy approach can still be used, with the addition of bone graft to neutralize the position of the talus under the tibia—for example, when erosion of the distal lateral tibia is present with valgus deformity.

- Correction of cavus foot deformity with the mini-arthrotomy fusion is not difficult. Be careful to position the heel correctly, because the forefoot tends to be brought out of equinus and the hindfoot is put in too much calcaneus. The deltoid ligament may need to be released for correction of severe varus deformity.

- Correction of a valgus deformity begins by realigning the ankle after debridement and inserting a guide pin medially from the medial malleolus into the talus. This procedure locks the medial ankle in the mortise.

- Weight bearing is contraindicated after ankle arthrodesis until fusion is evident on the plain radiograph. Adequacy of bone healing can be difficult to ascertain, because the articular apposition may be excellent early on, when fusion cannot have taken place. I therefore rely on the absence of swelling, induration, and warmth of the ankle to confirm that arthrodesis has been achieved. Use of a walking boot at this stage of healing is not recommended; instead, the foot should be kept in a cast until it is certain that fusion has occurred. I recommend use of a cast with an elevated rubber heel under the axis of the leg.

SUGGESTED READING

Gentchos CE, Bohay DR, Anderson JG: Technique tip: A simple method for ankle arthrodesis using solid screws, *Foot Ankle Int* 30:380–383, 2009.

Glick JM, Morgan CD, Myerson MS, et al: Ankle arthrodesis using an arthroscopic method: Long-term follow-up of 34 cases, *Arthroscopy* 12:428–434, 1996.

Levine SE, Myerson MS, Lucas P, Schon LC: Salvage of pseudoarthrosis after tibiotalar arthrodesis, *Foot Ankle Int* 18:580–585, 1997.

Muir DC, Amendola A, Saltzman CL: Long-term outcome of ankle arthrodesis, *Foot Ankle Clin* 7:703–708, 2002.

Myerson MS, Quill G: Ankle arthrodesis A comparison of an arthroscopic and an open method of treatment, *Clin Orthop* July, 1991, pp 84–95

Neufeld SK, Uribe J, Myerson MS: Use of structural allograft to compensate for bone loss in arthrodesis of the foot and ankle, *Foot Ankle Clin* 7:1–17, 2002.

Paremain GD, Miller SD, Myerson MS: Ankle arthrodesis: Results after the miniarthrotomy technique, *Foot Ankle Int* 17:247–252, 1996.

Paremain GD, Myerson MS: Vascularity of the ankle joint after arthrodesis: A cadaveric study, *Foot* 5:127–131, 1995.

Sealey RJ, Myerson MS, Molloy A, et al: Sagittal plane motion of the hindfoot following ankle arthrodesis: A prospective analysis, *Foot Ankle Int* 30:187–196, 2009.

CHAPTER 38

Tibiotalocalcaneal and Pan-Talar Arthrodesis

OVERVIEW

Whenever possible, it is preferable to perform a tibiotalocalcaneal (TTC) arthrodesis instead of a pan-talar arthrodesis. Including the transverse tarsal joint in the arthrodesis, which results in far more rigidity to the foot, is rarely necessary. When performing a talectomy and a tibiocalcaneal (TC) arthrodesis, I leave the navicular bone free of the anterior aspect of the remnant of the talus. With some deformities, the entire talus must be removed, and the anterior tibia will then abut the navicular. In patients with neuropathy and a Charcot deformity, including the navicular bone in this arthrodesis is tempting, because it will increase the surface area for the arthrodesis. In this manner, after a cheilectomy of the anterior distal tibia and debridement of the navicular, a tibionavicular arthrodesis can be added to the TC arthrodesis. In general, however, I do not consider this additional fusion to be advisable, because the function of the foot, particularly in the setting of a neuropathy, is better without it. Thus the only indications for a pan-talar arthrodesis are to address severe pan-talar arthritis and to correct a deformity of such magnitude that a TTC fusion alone will be inadequate.

The surgical approach for exposure in a pan-talar arthrodesis is almost identical to that for a combined ankle arthrodesis–triple arthrodesis. In fact, I start the procedure with exposure of the ankle joint using the mini-arthrotomy approach with two anterior incisions and then extend these distally once the ankle is completely debrided. The medial incision is extended distally from the ankle to expose the talonavicular joint. Laterally, however, if the incision for the ankle arthrodesis is extended distally, then one incision is placed slightly anterior or dorsal to the calcaneocuboid joint. A fibulectomy should not be performed, if possible. The same rationale applies with a pan-talar arthrodesis as with the ankle arthrodesis: Preservation of the fibula is desirable because the blood supply to the ankle is maintained. Likewise, preservation of the medial malleolus is preferable, although at times, correction of ankle deformity cannot be accomplished without either an osteotomy or a resection of the medial malleolus. An important case in point is that of a TTC arthrodesis with intramedullary (IM) rod fixation, in which slight medial translation of the foot under the tibia is helpful. This translation can be accomplished only if the medial malleolus is removed.

For fixation of the pan-talar arthrodesis, the approach is similar to that outlined for the screw technique used for a TTC arthrodesis. The only difference is that here the fixation of the talonavicular joint can be extended proximally into the tibia with screws started at the inferior pole of the navicular bone, which cross both the talonavicular and the tibiotalar joints into the back of the tibia.

TIBIOCALCANEAL AND TIBIOTALOCALCANEAL ARTHRODESIS

Fixation Alternatives

The fixation options for a TC arthrodesis are screws, a blade plate, and an IM rod. To some extent, the choice of fixation may depend on personal preference, but at times a more stable fixation with either a blade plate or an IM rod is preferable in the setting of significant bone loss and deformity. In my experience, when any erosive changes or avascular necrosis of the ankle is present, screws may not be strong enough, particularly with neuropathic deformity. Historically, a blade plate has been demonstrated to be biomechanically superior to an IM rod in torsion and bending strengths, but this finding was reported with use of an inferior IM rod device; by comparison, the current rod designs include capability for internal and external compression as well as locking mechanisms for the distal screws to create a fixed-angle device similar to the blade plate.

Thus, with the newer designs of the IM nail, rod fixation is preferable to use of a blade plate, provided that sufficient calcaneal bone is present. If the calcaneal bone is of poor quality, the posterior-to-anterior screw can be inserted across the calcaneocuboid joint into the cuboid bone. Postoperative weight-bearing status also may be a consideration. In patients in whom compliance with a non–weight-bearing regimen is in question, I prefer to use an IM rod that can be dynamized if necessary. Although the locking screws may break, a nonunion is not as worrisome in the setting of neuropathic deformity, provided that the foot remains axially aligned under the tibia.

I do sometimes use screws alone for a TTC fusion, but only when the bone quality is good, the alignment of the limb is not significantly abnormal, and focal arthritis is present without bone loss or avascular necrosis (Figures 38-1 to 38-4). I rarely use screws alone when the talus is missing and the overall alignment of the limb is not satisfactory. At present, therefore, for a TTC arthrodesis, I use screws for correction of minimal deformity in ankles with good bone quality and an IM rod in a majority of the remaining cases. A blade plate remains useful when tibia deformity is present, if an IM rod cannot be used or if a simultaneous tibia osteotomy cannot be performed for realignment.

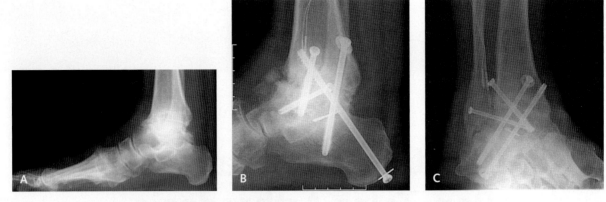

Figure 38-1 An attempt at tibiotalocalcaneal arthrodesis for correction of avascular necrosis of the talus, depicted in **A,** was followed by a nonunion, as shown in **B** and **C.**

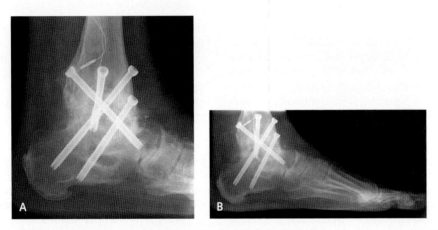

Figure 38-2 The screw pattern used for a tibiotalocalcaneal arthrodesis. **A,** Two screws are inserted in a manner similar to that for an ankle arthrodesis (from posterior tibia into anterior neck of talus, and from medial tibia into body of talus). **B,** Then two screws are inserted from the anterior tibia into the calcaneus.

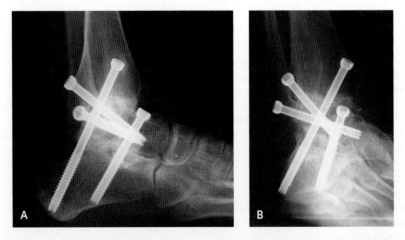

Figure 38-3 A and **B,** Cannulated screws were used to perform this tibiotalocalcaneal arthrodesis. The bone quality was good, alignment was not compromised, and no avascular necrosis was present.

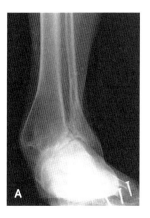 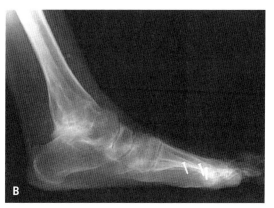 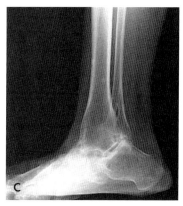

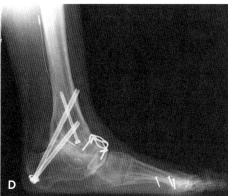 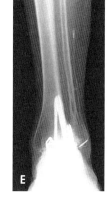

Figure 38-4 Screws and staples were used to convert this severely malunited ankle arthrodesis to a pan-talar arthrodesis. Although the hindfoot is in severe valgus. **A-C,** It was possible to correct the deformity by translating and rotating the calcaneus under the talus. This created a severe supination deformity of the transverse tarsal joint, which was then rotated and secured in position with staples. **D** and **E,** Although the use of staples was successful in this instance, it is not my preference for fixation; I would recommend insertion of one screw across the talonavicular joint supplemented by a small locking plate.

Surgical Approaches

A lateral transfibular approach to the ankle and hindfoot can be used for correction of severe deformity. Although this distal fibulectomy will devascularize the lateral ankle, an alternative often is unavailable for correction of severe deformity, particularly when the ankle is angulated and in varus and the fibula is prominent. The incision is made vertically, directly over the fibula, extending down distally over the sinus tarsi toward the inferior aspect of the calcaneus. The sural nerve must be identified and then retracted inferiorly with the peroneal tendons. A fibulectomy is performed with an acetabular reamer, which is used to completely denude and decorticate the fibula. The reamings that are obtained are preserved for later use as bone graft material (Figure 38-5).

If a blade plate is to be used for fixation, the distal 8 cm of the fibula must be removed, and following use of the reamer, the fibula is cut with a saw. I prefer to use a chisel and not a saw to denude the ankle and subtalar joints. If severe deformity is present, however, then the distal tibia may have to be cut at the plafond with a saw. Often the foot cannot be centered under the ankle because the medial malleolus blocks the shift of the talus. In such instances, the malleolus is removed with an oblique osteotomy made through a separate medial incision. The dissection in the sinus tarsi and subtalar joint is performed in the same manner as that described for a subtalar arthrodesis.

When a talectomy plus a TC arthrodesis is performed for avascular necrosis, the necrotic remnants of the talus are completely excised. A sizable defect remains; either it can be filled with bone graft or the talus can be apposed directly onto the calcaneus (Figure 38-6). Usually, despite the contouring of the posterior aspect of the calcaneus and the undersurface of the distal tibia, joint apposition cannot be easily obtained. It is difficult to appose the calcaneus flush up against the tibia, because the hindfoot tilts up into dorsiflexion,

leaving the hindfoot in a calcaneus position. A defect of variable size, depending on bone erosion, is always present between the undersurface of the tibia and the dorsal surface of the posterior facet; the shape of the defect may range from a trapezoid to a large triangle (Figure 38-7). At times, if the apposition between the tibia and the calcaneus is very good and the defect is not too large, it can be filled with cancellous graft only. Some bone graft is needed in the more anterior aspect of the arthrodesis to fill the defect properly. Here either cancellous graft or a tricortical structural allograft can be used; the choice will depend on the availability of large structural graft and the size of the defect. It is clearly easier to secure the posterior tibia to the dorsal calcaneus and then fill the defect with cancellous graft. Over the past several years, with the increased use of orthobiologic adjuvants, the latter has been my preferred technique (Figure 38-8). I use a structural graft when the height of the limb must be restored. In some circumstances, this structural graft has to be used between the tibia and the calcaneus. Of note, in performing a talectomy and TC arthrodesis, as the heel is pushed up against the tibia, the skin on either side of the ankle gets compressed, and closure can no longer be achieved without tension on the skin (the so-called accordion effect—as the structure is elongated, it narrows, and as it is compressed, it widens).

It is not easy to insert the structural graft and obtain compression as well as stability between the tibia and calcaneus. One method that works well is to align the calcaneus under the tibia and then secure this position with guide pins. With the foot now quite stable, it is forced into plantar flexion while the pins are in place. With the foot plantar flexed, the TC gap opens and the graft is inserted and tamped into place securely. The foot is now maximally dorsiflexed, and the bone graft is compressed between the calcaneus and the tibia, followed by definitive fixation.

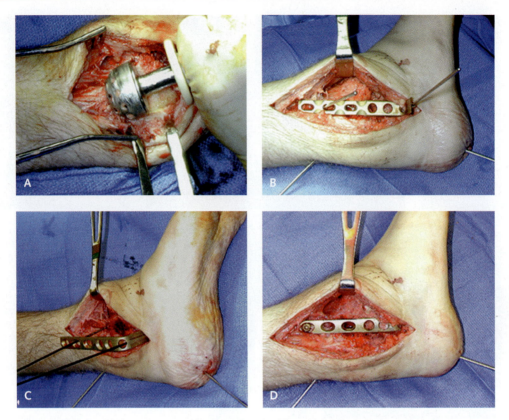

Figure 38-5 A, The acetabular reamer is used to decorticate and harvest the fibula for bone graft. **B,** Temporary guide pin fixation is used to maintain limb alignment, and the cannulated blade is applied with the flat plate surface apposed to the side of the ankle. **C,** Guide pins are inserted through the distal cannula and one of the screw holes. **D,** The plate is reversed and positioned over the preinserted guide pins and then tamped firmly into place.

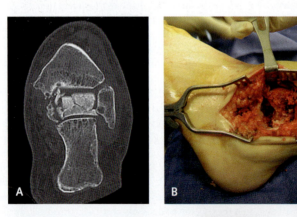

Figure 38-6 A, Avascular necrosis involving the entire talar body. **B,** Intra-operatively, a decision had to be made regarding use of a large structural bone graft versus the fusion of the tibia and the calcaneus, supplemented by cancellous graft. **C,** The latter technique was selected because the leg length discrepancy did not appear to be a significant concern for the patient.

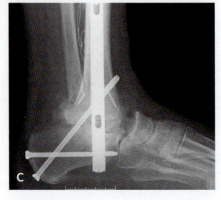

38

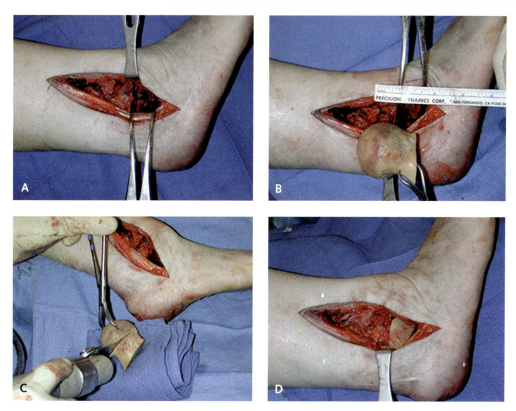

Figure 38-7 The steps in planning a tibiocalcaneal arthrodesis with interposition structural graft for a patient with avascular collapse of the talus. **A,** Note the laminar spreader in place that measures the size of the defect. **B** and **C,** The femoral head allograft was cut with a large saw into a trapezoid shape to fit the alignment of the calcaneus and the distal tibia. **D,** With dorsiflexion of the foot, the graft is well compressed.

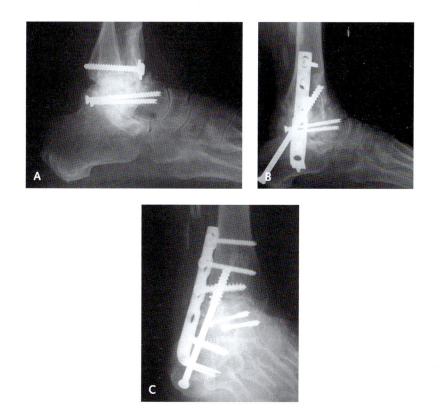

Figure 38-8 A, Avascular necrosis of the talus with collapse of the body only. **B** and **C,** A blade plate was used for arthrodesis. Note the use of an additional screw inserted from the calcaneus into the distal tibia, which is at times necessary to control rotation of the ankle.

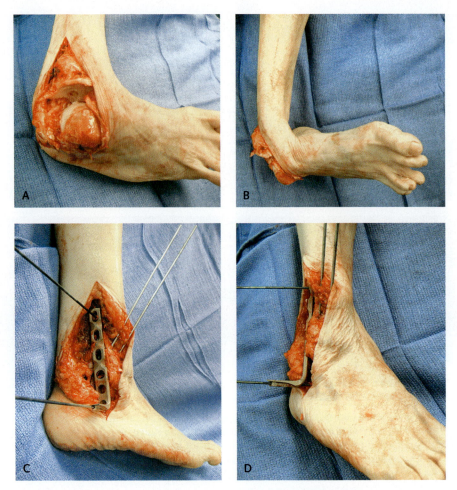

Figure 38-9 A and **B,** Neuromuscular equinovarus deformity. **C** and **D,** Stabilization was achieved with a blade plate inserted from slightly more posterior and lateral and directed anteriorly to gain maximum purchase in the calcaneus. The plate does not lie flat on the calcaneus when inserted in this manner, and the calcaneus must be notched to accept the contour of the plate.

Fixation Technique

Blade Plate Fixation

I first align and stabilize the hindfoot using percutaneous guide pins. The first guide pin is introduced from the plantar aspect of the heel into the anterior distal tibia, and the second pin is introduced from the posterior inferior tibia into the anterior midfoot. The alignment of the blade plate is now secured by placing it laterally against the calcaneus and the tibia. Guide pins are introduced through the cannulated holes or through the screw holes while the plate is in a reversed position, flush with the bone. The plate must be flush with the lateral aspect of the calcaneus and the distal tibia, which may have to be shaved or abraded with a saw for optimal apposition with the blade plate. The plate may have to be rotated or angulated to achieve maximum purchase in the calcaneus. If the blade enters the calcaneus perpendicular to its axis, then the blade must be under the subchondral plate of the posterior facet. Alternatively, the blade can be angled into the calcaneus from a more posterior-lateral position directed anteromedially into the sustentaculum tali. The plate is removed and reversed onto the guide pins and then is tamped securely into place using a large mallet. Care is taken to ensure that the blade enters the calcaneus in a smooth plane. Placing a small instrument under the plate is helpful to prevent its angulation while banging on the blade with the tamp. Once the plate is 1 cm from the bone, a tamp is used over the distal screw hole. Apposition of the

plate against the calcaneus and the tibia should be good. In addition to the screws through the plate, I may use supplemental cannulated screws for fixation from the inferior aspect of the calcaneus into the distal tibia or the distal tibia posteriorly into the navicular bone anteromedially (Figures 38-9 and 38-10).

Intramedullary Rod Fixation

The key to IM fixation is correct alignment of the foot under the tibia. Because the calcaneus is slightly lateral to the longitudinal axis of the tibia, insertion of the rod through the center of the calcaneus and in the center of the tibia at the same time is not physically possible. If a more medial position of the foot is perceived to be necessary, then the medial malleolus needs to undergo osteotomy, and the talus (if present) needs to be moved medially with the calcaneus. In this manner, a more vertical access to the tibia is possible.

Unique capabilities of the Biomet IM rod system include external and internal compression, control of rotation with posterior-to-anterior screws as well as lateral-to-medial screws in the talus and calcaneus, conversion of the rod to a fixed-angle device with an internal locking mechanism, and the option of inserting screws tangentially from the calcaneus into the tibia through an external guide system, thereby ensuring that the screws are not in the path of the rod. An additional option is to use a 10-mm dynamic compression slot in addition to a static screw for the proximal tibial fixation.

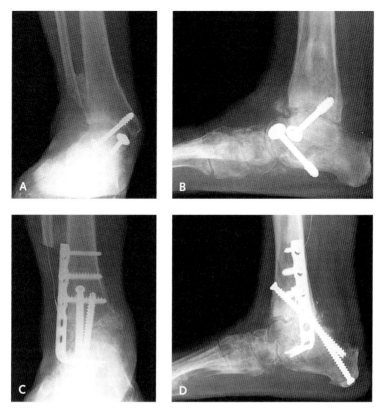

Figure 38-10 A and **B,** A tibiotalocalcaneal arthrodesis had been attempted to treat a flatfoot deformity, resulting in a nonunion and malunion of both joints. **C** and **D,** Two screws inserted in this manner do not provide ideal fixation. The repair was accomplished using a blade plate. **C** and **D,** Note that after compression with the blade plate, two fully threaded screws were used to supplement fixation, because further compression was not thought to be necessary.

One potential problem with all IM rod systems is that the trajectory of the posterior-to-anterior screw from the calcaneus through the rod cannot be anticipated. If the rod is, for example, externally rotated during insertion, the screws may appear radiographically to be in the calcaneus when in fact they are protruding medially into the soft tissue. Careful preoperative imaging is therefore essential, because the lateral radiograph usually obtained in such instances typically does not show the actual location of the posterior-to-anterior screw. The Biomet rod system has an alignment guide that can be attached to the targeting arm to indicate the exact location and trajectory of the posterior-to-anterior screw. Use of this radiolucent guide will ensure that the screw location and trajectory are correct *before* insertion of the proximal screws in the tibia, at which time no further control over rotation and location of the posterior-to-anterior calcaneal screw is possible. In the procedure illustrated in Figure 38-11, use of the Biomet Phoenix nail guide permitted accurate rotation of the nail to achieve correct alignment.

Each situation has to be monitored in accordance with the anatomy and the deformity. In placing the posterior-to-anterior screw, the orientation of the rod must be monitored, because the screw must enter the calcaneal tuberosity and not exit the soft tissues medially. If the rod is inserted medial to the calcaneus, it will not be possible to insert the posterior-to-anterior screw into the distal neck of the calcaneus unless the screw enters from posteromedial and is directed anterolaterally. Accordingly, an effort should be made to ensure that the rod is indeed in as much of the calcaneus

as possible, whether the locking screws are from lateral or from posterior-to-anterior inserted through the calcaneus.

The same principles apply with incision and exposure as with blade plate fixation. Once adequate debridement and alignment have been obtained, the IM guide pin is selected. A 2-cm incision is made on the plantar aspect of the hindfoot immediately anterior and slightly medial to the heel pad. Because the guide pin is close to the lateral plantar nerve, dissection with a clamp to the bone is useful. The plantar incision is made anterior to the fat pad slightly lateral to the midline, especially in the patient with significant preoperative valgus deformity.

Blunt dissection is carried down to the plantar fascia, which is split longitudinally. The intrinsic muscles are not visible but can be moved aside with a large clamp medially or laterally. The ideal position for the plantar calcaneal entry site is well anterior to the weight-bearing surface of the calcaneal tuberosity and approximately 2 cm posterior to the articulation of the calcaneus with the cuboid.

The guide pin is inserted through the inferomedial calcaneus through the talus (if present) and into the tibia; its position is then checked fluoroscopically. Before proceeding with the reaming, I use a large cannulated drill bit passed over the IM guide pin, followed by the reamers either the same diameter or 1 mm larger than the diameter of the rod selected. Generally, I select a rod 12 mm in diameter and 21 cm in length. The rod is now inserted and gradually tamped into place using the external alignment guide, and the inferior portion of the guide is used to gently tamp the rod into

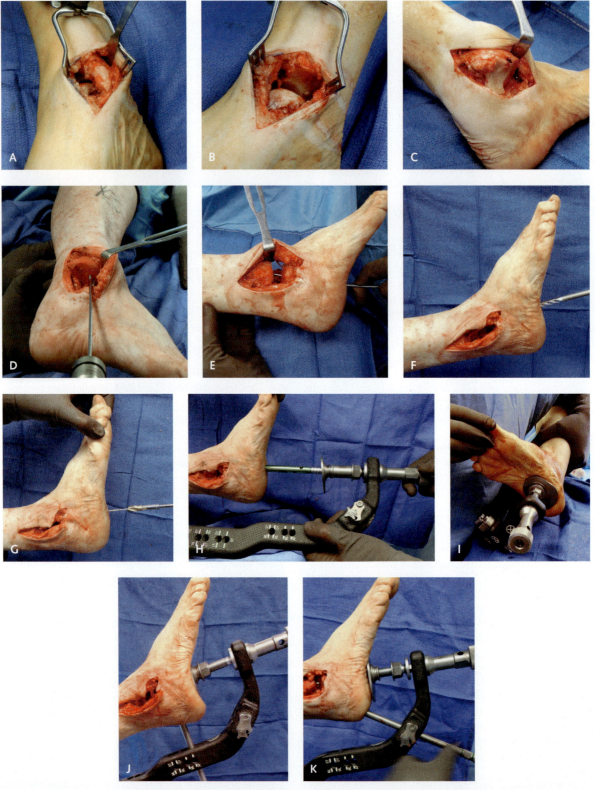

Figure 38-11 The surgical steps for a tibiotalocalcaneal arthrodesis with intramedullary rod fixation. **A** and **B,** Through a lateral transfibular incision, the medial malleolus is exposed and an osteotomy with removal of the malleolus is performed. **C,** The ankle is dislocated medially, and the tibial joint surface is cut perpendicular to the tibia with a saw. **D,** A drill guide is inserted directly into the tibia. **E** and **F,** A guide pin is inserted through the talus out the plantar foot, followed by repeated perforation of the talus with an 8-mm cannulated drill bit, which makes it easier to insert the guide from the plantar foot surface. **G** and **H,** Reaming commences, followed by insertion of the rod attached to the external alignment guide. **I,** Once rotation is set, the tibia screws are inserted, and external compression is applied through the heel plate. **J,** The posterior-to-anterior screw is inserted through the calcaneus. **K,** Once the calcaneal screws are in place, the oblique paramedian screws are inserted through the jig to complete the fixation.

position. The position of the rod must be checked fluoroscopically each step of the way to ensure correct positioning on the plantar surface of the heel. The proximal end of the nail should extend at least 4 cm above any potential cortical stress risers, such as from a tibial nonunion or fracture, an old osteotomy site, or cortical holes remaining after previous hardware removal. I try to countersink the nail approximately 10 mm in the plantar cortex of the calcaneus, to allow for the compression that will be subsequently required. The nail can of course be countersunk further, if warranted, such as with the anticipated requirement for a significant amount of compression.

The Biomet TTC nail provides internal compression of the fusion with 7.0 mm of inboard tibiotalar compression. Use of this system requires that a transverse screw be inserted across the talus from lateral to medial. The feasibility of transverse screw insertion depends on the amount of talus that is present and on the location of the transverse screw hole relative to the talus. Once the 5.0-mm screw is inserted through the talus, the internal compression system can be activated with a screwdriver inserted through the rod. The external compression device is a large pad attached to the rod, which fits well on the heel pad to safely accomplish compression across the subtalar and ankle joints. The distal end of the nail must obviously be countersunk in the calcaneal plantar surface to the desired amount of compression. Careful control of the amount of external compression, is essential to avoid leaving the distal end of the of the nail prominent. Once the calcaneal screws are finally locked, I insert additional oblique screws from the calcaneus into the tibia, as required. The unique design of the targeting arm allows an oblique screw to be inserted along the side of the nail but always missing the nail itself.

At my institution, the IM nail has been used successfully for management of massive defects of the distal tibia and talus, as, for example, after failed total ankle replacement. IM nailing requires a large structural allograft, frequently consisting of an entire femoral head. To enhance the rate of incorporation of the graft into the fusion, an iliac crest concentrate is injected into the femoral head after it has been well perforated with a 2-mm drill bit. For accurate insertion of the femoral head graft, the distal tibia and the calcaneus are prepared using an acetabular reamer. This instrument creates a more spherical defect, which is easier to fill with the structural graft when a femoral head is used for this purpose (Figure 38-12).

PAN-TALAR ARTHRODESIS

For the most part, the procedure for pan-talar arthrodesis involves an extension of the principles as well as the technique for a combined ankle-triple arthrodesis. The same can be said for a TTC arthrodesis to which a correction of the transverse tarsal joint is added. Ideally, I prefer to use the same incisions as for an ankle arthrodesis and then extend them down over the talonavicular joint medially and the subtalar and calcaneocuboid joints laterally. These incisions can, of course, be modified according to the presence of deformity, but, by and large, this approach as outlined is the one that I prefer to use. Occasionally, when the deformity is significant, a fibulectomy is performed through an extended lateral incision. Rarely, when the hindfoot exhibits severe varus deformity, the head of the talus is pointing laterally and barely articulating with the navicular bone. In such instances, a single lateral incision can be used to perform the arthrodesis. The head of the talus is visible in the sinus tarsi, and most of the talonavicular joint preparation and debridement can be performed from the lateral incision. At times, the posterior tibial tendon needs to be cut from its attachment to the navicular for correction, and this cutting can be done percutaneously. For practical purposes, however, the approach to the pantalar arthrodesis should include two incisions for maximal exposure and joint preparation (Figures 38-17 and 38-18).

TECHNIQUES, TIPS, AND PITFALLS

- Bone graft of some type is necessary to fill defects of any is present, particularly those associated with avascular necrosis. A decision has to be made whether to use cancellous or structural bone graft (Figures 38-13 and 38-14).

- A useful technique is to predrill the tibia before the guide pin is inserted from the heel. Predrilling makes insertion of the guide pin far easier but can be done only when the ankle can be dislocated to expose the joint (Figure 38-15).

- A locking plate is an alternative means of fixation for a TTC arthrodesis. Use of a locking plate is a good choice with multiplanar deformity (Figure 38-16).

- A fracture of the distal tibia can occur above a blade plate, a rod, or screws. A stress riser will be present at the tip of the hardware, and the chance of a fracture can be minimized with use of a longer rod.

- The lateral plantar nerve may be injured with the IM fixation. The potential for injury has been demonstrated anatomically. Nonetheless, even with the proximity of the rod to the nerve, I have rarely seen the nerve injured.

- Internal and external rotation of the foot and of the leg can become a problem with use of the IM rod system. This is purely a visual problem with the alignment of the foot relative to the leg and can be minimized with correct patient positioning for surgery; the supine position is preferable to the lateral decubitus position in this respect.

- If tension is present on the skin margins during closure, the skin flap has to be modified. Tension may occur because of compression across the ankle with an accordion or "concertina" effect on the skin. In addition to modification of the skin closure, the peroneal tendons can be transected and both tendons removed to facilitate wound closure.

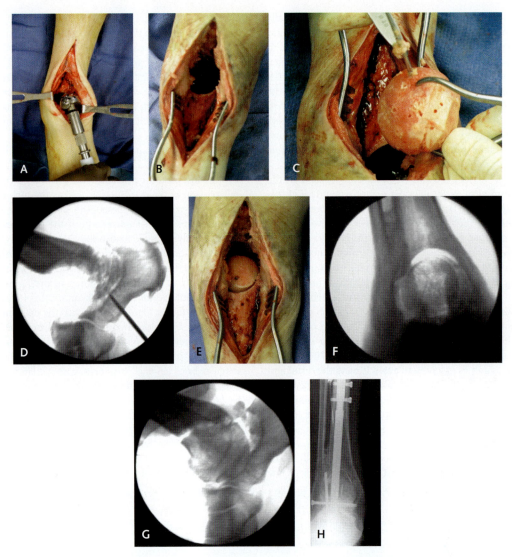

Figure 38-12 The technique for preparation of the joint for a large structural allograft. **A** and **B,** Preparation of the joint with an acetabular reamer. **C,** The femoral head graft is prepared with another reamer to match the contour of the defect. Before its insertion, the graft is perforated with a 2-mm drill bit and then injected with a concentrate of an iliac crest aspirate. **D,** The guide pin is inserted under fluoroscopic control, before insertion of the graft. **E-H,** The graft is inserted. Note the final radiograph at 4 months with good healing and good placement of the intramedullary rod.

38

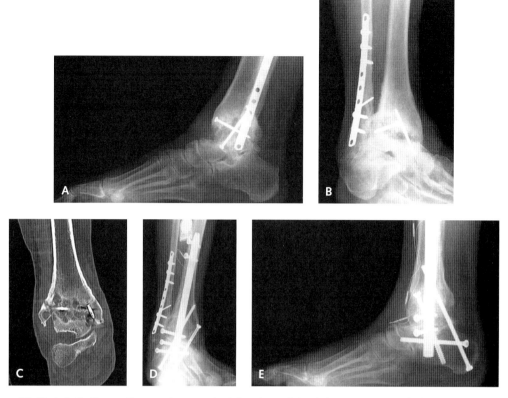

Figure 38-13 A-C, Posttraumatic avascular necrosis of the talus and distal tibia in a patient with diabetes and severe neuropathy. **D** and **E,** Treatment consisted of a tibiotalocalcaneal arthrodesis with structural bone grafting including an iliac aspirate concentrate and placement of an implantable bone stimulator.

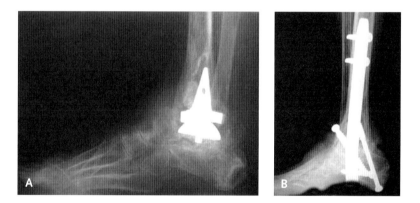

Figure 38-14 The patient presented with marked collapse of the entire talus after a total ankle replacement performed approximately 25 years previously. **A** and **B,** The tibiotalocalcaneal arthrodesis was performed with removal of the prosthesis, and cancellous bone grafting was followed by insertion of an intramedullary rod.

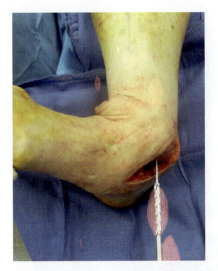

Figure 38-15 A useful technique is to predrill the tibia before the guide pin is inserted from the heel. Predrilling makes insertion of the guide pin far easier but can be used only when the ankle can be dislocated to expose the joint.

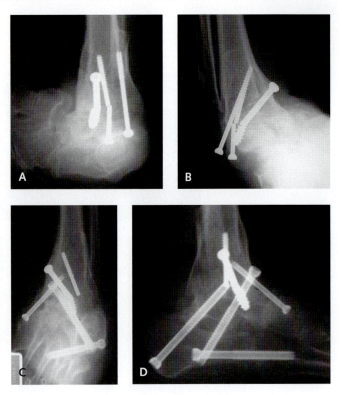

Figure 38-17 **A** and **B,** A severe equinovarus deformity that developed after attempted ankle arthrodesis in a patient with Charcot-Marie-Tooth disease. Although the ankle was fused, the foot position was not corrected. and subluxation of the transverse tarsal joint was present. **C** and **D,** A pan-talar arthrodesis was not sufficient for correction; muscle balance with appropriate tendon transfer was performed to create a plantigrade foot.

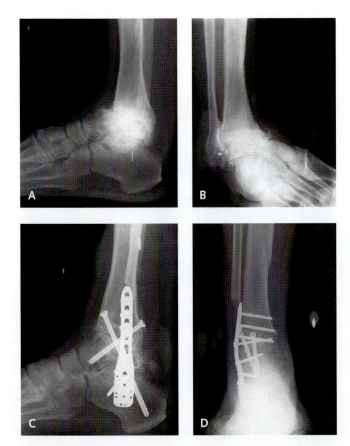

Figure 38-16 **A** and **B,** Marked varus deformity associated with avascular necrosis of the talus in a patient with Charcot-Marie-Tooth disease. **C** and **D,** Treatment was with a tibiotalocalcaneal arthrodesis with use of a locking plate supplemented by crossed screw fixation.

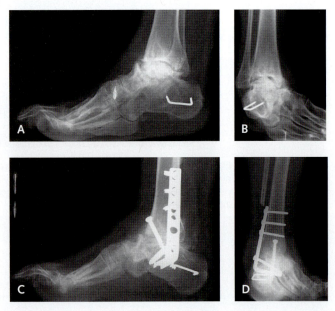

Figure 38-18 **A** and **B,** A previously attempted triple arthrodesis in a patient with Charcot-Marie-Tooth disease was not at all successful, and equinovarus deformity persisted, complicated by avascular necrosis of the talus associated with neuropathy. **C** and **D,** A pan-talar arthrodesis was performed using a blade plate for fixation. Resection of the fifth metatarsal was necessary to establish a plantigrade foot.

SUGGESTED READING

Ahmad J, Pour AE, Raikin SM: The modified use of a proximal humeral locking plate for tibiotalocalcaneal arthrodesis, *Foot Ankle Int* 28:977–983, 2007.

Levine SE, Myerson MS, Lucas P, Schon LC: Salvage of pseudoarthrosis after tibiotalar arthrodesis, *Foot Ankle Int* 18:580–585, 1997.

Myerson MS, Alvarez RG, Lam PW: Tibiocalcaneal arthrodesis for the management of severe ankle and hindfoot deformities, *Foot Ankle Int* 21:643–650, 2000.

Niinimäki TT, Klemola TM, Leppilahti JI: Tibiotalocalcaneal arthrodesis with a compressive retrograde intramedullary nail: A report of 34 consecutive patients, *Foot Ankle Int* 28:431–434, 2007.

Noonan T, Pinzur M, Paxinos O, et al: Tibiotalocalcaneal arthrodesis with a retrograde intramedullary nail: A biomechanical analysis of the effect of nail length, *Foot Ankle Int* 26:304–308, 2005.

Papa JA, Myerson MS: Pantalar and tibiotalocalcaneal arthrodesis for post-traumatic osteoarthrosis of the ankle and hindfoot, *J Bone Joint Surg Am* 74:1042–1049, 1992.

Papa J, Myerson M, Girard P: Salvage, with arthrodesis, in intractable diabetic neuropathic arthropathy of the foot and ankle, *J Bone Joint Surg Am* 75:1056–1066, 1993.

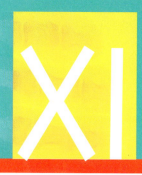

CHAPTER **39**

The Rheumatoid Foot and Ankle

FOREFOOT RECONSTRUCTION

The standard technique for correction of rheumatoid forefoot deformity has involved resection of the metatarsal heads with realignment of the lesser toe deformities and arthrodesis of the hallux metatarsophalangeal (MP) joint. Over the years, in my experience, this has been the most reliable procedure for correction of deformity, particularly that associated with erosive changes of the MP joint with destruction of bone, especially in the metatarsal head.

Modifications of the procedure may include resection of the lesser metatarsal heads with resection arthroplasty of the hallux MP joint (as an alternative to arthrodesis). This resection-based approach is certainly an option, although it does not appear to give as stable a result as that achieved with arthrodesis. Nevertheless, the resection arthroplasty can be considered in the presence of arthritis of both the MP and the interphalangeal (IP) joints of the hallux. If the arthritis is associated with deformity of both joints, then one alternative is to perform an arthrodesis of the IP joint in conjunction with a resection arthroplasty of the MP joint. I am, however, opposed to performing a resection arthroplasty of the hallux in the patient with rheumatoid arthritis and hallux valgus, because soft tissue laxity associated with erosive changes and ligamentous instability will lead to a recurrence of deformity. Some patients with these gross deformities are not symptomatic, and their function is acceptable. Which is preferred—form or function? Certainly, if function follows form, then the resection arthroplasty of the hallux (the Keller procedure) is not an ideal procedure, because the hallux is weak and unstable and the incidence of recurrent deformity is high.

Other options for correction of the deformity at the MP joint of the lesser toes include synovectomy and shortening osteotomies of the metatarsal head or shaft. Synovectomy is certainly an option to consider in the presence of severe synovitis associated with minimal joint deformity and the absence of metatarsalgia. Once subluxation or dislocation of the MP joints occurs, however, synovectomy is not of any benefit.

The concept of joint preservation of the MP joint is an important one in patients with inflammatory joint disease. The synovitis surprisingly decreases with mechanical off-loading of the MP joint as a result of the shortening osteotomy. Although the lesser metataral osteotomy is a reasonable procedure to be performed in a patient with rheumatoid arthritis, it is not easily accomplished because of the paucity of good bone around the metatarsal head, the erosive changes typically associated with joint subluxation and dislocation, and the difficulty of performing this operation while maintaining a salvageable joint. Nonetheless, in patients who have involvement of one or two joints without severe erosion, shortening osteotomy is an option. This procedure is indicated especially when one or two of the lesser MP joints are involved, and resection of all of the metatarsal heads is inadvisable for some reason (Figure 39-1).

Many intermediate stages of deformity of the rheumatoid forefoot exist in which arthrodesis of the MP joint may not be considered necessary. A good example is the presence of hallux valgus in an otherwise healthy joint. In this instance, a standard operation for correction of hallux valgus (e.g., bunionectomy and metatarsal osteotomy) may not be as successful as, for example, a tarsometatarsal arthrodesis (the modified Lapidus procedure) (Figure 39-2). If hallux valgus is not present initially and metatarsal head resections are performed, then the hallux deformity will always increase as a result of shortening of the lesser toes in the absence of a lateral buttress to the hallux. Preservation of the hallux MP joint is even more relevant if joint preservation osteotomy procedures of the lesser metatarsal heads are performed.

INCISIONS AND DISSECTION

The choice of incisions used for the metatarsal head resections or the metatarsal head osteotomies is determined by the magnitude of deformity. In general, I prefer two dorsal longitudinal incisions made in the second and fourth web spaces (Figure 39-3). The improved access with these incisions, however, must be balanced against the possibility of wound dehiscence and associated problems with skin

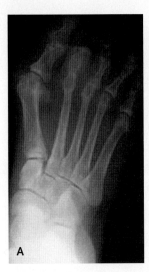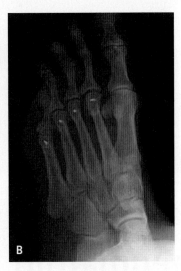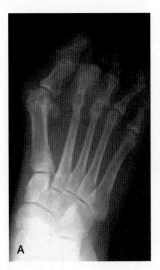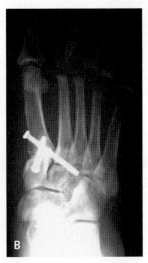

Figure 39-1 A and **B,** The patient was an ideal candidate for lesser metatarsophalangeal (MP) joint preservation, particularly because the hallux MP joint is relatively normal, although the interphalangeal joint is affected.

Figure 39-2 A, The patient had erosive disease of the lesser metatarsophalangeal (MP) joints but no involvement of the hallux MP joint. Arthritis of the hallux interphalangeal (IP) joint was present, and avoiding arthrodesis of the MP joint if the IP joint is already deformed is preferable. **B,** Although shortening osteotomies of the lesser metatarsals constituted an option, resection of the heads in conjunction with a Lapidus procedure was performed.

healing in this region. The option of a dorsal transverse incision is available, but not if dislocation of the MP joints is present with shortening and contracture of the soft tissues. Although the transverse incision is easier to perform and can be done with far less retraction than with two longitudinal incisions, the surgeon must be certain that sufficient bone has been resected to facilitate soft tissue closure. The other option is a plantar surface–based elliptical incision. Although I have used this incision on occasion, it is associated with problems with management of the contracted dorsal soft tissues, including the extensor tendons and capsule. I see no advantage to use of a plantar surface–based incision other than the proximity of the metatarsal heads. The hypertrophied soft tissue, callus, or bursae are always resorbed once the metatarsal heads have been resected, and the excision of an ellipse of tissue on the plantar surface does not seem warranted (Figures 39-4 and 39-5).

As noted, I generally use two dorsal longitudinal incisions made in the second and the fourth web spaces, with as wide a skin bridge as possible between them. The metatarsals are resected first, followed by the MP fusion. With this sequence, inadvertent manipulation of the hallux MP joint is avoided. Both incisions should be as long as possible and extend from the cleft of the web space proximally for approximately 4 cm. Care must be taken not to overretract the tissue, to prevent bruising and ecchymosis of the tissue during the dissection. When one side of the skin is retracted, the other is relaxed. I find it easier to start with the more lateral fourth web space incision, because the fifth metatarsal is always the easiest to remove. In each case, the extensor tendons of the toes are transected 2 cm proximal to the metatarsal neck and then clamped and pulled distally. This maneuver facilitates the exposure of the MP joint through retraction of the tendon all the way up to the dislocated joint.

The dissection is deepened, and a capsulectomy is performed until the MP joint is identified. This joint is not always easy to identify if it is dislocated, but this must be reduced before the osteotomy of the neck is performed. I use a curved periosteal elevator inserted over the dorsal surface of the MP joint; then, with plantar surface–directed pressure, the remnant of the metatarsal head is delivered into the dorsal surface of the wound. The proximal phalanx is depressed underneath the metatarsal head for further exposure. A problem encountered in this setting is the presence of soft

bone, which causes crushing of the metatarsal head when retracted with the elevator. The soft bone does not create a problem with the resection of the head, but remnants of the metatarsal head must be sought after it is removed. This problem also may arise at the base of the proximal phalanx, which can be fractured; retrieval of the bone fragments may be difficult here as well. I do not resect the base of the proximal phalanx, even with severe dislocation. This resection unnecessarily shortens the toe and adds to dorsal instability.

The metatarsal neck is cut with a saw at the level of the flare between the metaphysis and the diaphysis of the metatarsal. Use of an osteotome will fracture the metatarsal in an irregular manner, creating irregular bone spikes, and is therefore not recommended. The cut is made obliquely in a slightly plantar direction, to avoid creating any plantar spike, which will lead to metatarsalgia. I use a clamp or towel clip to hold, rotate, and then pull out the head, while cutting the collateral ligaments, and remnant of the plantar plate.

What should be done with the extensor tendons? As a matter of expedience, these can be simply left cut or repaired. Neither of these choices is my preference, however, because my aim here is to prevent the development of any dorsiflexion contracture postoperatively. I therefore perform a plantar tenodesis of the extensor tendons. Each extensor tendon is grasped with a hemostat and then passed underneath the metatarsal neck. A Kirschner wire (K-wire) is then passed in antegrade and then retrograde fashion across the MP joint and through the tendons into the metatarsal itself. This wire holds the extensor tendons under the metatarsal neck, and the tenodesis effect prevents dorsal extension contracture. The K-wires are never stable enough in osteopenic bone. Stability can be maximized, however, with insertion of the K-wire as proximal as possible into the cuneiforms or cuboid bone. Wound closure is performed with nylon sutures in the skin only, because the subcutaneous tissue is rarely thick enough to hold a suture. No tension at all should exist on the skin incisions.

The correction of the claw toe deformities often has been described as unnecessary. Of note, however, if the toes are left deformed at the proximal IP joint, MP joint deformity tends to

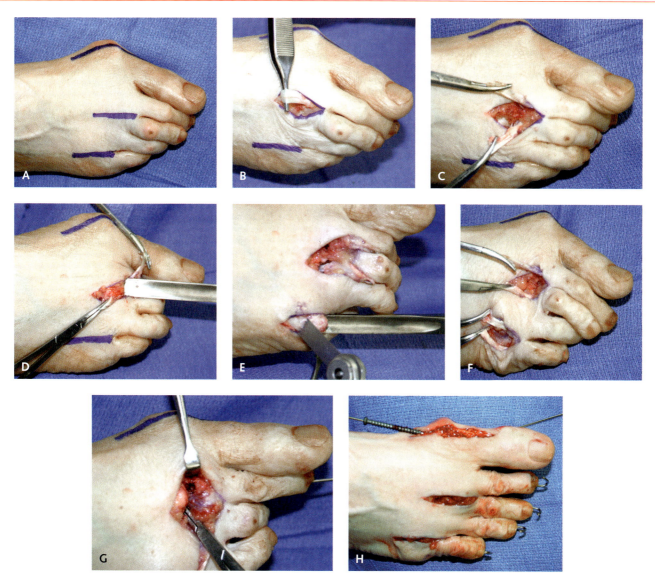

Figure 39-3 The forefoot reconstruction with arthrodesis of the hallux metatarsophalangeal (MP) joint and resection of the lesser metatarsal. **A,** The incisions are marked out as widely spaced as possible. **B** and **C,** The extensor tendons to the second toe are cut transversely and retracted. **D,** A curved periosteal elevator is inserted under the metatarsal head to expose the neck. **E,** Note the slightly oblique plane of resection of the fifth metatarsal. **F,** After resection of all of the metatarsal heads, the extensor tendons are clamped. **G,** The extensor tendon is then passed under the metatarsal neck, and a K-wire is passed through the extensor tendon into the metatarsal shaft. **H,** The arthrodesis of the MP joint is performed with cannulated 4-mm screws.

recur later as well. These contractures should be addressed with either manual manipulation of the joint or resection arthroplasty. Although a formal arthroplasty is my preferred procedure (Figure 39-6), manual manipulation of the joint occasionally will be successful in other than rigid contractures.

I prefer to leave the K-wires in for 6 weeks to gain as much stability as possible at the posterior interphalangeal (PIP) and MP joints. The K-wires are inserted as far posteriorly as possible, even into the cuneiforms, to prevent early loosening.

MANAGEMENT OF COMPLICATIONS OF TREATMENT

Management after failure of previous surgery is difficult, particularly when the toe deformities have worsened. Incorrectly performed metatarsal head resection is one of the more commonly encountered problems. The only alternative in such cases is to resect more bone and shorten the metatarsal(s) further (Figure 39-7). Generally, this outcome could have been avoided with the initial procedure, when one metatarsal typically was left significantly longer than another. More common than one long metatarsal is bone overgrowth on the tips of each metatarsal (Figure 39-8). Over the years I have tried numerous methods of bone resection to minimize this heterotopic bone formation, including the use of bone wax, cutting the bone with a bone cutter or a saw, and inserting the capsule into the joint. None of these seems to have made any difference in the outcome of the metatarsal head resection, because the overall rate of recurrence of metatarsalgia is approximately 10%.

More difficult to treat than the metatarsalgia is recurrent toe deformity (Figure 39-9). To some extent this is the result of excessive bone resection with the initial surgery; at times such deformity reflects inadequate correction of the lesser toe to begin with.

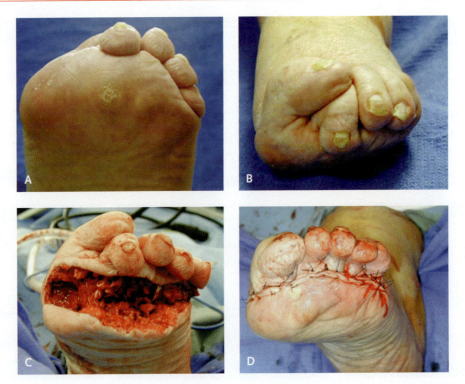

Figure 39-4 A and **B,** Approaching the metatarsal head resection from the plantar surface may be preferable in an elderly patient with severe deformity and potential ischemia. **C** and **D,** Although not conducive to a "cosmetic" reconstruction, removal of all of the metatarsal heads, including the first, was accomplished through the plantar incision, followed by resection of an ellipse of tissue.

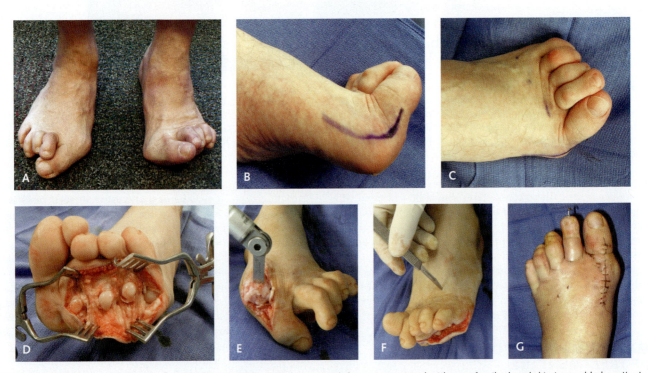

Figure 39-5 A-C, A plantar approach to metatarsal head resection for severe deformity associated with very fragile dorsal skin in an elderly patients. **D,** All of the metatarsal heads were exposed through an elliptical plantar incision. Resection of the heads was accomplished with a saw cut. **E,** The first metatarsal head was removed through a separate medial incision. **F,** Percutaneous extensor tenotomies were performed to further release the metatarsophalangeal joint contracture. **G,** Immediate postoperative appearance of the foot.

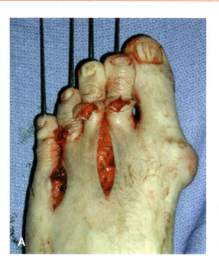 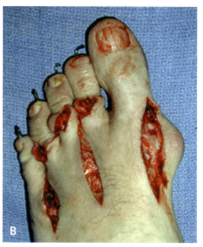

Figure 39-6 A, Correction of the lesser toe deformities was accomplished with a resection arthroplasty of the interphalangeal joints and K-wire fixation across the metatarsophalangeal (MP) joint. **B,** Appearance of the forefoot after pinning of the toes and the MP fusion.

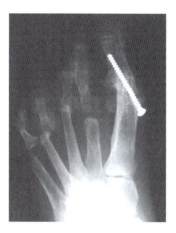

Figure 39-7 The alignment of the metatarsals is poor, and the original resection of the metatarsal heads was not performed correctly. Excessive bone was resected from the second metatarsal, and the forefoot parabola was not established, leading to recurrent metatarsalgia.

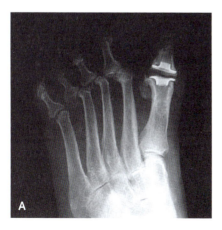 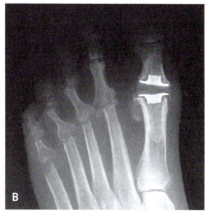

Figure 39-8 A, Recurrence of metatarsalgia was due in part to inadequate reduction of the joints. **B,** Bone overgrowth is not uncommon in such cases and is treated with revision of the metatarsal head resection.

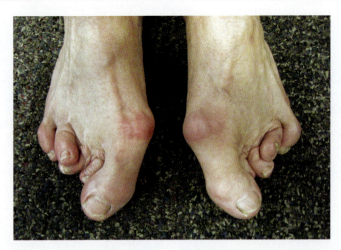

Figure 39-9 Recurrent deformity of the toes is very difficult to treat. In the feet shown here, although functional improvement can be achieved with an arthrodesis of the hallux metatarsophalangeal joint, the toes will remain deformed. Amputation is an option in such cases.

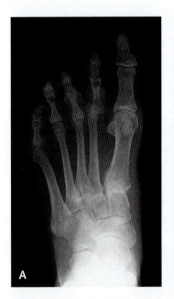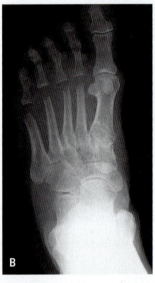

Figure 39-10 A, The hallux metatarsophalangeal joint was asymptomatic and well aligned. **B,** Treatment consisted of resection of the metatarsal heads alone. A better solution would have been to perform a joint preservation procedure with shortening osteotomies.

There are of course situations in which the hallux is not deformed at all, and the patient presents with metatarsalgia (Figure 39-10). The surgeon must then decide if the lesser toe MP joints can be salvaged without treating the hallux deformity. Ideally, preservation of the lesser MP joints should be attempted in such cases, rather than a more extensive metatarsal head resection, as in Figure 39-10. If recurrence of metatarsalgia or arthritis of the lesser toe MP joints then develops, proceeding with the head resection is always an option. Treatment of the recurrent deformity is never as easy as a well-performed primary procedure, particularly when hallux valgus occurs, creating scarring and further subluxation of the lesser toes. Nonetheless, from the standpoint of forefoot function, joint preservation is ideal.

Management of adjacent joint arthritis also can be problematic, whether in the hallux IP joint or the tarsometatarsal joint(s). With loading of the IP joint after MP arthrodesis, a high incidence of IP joint arthritis and deformity would be expected, yet this is not the case. Obviously such problems do occur, even when the hallux is fused in the correct position (Figure 39-11). Generally, the hallux will subluxate or hyperextend dorsally or deviate into valgus (Figure 39-12). If the toe hyperextends, then an interposition arthroplasty can be performed as an alternative to arthrodesis.

The arthroplasty is performed from a medial incision at the level of the IP joint. The joint is exposed, and the distal 6 mm is cut with a saw from medial to lateral. The plantar plate (which usually is quite attenuated) and the flexor hallucis longus are interposed in the joint by pulling the tissue dorsally, and the tendon and plantar plate are sutured to the distal phalanx. It usually is not necessary to insert a K-wire into the toe to maintain position, although this can be considered. At times the IP joint deformity can be quite severe; if it is caused by incorrect positioning of the MP joint arthrodesis, revision of the latter must be performed at the same time as the IP joint arthrodesis. An interposition arthroplasty of the hallux IP joint is not as successful for correction of valgus deformity, although it can still be considered. Arthritis of the tarsometatarsal joint occurs quite commonly but does not seem to be a consequence of the MP joint arthrodesis. At times, the arthritis is associated with quite marked deformity of the tarsometatarsal joint with dorsal instability and abduction of the forefoot, which needs to be corrected (Figure 39-13).

Failure of surgery to correct the hallux MP joint is the result of a malunion of an arthrodesis, failure of a resection arthroplasty (Keller), or development of complications following a joint replacement of some sort. Silicone joint replacement fortunately is performed less often nowadays. Although it certainly has its advantages in the patient with rheumatoid arthritis, the potential destructive effect on the joint and the adjacent bone is a significant concern. In a majority of patients with silicone erosive synovitis, I remove the implant and perform a soft tissue interposition arthroplasty (Figure 39-14). Considerable bone lysis around the joint is typical, and a solid fusion is difficult to obtain. I find it preferable to remove

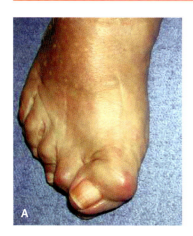

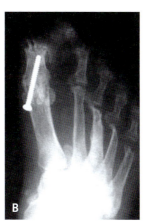

Figure 39-11 A, Recurrent deformity such as that shown difficult to treat. **B** and **C,** Hallux interphalangeal (IP) joint arthritis developed after arthrodesis and metatarsal head resection. In such cases, solid fusion of the IP joint is difficult to attain because of severe erosive joint disease, and a resection arthroplasty with interposition may be preferable to arthrodesis.

39

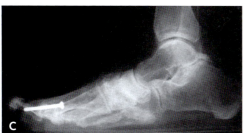

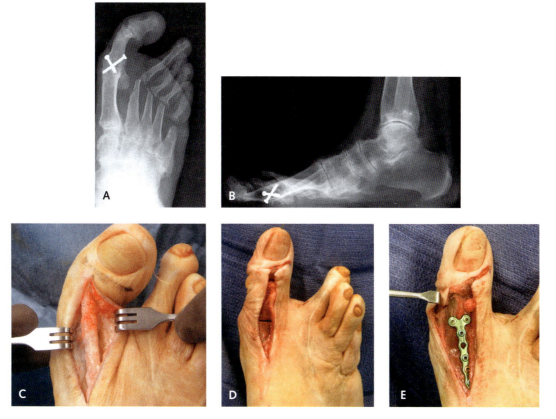

Figure 39-12 A and **B,** The recurrence of deformity in this foot probably was the result of positioning the hallux in neutral, creating stress on the interphalangeal (IP) joint. **C-E,** Simultaneous arthrodesis of the IP joint and revision of the metatarsophalangeal joint arthrodesis were performed.

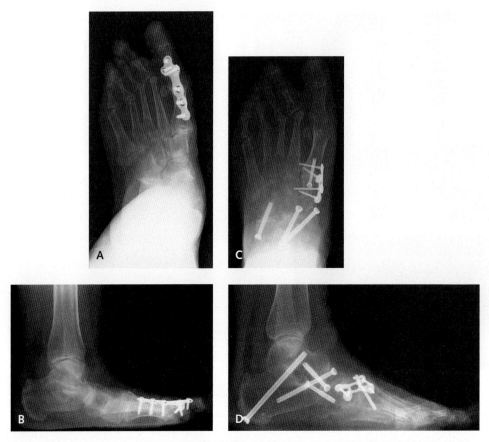

Figure 39-13 A and **B,** Deformity occurring more proximally after forefoot reconstruction. Such deformity is not the result of an abnormal load on the tarsometatarsal joint consequent to the metatarsophalangeal joint arthrodesis. **C** and **D,** Correction was obtained with a triple as well as a tarsometatarsal arthrodesis.

the implant, debride the synovial lining around the intramedullary canal, and then insert cancellous bone graft into the defect of the metatarsal and the proximal phalanx. The dorsal capsule, which usually is fairly thick, is then interposed in the joint. The bone graft gradually incorporates, so that if the arthroplasty fails, an arthrodesis performed at a later date will benefit from better bone quality. At times, implant failure is related specifically to pain, with less bone loss evident radiographically. In these instances, an interposition arthroplasty or an arthrodesis remains an option. Occasionally an in situ arthrodesis of the hallux is not sufficient to restore function and length; an arthrodesis is then performed with structural bone

grafting to lengthen the hallux (Figure 39-15). This is, however, rarely performed in the patient with rhematiod arthritis.

Complications after failure of a resection arthroplasty (Keller) usually require arthrodesis. At times, however, the deformity and bone loss are so severe that the best that can be expected is some improvement in alignment of the hallux. In such cases, I have found that an arthrodesis may not even be necessary, and the goal is to obtain better functional alignment. Generally, the bone is of poor quality, and the standard methods of fixation do not work; in my experience, a threaded Steinmann pin works quite well in these circumstances (Figure 39-16).

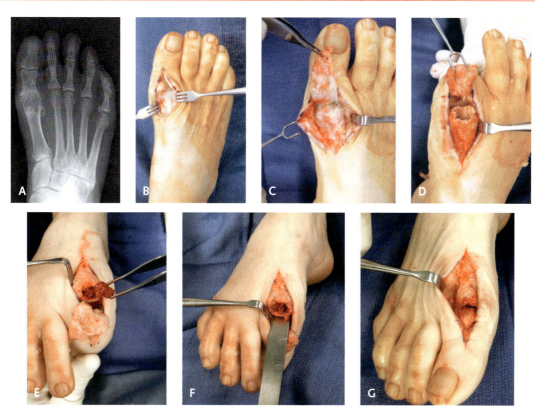

Figure 39-14 A and **B,** Severe bone lysis of the hallux and metatarsal associated with presence of a silicone implant. **C,** A soft tissue flap was elevated. **D,** The implant was removed. **E** and **F,** The defect in the metatarsal head and the phalanx was filled with cancellous bone graft. **G,** The soft tissue flap was inserted into the joint space.

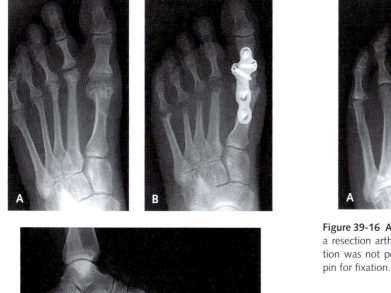

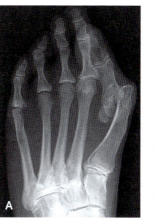

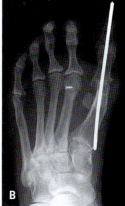

Figure 39-16 A, Marked bone loss of the hallux and first metatarsal after a resection arthroplasty. **B,** Arthrodesis with standard methods of fixation was not possible, necessitating use of a fully threaded Steinmann pin for fixation.

Figure 39-15 A, Erosion and lysis of bone associated with presence of a silicone implant. The bone quality was good, however, and the patient desired improved forefoot function. **B** and **C,** An arthrodesis was performed with structural grafting to lengthen the first ray.

TECHNIQUES, TIPS, AND PITFALLS

- Management of the toe deformity can be frustrating. Try to preserve as much length of the toe as possible. If severe deformity or contracture is present, the patient is far better off with an isolated toe amputation.

- The toes rarely function with any grip strength after head resection, and if recurrent contracture develops, it is more difficult to correct subsequently.

- If infection or ulceration under the metatarsal head is present, a more urgent operation is indicated. I use a similar approach to resect the metatarsal head(s) from the dorsal incisions but pass an antibiotic-soaked sponge through the incision from dorsal to plantar and then leave the plantar ulcer open but close the dorsal incision.

- With deformity of the hallux and the MP joint but minimal arthritis, a joint preservation procedure may be ideal. A modified Lapidus procedure is a good option that gives lasting relief and maintains alignment. This can be performed with either resection of the metatarsal heads or shortening osteotomies.

- Resection of the lesser metatarsal heads is a reliable procedure but should not be performed indiscriminately. Shortening osteotomies of the metatarsal relieve the pressure on the joint and decrease the pain from erosive disease. An interesting observation is that once the joints have been decompressed and the metatarsals have been shortened, joint function improves, along with the radiographic appearance of the articular surfaces. Such "improvement" is not always long-lasting, but with subsequent failure, the repair can be converted to an arthrodesis with resection of the metatarsal heads (Figure 39-17).

- For management of severe erosive deformity of the lesser toe MP joints, resection of all of the metatarsal heads can be performed through a transverse dorsal incision (Figure 39-18). This procedure will be successful, however, only if marked bone shortening is performed; otherwise, difficulty with skin closure will be encountered.

- With severe deformity featuring marked hallux valgus with dislocation of the MP joint, the soft tissue contracture is so severe laterally that even with an adequate lateral adductor and capsular release, the tension on the lateral soft tissue is still excessive so that tearing of the skin can occur. If the hallux does not reduce easily without tension laterally, then further bone should be resected.

- Fixation of the MP joint in patients with rheumatoid arthritis can be difficult because of associated osteopenia. If the screws are not likely to hold, a plate or large threaded pins should be added. Most of these patients have some IP joint disease as well, and crossing the IP joint with the Steinmann pins is not as problematic as in patients with a normal joint.

- Positioning the MP joint using large threaded pins is difficult. With this method of fixation, the declination angle of the first metatarsal has to be considered because the pins usually exit the metatarsal neck and do not engage the entire shaft of the metatarsal. If the hallux is plantar flexed to achieve better fixation with the threaded pins, a plantar flexion malunion, in which the hallux is too straight, will result, eventually leading to IP joint disease.

- Alignment of the hallux MP arthrodesis is important. If any valgus is present, subsequent IP joint arthritis is much more likely.

CORRECTION OF RHEUMATOID HINDFOOT AND ANKLE DEFORMITY

Arthrodesis is the predominant operation used for correction of rheumatoid hindfoot and ankle deformity (Figures 39-19 to 39-21). The complication rate in patients with such deformity is, however, significantly increased as a result of wound healing problems stemming from immune suppression, dysvascularity, skin fragility, and bone instability related to osteopenia. These potential complicating factors have to be taken into consideration, and efforts to prevent wound complications, infection, and ultimate failure including amputation must be undertaken at all times. Whenever possible, therefore, I try to use a single operation that carries a high rate of success. This is important, for example, in patients

with talonavicular arthritis, because I only occasionally use an isolated arthrodesis of this joint for correction of arthritis, even in the absence of deformity. Even if the arthritis is limited to the talonavicular joint, performing an isolated joint arthrodesis is not advantageous because the remaining minimal motion in the subtalar and calcaneal cuboid joints does not compensate for the potential for failure consequent to nonunion.

Currently, I use a single extensile medial incision for performing either a double or a triple arthrodesis, to avoid a lateral incision in a setting of severe deformity. Some patients have profound deformity with talonavicular dislocation, anterior subluxation of the talus, and associated rigid valgus deformity of the hindfoot. In these patients a lateral incision is more likely to lead to wound dehiscence because of the traction placed on the lateral foot as it is

39

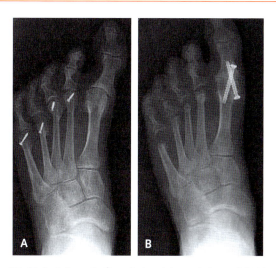

Figure 39-17 **A,** Failure of attempted metatarsophalangeal (MP) joint preservation. **B,** Revision surgery consisted of resection of the metatarsal heads and MP joint arthrodesis.

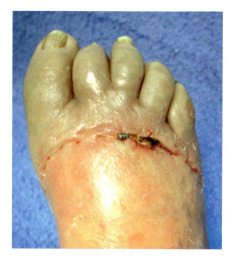

Figure 39-18 Immediate postoperative appearance after resection of all of the metatarsal heads, including the first, through a transverse incision, in an elderly patient who presented with a severe forefoot deformity. This procedure is an option for patients who are more debilitated and for whom the more prolonged recovery typically required after arthrodesis may not be appropriate. This incision should be used carefully when severe dislocations are present, out of concern for wound healing problems.

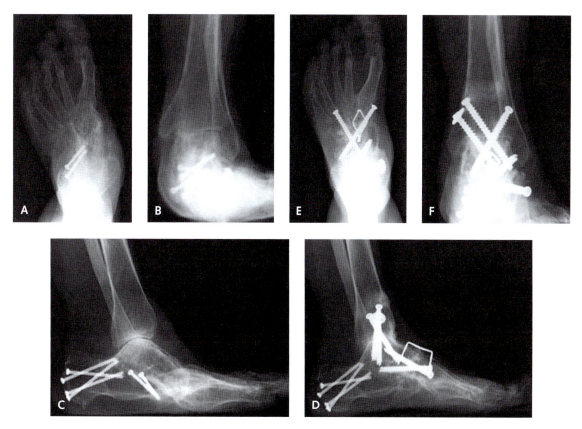

Figure 39-19 **A-C,** A pan-talar arthrodesis was performed to correct this recurrent and intractable deformity. The patient had undergone multiple previous surgeries including a triple arthrodesis and a calcaneus osteotomy. In **B,** note the stress fracture of the fibula, the result of chronic subfibular impingement from the flatfoot deformity. **D-F,** The alignment was markedly improved by revising the hindfoot arthrodesis and including the ankle joint in a pan-talar arthrodesis.

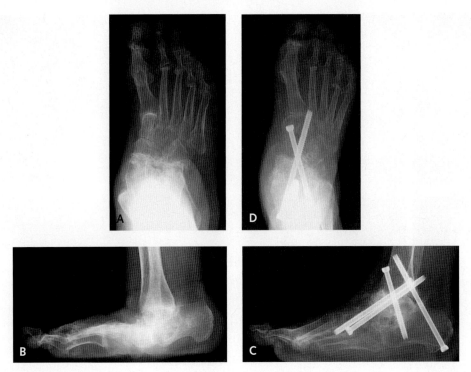

Figure 39-20 A-D, Long screws were inserted into the midfoot to obtain satisfactory fixation for this pan-talar arthrodesis. Note the restoration of the alignment of the hindfoot and midfoot, an important aspect of treatment in such cases.

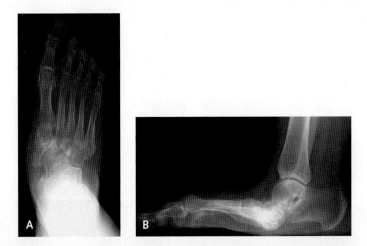

Figure 39-21 A and B, The midfoot is markedly collapsed, carrying a grave prognosis for cure unless alignment can be restored. The aim of treatment is to perform a wedge resection from the plantar aspect of the joint, to apply rigid plantar plate fixation on the tension side of the joint to enhance stability.

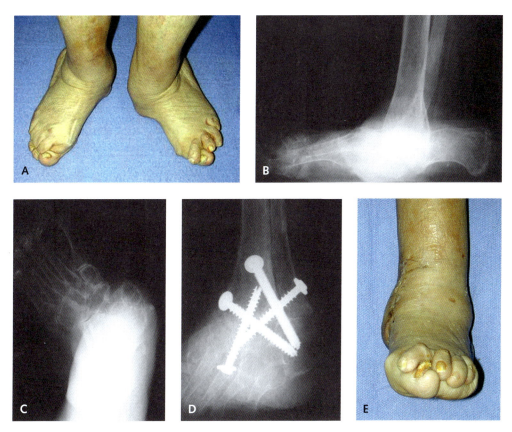

Figure 39-22 A-C, Dislocation of the talonavicular joint as well as ankle arthritis and deformity necessitated a pan-talar arthro-desis. **D,** Note the use of fully threaded screws for the arthrodesis. **E,** The final clinical alignment following arthrodesis.

corrected into neutral position. When I have any doubt about the likelihood of success of a hindfoot arthrodesis in the setting of associated ankle arthritis and deformity, I prefer to initiate treatment with a pan-talar arthrodesis, as depicted in Figure 39-22. In the case illustrated, fully threaded screws were used because the bone quality was particularly poor, and stability of fixation was more important than compression of the joints. This procedure is well tolerated in patients with debilitating deformity.

One of the problems with revision of a previous hindfoot arthrodesis in a patient with rheumatoid arthritis is the fixed deformity of the midfoot and forefoot that occurs simultaneously. If the ankle is eroded with a valgus deformity, then as the ankle deformity is corrected, whether with arthrodesis or joint replacement, the forefoot markedly supinates. This procedure should therefore commence with the ankle arthrodesis, and as the correct alignment is obtained, the revision or realignment of the hindfoot or midfoot is performed accordingly. In the example presented in Figure 39-19, once the ankle arthrodesis was performed, a marked forefoot supination resulted that required correction through the transverse tarsal joint with a revision of the previous arthrodesis. Because of the osteopenia associated with rheumatoid arthritis, care must be taken to ensure adequate fixation of any hindfoot or ankle arthrodesis, for which use of fully threaded screws may be advantageous. For the most part, alignment and stability are more important than compression for these fusions, as in Figure 39-19. At times, in order to increase the stability of fixation, the screws need to cross another joint, as demonstrated in Figure 39-20. In the case illustrated, a pan-talar arthrodesis was performed in a patient with profound osteopenia, so screws were inserted into the midfoot to increase bone stability.

These principles apply as well to revision hindfoot surgery in patients with rheumatoid arthritis. An important point is that an extended hindfoot arthrodesis will not be sufficient to correct fixed deformity if muscle imbalance exists. A good example is presented in Figure 39-23. In the case illustrated, the patient had undergone previous unsuccessful pan-talar arthrodesis. The hindfoot was in gross varus, with marked midfoot supination and fixed elevation of the first metatarsal. As a result of the fixed elevation of the first metatarsal, the hallux dropped into flexion, which was associated with contractures of the anterior tibial tendon, weakness of the peroneus longus, and contracture of the short flexors of the hallux. Although the alignment of the arthrodesis was not good to begin with, this case highlights the potential for recurrence of deformity when muscles are functioning distal to the point of the arthrodesis. In this patient, a revision of the pan-talar arthrodesis was performed in addition to a lateral transfer of the anterior tibial tendon and forefoot reconstruction (see Figure 39-23). Whenever possible, a tibiotalocalcaneal arthrodesis is preferable to a pan-talar arthrodesis. The remaining motion in the transverse tarsal joint is always desirable. Correction of deformity can be achieved with a tibiotalocalcaneal arthrodesis, and it is not always necessary to perform a pan-talar arthrodesis (Figure 39-24). In certain instances, no arthrodesis of any type can be contemplated, if contraindicated by bone loss, nature of the deformity, poor physical condition, or inability to comply with postoperative restrictions on weight bearing. If bracing fails or is not an option in these cases, insertion of a cement spacer with fully threaded Steinmann pins may be preferable for management of deformity. With secure fixation thus obtained, the patient may bear weight on the foot immediately (Figure 39-25).

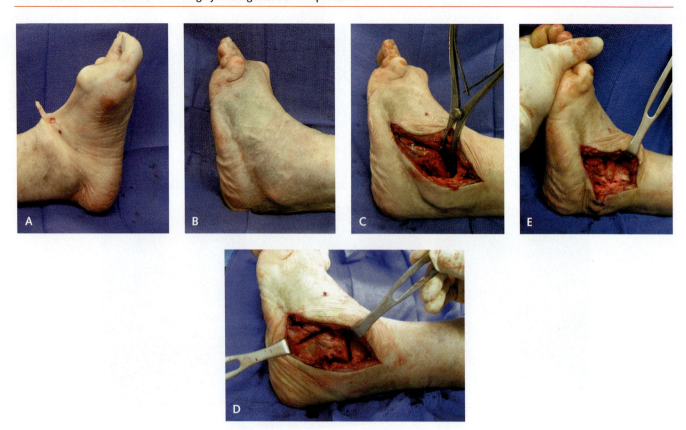

Figure 39-23 Revision of a previous pan-talar arthrodesis. **A** and **B,** Note the hindfoot varus and the fixed forefoot supination. **C-E,** The anterior tibial tendon was transferred laterally to the middle cuneiform, and a revision of the pan-talar arthrodesis performed. In **D,** note the removal of a biplanar wedge from the arthrodesis to correct the equinovarus deformity.

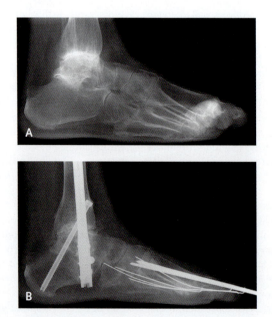

Figure 39-24 A, The patient had pan-talar arthritis that was most symptomatic in the ankle and subtalar joint. **B,** A tibiotalocalcaneal arthrodesis was performed.

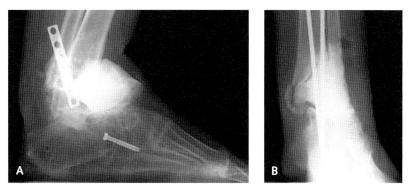

Figure 39-25 A, The patient was treated for ankle infection with a large bone block of antibiotic-impregnated cement. **B,** Eventually, however, the foot became severely unstable, at which time the cement was changed and large, fully threaded Steinmann pins were inserted to restore stability.

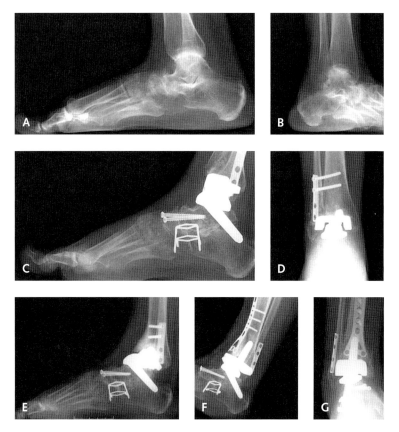

Figure 39-26 A and **B,** The patient had severe ankle and hindfoot deformity associated with painful arthritis. **C** and **D,** Treatment consisted of simultaneous triple arthrodesis and ankle replacement with a custom long-stem talus. **E,** Six months later, however, the tibial component crushed into the tibia. **F** and **G,** Revision was accomplished with cancellous bone grafting with insertion of a long-stem tibial component and application of an anterior plate to maintain the graft.

Although total ankle replacement has been performed successfully in patients with rheumatoid arthritis, caution is advised with use of this procedure because of an increased incidence of subsidence, fracture, and malalignment in the setting of osteopenia (Figure 39-26). For patients who have good limb alignment and have maintained the overall axis of the foot relative to the tibia, a total ankle replacement is a reasonable procedure. Total ankle replacement should not, however, be performed if a fixed hindfoot valgus deformity is present. Although I used to perform hindfoot correction and ankle replacement as staged procedures, I now perform the triple arthrodesis and ankle replacement simultaneously. The decision for staging of surgery in the patient with rheumatoid disease must be made judiciously. The repeated cessation of medication associated with the frequent and staged operations needed by persons with this disease leads to a flare-up of the arthritis, decreases mobility, and increases generalized debility. Osteopenia also worsens as a result of frequent periods of restricted weight bearing.

SUGGESTED READING

Bohay DR, Brage ME, Younger AS: Surgical treatment of the ankle and foot in patients with rheumatoid arthritis, *Instr Course Lect* 58:595–616, 2009.

Coughlin MJ: Rheumatoid forefoot reconstruction. A long-term follow-up study, *J Bone Joint Surg Am* 82:322–341, 2000.

Jeng C, Campbell J: Current concepts review: The rheumatoid forefoot, *Foot Ankle Int* 29:959–968, 2008.

Knupp M, Skoog A, Törnkvist H, Ponzer S: Triple arthrodesis in rheumatoid arthritis, *Foot Ankle Int* 29:293–297, 2008.

Molloy AP, Myerson MS: Surgery of the lesser toes in rheumatoid arthritis: Metatarsal head resection, *Foot Ankle Clin* 12:417–433, 2007.

Nassar J, Cracchiolo A III: Complications in surgery of the foot and ankle in patients with rheumatoid arthritis, *Clin Orthop Oct* (391):140–152, 2001.

Stockley I, Betts RP, Rowley I, et al: The importance of the valgus hindfoot in forefoot surgery in rheumatoid arthritis, *J Bone Joint Surg Br* 72:705–708, 1990.

Thordarson DB, Aval S, Krieger L: Failure of hallux MP preservation surgery for rheumatoid arthritis, *Foot Ankle Int* 23:486–490, 2002.

Toolan BC, Hansen ST Jr: Surgery of the rheumatoid foot and ankle, *Curr Opin Rheumatol* 10:116–119, 1998.

Weinfeld SB, Schon LC, Myerson MS: Controversies and perils: Fusions of the foot and ankle in patients with rheumatoid arthritis, *Tech Orthop* 11:224–235, 1996.

Index

Note: The letter *f* indicates a figure, *b* indicates a box.